Quick Find Guide

Foundations of Periodontics for the Dental Hygienist

Third Edition

Jill S. Nield-Gehrig, RDH, MA
Dean Emeritus, Division of Allied Health & Public Service Education
Asheville-Buncombe Technical Community College
Asheville, North Carolina

Donald E. Willmann, DDS, MS
Professor Emeritus, Department of Periodontics
University of Texas Health Science Center at San Antonio Dental School
San Antonio, Texas

Wolters Kluwer | Lippincott Williams & Wilkins
Health
Philadelphia · Baltimore · New York · London
Buenos Aires · Hong Kong · Sydney · Tokyo

Acquisitions Editor: Peter Sabatini
Product Manager: Kristin Royer
Marketing Manager: Allison Powell
Editorial Assistant: Rachel Stark
Design Coordinator: Teresa Mallon
Art Director: Jennifer Clements
Manufacturing Coordinator: Margie Orzech
Prepress Vendor: SPi Technologies

Copyright © 2011 Wolters Kluwer Health | Lippincott Williams & Wilkins.

Printed in China

Library of Congress Cataloging-in-Publication Data
Nield-Gehrig, Jill S. (Jill Shiffer)
    Foundations of periodontics for the dental hygienist / Jill S. Nield-Gehrig,
Donald E. Willmann.—3rd ed.
        p. ; cm.
    Includes bibliographical references and index.
    ISBN 978-1-60547-573-8 (alk. paper)
    1. Periodontics. 2. Dental hygienists. I. Willmann, Donald E. II. Title.
    [DNLM: 1. Periodontics. 2. Dental Hygienists. WU 240]

RK361.F675 2011
617.6'32—dc22

2010027962

Care has been taken to confirm the accuracy of the information presented and to describe generally accepted practices. However, the author, editors, and publisher are not responsible for errors or omissions or for any consequences from application of the information in this book and make no warranty, expressed or implied, with respect to the currency, completeness, or accuracy of the contents of the publication. Application of this information in a particular situation remains the professional responsibility of the practitioner; the clinical treatments described and recommended may not be considered absolute and universal recommendations.

The author, editors, and publisher have exerted every effort to ensure that drug selection and dosage set forth in this text are in accordance with the current recommendations and practice at the time of publication. However, in view of ongoing research, changes in government regulations, and the constant flow of information relating to drug therapy and drug reactions, the reader is urged to check the package insert for each drug for any change in indications and dosage and for added warnings and precautions. This is particularly important when the recommended agent is a new or infrequently employed drug.

Some drugs and medical devices presented in this publication have Food and Drug Administration (FDA) clearance for limited use in restricted research settings. It is the responsibility of the health care provider to ascertain the FDA status of each drug or device planned for use in his or her clinical practice.

LWW.com

9 8 7 6 5 4 3 2

Liability Statement

This textbook endeavors to present an evidence-based discussion of periodontology based on information from recent research. Periodontology, however, is a rapidly changing science. The authors, editors, and publisher have made every effort to confirm the accuracy of the information presented and to describe generally accepted practices at the time of publication. However, as new information becomes available, changes in treatment may become necessary. The reader is encouraged to keep up with dental and medical research through the many peer-reviewed journals available to verify information found here and to determine the best treatment for each individual patient. The authors, contributors, editors, and publisher are not responsible for errors or omissions or for any consequences from application of the information in this book and make no warranty, express or implied, with respect to the contents of this publication.

Contents

PART 3: ETIOLOGY OF PERIODONTAL DISEASES

PART 7: IMPLEMENTATION OF THERAPY

Contributors

Ralph M. Arnold, DDS
Associate Professor, Retired
Department of Periodontics
University of Texas Health Science
    Center at San Antonio
San Antonio, Texas

Elizabeth Carr, RDH, BS
Department of Dental Hygiene
University of Mississippi Medical
    Center
Jackson, Mississippi

Delwyn Catley, PhD
Associate Professor and Director of
    Clinical Training
Department of Psychology
University of Missouri – Kansas City
Kansas City, Missouri

Teresa Butler Duncan, RDH, BS
Department of Dental Hygiene
School of Health Related Professions
The University of Mississippi Medical
    Center
Jackson, Mississippi

Richard Foster, DMD
Dental Director
Guilford Technical Community College
Jamestown, North Carolina

Carol A. Jahn, BSDH, MS
Manager, Professional Education &
    Communications
WaterPik Technologies, Inc.
Fort Collins, Colorado

Archie A. Jones, MBA, DDS
Associate Professor
Department of Periodontics
University of Texas Health Science
    Center at San Antonio
San Antonio, Texas

Margaret Lemaster, BSDH, MS
School of Dental Hygiene
Old Dominion University
Norfolk, Virginia

Sharon Logue, RDH, MPH
Virginia Department of Health
Division of Dental Health
Richmond, Virginia

Deborah P. Milliken, BS, DMD
Professor, Dental Hygiene
South Florida Community College
Avon Park, Florida

William S. Moore, DDS, MS
Assistant Professor and Clinic
    Director
Division of Oral & Maxillofacial
    Radiology
Department of Dental Diagnostic
    Science
University of Texas Health Science
    Center at San Antonio
San Antonio, Texas

John Preece, DDS, MS
Professor, Division of Oral &
    Maxillofacial Radiology
Department of Dental Diagnostic
    Science
University of Texas Health Science
    Center at San Antonio
San Antonio, Texas

Christoph A. Ramseier, MAS Dr. Med. Dent.
Assistant Professor
Department of Periodontology
University of Berne, School of Dental
    Medicine
Bern, Switzerland

Carol Southard, RN, MSN
Tobacco Cessation Specialist
Northwestern Memorial Hospital
Wellness Institute
Chicago, Illinois

Rebecca Sroda, RDH, MS
Associate Dean
Allied Health
South Florida Community College
Avon Park, Florida

Clemens Walter, DDS
Assistant Professor
Department of Periodontology,
    Endodontology, & Cariology
University of Basel Dental School
Basel, Switzerland

Dianne Glasscoe Watterson, RDH, MBA, CEO
Professional Dental Management,
    Inc.
www.professionaldentalmgmt.com
Frederick, Maryland

Karen Williams, RDH, MS, PhD
Professor
Department of Dental Hygiene and
    Dental Public Health and
    Behavioral Sciences
University of Missouri – Kansas City
Kansas City, Missouri

Erin Waugh, BSDH, MS
School of Dental Hygiene
Old Dominion University
Norfolk, Virginia

Reviewers

Gail Aamodt, RDH, MS
Clinical Coordinator
School of Dental Health Science
Pacific University
Hillsboro, Oregon

Joanna Allaire, BSDH
Clinical Assistant Professor
Periodontics/Dental Hygiene
The University of Texas Dental
   Branch
Houston, Texas

Jean Byrnes-Ziegler, RDH, MS
Professor and Program Director
Dental Hygiene
Harcum College
Bryn Mawr, Pennsylvania

Elizabeth Di Silvio, RDH, MEd
Associate Professor
Dental Hygiene
Northern Virginia Community
   College
Springfield, Virginia

Marie Gillis, RDH, MS
National Dean
Dental Programs
Education Affiliates
Washington, District of Columbia

Susan Gorman RDH, BS Ed, MEd (C)
Director
Dental Hygiene
Tri-State Institute
Birmingham, Alabama

Stephanie Harrison, RDH, MA
Director
Dental Hygiene
Community College of Denver,
Denver, Colorado

Sharon Logue, RDH, MPH
Division of Dental Health
Virginia Department of Health
Richmond, Virginia

Susan Long, RDH, EdD
Chairman and Professor
Dental Hygiene
University of Arkansas for Medical
   Sciences
Little Rock, Arkansas

Susan Nichols, RDH, EFDA, BIS
Periodontology Instructor
Department of Dental Hygiene
Owens Community College
Toledo, Ohio

Amilia Peskir, Dip. DH, BSc
Instructor
Dental Hygiene
John Abbott College
Ste. Anne de Bellevue, Québec

Kelli Shaffer, RDH, MA Ed
Full-Time Faculty
Dental Health Science
Pacific University
Hillsboro, Oregon

Alla Wheeler, RDH, BA, MPA
Professor
Dental Hygiene
New York University College of
   Dentistry
New York, New York

Preface for Course Instructors

Foundations of Periodontics for the Dental Hygienist, 3rd edition, is written with two primary goals in mind. First and foremost, this textbook focuses on the dental hygienist's role in periodontics. Our second goal was to develop a book with an instructional design that facilitates the teaching and learning of the complex subject of periodontics—as it relates to dental hygiene practice—without omitting salient concepts or "watering down" the material. Written primarily for dental hygiene students, *Foundations of Periodontics for the Dental Hygienist* also would be a valuable resource on current concepts in periodontics for the practicing dental hygienist or general dentist.

INSTRUCTOR TEACHING RESOURCES

Follow the steps in Box 1 to access the online instructor resources.

Box 1 Accessing Online Instructor Resources

1. Open an internet browser and select: http://thePoint.lww.com
2. Existing users: log on. Skip to step 4 in this list.
3. New users: select "Register a New Account." Complete all required fields on the online access request form. Select "Submit Adoption Form" button. Once the form is submitted in good order, you will receive an approval notice. U.S. and Canadian educators, please allow three business days for a reply. Note: the access codes that come in the textbook provide students with access to the full online text and chapter review questions only.
4. Locate "Foundations of Periodontics for the Dental Hygienist." Select "Instructor Resources."

TEXTBOOK FEATURES

The third edition of *Foundations of Periodontics for the Dental Hygienist* has many features designed to facilitate learning and teaching.

1. **Module Overview and Outline.** Each module begins with a concise overview of the module content. The module outline makes it easier to locate material within the module. The outline provides the reader with an organizational framework with which to approach new material.

2. **Learning Objectives and Key Terms.** Learning objectives assist students in recognizing and studying important concepts in each chapter. Key terms are listed at the beginning of each chapter. One of the most challenging tasks for any student is learning a whole new dental vocabulary and gaining the confidence to

use new terms with accuracy and ease. The key terms list assists students in this task by identifying important terminology and facilitating the study and review of terminology in each chapter. Terms are highlighted and clearly defined within the chapter.

3. **Instructional Design**
   * Each chapter is subdivided into sections to help the reader recognize major content areas.
   * Chapters are written in an expanded outline format that makes it easy for students to identify, learn, and review key concepts.
   * Material is presented in a manner that recognizes that students have different learning styles. Hundreds of illustrations and clinical photographs visually reinforce chapter content.
   * Chapter content is supplemented in a visual format with boxes, tables, and flow charts.

4. **Focus on Patients.** The *"Focus on Patients"* items allow the reader to apply chapter content in the context of clinical periodontal care. The cases provide opportunities for students to integrate knowledge into their clinical work.

5. **Chapter Review Questions.** Chapter Review Questions provide a quick review of chapter content. The chapter review questions are available to students on the companion website at http://thePoint.lww.com.

6. **Internet Resources in Periodontics.** Chapter 38 provides an extensive list of Internet resources. Students should be encouraged to develop skills in online information gathering. With the rapid explosion of knowledge in the dental and medical sciences, a student can no longer expect to learn everything that he or she needs to know, now and forever, in a few years of professional training. Students must learn how to retrieve accurate information quickly from reliable Internet sites, such as MEDLINE. Chapter 38, *Periodontal Resources in Dental Literature and on the Internet*, is available to students on the companion website at http;//thePoint. lww.com.

7. **Comprehensive Patient Cases.** Chapter 36 presents three fictitious patient cases. Patient assessment data pertinent to the periodontium challenge the student to interpret and use the information in periodontal care planning for the patient.

8. **Glossary.** The glossary provides quick assess to common periodontal terminology.

CONTENT SEQUENCING

The book is divided into nine major content areas:

Part 1: The Periodontium in Health

Part 2: Classification and Tissue Destruction in Periodontal Diseases

Part 3: Etiology of Periodontal Diseases

Part 4: Gingival Disease

Part 5: Periodontitis

Part 6: Assessment for Clinical Decision Making

Part 7: Implementation of Therapy

Foundations of Periodontics for the Dental Hygienist, 3rd edition, strives to present the complex subject of periodontics in a reader-friendly manner. The authors greatly appreciate the comments and suggestions from educators and students. It is our sincere hope that this textbook will help students and practitioners alike to acquire knowledge that will serve as a foundation for the prevention and management of periodontal diseases.

Jill S. Nield-Gehrig, RDH, MA
Donald E. Willmann, DDS, MS

Acknowledgments

It is a great pleasure to acknowledge the following individuals whose assistance was indispensable to this third edition:

- **Charles D. Whitehead** and **Holly R. Fischer,** MFA the highly skilled medical illustrators, who created all the wonderful illustrations for the book.
- **Kevin Dietz,** a colleague and friend for his vision and guidance for all three editions of this book.
- And with great thanks to our wonderful team at Lippincott Williams & Wilkins without whose expertise and support this book would not have been possible: **John Goucher, Kristin Royer, Peter Sabatini,** and **Jennifer Clements.**

Jill S. Nield-Gehrig, RDH, MA
Donald E. Willmann, DDS, MS

Chapter 1

Periodontium: The Tooth-Supporting Structures

Learning Objectives

- List and recognize the clinical features of periodontal health.

- Describe the function that each tissue serves in the periodontium, including the gingiva, periodontal ligament, cementum, and alveolar bone.

- In a clinical setting, identify the following anatomical areas of the gingiva in the oral cavity: free gingiva, gingival sulcus, interdental gingiva, and attached gingiva.

- Identify the tissues of the periodontium on an unlabeled drawing depicting the periodontium in cross section.

- In a clinical setting, identify the following boundaries of the gingiva in the oral cavity: gingival margin, free gingival groove, and mucogingival junction. If the free gingival groove is not visible clinically, determine the apical boundary of the free gingiva by inserting a probe to the base of a sulcus on an anterior tooth.

- In a clinical setting, identify the free gingiva on an anterior tooth by inserting a periodontal probe to the base of the sulcus.

- In a clinical setting, contrast the coral pink tissue of the attached gingiva with the darker, shiny tissue of the alveolar mucosa.

- In a clinical setting, use compressed air to detect the presence or absence of stippling of the attached gingiva.

- Identify the alveolar process (alveolar bone) on a human skull.

- Describe the position and contours of the alveolar crest of the alveolar bone in health.

- Describe the nerve and blood supply to the periodontium.

- Explain the role of the lymphatic system in the health of the periodontium.

- Define the key terms in this chapter.

- Demonstrate knowledge of the tissues of the periodontium by applying concepts from this chapter to the cases found in the section "Focus on Patients" of this chapter.

Key Terms

Periodontium

Gingiva

Periodontal ligament

Cementum

Alveolar bone

Gingival margin

Alveolar mucosa

Free gingival groove

Mucogingival junction

Free gingiva

Attached gingiva

Stippling

Interdental gingiva

Papillae

Col

Gingival sulcus

Gingival crevicular fluid

Alveolar process

Alveolar bone

Alveolar bone proper

Alveolus

Cortical bone

Alveolar crest

Cancellous bone

Periosteum

Innervation

Trigeminal nerve

Anastomose

Lymphatic system

Lymph nodes

Section 1
Tissues of the Periodontium

The periodontium (peri = around and odontos = tooth) is the functional system of tissues that surrounds the teeth and attaches them to the jaw bone (Figs. 1-1 and 1-2). The periodontium is also called the "supporting tissues of the teeth" and "the attachment apparatus." The tissues of the periodontium include the

1. Gingiva—the tissue that covers the cervical portions of the teeth and the alveolar processes of the jaws.
2. Periodontal ligament (PDL)—the fibers that surround the root of the tooth. These fibers attach to the bone of the socket on one side and to the cementum of the root on the other side.
3. Cementum—the thin layer of mineralized tissue that covers the root of the tooth.
4. Alveolar bone—the bone that surrounds the roots of the teeth. It forms the bony sockets that support and protect the roots of the teeth.

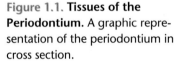

Figure 1.1. Tissues of the Periodontium. A graphic representation of the periodontium in cross section.

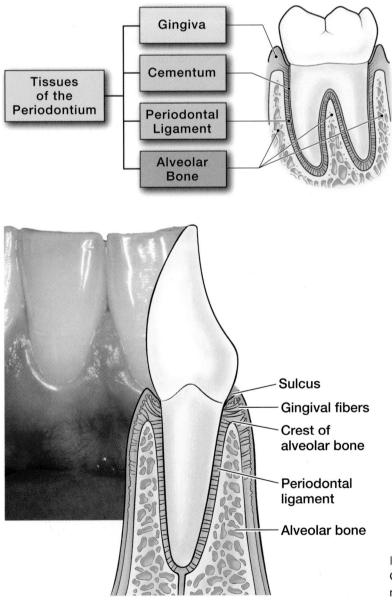

Figure 1.2. Healthy Periodontium. Clinical photograph and drawing of the major structures of the periodontium.

TABLE 1-1. The Periodontium	
Structure	**Brief Description of Its Function**
Gingiva	Provides a tissue seal around the cervical portion (neck) of the tooth
	Covers the alveolar processes of the jaws
	Holds the tissue against the tooth during mastication
Periodontal ligament	Suspends and maintains the tooth in its socket
Cementum	Anchors the ends of the periodontal ligament fibers to the tooth so that the tooth stays in its socket
	Protects the dentin of the root
Alveolar bone	Surrounds and supports the roots of the tooth

Each of the tissues of the periodontium plays a vital role in maintaining the health and function of the periodontium (Table 1-1). Knowledge of the periodontal tissues in health is a necessary foundation for understanding the concepts of (1) normal function of the periodontium, (2) disease prevention, and (3) the periodontal disease process.

Dental hygiene students usually are introduced to the tissues of the periodontium during the first semester or quarter of the dental hygiene curriculum. In the preclinical stages of the curriculum, mastering dental terminology and anatomy can sometimes be overwhelming and confusing. This chapter provides an opportunity to review this complex system of tissues known as the periodontium.

THE GINGIVA

1. **Overview of the Gingiva**
   A. **Description.** The gingiva is the part of the mucosa that surrounds the cervical portions of the teeth and covers the alveolar processes of the jaws (FIGS. 1-3, 1-4).
      1. The gingiva ends coronal to the cementoenamel junction (CEJ) of each tooth and attaches to the tooth by means of a specialized type of epithelial tissue (junctional epithelium).
      2. It is composed of a thin outer layer of epithelium and an underlying core of connective tissue.
      3. The gingiva is divided into four anatomical areas (FIG. 1-3).
         a. Free gingiva
         b. Gingival sulcus
         c. Interdental gingiva
         d. Attached gingiva
   B. **Function.** The gingiva protects the underlying tooth-supporting structures of the periodontium from the oral environment. The oral environment is exposed to a wide range of temperatures in food and drink, mechanical forces, and a large number of oral bacteria. To accomplish these functions, the gingiva has several defense mechanisms, including the saliva and immune system defense mechanisms.

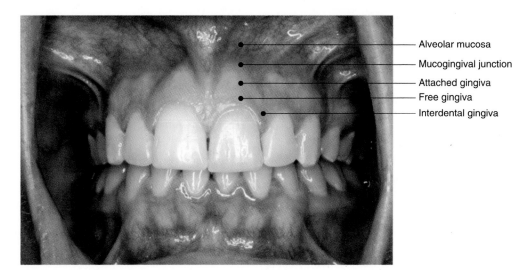

— Alveolar mucosa
— Mucogingival junction
— Attached gingiva
— Free gingiva
— Interdental gingiva

Figure 1.3. The Gingival Tissues. Photograph of healthy gingival tissues showing the free, attached, and interdental gingiva.

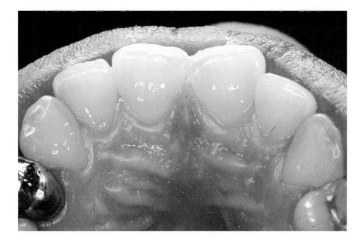

Figure 1.4. Gingival Tissue of the Palate. On the palate, the lingual gingiva is directly continuous with the keratinized masticatory mucosa of the gingiva.

C. **Boundaries of the Gingiva**
1. The coronal boundary of the gingiva is the gingival margin (FIG. 1-5).
2. The apical boundary of the gingiva is the alveolar mucosa. The alveolar mucosa can be distinguished easily from the gingiva by its dark red color and smooth, shiny surface.

D. **Demarcations of the Gingiva**
1. The free gingival groove is a shallow linear depression that separates the free and attached gingiva (FIG. 1-5). This line may be visible clinically but is not obvious in many instances.
2. The mucogingival junction is the clinically visible boundary where the pink attached gingiva meets the red, shiny alveolar mucosa (FIG. 1-5). Clinically visible means that this landmark can be seen in the oral cavity.

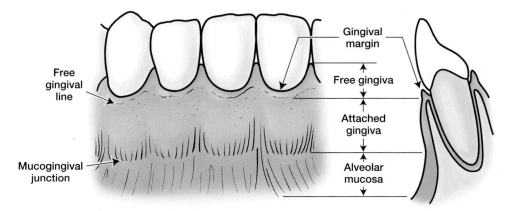

Figure 1.5. **Boundaries of the Gingiva.** Illustration showing the boundaries and anatomical areas of the gingiva.

2. **Free Gingiva.** The free gingiva is the unattached portion of the gingiva that surrounds the tooth in the region of the CEJ (FIG. 1-5). The free gingiva is also known as the unattached gingiva or the marginal gingiva.
    A. **Location of the Free Gingiva**
        1. The free gingiva is located coronal to (above) the CEJ.
        2. It surrounds the tooth in a turtleneck or cufflike manner.
        3. The free gingiva attaches to the tooth by means of a specialized epithelium—the junctional epithelium.
    B. **Characteristics of the Free Gingiva**
        1. The tissue of the free gingiva fits closely around the tooth but is not directly attached to it.
        2. This tissue, because it is unattached, may be gently stretched away from the tooth surface with a periodontal probe.
        3. The free gingiva also forms the soft tissue wall of the gingival sulcus.
    C. **Contour of the Free Gingival Margin**
        1. The tissue of the free gingiva meets the tooth in a thin rounded edge called the gingival margin (FIG. 1-5).
        2. The gingival margin follows the contours of the teeth, creating a scalloped (wavy) outline around them.
3. **Attached Gingiva.** The attached gingiva is the part of the gingiva that is tightly connected to the cementum on the cervical third of the root and to the periosteum (connective tissue cover) of the alveolar bone.
    A. **Location of the Attached Gingiva.** The attached gingiva lies between the free gingiva and the alveolar mucosa (FIG. 1-6).
    B. **Width of the Attached Gingiva**
        1. The attached gingiva is widest in the incisor and molar regions, ranging from 3.3 to 3.9 mm on the mandible and 3.5 to 4.5 mm on the maxilla (FIG. 1-7).
        2. The attached gingiva is narrowest in premolar regions (1.8 mm on mandible and 1.9 mm on maxilla).
        3. The width of the attached gingiva is not measured on the palate since clinically it is not possible to determine where the attached gingiva ends and the palatal mucosa begins (see FIG. 1-4).
        4. It was once believed that a minimum 2-mm width of the attached gingiva is necessary to maintain the health of the periodontium; this concept is not accepted today [1].

C. Color of the Attached Gingiva
   1. In health, the attached gingiva is pale or coral pink (Fig. 1-8).
   2. The attached gingiva may be pigmented (Fig. 1-8).
      a. Pigmentation occurs more frequently in dark-skinned individuals [2].
      b. The pigmented areas of the attached gingiva may range from light brown to black.

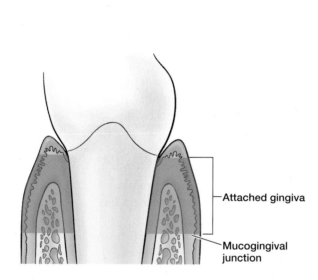

Figure 1.6. Location of the Attached Gingiva. The attached gingiva extends from the free gingival groove to the mucogingival junction.

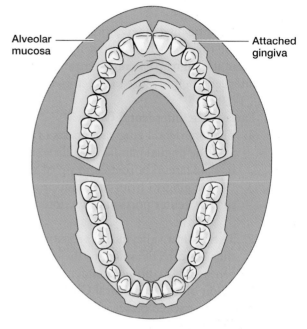

Figure 1.7. Mean Width of the Attached Gingiva. The attached gingiva is widest in the incisor and molar regions and narrowest in premolar regions.

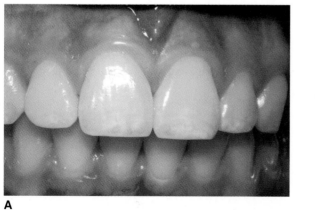

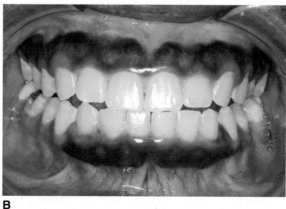

A   **B**

Figure 1.8. Color Variations of Normal Gingiva. The color of the normal gingiva varies among different persons. **A.** The color is a lighter, coral pink in individuals with a fair complexion. **B.** In individuals with dark skin and hair, the gingiva may be pigmented. (Courtesy of Elizabeth Carr, University of Mississippi Medical Center, Jackson, MS.)

D. **Texture of the Attached Gingiva.** In health, the surface of the attached gingiva may have a dimpled appearance similar to the skin of an orange peel. This dimpled appearance is known as stippling (FIG. 1-9). Healthy tissue may or may not exhibit a stippled appearance as the presence of stippling varies greatly from individual to individual. Stippling is present in 40% of adults.

E. **Function of the Attached Gingiva**
   1. The attached gingiva allows the gingival tissue to withstand the mechanical forces created during activities such as mastication, speaking, and tooth-brushing.
   2. The attached gingiva prevents the free gingiva from being pulled away from the tooth when tension is applied to the alveolar mucosa.

4. **Interdental Gingiva.** The interdental gingiva is the portion of the gingiva that fills the interdental embrasure between two adjacent teeth apical to the contact area (FIG. 1-10).

A. **Parts of the Interdental Gingiva**
   1. The interdental gingiva consists of two interdental papillae—one facial papilla and one lingual papilla (papilla = singular noun; papillae = plural noun).
      a. The lateral borders and tip of an interdental papilla are formed by the free gingiva from the adjacent teeth.
      b. The center portion of the interdental papilla is formed by the attached gingiva.
   2. The **col** is a valleylike depression in the portion of the interdental gingiva that lies directly apical to the contact area. The col is not present if the adjacent teeth are not in contact or if the gingiva has receded (FIG. 1-11).

B. **Function of the Interdental Gingiva.** The interdental gingiva prevents food from becoming packed between the teeth during mastication.

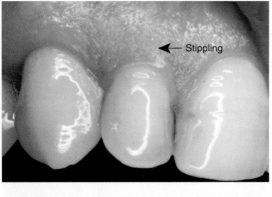

Figure 1.9. **Gingival Stippling.** In health, the surface of the attached gingiva may have a dimpled appearance known as gingival stippling.

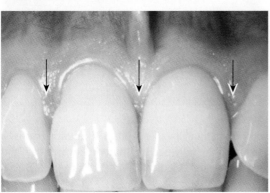

Figure 1.10. **The Interdental Gingiva.** The interdental tissue fills the area between two adjacent teeth.

5. Gingival Sulcus. The gingival sulcus is the *space* between the free gingiva and the tooth surface (FIG. 1-12).

    A. Description. The sulcus is a V-shaped, shallow space around the tooth [3].

        1. The depth of a clinically normal gingival sulcus is from 1 to 3 mm, as measured using a periodontal probe.

        2. Base of Sulcus. The base of the sulcus is formed by the junctional epithelium (a specialized type of epithelium that attaches to the tooth surface).

    B. Gingival Crevicular Fluid. The gingival crevicular fluid, also called the gingival sulcular fluid, is a fluid that seeps from the underlying connective tissue into the sulcular space.

        1. Little or no fluid is found in the healthy gingival sulcus, but the fluid flow increases in the presence of dental plaque biofilm and the resulting gingival inflammation [4].

        2. Fluid flow increases in response to toothbrushing, mastication, or other stimulation of the gingivae. The flow is greatly increased when the gingivae are inflamed.

        3. If a filter strip is inserted into the sulcus, it aborbs the fluid in the sulcus. Using the filter strip, the amount of gingival crevicular fluid can be measured and used as an index of gingival inflammation.

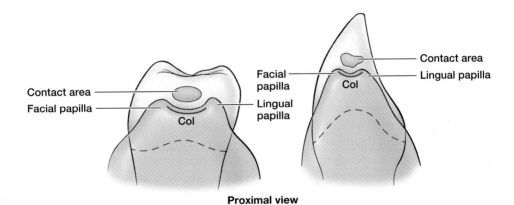

Proximal view

Figure 1.11. Interdental Col. A drawing of the interdental col, located between the facial and the lingual papillae and beneath the contact area of the tooth.

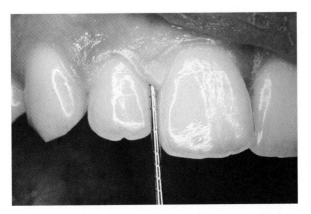

Figure 1.12. Gingival Sulcus. This photograph shows a periodontal probe inserted into the gingival sulcus, the space between the free gingiva and the tooth.

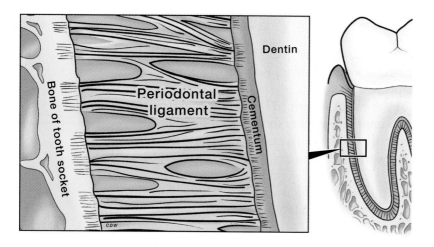

Figure 1.13. Periodontal Ligament.

- On the bone side, the ends of the periodontal ligament fibers are anchored in the alveolar bone of the tooth socket.
- On tooth side, the ends of the periodontal ligament fibers are anchored in the cementum of the root.

PERIODONTAL LIGAMENT

1. **Description**
   A. The periodontal ligament is a layer of soft connective tissue that covers the root of the tooth and attaches it to the bone of the tooth socket (Fig. 1-13).
      1. The periodontal ligament is composed mainly of dense fibrous connective tissue [3].
      2. The fibers of the periodontal ligament attach on one side to the root cementum and on the other side to the alveolar bone of the tooth socket [5].
   B. The periodontal ligament not only connects the tooth to the alveolar process but also supports the tooth in the socket and absorbs mechanical loads placed on the tooth, thus protecting the tooth in its socket.
2. **Functions.** The periodontal ligament has five functions in the periodontium:
   A. Supportive function—suspends and maintains the tooth in its socket.
   B. Sensory function—provides sensory feeling to the tooth, such as pressure and pain sensations.
   C. Nutritive function—provides nutrients to the cementum and bone.
   D. Formative function—builds and maintains cementum and the alveolar bone of the tooth socket.
   E. Resorptive function—can remodel the alveolar bone in response to pressure, such as that applied during orthodontic treatment (braces).

ROOT CEMENTUM

1. **Description.** Cementum is a thin layer of hard, mineralized connective tissue that covers the surface of the tooth root (Fig. 1-14).
2. **Characteristics of Cementum**
   A. Cementum overlies and is attached to the dentin of the root. It is light yellow in color and softer than dentin or enamel.
   B. Cementum is a bonelike tissue that is more resistant to resorption than bone [6].
      1. Resistance to resorption (loss of substance) is an important characteristic of cementum that makes it possible for the teeth to be moved during orthodontic treatment [7].

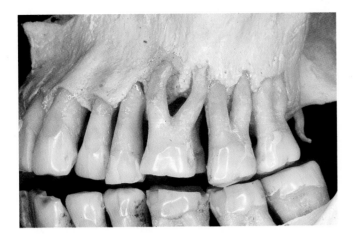

Figure 1.14. Cementum. Cementum is mineralized connective tissue that covers the root of the tooth; it is light yellow in color.

    2. The high resistance of cementum to resorption allows the pressure applied during orthodontics to cause resorption of the alveolar bone, for tooth movement, without resulting in root resorption.

  C. Cementum is formed slowly throughout life. There are two main types of cementum: cellular and acellular.

  D. Cementum does not have its own blood or nutrient supply; it receives its nutrients from the periodontal ligament.

3. Functions of Cementum in the Periodontium. Cementum performs several important roles in the periodontium, and, therefore, conservation of cementum should be a goal of periodontal instrumentation.

  A. The primary function of cementum is to give attachment to the collagen fibers of the periodontal ligament. Cementum anchors the ends of the periodontal ligament fibers to the tooth; without cementum, the tooth would fall out of its socket.

  B. The outer layer of cementum protects the underlying dentin and seals the ends of the open dentinal tubules.

  C. Cementum formation compensates for tooth wear at the occlusal or incisal surface due to attrition. Cementum is formed at the apical area of the root to compensate for occlusal attrition.

ALVEOLAR BONE

1. Description

  A. The alveolar process or alveolar bone is the bone of the upper or lower jaw that surrounds and supports the roots of the teeth (FIG. 1-15).

  B. The alveolar bone is mineralized connective tissue and consists, by weight, of about 60% inorganic material, 25% inorganic material, and about 15% water.

  C. The existence of the alveolar bone is dependent on the presence of teeth; when teeth are extracted, in time, the alveolar bone resorbs. If teeth do not erupt, the alveolar bone does not develop.

2. Function of the Alveolar Bone in the Periodontium. The alveolar bone forms the bony sockets that provide support and protection for the roots of the teeth.

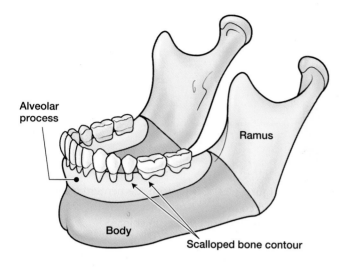

Alveolar process

Ramus

Body

Scalloped bone contour

Figure 1.15. Alveolar Process. The alveolar process is the bone that surrounds and supports the roots of the teeth.

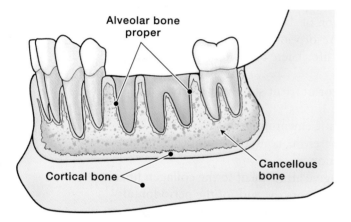

Alveolar bone proper

Cortical bone

Cancellous bone

Figure 1.16. Layers of the Alveolar Process. A lateral section of the mandible reveals the three bony layers: the alveolar bone proper, cancellous bone, and cortical bone.

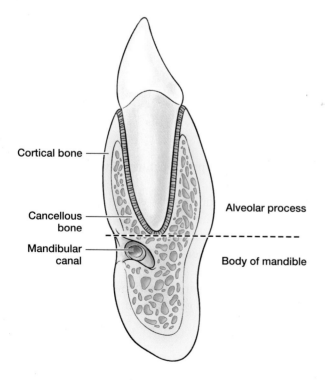

Cortical bone

Cancellous bone

Mandibular canal

Alveolar process

Body of mandible

Figure 1.17. Cross Section of the Mandible. The dotted line indicates the boundary of the alveolar process with the body of the mandible.

3. **Layers that Compose the Alveolar Process.** When viewed in cross section, the alveolar process is composed of three layers of hard tissue and covered by a thin layer of connective tissue (Figs. 1-16 and 1-17).
   A. The alveolar bone proper (or cribriform plate) is the thin layer of bone that lines the socket to surround the root of the tooth.
      1. The alveolus is the bony socket, a cavity in the alveolar bone that houses the root of a tooth (alveolus = singular; alveoli = plural) (FIG. 1-18).
      2. The alveolar bone proper has numerous holes that allow blood vessels from the cancellous bone to connect with the vessels of the periodontal ligament space.
      3. The ends of the periodontal ligament fibers are embedded in the alveolar bone proper.
   B. The cortical bone is a layer of compact bone that forms the hard, outside wall of the mandible and maxilla on the facial and lingual aspects. This cortical bone surrounds the alveolar bone proper and gives support to the socket.
      1. The buccal cortical bone is thin in the incisor, canine, and premolar regions; cortical bone is thicker in molar regions.
      2. Since the cortical plate is only on the facial and lingual sides of the jaw, it will not show up in a radiograph; only the cancellous bone and the alveolar bone proper can be seen on a radiograph.
      3. The alveolar crest is the most coronal portion of the alveolar process.
         a. In health, the alveolar crest is located 1 to 2 mm apical to (below) the CEJ of the teeth (FIG. 1-19).
         b. When viewed from the facial or lingual aspect, the alveolar crest meets the teeth in a scalloped (wavy) line that follows the contours of the CEJs (FIG. 1-9).
   C. The cancellous bone (or spongy bone) is the latticelike bone that fills the interior portion of the alveolar process (between the cortical bone and the alveolar bone proper). The cancellous bone is oriented around the tooth to form support for the alveolar bone proper.
   D. The periosteum is a layer of connective soft tissue covering the outer surface of bone; it consists of an outer layer of collagenous tissue and an inner layer of fine elastic fibers.

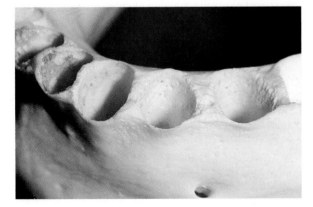

Figure 1.18. **Alveoli of the Mandible.** The alveoli are the sockets in the alveolar bone that house the roots of the teeth. (Courtesy of Dr Don Rolfs, Periodontal Foundations, Wenatchee, WA.)

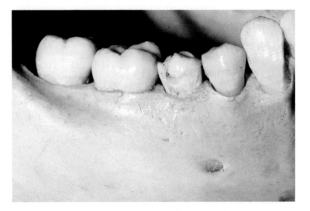

Figure 1.19. **Bony Contours.** The alveolar crest meets the teeth in a scalloped line that follows the contours of the CEJs. (Courtesy of Dr Don Rolfs, Periodontal Foundations, Wenatchee, WA.)

Section 2
Nerve Supply, Blood Supply, and Lymphatic System

NERVE SUPPLY TO THE PERIODONTIUM

1. **Description.** The innervation of the periodontium—nerve supply to the periodontium—occurs via the branches of the trigeminal nerve (FIG. 1-20). Innervation to the maxilla (FIG. 1-21) is by the second branch of the trigeminal nerve (the maxillary nerve) and the mandible by the third branch (the mandibular nerve).
   A. The trigeminal nerves have sensory, motor, and intermediate roots that attach directly to the brain.
   B. The trigeminal nerve is responsible for the sensory sensibility of most of the skin of the front part of the face and head, the teeth, oral cavity, maxillary sinus, and nasal cavity.
   C. The motor function of the trigeminal nerve is essential for the act of chewing.

2. **Functions of the Nerve Supply to the Periodontium**
   A. Nerve receptors in the gingiva, alveolar bone, and periodontal ligament register pain, touch, and pressure.
   B. Nerves in the periodontal ligament provide information about movement and tooth position. These nerves provide the sensations of light touch or pressure against the teeth and play an important role in the regulation of chewing forces and movements. When biting down on something hard, it is the nerves of the periodontal ligament that are stimulated, allowing the individual to experience a sense of pressure with the teeth against the hard object.

3. **Innervation of the Periodontium**
   A. Innervation of the Gingiva
      1. Innervation of the gingiva of the maxillary arch is from the superior alveolar nerves (anterior, middle, and posterior branches), infraorbital nerve, and the greater palatine and nasopalatine nerves (FIG. 1-21).
      2. Innervation of the gingiva of the mandibular arch is from the mental nerve, buccal nerve, and the sublingual branch of the lingual nerve (FIG. 1-22).
   B. Innervation of the Teeth and Periodontal Ligament
      1. Innervation of the teeth and periodontal ligament of the maxillary arch is from the superior alveolar nerves (anterior, middle, and posterior branches).
      2. Innervation of the teeth and periodontal ligament of the mandibular arch is from the inferior alveolar nerve.

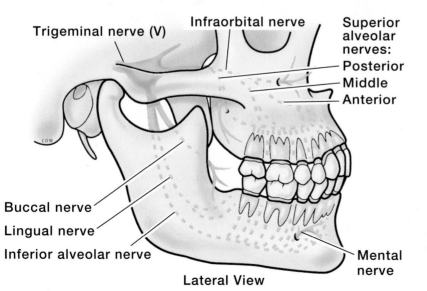

Figure 1.20. Nerve Supply to the Periodontium (Lateral View). The nerve supply to the periodontium is derived from the branches of the trigeminal nerve.

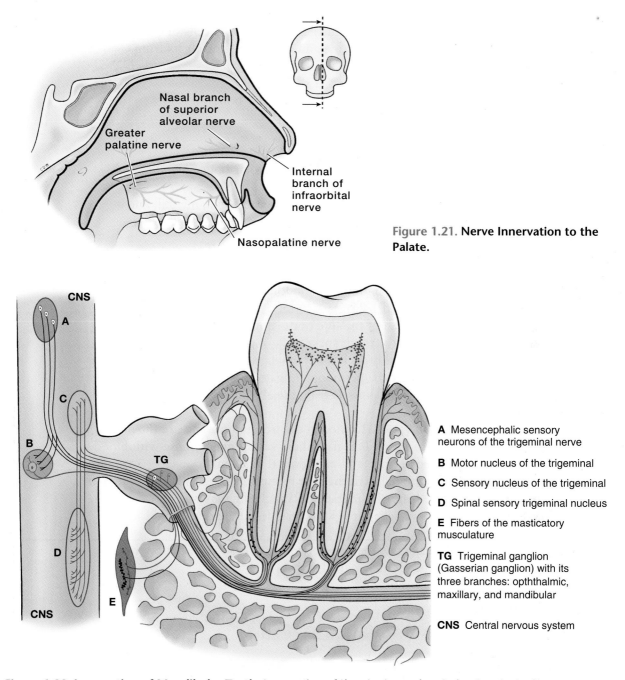

Figure 1.21. Nerve Innervation to the Palate.

A Mesencephalic sensory neurons of the trigeminal nerve

B Motor nucleus of the trigeminal

C Sensory nucleus of the trigeminal

D Spinal sensory trigeminal nucleus

E Fibers of the masticatory musculature

TG Trigeminal ganglion (Gasserian ganglion) with its three branches: opththalmic, maxillary, and mandibular

CNS Central nervous system

Figure 1.22. Innervation of Mandibular Teeth. Innervation of the gingiva and periodontium is via the mandibular nerve.

BLOOD SUPPLY TO THE PERIODONTIUM

1. **Description.** The vessels of the periodontium **anastomose** (join together) to create a complex *system of blood vessels* that supply blood to the periodontal tissues.
   A. This network of blood vessels acts as a unit, supplying blood to the soft and hard tissues of the maxilla and mandible.
   B. It is the proliferation of this rich blood supply to the gingiva that accounts for the dramatic color changes that are seen in gingivitis.

2. **Function.** The major function of the complex network of blood vessels of the periodontium is to transport oxygen and nutrients to the tissue cells of the periodontium and to remove carbon dioxide and other waste products from the cells for elimination.

3. **Vascular Supply to the Periodontium** (FIG. 1-23)
   A. Maxillary gingiva, periodontal ligament, and alveolar bone
      1. Anterior and posterior superior alveolar arteries
      2. Infraorbital artery
      3. Greater palatine artery
   B. Mandibular gingiva, periodontal ligament, and alveolar bone
      1. Inferior alveolar artery
      2. Branches of the inferior alveolar artery: the buccal, facial, mental, and sublingual arteries

4. **Vascular Supply to the Teeth and Periodontal Tissues**
   A. The major arteries
      1. Superior alveolar arteries—maxillary periodontal tissues
      2. Inferior alveolar artery—mandibular periodontal tissues
   B. Branch arteries (Figs. 1-24 and 1-25)
      1. The dental artery: a branch of the superior or inferior alveolar artery
      2. Intraseptal artery: enters the tooth socket
      3. Rami perforantes: terminal branches of the intraseptal artery; they penetrate the tooth socket and enter the periodontal ligament space where they anastomose (join) with the blood vessels from the alveolar bone and periodontal ligament
      4. Supraperiosteal blood vessels: located in the free gingiva and are the main supply of the blood to the free gingiva; these vessels anastomose with blood vessels from the alveolar bone and periodontal ligament
      5. Subepithelial plexus: branches of the supraperiosteal blood vessels located in the connective tissue beneath the free and attached gingiva
      6. Periodontal ligament vessels: supply the periodontal ligament and form a complex network of vessels that surrounds the root
      7. Dentogingival plexus: a fine-meshed network of blood vessels located in the connective tissue beneath the gingival sulcus

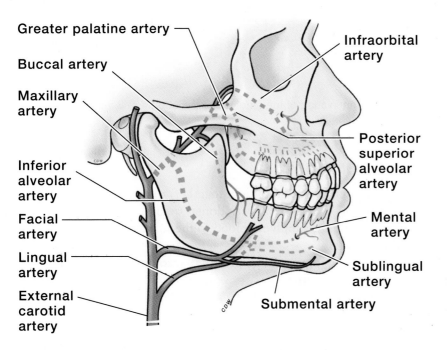

Figure 1.23. **Vascular Supply to the Periodontium.** A complex network of blood vessels supplies blood to the periodontium.

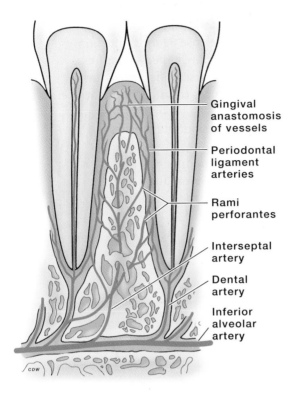

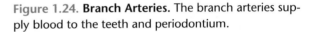

Figure 1.24. **Branch Arteries.** The branch arteries supply blood to the teeth and periodontium.

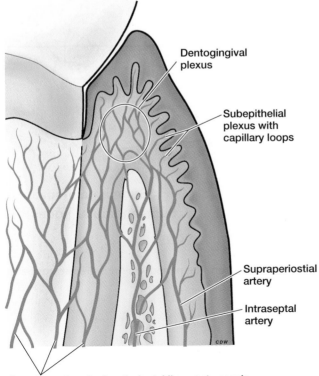

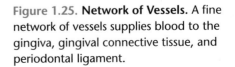

Figure 1.25. **Network of Vessels.** A fine network of vessels supplies blood to the gingiva, gingival connective tissue, and periodontal ligament.

LYMPHATIC SYSTEM AND THE PERIODONTIUM

1. **Description.** The lymphatic system is a network of lymph nodes connected by lymphatic vessels that plays an important role in the body's defense against infection.
2. **Function.** Lymph nodes (pronounced: limf nodes) are small bean-shaped structures located on either side of the head, neck, armpits, and groin. These nodes filter out and trap bacteria, fungi, viruses, and other unwanted substances to safely eliminate them from the body.
3. **Lymph Drainage of the Periodontium.** The lymph from the periodontal tissues is drained to the lymph nodes of the head and neck (FIG. 1-26).
   A. Submandibular lymph nodes—drain most of the periodontal tissues
   B. Deep cervical lymph nodes—drain the palatal gingiva of the maxilla
   C. Submental lymph nodes—drain the gingiva in the region of the mandibular incisors
   D. Jugulodigastric lymph nodes—drain the gingiva in the third molar region

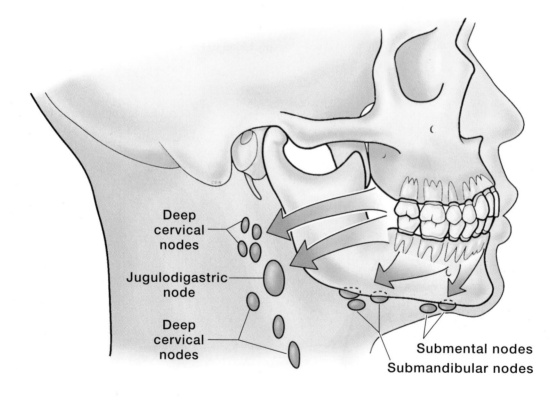

Figure 1.26. Lymphatic System of the Periodontium. The lymph from the periodontium is drained to the lymph nodes of the head and neck.

Chapter Summary Statement

The gingiva, periodontal ligament, cementum, and alveolar bone make up a system of tissues that surround the teeth and attach them to the alveolar bone. Each tissue of the periodontium plays a vital role in the functioning and retention of the teeth.

- The gingiva provides a tissue seal around the cervical portion of the teeth and covers the alveolar process.
- The periodontal ligament supports the tooth in its socket, provides nutrients and sensory feeling to the tooth, and maintains cementum and the alveolar bone of the tooth socket.
- The cementum anchors the periodontal ligament to the tooth and seals the ends of the open dentinal tubules. Cementum formation compensates for tooth wear due to occlusal attrition.
- The alveolar bone forms the bony sockets that provide support and protection for the roots of the teeth.

Section 3
Focus on Patients

Case 1

A patient involved in an automobile accident receives a penetrating wound involving the oral cavity. The wound enters the alveolar mucosa near the apex of a lower premolar tooth and extends from the surface mucosa all the way through the tissues to the premolar tooth root. List periodontal tissues most likely injured by this penetrating wound.

Case 2

A patient who has lost a maxillary lateral incisor tooth is scheduled to have a dental implant placed. The dental implant placement will require the clinician to prepare a hole with a drill in the bone formerly occupied by the lateral incisor tooth. Name the types of bone that will most probably be penetrated by the drill.

Case 3

A dentist injects a local anesthetic before working on a maxillary molar tooth. The injection results in complete loss of sensation in the molar tooth and in most of the gingiva surrounding the molar tooth. Name the nerves that most likely have been affected by the injection of the local anesthetic.

References

1. Lang NP, Loe H. The relationship between the width of the keratinized gingiva and gingival health. *J Periodontol.* 1972;43:623–627.
2. Ainamo J, Loe H. Anatomical characteristics of gingiva. A clinical and microscopic study of the free and attached gingiva. *J Periodontol.* 1966;37(1):5–13.
3. Cho MI, Garant PR. Development and general structure of the periodontium. *Periodontology 2000.* 2000;24:9–27.
4. Cimasoni G. Crecicular fluid updated. *Monogr Oral Sci.* 1983;12:III–VII, 1–152.
5. Saygin NE, Giannobile WV, Somerman MJ. Molecular and cell biology of cementum. *Periodontology 2000.* 2000;24:73–98.
6. Diekwisch TG. The developmental biology of cementum. *Int J Dev Biol.* 2001;45(5–6):695–706.
7. Sodek J, McKee MD. Molecular and cellular biology of alveolar bone. *Periodontology 2000.* 2000;24:99–126.

Suggested Readings

Alvarez-Perez MA, Alvarez-Fregoso MA, Ortiz-Lopez J, Arzate, H. X-ray microanalysis of human cementum. *Microsc Microanal.* 2005;11(4):313–318.

Attstrom R, Graf-de Beer M, Schroeder HE. Clinical and histologic characteristics of normal gingiva in dogs. *J Periodontal Res.* 1975;10(3):115–127.

Bilgin E, Gurgan CA, Arpak, MN, Bostanci HS, Guven K. Morphological changes in diseased cementum layers: a scanning electron microscopy study. *Calcif Tissue Int.* 2004;74(5):476–485.

Cleaton-Jones P, Buskin SA, Volchansky A. Surface ultrastructure of human gingiva. *J Periodontal Res.* 1978;13(4): 367–371.

Dale BA. Periodontal epithelium: a newly recognized role in health and disease. *Periodontology 2000.* 2002;30:70–78.

Gokhan K, Keklikoglu N, Buyukertan M. The comparison of the thickness of the cementum layer in Type 2 diabetic and non-diabetic patients. *J Contemp Dent Pract.* 2004;5(2):124–133.

Listgarten MA. Electron microscopic study of the gingivo-dental junction of man. *Am J Anat.* 1966;119(1):147–177.

Pinchi V, Forestieri AL, Calvitti M. Thickness of the dental (radicular) cementum: a parameter for estimating age. *J Forensic Odontostomatol.* 2007;25(1):1–6.

Popowics T, Foster BL, Swanson EC, et al. Defining the roots of cementum formation. *Cells Tissues Organs.* 2005;181(3–4):248–257.

Sabag N, Saglie R, Mery C. Ultrastructure of the normal human epithelial attachment to the cementum root surface. *J Periodontol.* 1981;52(2):94–95.

Schroeder HE, Listgarten MA. The gingival tissues: the architecture of periodontal protection. *Periodontology 2000.* 1997;13:91–120.

Chapter 2

Microscopic Anatomy of the Periodontium

Learning Objectives

- Define the term epithelial tissue and describe its function in the body.

- List and define the layers that comprise the stratified squamous epithelium of the skin.

- Define keratin and describe its function in the epithelium.

- Define the term cell junction and describe its function in the epithelial tissues.

- Compare and contrast the terms desmosome and hemidesmosome.

- Describe the epithelium–connective tissue interface found in most tissues of the body, such as the interface between the epithelium and connective tissues of the skin.

- Describe the function of connective tissue in the body.

- List and recognize the histologic features of periodontal health.

- List and define the layers that comprise the stratified squamous epithelium of the gingiva.

- Identify the three anatomical areas of the gingival epithelium on an unlabeled drawing of the anatomical areas of the gingival epithelium.

- Define the term oral epithelium and describe its location and function in the gingival epithelium.

- Define the term sulcular epithelium and describe its location and function in the gingival epithelium.

- Define the term junctional epithelium and describe its location and function in the gingival epithelium.

- State which of the anatomical areas of the gingival epithelium have an uneven, wavy epithelium–connective tissue interface in health and which have a smooth junction in health.

- State the level of keratinization present in each of the three anatomical areas of the gingival epithelium (keratinized, nonkeratinized, or parakeratinized).

- Identify the enamel, gingival connective tissue, junctional epithelium, internal basal lamina, external basal lamina, epithelial cells, desmosomes, and hemidesmosomes on an unlabeled drawing depicting the microscopic anatomy of the junctional epithelium and surrounding tissues.

- Describe the function of the gingival connective tissue.

- Define the term supragingival fiber bundles and describe their function in the periodontium.

- Define the term periodontal ligament and describe is function in the periodontium.

- Identify the principle fiber groups of the periodontal ligament on an unlabeled drawing.

- Define the term Sharpey fibers.

- Define the term cementum and describe its function in the periodontium.

- State the three relationships that the cementum may have in relation to the enamel at the cementoenamel junction.

- Define the term alveolar bone and describe its function in the periodontium.

Key Terms

Histology

Tissue

Cells

Extracellular matrix

Epithelial tissue

Stratified squamous epithelium

Basal lamina

Keratinization

Keratinized epithelial cells

Nonkeratinized epithelial cells

Connective tissue

Epithelial–connective tissue interface

Epithelial ridges

Connective tissue papillae

Cell junctions

Desmosome

Hemidesmosome

Gingival epithelium

Oral epithelium (OE)

Sulcular epithelium (SE)

Junctional epithelium (JE)

Parakeratinized

Keratin

Gingival crevicular fluid

Internal basal lamina

External basal lamina

Supragingival fiber bundles

Collagen fibers

Dentogingival unit

Periosteum

Periodontal ligament (PDL)

Fiber bundles of the PDL

Sharpey fibers

Cementum

OMG (overlap, meet, gap)

Alveolar process

Section 1
Histology of the Body's Tissues

Histology is a branch of anatomy concerned with the study of the microscopic structures of tissues. Knowledge of the microscopic characteristics of tissues is a prerequisite for understanding the microscopic anatomy of the periodontium. The first section reviews the microscopic anatomy of the epithelial and connective tissues of the body.

MICROSCOPIC ANATOMY OF A TISSUE

A tissue is a group of interconnected cells that perform a similar function within an organism. For example, muscle cells group together to form muscle tissue that functions to move parts of the body. **The tissues of the body consist of cells and an extracellular matrix.**

1. Cells
   A. Cells are the smallest structural unit of living matter capable of functioning independently.
   B. Cells group together to form a tissue.
   C. The four basic types of tissue are epithelial, connective, nerve, and muscle tissues.
2. **Extracellular Matrix.** Tissues are not made up solely of cells. A gel-like substance containing interwoven protein fibers surrounds most cells.
   A. The extracellular matrix is a meshlike material that surrounds the cells (FIG. 2-1). It is like scaffolding for the cells. This material helps to hold cells together and provides a framework within which cells can migrate and interact with one another.
   B. The extracellular matrix consists of ground substance and fibers.
      1. The ground substance is a gel-like material that fills the space between the cells.
      2. The fibers consist of collagen, elastin, and reticular fibers. Collagens are the major proteins of the extracellular matrix.
   C. Amount of Extracellular Matrix
      1. In epithelial tissue, the extracellular matrix is scanty, consisting mainly of a thin mat called the basal lamina, which underlies the epithelium.
      2. In connective tissue, the extracellular matrix is more plentiful than the cells that it surrounds.

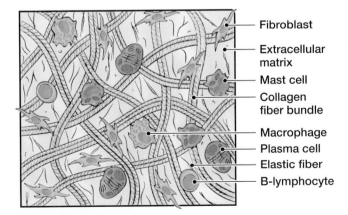

- Fibroblast
- Extracellular matrix
- Mast cell
- Collagen fiber bundle
- Macrophage
- Plasma cell
- Elastic fiber
- B-lymphocyte

Figure 2.1. Extracellular Matrix. The extracellular matrix surrounds the cells of a tissue and consists of fibers and a gel-like substance.

MICROSCOPIC ANATOMY OF EPITHELIAL TISSUE

1. **Description.** The epithelial tissue is the tissue that makes up the outer surface of the body (skin) and lines the body cavities such as the mouth, stomach, and intestines (mucosa). The skin and mucosa of the oral cavity are made up of stratified squamous epithelium—a type of epithelium that is composed of flat cells arranged in several layers.

2. **Composition of Epithelial Tissue**
   A. **Plentiful Cells.** Most of the volume of epithelial tissue consists of many closely packed epithelial cells (FIG. 2-2). Epithelial cells are bound together into sheets.
   B. **Sparse Extracellular Matrix**
      1. The extracellular matrix component of epithelial tissue is small, consisting mainly of a thin mat called the basal lamina, which underlies the epithelium.
      2. Beneath the basal lamina lies the connective tissue.

3. **Keratinization.** Keratinization—the process by which epithelial cells on the surface of the skin become stronger and waterproof.
   A. **Keratinized Epithelial Cells**
      1. Keratinized epithelial cells have no nuclei and form a tough, resistant layer on the surface of the skin.
      2. The most heavily keratinized epithelium of the body is found on the palms of the hands and soles of the feet.
   B. **Nonkeratinized Epithelial Cells**
      1. Nonkeratinized epithelial cells have nuclei and act as a cushion against mechanical stress and wear. Nonkeratinized epithelial cells are softer and more flexible.
      2. Nonkeratinized epithelium is found in areas such as the mucosal lining of the cheeks—permitting the mobility needed to speak, chew, and make facial expressions.

4. **Blood Supply.** Epithelial tissues do not contain blood vessels; nourishment is received from blood vessels contained in the underlying connective tissue (FIG. 2-2).

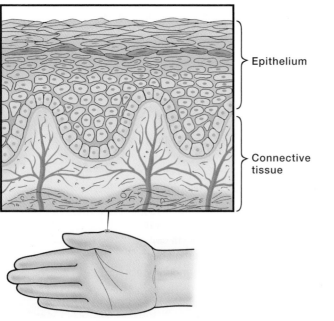

Epithelium

Connective tissue

Figure 2.2. Stratified Squamous Epithelium and Connective Tissue of the Skin. The epithelium of the skin consists of many closely packed epithelial cells and a thin basal lamina. The epithelium of the skin rests on a supporting bed of connective tissue. The epithelium does not contain blood vessels; nourishment is received from blood vessels in the underlying connective tissue.

MICROSCOPIC ANATOMY OF CONNECTIVE TISSUE

1. **Description.** Connective tissue fills the spaces between the tissues and organs in the body. It supports and binds other tissues. Connective tissue consists of cells separated by abundant extracellular substance.
2. **Composition of Connective Tissue**
   A. **Sparse Cells.** Connective tissue cells are sparsely distributed in the extracellular matrix.
      1. Fibroblasts ("fiber builders")—cells that form the extracellular matrix (fibers and ground substance) and secrete it into the intercellular spaces
      2. Macrophages and neutrophils—phagocytes ("cell eaters") that devour dying cells and microorganisms that invade the body
      3. Lymphocytes—cells that play a major role in the immune response
   B. **Plentiful Extracellular Matrix.** The extracellular matrix—a rich gel-like substance containing a network of strong fibers—is the major component of connective tissue. The network of fiber matrix, rather than the cells, gives connective tissue the strength to withstand mechanical forces.
3. **Dental Connective Tissue**
All dental tissues of the tooth—cementum, dentin, alveolar bone, and the pulp—are specialized forms of connective tissue *except enamel*. Enamel is an epithelial tissue.

EPITHELIAL–CONNECTIVE TISSUE BOUNDARY

1. **Description.** The epithelial–connective tissue interface is the boundary where the epithelial and connective tissues meet.
2. **Characteristics of the Epithelial–Connective Tissue Boundary**
   A. **Wavy Boundary.** In most places in the body, the epithelium meets the connective tissue in a wavy, uneven manner (FIG. 2-3).
      1. Epithelial ridges—deep extensions of epithelium that reach down into the connective tissue. The epithelial ridges are also known as rete pegs (FIG. 2-3).
      2. Connective tissue papillae—fingerlike extensions of connective tissue that extend up into the epithelium (FIG. 2-3).
   B. **Smooth Boundary**
      1. Some specialized epithelial tissues in the body meet the connective tissue in a smooth interface that has no epithelial ridges or connective tissue papillae.
      2. Some anatomical areas of the gingiva have an epithelial–connective tissue interface that is smooth.

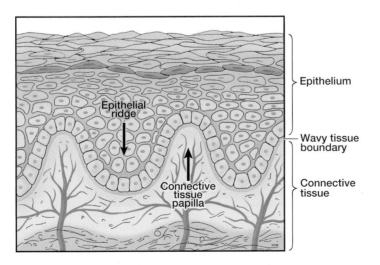

Epithelium

Epithelial ridge

Wavy tissue boundary

Connective tissue papilla

Connective tissue

Figure 2.3. Wavy Epithelial–Connective Tissue Interface. In most cases, the epithelium meets the connective tissue at an uneven, wavy border. Epithelial ridges extend down into the connective tissue. Connective tissue papillae extend upward into the epithelium.

3. **Function of the Wavy Tissue Boundary**
    A. **Enhances Adhesion.** The wavy tissue interface enhances the adhesion of the epithelium to the connective tissue by increasing the surface area of the junction between the two tissues. This strong adhesion of the epithelium allows the skin to resist mechanical forces.
    B. **Provides Nourishment.** The wavy junction between the epithelium and the connective tissue also increases the area from which the epithelium can receive nourishment from the underlying connective tissue. The epithelium does not have its own blood supply; blood vessels are carried close to the epithelium in the connective tissue papillae.

EPITHELIAL CELL JUNCTIONS

Neighboring epithelial cells attach to one another by specialized cell junctions that give the tissue strength to withstand mechanical forces and to form a protective barrier.

1. **Definition.** Cell junctions are cellular structures that mechanically attach a cell and its cytoskeleton to its neighboring cells or to the basal lamina.
2. **Purpose.** Cell junctions bind cells together so that they can function as a strong structural unit. Tissues, such as the epithelium of the skin that must withstand severe mechanical stresses, have the most abundant number of cell junctions.
3. **Forms of Epithelial Cell Junctions**
    A. Desmosome—a specialized cell junction that connects two neighboring epithelial cells and their cytoskeletons together. You might think of desmosomes as being like the snaps used to close a denim jacket. Instead of fastening the front of a jacket together, desmosomes fasten cells together (FIG. 2-4).
        1. A cell-to-cell connection
        2. An important form of cell junction found in the gingival epithelium.
    B. Hemidesmosome—a specialized cell junction that connects the epithelial cells to the basal lamina (FIG. 2-4).
        1. A cell-to-basal lamina connection
        2. An important form of cell junction found in the gingival epithelium.

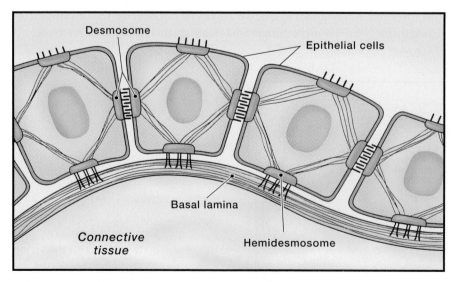

Figure 2.4. Epithelial Cell Junctions. Epithelial cells attach to each other with specialized cell junctions called desmosomes. Hemidesmosomes attach the epithelial cells to the basal lamina.

Section 2
Histology of the Gingiva

Knowledge of the microscopic anatomy of the gingiva is a prerequisite for understanding the periodontium in health and in disease. At first glance, the microscopic anatomy of the periodontium may seem to be impossibly complicated. The anatomy of the periodontium, however, is much like that of tissues elsewhere in the body. **The gingiva consists of an epithelial layer and an underlying connective tissue layer.** This section reviews the microscopic anatomy of the gingival epithelium, junctional epithelium (JE), and gingival connective tissues.

MICROSCOPIC ANATOMY OF GINGIVAL EPITHELIUM

The gingival epithelium is a specialized stratified squamous epithelium that functions well in the wet environment of the oral cavity [1]. The microscopic anatomy of the gingival epithelium is similar to the epithelium of the skin. The gingival epithelium may be differentiated into three anatomical areas (FIG. 2-5):

1. Oral Epithelium (OE): epithelium that faces the oral cavity.
2. Sulcular Epithelium (SE): epithelium that faces the tooth surface *without being in contact with the tooth surface.*
3. Junctional Epithelium (JE): epithelium that attaches the gingiva to the tooth.

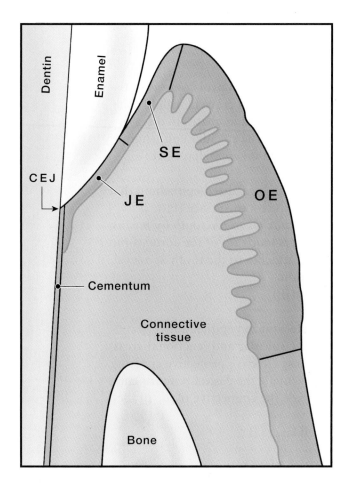

Figure 2.5. **Three Areas of the Gingival Epithelium.** The gingival epithelium has three distinct areas:

- JE—junctional epithelium at the base of the sulcus
- SE—sulcular epithelium that lines the sulcus
- OE—oral epithelium covering the free and attached gingiva

1. **Oral epithelium (OE).** The oral epithelium covers the outer surface of the free gingiva and attached gingiva; it extends from the crest of the gingival margin to the mucogingival junction. The OE is the only part of the periodontium that is visible to the unaided eye (Fig. 2-5).
    A. **Cellular Structure of the Oral Epithelium (OE)**
        1. The OE may be keratinized or parakeratinized (partially keratinized). Keratin is a tough, fibrous structural protein that occurs in the outer layer of the skin and the OE.
        2. The OE is a stratified squamous epithelium that can be divided into the following cell layers (Fig. 2-6):
            a. Basal cell layer: cube-shaped cells
            b. Prickle cell layer: spinelike cells with large intercellular spaces. The cells of both the basal and prickle cell layers attach to each other with desmosomes.
            c. Granular cell layer: flattened cells and increased intracellular keratin.
            d. Keratinized cell layer: flattened cells with extensive intracellular keratin.
    B. **Interface with Gingival Connective Tissue.** In health, OE joins with the connective tissue in a *wavy interface* with epithelial ridges (Figs. 2-5 and 2-7).
2. **Sulcular Epithelium.** Sulcular epithelium (SE) is the epithelial lining of the gingival sulcus. It extends from the crest of the gingival margin to the coronal edge of the JE (Fig. 2-5).
    A. **Cellular Structure of the Sulcular Epithelium (SE)**
        1. The SE is a thin, nonkeratinized epithelium [2].
        2. The SE has three cellular layers (Fig. 2-6):
            a. Basal cell layer
            b. Prickle cell layer
            c. Superficial cell layer: flattened cells without keratin
        3. The SE is permeable allowing fluid to flow from the gingival connective tissue into the sulcus. This fluid is known as the gingival crevicular fluid. The flow of gingival crevicular fluid is slight in health and increases in disease.
    B. **Interface with Gingival Connective Tissue.** In health, the sulcular epithelium joins the connective tissue at a *smooth interface* with no epithelial ridges (no wavy junction) (Fig. 2-5).
3. **Junctional Epithelium.** Junctional epithelium (JE) is the specialized epithelium that forms the base of the sulcus and joins the gingiva to the tooth surface (Fig. 2-5). *The gingiva surrounds the cervix of the tooth and attaches to the tooth by means of the junctional epithelium. The base of the sulcus is made up of the coronal-most cells of the junctional epithelium.* In health, the JE attaches to the tooth at a level that is slightly coronal to the cementoenamel junction.
    A. **Cellular Structure of the Junctional Epithelium (JE)**
        1. Keratinization of JE
            a. The junctional epithelium is a thin, nonkeratinized epithelium.
            b. Nonkeratinized epithelial cells of both the sulcular and junctional areas of the gingival epithelium make them a less effective protective covering. Thus, the sulcular and junctional areas provide the easiest point of entry for bacteria or bacterial products to invade the connective tissue of the gingiva.
        2. The junctional epithelium has only two cell layers (Fig. 2-6):
            a. Basal cell layer
            b. Prickle cell layer

   3. Length and width of JE
      a. The junctional epithelium ranges from 0.71 to 1.35 mm in length [3].
      b. The JE is about 15 to 30 cells thick at the coronal zone—the zone that attaches highest on the crown of the tooth.
      c. The JE tapers to 4- to 5-cell thickness at the apical zone.
   B. JE Interface with Gingival Connective Tissue. In health, the junctional epithelium has a *smooth tissue interface* with the connective tissue (no wavy junctions) (FIG. 2-5).

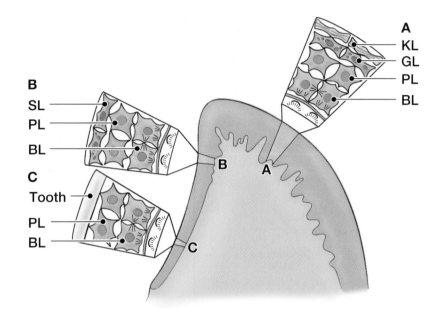

Figure 2.6. Cell Layers of the Gingival Epithelium. The cell layers of the OE, SE, and JE. *Illustration key:* A, oral epithelium; B, sulcular epithelium; C, junctional epithelium; KL, keratinized cell layer; GL, granular cell layer; SL, superficial cell layer; PL, prickle cell layer; BL, Basal cell layer.

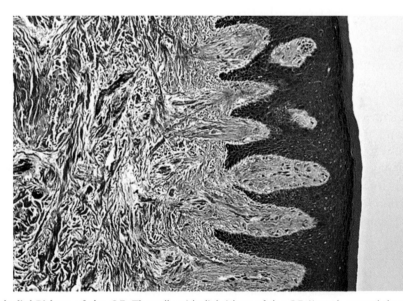

Figure 2.7. Epithelial Ridges of the OE. The tall epithelial ridges of the OE (*in red*) extend down into the underlying connective tissue. A dense network of collagen fibers (*in blue*) tightly anchors the epithelium. Used with permission from Mills SE. *Histology for Pathologists.* 3rd ed. Philadelphia: Lippincott Williams & Wilkins; 2006; Figure 15-33, p 419.

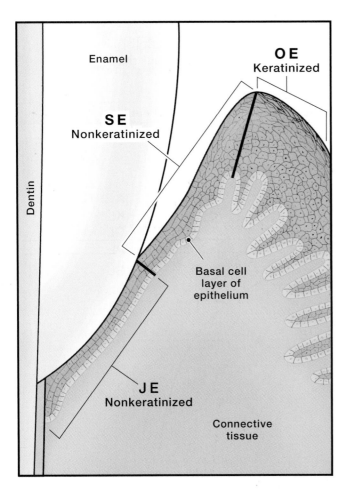

Figure 2.8. Microscopic Anatomy of the Three Areas of the Gingival Epithelium. Interface with Connective Tissue.

- OE (oral epithelium)—these epithelial cells form the outer layer of the free and attached gingiva.
- SE (sulcular epithelium)—these epithelial cells extend from the edge of the junctional epithelium coronally to the crest of the gingival margin.
- JE (junctional epithelium)—these epithelial cells join the gingiva to the tooth surface at the base of the sulcus.

WHY THE TEETH NEED A JUNCTIONAL EPITHELIUM

1. **The Teeth Create a Break in the Epithelial Protective Covering**
   A. **Protective Epithelial Sheet Covers the Body**
      1. A continuous sheet of epithelium protects the body by covering its outer surfaces and lining the body's cavities, including the oral cavity.
      2. The teeth penetrate this protective covering by erupting through the epithelium, thus creating an opening through which microorganisms can enter the body.
   B. **The Teeth Puncture the Protective Epithelial Sheet**
      1. The body attempts to seal the opening created when a tooth penetrates the epithelium by attaching the epithelium to the tooth.
      2. The word "junction" means "connection"; thus, the epithelium that is connected to the tooth is termed the "junctional epithelium."
2. **Functions of Junctional Epithelium**
   A. **Epithelial Attachment.** The JE provides an attachment between the gingiva and the tooth surface, thus providing a seal at the base of the gingival sulcus or periodontal pocket (FIG. 2-8).
   B. **Barrier.** The junctional epithelium provides a protective barrier between the plaque biofilm and the connective tissue of the periodontium.
   C. **Host Defense.** The epithelial cells play a role in defending the periodontium from bacterial infection by signaling the immune response [4].

ATTACHMENT OF THE CELLS OF THE JUNCTIONAL EPITHELIUM

1. **Microscopic Anatomy of the Junctional Epithelium**
    A. **Components of the junctional epithelium (JE).** The junctional epithelium consists of
        1. Plentiful cells
            a. Layers of closely packed epithelial cells
            b. Desmosomes and hemidesmosomes—specialized cell junctions
        2. A sparse extracellular matrix
            a. Internal basal lamina—a thin mat of extracellular matrix between the epithelial cells of the junctional epithelium and the tooth surface.
            b. External basal lamina—a thin mat of extracellular matrix between the epithelial cells of the junctional epithelium and the gingival connective tissue.
2. **Attachment of the Junctional Epithelium to the Tooth Surface**
    A. **Attachment to the Tooth Surface**
        1. The JE cells next to the tooth surface form *hemidesmosomes* that enable these cells to attach to the *internal basal lamina* and the surface of the tooth [5–8].
        2. The internal basal lamina is a thin sheet of extracellular matrix adjacent to the tooth surface.
        3. The epithelial cells physically attach to the tooth surface by four to eight hemidesmosomes per micron at the coronal zone and two hemidesmosomes per micron in the apical zone of the junctional epithelium [9,10]. The apical zone is the area of the junctional epithelium with the least adhesiveness (Figs. 2-9 and 2-10).
        4. The attachment of the hemidesmosomes and internal basal lamina to the tooth surface is not static; rather, the cells of the junctional epithelium appear to be capable of moving along the tooth surface.
    B. **Attachment to the Underlying Gingival Connective Tissue**
        1. The epithelial cells of the junctional epithelium attach to the underlying *gingival connective tissue* via *hemidesmosomes* and the *external basal lamina* (Fig. 2-9) [7,8,11].
        2. In health, the junctional epithelium has a *smooth tissue interface* with the connective tissue (no wavy junctions).

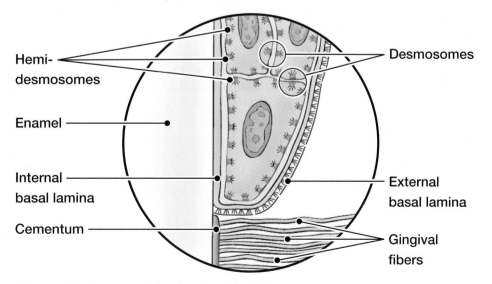

Figure 2.9. Microscopic Anatomy of the Junctional Epithelium (JE). Microscopic structures of the JE include the epithelial cells, desmosomes, external and internal basal laminae, and hemidesmosomes.

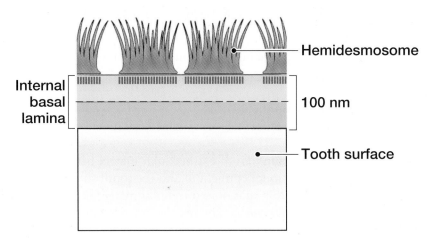

Figure 2.10. Hemidesmosomes. The epithelial cells next to the tooth surface form hemidesmosomes that attach to the internal basal lamina and the tooth surface.

MICROSCOPIC ANATOMY OF GINGIVAL CONNECTIVE TISSUE

1. **Function of Gingival Connective Tissue.** The gingival connective tissue of the free and attached gingiva provides solidity to the gingiva and attaches the gingiva to the cementum of the root and the alveolar bone. The gingival connective tissue is also known as the lamina propria [1,12].
2. **Components of the Gingival Connective Tissue**
   A. **Cells**
   1. In contrast to the gingival epithelium (which has an abundance of cells and sparse extracellular matrix), the gingival connective tissue has an abundance of extracellular matrix and few cells (Fig. 2-11).
   2. Cells comprise about 5% of the gingival connective tissue.
   3. The different types of cells present in the gingival connective tissue include
      a. Fibroblasts
      b. Mast cells
      c. Immune cells, such as macrophages, neutrophils, and lymphocytes.
   4. The fibers of the connective tissue are produced by the fibroblasts.
   B. **Extracellular Matrix**
   1. The major components of the connective tissue are protein fibers, fibroblasts, vessels, and nerves that are embedded in the extracellular matrix. The matrix of the connective tissue is produced mainly by the fibroblasts.
   2. The matrix is the medium in which the connective tissue cells are embedded and it is essential for the maintenance of the normal function of the connective tissue. The transportation of water, nutrients, metabolites, oxygen, etc., to and from the individual connective tissue cells occurs within the matrix.
   3. Protein fibers account for about 55% to 65% of the gingival connective tissue. Most of these are collagen fibers that form a dense network of strong, ropelike cables that secure and hold the gingival connective tissues together [13].
   4. The collagen fibers enable the gingiva to form a rigid cuff around the tooth.
   5. Gel-like material between the cells makes up about 30% to 35% of the gingival connective tissue. This gel-like material helps to hold the tissue together.

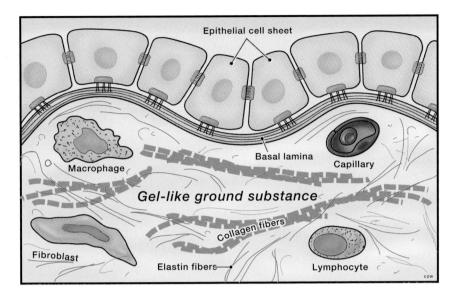

Figure 2.11. **Microscopic Anatomy of Gingival Connective Tissue.** The gingival connective tissue comprises a gel-like substance, protein fibers, and cells.

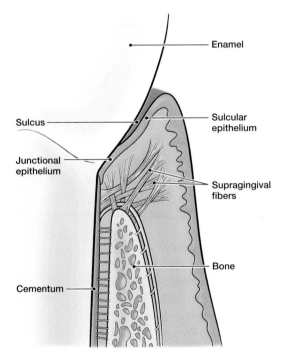

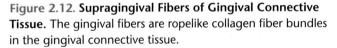

Figure 2.12. **Supragingival Fibers of Gingival Connective Tissue.** The gingival fibers are ropelike collagen fiber bundles in the gingival connective tissue.

3. **The Supragingival Fiber Bundles of the Gingival Connective Tissue.** The **supragingival fiber bundles (gingival fibers)** are a network of ropelike collagen fiber bundles in the gingival connective tissue (FIG. 2-12). These fibers are located coronal to (above) the crest of the alveolar bone (FIG. 2-13).
   A. **Characteristics of the Fiber Bundles**
      1. The fiber bundles are embedded in the gel-like extracellular matrix of the gingival connective tissue.
      2. The supragingival fiber bundles strengthen the attachment of the JE to the tooth by bracing the gingival margin against the tooth surface.
      3. Together the JE and the gingival fibers are referred to as the dentogingival unit. The dentogingival unit acts to provide structural support to the gingival tissue.

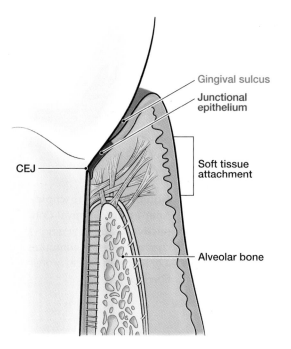

Figure 2.13. **Location of the Supragingival Fibers.** The supragingival fibers of the gingival tissue form a soft tissue attachment coronal to the alveolar bone.

B. **Functions of the Gingival Fiber Bundles**
1. Brace the free gingiva firmly against the tooth and reinforce the attachment of the JE to the tooth.
2. Provide the free gingiva with the rigidity needed to withstand the frictional forces that result during mastication.
3. Unite the free gingiva with the cementum of the root and alveolar bone.
4. Connect adjacent teeth to one another to control tooth positioning within the dental arch.

C. **Classification of Gingival Fiber Groups.** The supragingival fiber bundles are classified based on their orientation, sites of insertion, and the structures that they connect (FIGS. 2-14 and 2-15).
1. **Alveologingival fibers**—extend from the periosteum of the alveolar crest into the gingival connective tissue (FIG. 2-14). These fiber bundles attach the gingiva to the bone. (The periosteum is a dense membrane composed of fibrous connective tissue that closely wraps the outer surface of the alveolar bone.)
2. **Circular fibers**—encircle the tooth in a ringlike manner coronal to the alveolar crest and are not attached to the cementum of the tooth (FIGS. 2-14 and 2-15). These fiber bundles connect adjacent teeth to one another.
3. **Dentogingival fibers**—embedded in the cementum near the CEJ and fan out into the gingival connective tissue (FIGS. 2-14 and 2-15). These fibers act to attach the gingiva to the teeth.
4. **Periostogingival fibers**—extend laterally from the periosteum of the alveolar bone. These fibers attach the gingiva to the bone (FIG. 2-14).
5. **Intergingival fibers**—extend in a mesiodistal direction along the entire dental arch and around the last molars in the arch. These fiber bundles link adjacent teeth into a dental arch unit (FIG. 2-15).
6. **Intercircular fibers**—encircle several teeth. These fiber groups link adjacent teeth into a dental arch unit.
7. **Interpapillary fibers**—are located in the papillae coronal to (above) the transseptal fiber bundles. These fiber groups connect the oral and vestibular interdental papillae of posterior teeth (FIG. 2-15).

8. **Transgingival fibers**—extend from the cementum near the CEJ and run horizontally between adjacent teeth (FIG. 2-15). These fiber bundles link adjacent teeth into a dental arch unit.
9. **Transseptal**—pass from the cementum of one tooth, over the crest of alveolar bone, to the cementum of the adjacent tooth (FIG. 2-15). These fiber bundles connect adjacent teeth to one another and secure alignment of teeth in the arch.

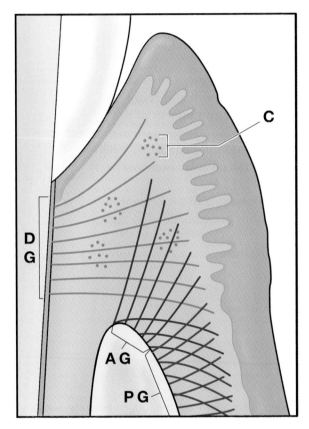

Figure 2.14. Supragingival Fiber Groups.

- C—circular
- AG—alveologingival
- DG—dentogingival
- PG—periostogingival

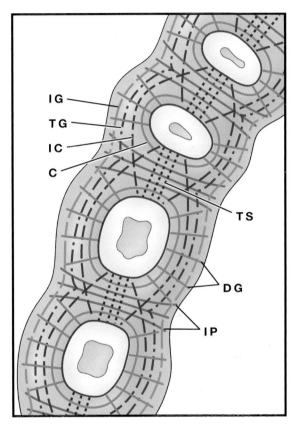

Figure 2.15. Supragingival Fiber Groups of the Mandibular Arch (Occlusal View, Looking Down on the Mandibular Arch).

- C—circular
- IG—intergingival
- IC—intercircular
- IP—interpapillary
- DG—dentogingival
- TG—transgingival
- TS—transseptal

4. **The periodontal ligament Fibers of the Gingival Connective Tissue.**
    A. **Definition.** The periodontal ligament (PDL) is a thin sheet of fibrous connective tissue that surrounds the roots of the teeth and joins the root cementum with the socket wall. The thickness of the periodontal ligament ranges from 0.05 to 0.25 mm depending on the age of the patient and the function of the tooth [14].
    B. **Components of the Periodontal Ligament.** The periodontal ligament consists of connective tissue fibers, cells, and extracellular matrix.
        1. Cells. The cells of the periodontal ligament are mainly fibroblasts with some cementoblasts and osteoblasts.
        2. Extracellular Matrix.
            a. The extracellular matrix of the periodontal ligament is similar to the extracellular matrix of other connective tissue. This rich gel-like substance contains specialized connective fibers.
            b. Fiber Bundles. The fiber bundles of the periodontal ligament are a specialized connective tissue that surrounds the root of the tooth and connects it with the alveolar bone. These fibers are the largest component of the periodontal ligament.
                1) The ropelike collagen fiber bundles of the periodontal ligament stretch across the space between the cementum and the alveolar bone of the tooth socket (FIG. 2-16).
                2) The collagen fiber bundles are anchored on one side in the cementum covering the tooth root; on the other side, they are embedded in the bone of the tooth socket.
        3. Blood vessels and nerve supply. The periodontal ligament has a rich supply of nerves and blood vessels.

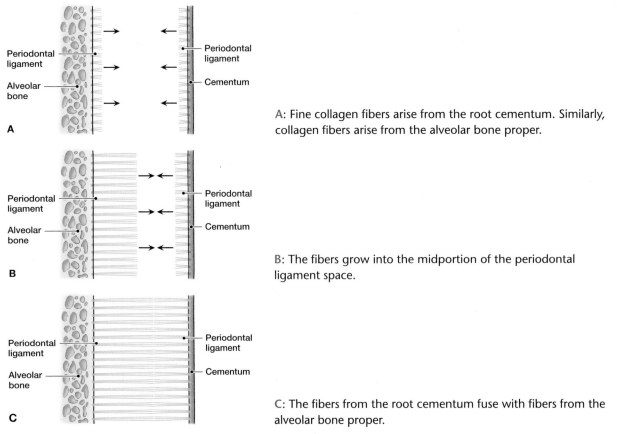

A: Fine collagen fibers arise from the root cementum. Similarly, collagen fibers arise from the alveolar bone proper.

B: The fibers grow into the midportion of the periodontal ligament space.

C: The fibers from the root cementum fuse with fibers from the alveolar bone proper.

Figure 2.16. **Development of the Periodontal Ligament Fibers.**

C. **Functions of the Periodontal Ligament**
1. Supportive function—the major function of the periodontal ligament is to anchor the tooth to its bony socket and to separate the tooth from the socket wall, so that the root does not collide with the bone during mastication.
2. Sensory function—the periodontal ligament is supplied with nerve fibers that transmit tactile pressure (such as a tap with dental instrument against tooth) and pain sensations.
3. Nutritive function—the periodontal ligament is supplied with blood vessels that provide nutrients to the cementum and bone.
4. Formative function—the periodontal ligament contains cementoblasts ("cementum builders") that produce cementum throughout the life of the tooth, while the osteoblasts ("bone builders") maintain the bone of the tooth socket.
5. Resorptive function—in response to severe pressure, cells of the periodontal ligament (osteoclasts) can produce rapid bone resorption and, sometimes, resorption of cementum.

D. **Principal Fiber Groups of the Periodontal Ligament.** The tooth is joined to the bone by bundles of collagen fibers that can be divided into the five groups based on their location and orientation (FIG. 2-17).
1. **Alveolar crest fiber group**—extend from the cervical cementum, running downward in a diagonal direction, to the alveolar crest. This fiber group resists horizontal movements of the tooth.
2. **Horizontal fiber group**—located apical to the alveolar crest fibers. They extend from the cementum to the bone at right angles to the long axis of the root. This fiber group resists horizontal pressure against the crown of the tooth
3. **Oblique fiber group**—located apical to the horizontal group. They extend from the cementum to the bone, running in a diagonal direction. This fiber group resists vertical pressures that threaten to drive the root into its socket.
4. **Apical fiber group**—extend from the apex of the tooth to the bone. This fiber group secures the tooth in its socket and resists forces that might lift the tooth out of the socket.
5. **Interradicular fiber group** (present only in multirooted teeth)—extend from the cementum in the furcation area of the tooth to the interradicular septum of the alveolar bone. These fiber groups help stabilize the tooth in its socket.

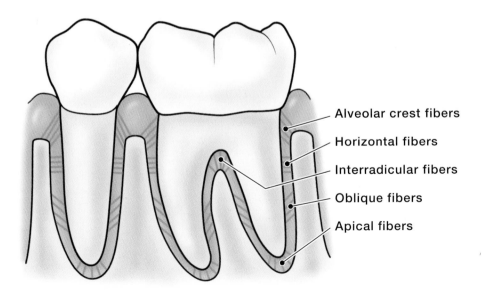

Alveolar crest fibers

Horizontal fibers

Interradicular fibers

Oblique fibers

Apical fibers

Figure 2.17. **Principal Fiber Groups of the Periodontal Ligament.** The fibers of the periodontal ligament are classified as the alveolar crest, horizontal, interradicular, oblique, and apical.

E. Sharpey Fibers of the Periodontal Ligament
1. The ends of the periodontal ligament fibers that are embedded in the cementum and alveolar bone are known as Sharpey fibers (FIG. 2-18).
2. The attachment of the fiber bundles occurs when the cementum and bone are forming. As cementum forms, the tissue hardens around the ends of the periodontal fibers (Sharpey fibers) surrounding them with cementum. The same process occurs during bone formation. As the bony wall of the tooth socket hardens, it surrounds the ends of the periodontal fibers with bone. The ends of the fiber bundles become trapped in the bone that forms around them.

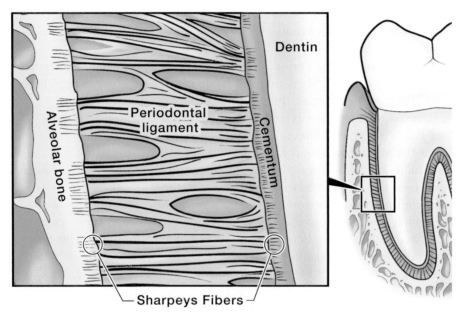

Figure 2.18. Sharpey Fibers. The ends of the periodontal ligament fibers that are embedded in the alveolar bone and the cementum are known as Sharpey Fibers.

Section 3
Histology of Root Cementum and Alveolar Bone

The third section reviews the microscopic anatomy of the cementum and alveolar bone. Knowledge of the microscopic anatomy of these structures is a prerequisite to understanding the function of these structures in health and the alterations in disease.

MICROSCOPIC ANATOMY OF CEMENTUM

1. **Definition.** Cementum is a mineralized layer of connective tissue that covers the root of the tooth. Anatomically, cementum is part of the tooth; however, it also part of the periodontium.
   A. **Functions of Cementum**
      1. Seals and covers the open dentinal tubules and acts to protect the underlying dentin (FIG. 2-19).
      2. Attaches the periodontal fibers to the tooth.
      3. Compensates for attrition of teeth at their occlusal or incisal surfaces. Over time, teeth experience wear at their occlusal or incisal surfaces. Cementum is formed at the apical areas of the roots to compensate for loss of tooth tissues due to attrition.
   B. **Conservation of Cementum During Periodontal Instrumentation.**
      1. Conservation of cementum is ideal since loss of cementum is accompanied by exposure of the dentinal tubules and by a loss of attachment of periodontal ligament fibers to the root surface.

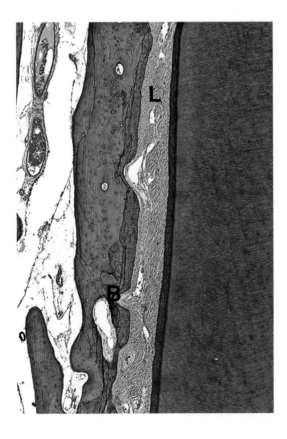

Figure 2.19. Cementum and Tooth Supporting Structures. A thin layer of cementum (appearing as a *blue band*) covers the dentin of the root. The periodontal ligament (L) holds the tooth in the bony socket of the alveolar bone (B). (Used with permission from Mills SE. *Histology for Pathologists*. 3rd ed. Philadelphia: Lippincott Williams & Wilkins; 2006.)

2. Until recently, intentional aggressive removal of cementum was the standard of care for treatment during instrumentation of root surfaces exposed by the apical migration of the junctional epithelium.
   a. Intentional removal of cementum on the coronal half of the root should be avoided, as the cementum is important to the health of the periodontium.
   b. Over the course of many years, overzealous instrumentation can result in removal of all cementum and exposure of the underlying dentin.

2. **Components of Mature Cementum.** Cementum contains collagen fibers embedded in an organic matrix [15].
   A. **Collagen Fibers.** The organic matrix of cementum is composed of a framework of densely packed collagen fibers held together by the gel-like extracellular ground substance. These fibers are oriented more or less parallel to the long axis of the tooth.
   B. **Mineralized Portion.** The mineralized portion of cementum is made up of hydroxyapatite crystals (calcium and phosphate).
   C. **Vessels and Innervation.** Cementum contains no blood vessels or nerves. (Hypersensitivity of the root surface occurs when the cementum is removed exposing the dentin. It is the dentin that is sensitive to brushing or the touch of a dental instrument.)

3. **Types of Cementum**
   A. **Acellular Cementum.** Acellular cementum is primarily responsible for attaching the tooth to the alveolar bone (FIG. 2-20).
      1. Contains no living cells within its mineralized tissue
      2. First to be formed and covers approximately the cervical third or half of the root
      3. No new acellular cementum is produced during the life of the tooth
      4. Thickness ranges from 30 to 60 µm
      5. Sharpey fibers make up most of the structure of acellular cementum
   B. **Cellular Cementum**
      1. Contains cementoblasts and fibroblasts within its mineralized tissue (FIG. 2-20)
      2. Formed after the tooth has erupted and is less calcified than acellular cementum
      3. Deposited in intervals throughout the life of the tooth (thickness increases with age)
      4. Thickness ranges from 150 to 200 µm
      5. Sharpey fibers make up a smaller portion of cellular cementum.

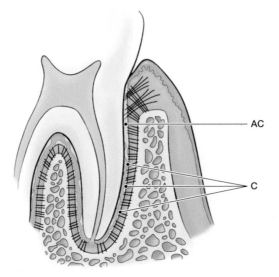

Figure 2.20. Types of Cementum. Acellular cementum (AC) covers approximately the cervical third or half of the root. New acellular cementum normally is not produced during the life of the tooth. Cellular cementum (C) covers the apical half of the root. It is deposited throughout the life of the tooth and increases in thickness with age.

4. **Relationship of Cementum to Enamel at the CEJ.** The cementum covering the root may have any one of three relationships with the enamel of the tooth crown. In the order of frequency, the cementum may overlap the enamel, meet the enamel, or there is a gap between the cementum and the enamel. This order of frequency is known as the **OMG** (overlap, meet, gap) (Fig. 2-21).
   A. **Overlap**—in 60% of all cases, the cementum overlaps the enamel for a short distance.
   B. **Meet**—in 30% of all cases, the cementum meets the enamel.
   C. **Gap**—in 10% of all cases, there is a small gap between the cementum and the enamel (exposing the dentin in this area). The patient may experience discomfort (dentinal sensitivity) during instrumentation. The use of local anesthesia may be helpful during instrumentation, and desensitization of sensitive areas should be performed following instrumentation.

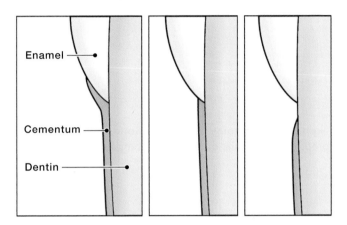

Figure 2.21. **Relationship of Cementum to Enamel at the Cementoenamel Junction.** In the order of frequency, the cementum may (1) overlap the enamel, (2) meet the enamel, or (3) not meet, leaving a gap between the cementum and the enamel.

MICROSCOPIC ANATOMY OF ALVEOLAR BONE

1. **Definition.** The alveolar process or alveolar bone is the part of the maxilla and mandible that form and support the sockets of the teeth (Fig. 2-22).
2. **Function of Alveolar Bone in the Periodontium**
   A. **Protects Roots of Teeth.** The alveolar bone forms the bony sockets that provide support and protection for the roots of the teeth.
   B. **Remodels in Response to Mechanical Forces and Inflammation.** Alveolar bone constantly undergoes periods of bone formation and resorption (loss) in response to mechanical forces on the tooth and inflammation of the periodontium.
3. **Characteristics of Alveolar Bone**
   A. **Components.** Alveolar bone is mineralized connective tissue made by cells called osteoblasts ("bone builders") [16].
      1. Major cell types
         a. Osteoblasts—bone-forming cells—produce the bone matrix consisting of collagen fibers and other protein fibers.
         b. Osteoclasts—bone consumers—cells that remove the mineral materials and organic matrix of alveolar bone.
      2. Extracellular matrix
         a. Collagen fibers and gel-like substance forms the major component of the alveolar bone
         b. The bone matrix is rigid because it undergoes mineralization by the deposition of minerals such as calcium and phosphate, which are subsequently transformed into hydroxyapatite (Fig. 2-23).
   B. **Vessels and Innervation.** The alveolar bone has blood vessels and nerve innervation.

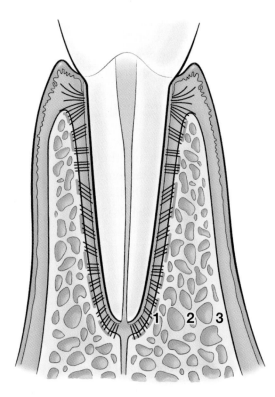

Figure 2.22. Anatomy of Alveolar Bone. *1*, Alveolar bone proper, *2*, trabecular bone, and *3*, compact bone.

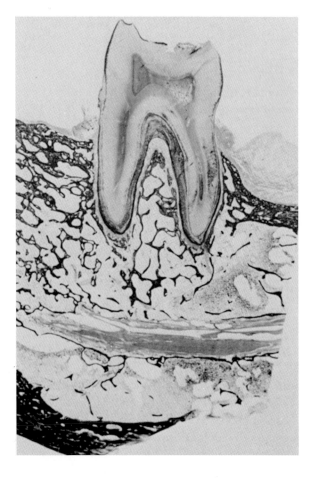

Figure 2.23. Histology of Alveolar Bone. A histologic section through a mandibular first molar and its alveolar process. (Used with permission from Melfi RC. *Permar's Oral Embryology and Microscopic Anatomy*. 10th ed. Philadelphia: Lippincott Williams & Wilkins; 2000; Figure 9-20, p 215.)

Chapter Summary Statement

Knowledge of the microscopic anatomy of the periodontium is fundamental in understanding the (1) function of the periodontium in health and (2) changes that occur during the periodontal disease process. The JE plays an important role in the health of the periodontium by attaching the gingival epithelium to the tooth via hemidesmosomes and an internal basal lamina. In health, the periodontal ligament, cementum, and alveolar bone act as a functional unit to support and maintain the teeth in the oral cavity.

Section 4
Focus on Patients

Case 1

A clinician penetrates the oral mucosa with a needle before injecting a local anesthetic. The needle tip stops in the loose connective tissue underlying the surface structures. Name the layers of epithelium that have been penetrated by the needle.

Case 2

A clinician finds it necessary to use a unique type of injection to achieve total anesthesia of a tooth being treated. The injection involves sliding a small-diameter needle into the periodontal ligament space to a point halfway down the tooth root. Name the periodontal ligament fibers most likely encountered by the needle tip during insertion.

Case 3

Recession of the gingival margin exposes a portion of tooth root on a maxillary canine tooth. Microscopic examination of the cementum in the area of the crown margin on the canine will reveal what possible relationships exist between the level of cementum and the level of the tooth crown.

References

1. Bartold PM, Walsh LJ, Narayanan AS. Molecular and cell biology of the gingiva. *Periodontol 2000*. 2000;24:28–55.
2. Weinmann JP, Meyer J. Types of keratinization in the human gingiva. *J Invest Dermatol*. 1959;32(2 Part 1):87–94.
3. Listgarten MA. Electron microscopic study of the gingivo-dental junction of man. *Am J Anat*. 1966;119(1):147–177.
4. Dale BA. Periodontal epithelium: a newly recognized role in health and disease. *Periodontol 2000*. 2002;30:70–78.
5. Thilander H, Bloom GD. Cell contacts in oral epithelia. *J Periodontal Res*. 1968;3(2):96–110.
6. Listgarten MA. Electron microscopic study of the gingivo-dental junction of man. *Am J Anat*. 1966;119(1):147–177.
7. Schroeder HE, Listgarten MA. The gingival tissues: the architecture of periodontal protection. *Periodontol 2000*. 1997;13:91–120.
8. Schroeder HE, Listgarten MA. The junctional epithelium: from strength to defense. *J Dent Res*. 2003;82(3):158–161.
9. Sabag N, Saglie R, Mery C. Ultrastructure of the normal human epithelial attachment to the cementum root surface. *J Periodontol*. 1981;52(2):94–95.
10. Pollanen MT, Salonen JI, Uitto VJ. Structure and function of the tooth-epithelial interface in health and disease. *Periodontol 2000*. 2003;31:12–31.
11. Schroeder HE, Theilade J. Electron microscopy of normal human gingival epithelium. *J Periodontal Res*. 1966;1(2):95–119.
12. Bartold PM. Connective tissues of the periodontium. Research and clinical implications. *Aust Dent J*. 1991;36(4):255–268.
13. Ho SP, et al. The tooth attachment mechanism defined by structure, chemical composition and mechanical properties of collagen fibers in the periodontium. *Biomaterials*. 2007;28(35):5238–5245.
14. Beertsen W, McCulloch CA, Sodek J. The periodontal ligament: a unique, multifunctional connective tissue. *Periodontol 2000*. 1997;13:20–40.
15. Saygin NE, Giannobile WV, Somerman MJ. Molecular and cell biology of cementum. *Periodontol 2000*. 2000;24:73–98.
16. Sodek J, McKee MD. Molecular and cellular biology of alveolar bone. *Periodontol 2000*. 2000;24:99–126.

Suggested Readings

Bartold PM. Connective tissues of the periodontium. Research and clinical implications. *Aust Dent J*. 1991;36(4):255–268.

Bartold PM, Walsh LJ, and Narayanan, AS. Molecular and cell biology of the gingiva. *Periodontol 2000*. 2000;24:28–55.

Beertsen W, McCulloch CA, and Sodek, J. The periodontal ligament: a unique, multifunctional connective tissue. *Periodontol 2000*. 1997;13:20–40.

Bosshardt DD, Lang NP. The junctional epithelium: from health to disease. *J Dent Res*. 2005;84(1):9–20.

Bosshardt DD, Schroeder HE. Establishment of acellular extrinsic fiber cementum on human teeth. A light- and electron-microscopic study. *Cell Tissue Res*. 1991;263(2):325–336.

Bosshardt DD, Selvig KA. Dental cementum: the dynamic tissue covering of the root. *Periodontol 2000*. 1997;13:41–75.

Caillon P, Saffar JL. Improvement of gingival and alveolar bone status in periodontitis-affected hamsters treated with 15-methyl prostaglandin E1. *J Periodontal Res*. 1994;29(2):138–145.

Dale BA. Periodontal epithelium: a newly recognized role in health and disease. *Periodontol 2000*. 2002;30:70–78.

Ekuni D, Tomofuji T, Yamanaka, R, et al. Initial apical migration of junctional epithelium in rats following application of lipopolysaccharide and proteases. *J Periodontol*. 2005;76(1):43–48.

Green KJ, Jones JC. Desmosomes and hemidesmosomes: structure and function of molecular components. *Faseb J*. 1996;10(8):871–881.

Hormia M, Owaribe K, and Virtanen, I. The dento-epithelial junction: cell adhesion by type I hemidesmosomes in the absence of a true basal lamina. *J Periodontol*. 2001;72(6):788–797.

Jones JC, Asmuth J, Baker, SE, et al. Hemidesmosomes: extracellular matrix/intermediate filament connectors. *Exp Cell Res.* 1994;213(1):1–11.

Jones JC, Hopkinson SB, and Goldfinger, LE. Structure and assembly of hemidesmosomes. *Bioessays.* 1998;20(6):488–494.

Listgarten MA. The ultrastructure of human gingival epithelium. *Am J Anat.* 1964;114:49–69.

Listgarten MA. Electron microscopic study of the gingivo-dental junction of man. *Am J Anat.* 1966;119(1):147–177.

Pollanen MT, Salonen JI, and Uitto, VJ. Structure and function of the tooth-epithelial interface in health and disease. *Periodontol 2000.* 2003;31:12–31.

Saygin NE, Giannobile WV, and Somerman, MJ. Molecular and cell biology of cementum. *Periodontol 2000.* 2000;24:73–98.

Schroeder HE. Ultrastructure of the junctional epithelium of the human gingiva. *Helv Odontol Acta.* 1969;13(2):65–83.

Schroeder HE, Listgarten MA. The gingival tissues: the architecture of periodontal protection. *Periodontol 2000.* 1997;13:91–120.

Schroeder HE, Theilade J. Electron microscopy of normal human gingival epithelium. *J Periodontal Res.* 1966;1(2):95–119.

Sodek J, McKee MD. Molecular and cellular biology of alveolar bone. *Periodontol 2000.* 2000;24:99–126.

Thilander H, Bloom GD. Cell contacts in oral epithelia. *J Periodontal Res.* 1968;3(2):96–110.

Weinmann JP, Meyer J. Types of keratinization in the human gingiva. *J Invest Dermatol.* 1959;32 (2 Part 1):87–94.

The Progression of Periodontal Disease

Learning Objectives

- Define the term pathogenesis.

- Define the term periodontal disease and contrast it with the term periodontitis.

- Name and define the two types of periodontal disease.

- Compare and contrast the clinical and histologic characteristics of the periodontium in health, gingivitis, and periodontitis.

- In the clinical setting, point out to your clinical instructor visible clinical signs of health, gingivitis, and/or periodontal disease.

- In the clinical setting, point out to your clinical instructor any visible clinical signs of periodontal disease. Using a periodontal probe, measure the depth of the sulci or pockets on the facial aspect of one sextant of the mouth. Using the information gathered visually and with the periodontal probe, explain whether this patient's disease is gingivitis or periodontitis.

- Describe the sequential development of inflammatory periodontal disease.

- Describe the position of the crest of the alveolar bone in gingivitis.

- Describe the position of the junctional epithelium in health, gingivitis, and periodontitis.

- Describe the epithelial–connective tissue junction in health, gingivitis, and periodontitis.
- Explain why there is a band of intact transseptal fibers even in the presence of severe bone loss.
- Describe the progressive destruction of alveolar bone loss that occurs in periodontitis.
- Compare and contrast horizontal and vertical bone loss.
- Describe the pathway of inflammation that occurs in horizontal bone loss.
- Describe the pathway of inflammation that occurs in vertical bone loss.
- Define the terms active disease site and inactive disease site.
- Define the term attachment loss.
- Define the term gingival pocket. Explain why a gingival pocket sometimes is referred to as a false pocket.
- Define the term periodontal pocket.
- Name the two types of periodontal pockets.
- Given a drawing of a periodontal pocket, determine whether the pocket illustrated is a suprabony or infrabony pocket.

Key Terms

Pathogenesis
Gingivitis
Acute gingivitis
Chronic gingivitis
Reversible (tissue damage)
Periodontitis
Apical migration of the junctional
   epithelium
Inflammation
Alveolar bone loss
Horizontal bone loss
Vertical bone loss

Osseous defect
Infrabony defect
Osseous crater
Furcation involvement
Attachment loss
Disease site
Inactive disease site
Active disease site
Gingival pocket
Periodontal pocket
Suprabony pocket
Infrabony pocket

Section 1
The Periodontium in Health and Disease

THREE BASIC STATES OF THE PERIODONTIUM

Pathogenesis is the sequence of events that occur during the development of a disease or abnormal condition. The periodontium exists in three basic states: health, gingivitis, and periodontitis (FIGS. 3-1 and 3-2). It is important to recognize the differences among health, gingivitis, and periodontitis (TABLE 3-1). This section provides an overview of these three basic states at the clinical and microscopic levels.

The term *periodontal disease* should not be confused with the term *periodontitis*. Gingivitis and periodontitis are the two basic categories of periodontal disease.

- Gingivitis is a bacterial infection that is confined to the gingiva. The tissue damage that occurs in gingivitis results in reversible destruction to the tissues of the periodontium (FIG. 3-3).
- Periodontitis is a bacterial infection of all parts of the periodontium including the gingiva, periodontal ligament, bone, and cementum. The tissue damage that occurs in periodontitis results in irreversible destruction to the tissues of the periodontium (FIG. 3-4).

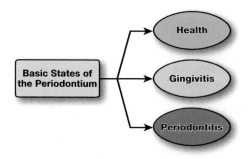

Figure 3.1. **Three Basic States of the Periodontium.** In the absence of disease, the periodontium is healthy. The two basic categories of periodontal disease are gingivitis and periodontitis.

TABLE 3-1. Histologic Changes in Gingivitis and Periodontitis

State	Junctional Epithelium	Connective Tissue Attachment	Periodontal Ligament Fibers	Alveolar Bone
Health	JE coronal to CEJ; Tight intercellular junctions	Intact; supragingival fiber bundles provide support to the gingiva and JE	Intact; attach root to the bone of the tooth socket	Intact; supports and protects the root of the tooth
Gingivitis	JE at CEJ Widened intercellular junctions; epithelial extensions into connective tissue	Connective tissue damage	Intact	Intact
Periodontitis	JE apical to CEJ Widened intercellular junctions; epithelial extensions into connective tissue	Destruction of supragingival fiber bundles	Destruction of periodontal ligament fibers; Exposure of cementum to pocket environment	Destruction of bone Eventual tooth loss

JE, junctional epithelium; CEJ, cementoenamel junction.

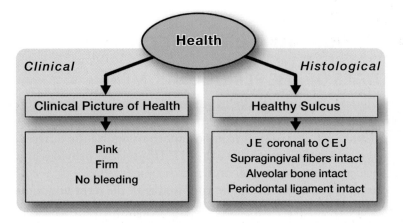

Figure 3.2. Characteristics of the Healthy Periodontium. The clinical and histologic characteristics of the tissues of the periodontium in health.

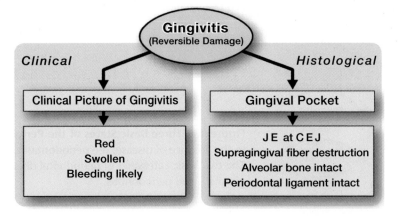

Figure 3.3. Characteristics of Gingivitis. The clinical and histologic characteristics of gingivitis. Some reversible tissue damage occurs in gingivitis.

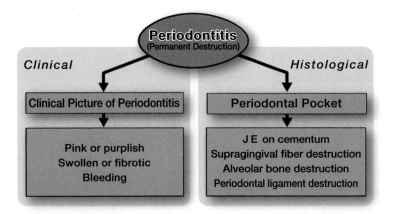

Figure 3.4. Characteristics of Periodontitis. The clinical and histologic characteristics of periodontitis. Permanent tissue damage occurs in periodontitis.

PERIODONTIUM IN HEALTH

1. **Clinical Picture of Healthy Gingiva**
   A. **Color:** Pink, may be pigmented, and is resilient in consistency.
   B. **Gingival Margin**
      1. Scalloped outline
      2. Located coronal to (above) the cementoenamel junction (CEJ).
   C. **Interdental Papillae:** Firm and occupy the embrasure spaces apical to the contact areas.
   D. **Absence of Bleeding:** No bleeding upon probing.
   E. **Sulcus:** Probing depths range from 1 to 3 mm.
2. **The Microscopic Picture of Healthy Gingiva** (FIG. 3-5)
   A. **Junctional Epithelium:** The JE is firmly attached by hemidesmosomes to the enamel slightly coronal to (above) the cementoenamel junction (CEJ).
   B. **Epithelial–Connective Tissue Junction:** In health, the junctional epithelium has no epithelial ridges.
   C. **Gingival Fibers:** Intact supragingival fiber bundles support the junctional epithelium.
   D. **Alveolar Bone:** The crest of the alveolar bone is intact and located 2 to 3 mm apical to (below) the base of the junctional epithelium.
   E. **Periodontal Ligament Fibers:** Intact periodontal ligament fiber bundles stretch between the bony walls of the tooth socket to the cementum of the root.
   F. **Cementum:** Cementum is normal.

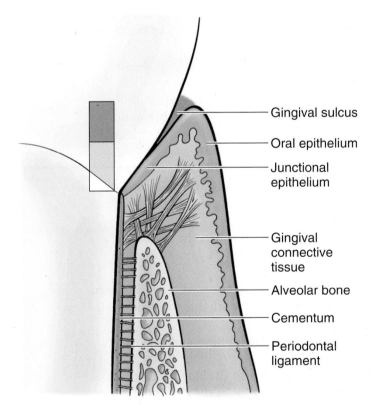

Gingival sulcus

Oral epithelium

Junctional epithelium

Gingival connective tissue

Alveolar bone

Cementum

Periodontal ligament

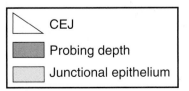

CEJ

Probing depth

Junctional epithelium

Figure 3.5. The Healthy Periodontium.

- **Plaque biofilm:** light accumulation
- **Junctional epithelium:** slightly coronal to the CEJ, no epithelial ridge formation
- **Supragingival fibers:** intact
- **Periodontal ligament fibers:** intact
- **Alveolar bone:** intact

GINGIVITIS—REVERSIBLE TISSUE DAMAGE

1. **Characteristics of Gingivitis.** Gingivitis is *a type of periodontal disease* characterized by changes in the color, contour, and consistency of the gingival tissues (FIG. 3-6).
   A. **Onset of Gingivitis.** Gingivitis is observed clinically from 4 to 14 days after plaque biofilm accumulates in the gingival sulcus.
      1. Acute gingivitis is a gingivitis that lasts for a short period of time. Acute gingivitis often is characterized by fluid in the gingival connective tissues that results in swollen gingiva.
      2. Chronic gingivitis is a gingivitis that lasts for months or years.
         a. When gingivitis is chronic, the body may attempt to repair the tissue damage by forming new collagen fibers in the gingival connective tissue.
         b. Excess collagen fibers lead to gingival tissues that are enlarged and fibrotic (leathery) in consistency.
         c. The excess collagen fibers conceal the redness caused by the increased blood flow, making the tissue appear less red.
   B. **Tissue Enlargement.** Gingival enlargement may be caused by swelling (acute gingivitis) or fibrosis (chronic gingivitis).
      1. Tissue enlargement causes the gingival margin to cover more of the crown of the tooth and results in deeper probing depths.
      2. This enlargement of the gingival tissue is said to produce a false or gingival pocket.
      3. A gingival pocket has a sulcus depth over 3 mm. This increased probing depth is caused solely by enlarged gingival tissue. Microscopically, the junctional epithelium remains in its normal position coronal to the CEJ on the tooth in a gingival pocket.
   C. **Reversible Tissue Damage.** *The tissue damage in gingivitis is reversible*—that is, with good patient self-care, the body can repair the damage.
   D. **Duration of Gingivitis.** In many cases, gingivitis may persist for years without ever progressing to the next stage, periodontitis. In some cases, a combination of risk factors may result in gingivitis progressing to periodontitis.
2. **Clinical Picture of Gingivitis**
   A. **Color:** In gingivitis, the gingival tissue usually is red or reddish blue in color.
      1. The blood flow increases in the gingival connective tissue and the gingival blood vessels become engorged with blood, causing the gingiva to appear red.
      2. If the gingivitis persists, the gingival blood vessels may become congested. This slow-moving blood flow causes the gingiva to have a bluish color.
   B. **Gingival Margin**
      1. The gingival margin is swollen and loses its knife-edge adaptation to the tooth.
      2. Gingival tissue may cover more of the crown of the tooth due to tissue swelling or fibrosis.
   C. **Interdental Papillae:** The interdental papillae often are bulbous and swollen.
   D. **Bleeding:** There is bleeding upon gentle probing.
   E. **Sulcus:** Probing depths may be greater than 3 mm due to swelling of the tissues. It is important to note that *there is NO apical migration of the junctional epithelium* in gingivitis.
3. **The Microscopic Picture of Gingivitis**
   A. **Junctional Epithelium:** The hemidesmosomes still attach to the enamel coronal to the cementoenamel junction (FIG. 3-6 and TABLE 3-2).

B. **Epithelial–Connective Tissue Junction**
  1. The junctional epithelium extends epithelial ridges down into the connective tissue.
  2. *Such extension of the epithelial ridges only can occur because destruction of the gingival fibers creates space for the growing epithelium.*
C. **Gingival Fibers:** Damage has occurred to the supragingival fiber bundles. This damage is reversible if the bacterial infection is brought under control.
D. **Alveolar Bone:** The bacterial infection has not progressed into the alveolar bone. There is no destruction of alveolar bone.
E. **Periodontal Ligament Fibers:** The bacterial infection has not progressed into the periodontal ligament fibers.
F. **Cementum:** The cementum covering the root of the tooth is normal.

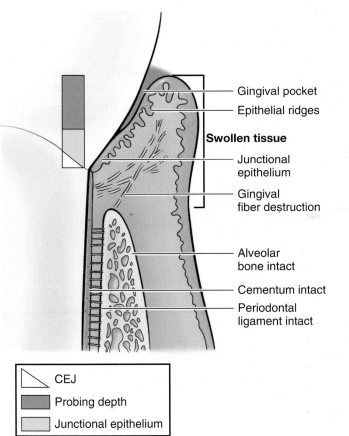

Figure legend labels:
- Gingival pocket
- Epithelial ridges
- **Swollen tissue**
- Junctional epithelium
- Gingival fiber destruction
- Alveolar bone intact
- Cementum intact
- Periodontal ligament intact

Legend box:
- CEJ
- Probing depth
- Junctional epithelium

Figure 3.6. Gingivitis.

- **Plaque biofilm:** increased numbers of bacteria
- **Junctional epithelium:** slightly coronal to the CEJ; the coronal portion of the JE detaches from the tooth; probing depth increases; epithelial ridges extend down into gingival connective tissue
- **Supragingival fibers:** some fiber destruction
- **Periodontal ligament fibers:** intact
- **Alveolar bone:** intact

PERIODONTITIS—PERMANENT TISSUE DESTRUCTION

1. **Characteristics of Periodontitis**
   A. **Extent of Tissue Destruction**
      1. Periodontitis is *a type of periodontal disease* that is characterized by the (1) apical migration of the junctional epithelium, (2) loss of connective tissue attachment, and (3) loss of alveolar bone.
      2. The tissue damage of periodontitis is permanent.

B. Process of Tissue Destruction
1. The tissue destruction of periodontitis is not a continuous process. Rather, the disease process occurs in an intermittent manner with extended periods of disease inactivity followed by short periods of destruction.
2. Tissue destruction progresses at different rates throughout the mouth. Destruction does not occur in all parts of the mouth at the same time, but instead, destruction usually occurs in only a few specific sites (tooth surfaces) at a time.

2. Clinical Picture of Periodontitis
   A. Color: The gingival tissue shows visible alternations color, contour, and consistency.
   1. Edematous tissue (spongy tissue)—bluish- or purplish-red with a smooth, shiny appearance.
   2. Fibrotic tissue (firm, nodular tissue)—light pink with a leathery consistency. Beginning clinicians often mistakenly interpret this light pink color as a sign of tissue health.

   B. Gingival Margin
   1. The gingival margin may be swollen or fibrotic and does not have a close knife-edged adaptation to the tooth.
   2. The position of the gingival margin varies greatly in periodontitis. The margin may be apical to the cementoenamel junction (recession) resulting in a portion of the root being visible in the mouth.

   C. Interdental Papillae: The interdental papillae may not fill the interdental embrasure spaces.

   D. Bleeding: There often is bleeding upon probing, and suppuration (a discharge of pus) may be visible.

   E. Pocket: Probing depths are 4 mm or greater because the junctional epithelium is attached to the root surface.
   1. Pus may be evident upon probing.
   2. Pain is usually absent; however, probing may cause some pain due to ulceration of the pocket epithelium.

3. The Microscopic Picture of Periodontitis
   A. Junctional Epithelium
   1. The junctional epithelium is located on the cementum, apical to—below—its normal location. Movement of the junctional epithelium apical to its normal location is termed the apical migration of the junctional epithelium.
   2. The coronal-most portion of the junctional epithelium detaches from the tooth surface. As the bacterial infection progresses, the apical portion of the junctional epithelium moves further in an apical direction along the root surface creating a periodontal pocket (Fig. 3-7 and Table 3-2).
   3. The extracellular matrix of the gingiva and the attached collagen fibers at the apical edge of the junctional epithelium are destroyed.

   B. Epithelial–Connective Tissue Junction
   1. The *junctional* epithelium proliferates and extends epithelial ridges into the connective tissue.
   2. The *sulcular* epithelium of the pocket wall thickens and extends epithelial ridges deep into the connective tissue. Small ulcerations of the pocket epithelium expose the underlying inflamed connective tissue.

C. **Gingival Connective Tissue**
   1. Changes in the gingival connective tissue are severe. Collagen destruction in the area of inflammation is almost complete.
   2. There is widespread destruction of the supragingival fiber bundles, reducing them to fiber fragments. The destruction of the periodontal ligament fiber bundles makes it easier for the junctional epithelium to migrate apically along the root surface.
   3. The transseptal fiber bundles, however, are regenerated continuously across the crest of bone. A band of intact transseptal fibers separates the site of inflammation from the remaining alveolar bone even in cases of extensive bone loss (FIG. 3-8).
   4. Epithelium grows over the root surface in areas where the fiber bundles have been destroyed. *The loss of fiber attachment is permanent because the epithelium growing over the root surface prevents the reinsertion of the periodontal ligament fibers in the cementum.*

D. **Alveolar Bone:** There is permanent destruction of the alveolar bone that supports the teeth. Tooth mobility may be present.

E. **Periodontal Ligament Fibers:** There is permanent destruction of some or all of the periodontal ligament fiber bundles.

F. **Cementum:** Cementum within the periodontal pocket is exposed to dental plaque biofilm.

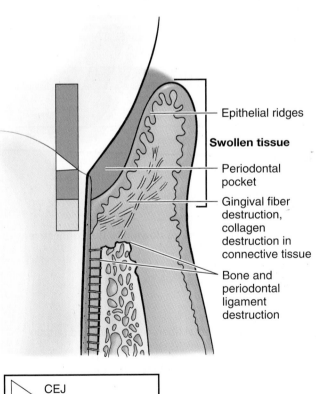

Epithelial ridges

Swollen tissue

Periodontal pocket

Gingival fiber destruction, collagen destruction in connective tissue

Bone and periodontal ligament destruction

☐ CEJ
☐ Probing depth
☐ Junctional epithelium

Figure 3.7. Periodontitis.

- **Plaque biofilm:** vast numbers of bacteria
- **Junctional epithelium:** apical to the CEJ with attachment on cementum; a remnant of the JE persists at the base of the periodontal pocket: epithelial ridges extend down into gingival connective tissue
- **Supragingival fibers:** fiber destruction
- **Periodontal ligament fibers:** fiber destruction
- **Alveolar bone:** portions of alveolar bone destroyed

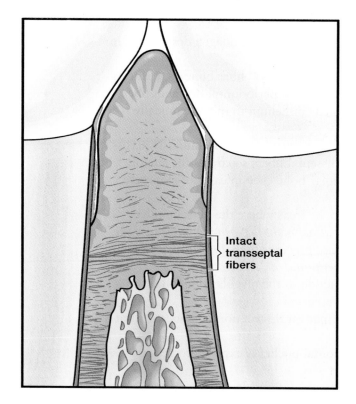

Figure 3.8. Band of Intact Transseptal Fibers. Even in the presence of severe horizontal bone loss, there is an intact band of transseptal fibers above the remaining alveolar bone.

TABLE 3-2.   Histologic Changes in Disease

Disease State	Histology
Gingivitis	Epithelial ridges extend down into connective tissue
	Destruction of supragingival fiber bundles
Periodontitis	Changes in epithelial tissues:
	• Junctional epithelium located apical to the cementoenamel junction
	• Junctional epithelium grows along the root surface
	• Sulcular epithelium thickens and extends epithelial ridges down into the connective tissue
	Changes in connective tissues and alveolar bone:
	• Collagen destruction
	• Destruction of supragingival fiber bundles
	• Destruction of periodontal ligament fibers; transseptal fibers regenerate and remain intact
	• Junctional epithelium grows over the root surface in areas where the periodontal ligament fibers are destroyed
	• Root cementum is exposed to the plaque biofilm
	• Destruction of alveolar bone

Section 2
Pathogenesis of Bone Destruction

Inflammation is the body's reaction to injury or invasion by disease-producing organisms. The inflammatory process that occurs in periodontitis results in permanent destruction to the tissues of the periodontium, including the destruction of gingival connective tissue, periodontal ligament, and alveolar bone. Alveolar bone loss is the resorption of alveolar bone as a result of periodontitis. This section discusses the patterns of bone destruction that occur in periodontitis. *The pattern of bone destruction that occurs depends on the pathway of inflammation as it spreads from the gingiva into the alveolar bone.* It is important to understand the changes that occur in the alveolar bone because it is the reduction in bone height that eventually results in tooth loss.

CHANGES IN ALVEOLAR BONE HEIGHT IN DISEASE

1. **Reduction in Bone Height**
    A. **Bone Height in Health and Gingivitis.** In health and gingivitis, the crest of the alveolar bone is located approximately 2 mm apical to (below) the CEJs of the teeth (FIG. 3-9).
    B. **Bone Height in Periodontitis.** In periodontitis, the bone destruction may be severe (FIG. 3-10). As periodontal disease progresses (worsens), tooth loss may occur from lack of alveolar bone support (FIG. 3-11).

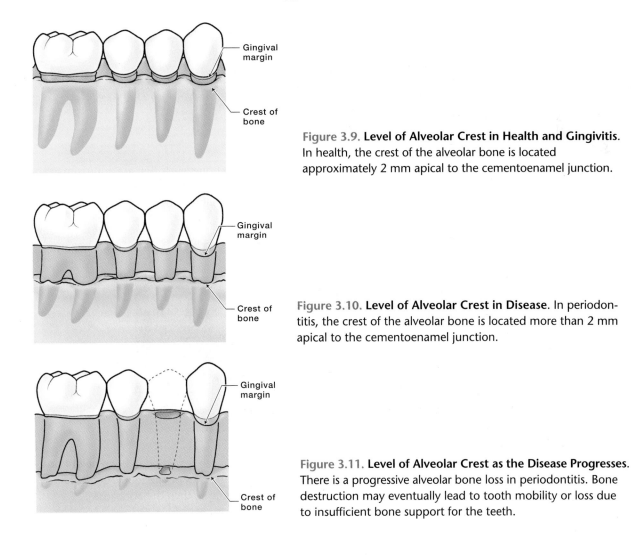

Figure 3.9. **Level of Alveolar Crest in Health and Gingivitis.** In health, the crest of the alveolar bone is located approximately 2 mm apical to the cementoenamel junction.

Figure 3.10. **Level of Alveolar Crest in Disease.** In periodontitis, the crest of the alveolar bone is located more than 2 mm apical to the cementoenamel junction.

Figure 3.11. **Level of Alveolar Crest as the Disease Progresses.** There is a progressive alveolar bone loss in periodontitis. Bone destruction may eventually lead to tooth mobility or loss due to insufficient bone support for the teeth.

PATTERNS OF BONE LOSS IN PERIODONTITIS

1. **Patterns of Bone Loss.** The two types of bone loss are (1) horizontal and (2) vertical bone loss.
   A. **Horizontal Bone Loss**
      1. Horizontal bone loss is the most common pattern of bone loss (FIG. 3-12).
      2. This type of bone loss results in a fairly even, overall reduction in the height of the alveolar bone.
      3. The alveolar bone is reduced in height, but the margin of the alveolar crest remains more or less perpendicular to the long axis of the tooth.
   B. **Vertical Bone Loss**
      1. Vertical bone loss is a less common pattern of bone loss (FIG. 3-13). Vertical bone loss is also known as angular bone loss.
      2. This type of bone loss results in an uneven reduction in the height of the alveolar bone.
      3. In vertical bone loss, the resorption progresses *more rapidly* in the bone next to the root surface. This uneven pattern of bone loss leaves a trenchlike area of missing bone alongside the root.

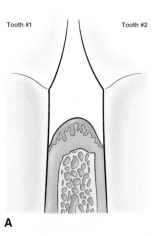
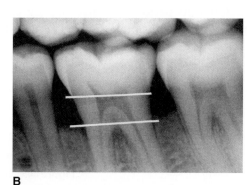

Figure 3.12. Horizontal Pattern of Bone Loss. Horizontal bone loss results in bone levels that are approximately at the same height on adjacent tooth roots. On a radiograph, if an imaginary line drawn between the CEJs of adjacent teeth is approximately parallel, then the bone loss is described as horizontal bone loss.

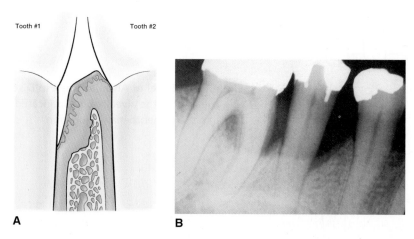

Figure 3.13. Vertical Pattern of Bone Loss. Vertical bone loss results in an uneven reduction in bone height on adjacent tooth roots, resulting in a trenchlike area of missing bone alongside the root of one tooth. On a radiograph, if an imaginary line drawn between the CEJs of adjacent teeth is not parallel, then the bone loss is described as vertical bone loss.

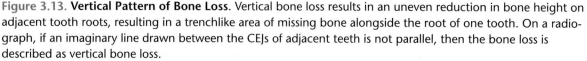

2. Pathways of Inflammation into the Alveolar Bone
   A. **Pathway of Inflammation in Horizontal Bone Loss**
      1. In horizontal bone loss, inflammation spreads into the tissues in this order: (1) within the gingival connective tissue along the connective tissue sheaths surrounding the blood vessels, (2) into the alveolar bone, and (3) finally, into the periodontal ligament space (FIG. 3-14A).
      2. Inflammation usually spreads in this manner because it is the *path of least resistance*. The periodontal ligament fiber bundles act as an effective barrier to the spread of inflammation. Thus, the inflammation spreads into the alveolar bone and then into the periodontal ligament space.
   B. **Pathway of Inflammation in Vertical Bone Loss**
      1. In vertical bone loss, inflammation spreads into the tissues in this order: (1) within the gingival connective tissue, (2) directly into the periodontal ligament space and (3) finally, into the alveolar bone (FIG. 3-14B).
      2. Inflammation spreads in this manner whenever the crestal periodontal ligament fiber bundles are weakened and no longer present an effective barrier. Prior events such as occlusal trauma can be responsible for the weakened condition of the fiber bundles.

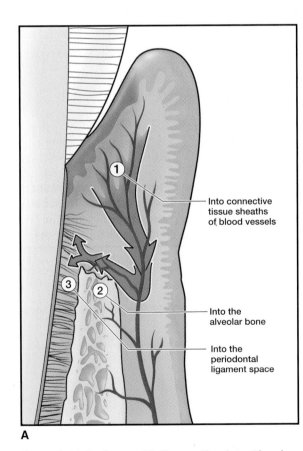

A

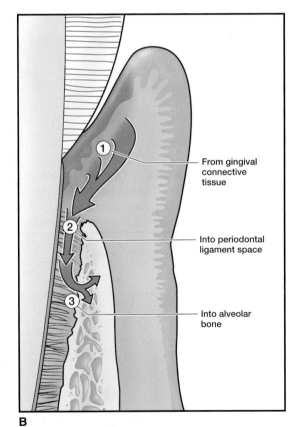

B

Figure 3.14. **Pathway of Inflammation into Alveolar Bone.** A: In horizontal bone loss, inflammation spreads through the tissues in this order:

1—into the gingival connective tissue
2—into the alveolar bone
3—finally, into the periodontal ligament

B: In vertical bone loss, inflammation spreads through the tissues in this order:

1—into the gingival connective tissue
2—into the periodontal ligament
3—finally, into the alveolar bone

3. **Bone Defects in Periodontal Disease.** Periodontitis results in different types of defects in the alveolar bone. These bony defects are called osseous defects.
   A. **Infrabony Defects**
      1. Infrabony defects result when bone resorption occurs in an uneven, oblique direction. In infrabony defects, the bone resorption primarily affects one tooth.
      2. Classification of Infrabony Defects. Infrabony defects are classified on the basis of the number of osseous walls. Infrabony defects may have one, two, or three walls (Fig. 3-15).
   B. **Osseous Craters.** An osseous crater is a bowl-shaped defect in the interdental alveolar bone, with bone loss nearly equal on the roots of two adjacent teeth (Figs. 3-16A, B).
      1. Whereas infrabony defects primarily affect one tooth, in craters the defect affects two adjacent root surfaces to a similar extent.
      2. The presence of an osseous crater causes dental plaque biofilm to collect and makes it difficult to clean the interdental area.

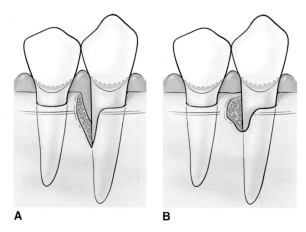

A   B

Figure 3.15. **Osseous Defects**. A: One-wall infrabony defect. Looking from the canine tooth root distally toward the premolar, there is only "one" wall of bone remaining and that is on the mesial surface of the premolar. The facial plate and lingual plate of bone are missing. B: Two-wall infrabony defect with facial plate of bone missing. The "two walls" of the bone surrounding this defect are the remaining lingual plate and bone on the mesial surface of the premolar tooth root.

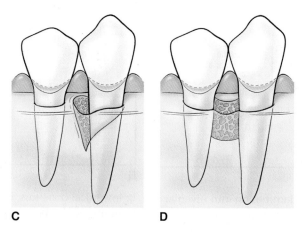

C   D

C: **Three-wall** infrabony defect. The "three walls" of remaining bone that surround this defect are the lingual plate, facial plate, and the bone on the mesial surface of the adjacent premolar root. D: Interproximal osseous crater with intact lingual plate and facial plate of bone remaining. The bone between these plates is missing resulting in bone being lost on the mesial surface of the premolar and the distal surface of the adjacent canine. The term crater refers to the dip in the contour of the interproximal bone between the facial and lingual plates.

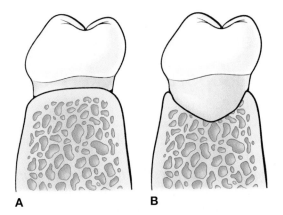

A   B

Figure 3.16. Contour of Interdental Bone. A: Normal contour of the alveolar bone on the proximal (mesial or distal) surface of a posterior tooth. Note that the bone contour from the facial to lingual is a relatively flat inter-proximal contour. **B:** Osseous crater on the proximal surface of a posterior tooth. Note that the contour of the bone from the facial to the lingual dips apically and forms what is described as a "crater" between the facial and lingual bone margins.

C. Bone Loss in Furcation Areas

1. **Furcation involvement** occurs on a multirooted tooth when periodontal infection invades the area between and around the roots, resulting in a loss of alveolar bone between the roots of the teeth.

2. Bone loss in the furcation area may be hidden by the gingival tissue or may be clinically visible in the mouth (FIG. 3-17).

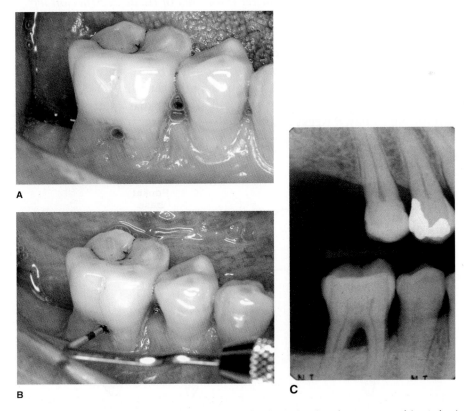

A

B   C

Figure 3.17. Furcation Involvement. A: Due to recession, the furcation involvement on this molar is clinically evident. **B:** A periodontal probe easily can be inserted between the two roots of this mandibular molar. **C:** A radiograph shows the extensive bone loss around this molar. (Images courtesy of Dr Richard J. Foster, Guilford Technical Community College, Jamestown, NC.)

Section 3
Periodontal Pockets

CHARACTERISTICS OF PERIODONTAL POCKETS

1. **Attachment Loss in Periodontal Pockets**
   A. Attachment loss is the destruction of the fibers and bone that support the teeth.
   B. Tissue destruction spreads not only in an apical (vertical) direction but also in a lateral (side-to-side) direction.
   C. *A pocket on different root surfaces of the same tooth can have different depths.* The loss of attachment may vary from surface to surface of the tooth, with the base of the pocket exhibiting very irregular patterns of tissue destruction (FIG. 3-18).
2. **Disease Sites.** A disease site is an area of tissue destruction. A disease site may involve only a single surface of a tooth, for example, the distal surface of a tooth. The disease site may involve several surfaces of the tooth or all four surfaces (mesial, distal, facial, and lingual).
   A. Inactive disease site—a disease site that is stable, with the attachment level of the JE remaining the same over time.
   B. Active disease site—a disease site that shows continued apical migration of the JE over time.
   C. **Assessment of Disease Activity.** The disease activity of each site in the mouth should be assessed using a periodontal probe and recorded in the patient chart at regular intervals (scheduled checkup appointments).
   D. **Periodontal Pockets.** *A periodontal pocket is an area of tissue destruction left by the disease process.* The pocket is much like a demolished home that is left after a hurricane.
      1. The presence of a periodontal pocket does not indicate necessarily that there is active disease at that site. Likewise, a demolished house does not necessarily indicate that a hurricane still is pounding the shoreline. A demolished house may indicate that the hurricane is still active or that a hurricane passed through a day, a week, or a year ago.
      2. *The majority of pockets in most adult patients with periodontitis are inactive disease sites.*

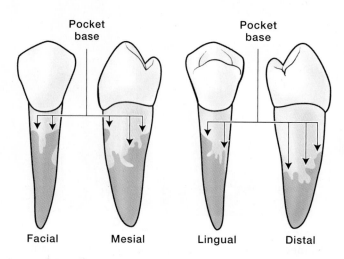

Pocket base   Pocket base

Facial   Mesial   Lingual   Distal

Figure 3.18. Irregular Pattern of Attachment Loss. The amount of attachment loss can vary greatly on different surfaces of the same tooth. The base of a pocket may exhibit very irregular patterns of destruction.

POCKET FORMATION

1. **Gingival Sulcus.** In health, the sulcus is 0.5 to 3 mm in depth. The junctional epithelium is coronal to the CEJ and *attaches along its entire length to the enamel of the tooth*. (FIG. 3-19).

2. **Gingival Pockets.** A gingival pocket is a deepening of the gingival sulcus as a result of swelling or enlargement of the gingival tissue (FIG. 3-20).

    A. **False Pocket.** Also known as a "pseudopocket," meaning "false pocket," because there is no destruction of the periodontal ligament fibers or alveolar bone in a gingival pocket.

    B. **No Apical Migration.** *There is no apical migration of the junctional epithelium in a gingival pocket.*

        1. The junctional epithelium remains coronal to the CEJ.

        2. *In gingivitis, however, the <u>coronal portion</u> of the junctional epithelium detaches from the tooth resulting in a slight increase in probing depths.*

    C. **Increased Probing Depths.** The increased probing depth seen in a gingival pocket is due to (1) detachment of the coronal portion of the JE from the tooth and (2) increased tissue size due to (a) swelling of the tissue or (b) tissue enlargement due to increased collagen fibers in the connective tissue.

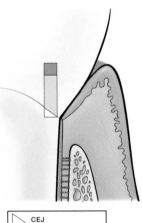

◣	CEJ
▨	Probing depth
▨	Junctional epithelium

Figure 3.19. Gingival Sulcus. In health, the gingival sulcus has a shallow probing depth ranging from 0.5 to 3 mm. *The junctional epithelium attaches along its entire length to the enamel of the tooth.*

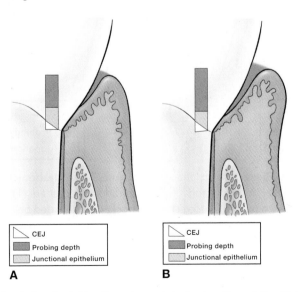

◣	CEJ
▨	Probing depth
▨	Junctional epithelium

A

◣	CEJ
▨	Probing depth
▨	Junctional epithelium

B

Figure 3.20. Gingival Pockets. A: In gingivitis, there is no apical migration of the JE. **B:** In some cases the gingival tissue swells, resulting in a pseudopocket.

3. **Periodontal Pockets**
    A. A periodontal pocket is a pathologic deepening of the gingival sulcus.
        1. Pocket formation occurs as the result of the (1) apical migration of the junctional epithelium, (2) destruction of the periodontal ligament fibers, and (3) destruction of alveolar bone.
        2. Apical migration is the movement of the cells of the JE from their normal position—coronal to the CEJ—to a position apical to the CEJ. In health, the junctional epithelium cells attach to the enamel of the tooth crown. In periodontitis, the JE cells attach to the cementum of the tooth root.
    B. **Two Types of Periodontal Pockets. The type of periodontal pocket is determined based on *the relationship of the JE to the crest of the alveolar bone.***
        1. **Suprabony pocket**
            a. Suprabony pockets occur when there is horizontal bone loss (FIG. 3-21).
            b. The JE, forming the base of the pocket, is located *coronal* to (above) the crest of the alveolar bone.
        2. **Infrabony pocket**
            a. Infrabony pockets occur when there is vertical bone loss (FIG. 3-22).
            b. The junctional epithelium, forming the base of the pocket, is located *apical* to (below) the crest of the alveolar bone. The base of the pocket is located within the cratered-out area of the bone alongside of the root surface.

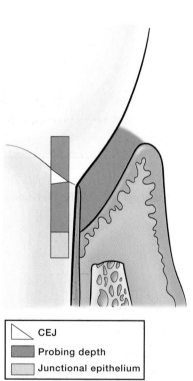

	CEJ
	Probing depth
	Junctional epithelium

	CEJ
	Probing depth
	Junctional epithelium

Figure 3.21. Suprabony Pocket. Characteristics of a suprabony pocket are (1) horizontal bone loss and (2) a pocket base located coronal to (above) the crest of the alveolar bone.

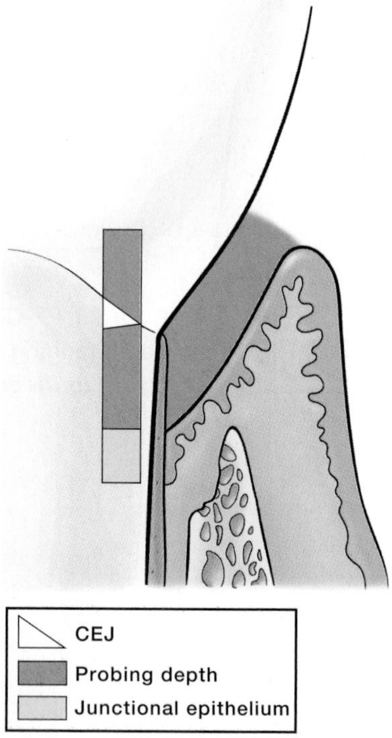

Figure 3.22. Infrabony Pocket. Characteristics of an infrabony pocket are (1) vertical bone loss and (2) a pocket base located below the crest of the alveolar bone within a trenchlike area of the bone.

Chapter Summary Statement

Periodontal pathogenesis is the sequence of events that occur during the development of periodontal disease. The two types of periodontal disease are gingivitis and periodontitis.

- Gingivitis is a *reversible condition* that is characterized by changes in the color, contour, and consistency of the gingiva. There is no apical migration of the JE or bone loss in gingivitis.
- Periodontitis results in some extent of *permanent tissue destruction* characterized by pocket formation, destruction of the periodontal ligament fibers, and resorption of alveolar bone. The pattern of alveolar bone loss and periodontal ligament destruction depends on the pathway that the inflammatory process takes as it spreads from the gingiva into the alveolar bone. It is the destruction of periodontal ligament fibers and resorption of alveolar bone that lead to tooth mobility and the possibility of tooth loss.

Section 4
Focus on Patients

Case 1

Examination of a patient reveals swelling and redness of the gingival margin. In addition, gingival papillae are slightly enlarged. Gentle probing elicits bleeding, and probing depths measure 4 to 5 mm in some sites. What additional information would you need about the condition of this patient to assign a diagnosis of either gingivitis or periodontitis?

Case 2

Your patient has 6 to 7 mm attachment loss on all surfaces of the maxillary first molar. Which of the tissues of the periodontium have experienced tissue destruction surrounding this tooth?

Case 3

Your dental team provides appropriate therapy for a patient with periodontitis. When you began treatment, your initial findings were redness and edema (swelling) of the gingiva, bleeding on probing, periodontal pockets, and attachment loss. Successful control of the periodontal disease in the patient should **not** be expected to result in elimination of which of these initial clinical findings?

Suggested Readings

The pathogenesis of periodontal diseases. *J Periodontol*. 1999;70(4):457–470.

Akiyoshi M, Mori K. Marginal periodontitis: a histological study of the incipient stage. *J Periodontol*. 1967;38(1):45–52.

Brecx MC, Gautschi M, Gehr P, et al. Variability of histologic criteria in clinically healthy human gingiva. *J Periodontal Res*. 1987;22(6):468–472.

Listgarten MA. Pathogenesis of periodontitis. *J Clin Periodontol*. 1986;13(5):418–430.

Offenbacher S. Periodontal diseases: pathogenesis. *Ann Periodontol*. 1996;1(1):821–878.

Page RC, Offenbacher S, Schraeder HE, et al. Advances in the pathogenesis of periodontitis: summary of developments, clinical implications and future directions. *Periodontol 2000*. 1997;14:216–248.

Page RC, Schroeder HE. Pathogenesis of inflammatory periodontal disease. A summary of current work. *Lab Invest*. 1976;34(3):235–249.

Payne WA, Page RC, Ogilvie AL. Histopathologic features of the initial and early stages of experimental gingivitis in man. *J Periodontal Res*. 1975;10(2):51–64.

Takata T, Donath K. The mechanism of pocket formation. A light microscopic study on undecalcified human material. *J Periodontol*. 1988;59(4):215–221.

Van Dyke TE, Serhan CN. Resolution of inflammation: a new paradigm for the pathogenesis of periodontal diseases. *J Dent Res*. 2003;82(2):82–90.

Waerhaug J. Anatomy, physiology and pathology of the gingival pocket. *Rev Belge Med Dent*. 1966;21(1):9–15.

Waerhaug J. The angular bone defect and its relationship to trauma from occlusion and downgrowth of subgingival plaque. *J Clin Periodontol*. 1979;6(2):61–82.

Chapter 4

Classification of Periodontal Diseases

Learning Objectives

- List, describe, and differentiate the various periodontal diseases according to the 1999 classification system established by the American Academy of Periodontology.

- Define and contrast the terms gingival disease, periodontal disease, and periodontitis.

- Define and contrast the terms plaque-induced gingival diseases and non–plaque-induced gingival lesions.

- Define and contrast the terms chronic periodontitis and aggressive periodontitis.

Key Terms

Classification
Gingivitis
Periodontitis
Periodontal disease
American Academy of Periodontology
Plaque-induced gingival diseases
Non–plaque-induced gingival lesions
Chronic periodontitis

Aggressive periodontitis
Periodontitis as a manifestation of
systemic diseases
Necrotizing periodontal diseases
Tissue necrosis
Periodontal abscess
Periodontitis associated with endodontic
lesions

Section 1
Introduction to Disease Classification

"Periodontal disease" is a broad term used to refer to a bacterial infection of the periodontium, just as "heart disease" is a general term. There are many different diseases of the heart, such as coronary artery disease, congestive heart failure, valvular disease, rheumatic heart disease, and infectious endocarditis. As with heart disease, there are many specific periodontal diseases that affect the gingival tissues, periodontal connective tissues, and/or the supporting alveolar bone.

This chapter outlines a periodontal disease classification adopted in 1999 at the International Workshop for a Classification of Periodontal Diseases and Conditions.

MAJOR DIAGNOSTIC CATEGORIES OF PERIODONTAL DISEASE

A classification is a systematic arrangement into groups or categories based on common attributes. An everyday example is classifying vehicles into categories such as passenger cars, sport utility vehicles, and trucks. Classification systems provide a tool to study the etiology, pathogenesis, and treatment of periodontal diseases in an orderly manner. Periodontal diseases are divided into types, or classifications, based on their specific bacterial etiology, development, and clinical manifestations.

1. **Classifying Periodontal Diseases**
    A. **Purposes of Classifying Periodontal Diseases.** A periodontal classification system provides information necessary in
        1. Communicating clinical findings accurately to other dental healthcare providers and to dental insurance providers.
        2. Presenting information to the patient about his or her disease.
        3. Formulating individualized treatment plans.
        4. Predicting treatment outcomes.
    B. **Major Diagnostic Categories of Periodontal Disease.** The two basic diagnostic categories of periodontal disease are (1) gingivitis and (2) periodontitis (FIG. 4-1).
        1. Gingivitis is inflammation of the periodontium that is confined to the gingiva. It results in damage to the gingival tissue that is reversible.
        2. Periodontitis is an inflammatory disease of the supporting structures of the periodontium including the gingiva, periodontal ligament, bone, and cementum. It results in irreversible destruction to the tissues of the periodontium.
        3. It is important to recognize the differences among health, gingivitis, and periodontitis (FIG. 4-2).
            a. In health, no clinical signs of inflammation are present.
            b. In gingivitis, there are clinical signs of inflammation such as bleeding, redness, and swelling.
                1) There is no attachment loss in gingivitis. Attachment loss refers to the apical migration of the junctional epithelium and the destruction of connective tissue, periodontal ligament fibers, and alveolar bone.
                2) The tissue destruction in gingivitis can be reversed with professional treatment and good self-care by the patient.
            c. Periodontitis is characterized by inflammation, apical migration of the junctional epithelium, and attachment loss. In periodontitis, there is irreversible tissue destruction including destruction of connective tissue, periodontal ligament fibers, and alveolar bone.

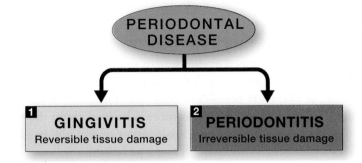

Figure 4.1. **Periodontal Disease.** There are two major categories of periodontal disease: (1) gingivitis and (2) periodontitis.

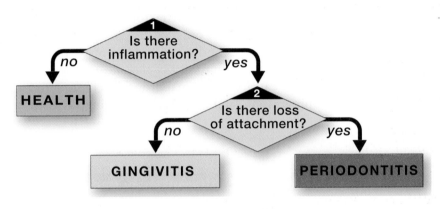

Figure 4.2. **Decision Tree.** Is it health, gingivitis, or periodontitis?

2. Terminology: *Periodontal Disease* Versus *Periodontitis*
   A. Many beginning clinicians confuse the meaning of the terms "*periodontal disease*" and "*periodontitis*." Often these terms are used interchangeably, as if they mean the same thing. They do not.
   B. Periodontal disease refers to inflammation of the periodontium.
      1. Periodontal disease that is limited to an inflammation of the gingival tissues is called gingivitis.
      2. Periodontal disease that involves all the structures of the periodontium is called periodontitis.
   C. **Correct Terminology.** It is important to understand that the terms "*periodontal disease*" and "*periodontitis*" are not identical in their meaning and not interchangeable in their use.
      1. When a dental hygienist says to the dentist, "My patient has periodontal disease," the hygienist is conveying the general information that the patient has an inflammation of the periodontium that could be gingivitis or periodontitis.
      2. When the hygienist says, "My patient has periodontitis," the hygienist is conveying the specific information that the patient has a bacterial infection that involves all tissues of the periodontium including the periodontal ligament, cementum, and alveolar bone.

Section 2
Classification Systems

Over time, classification systems have changed in response to new scientific knowledge about the etiology and pathogenesis of periodontal diseases and conditions. In recent years, there have been several attempts to classify periodontal diseases. There has never been a perfect disease classification of periodontal diseases; as more is learned about the nature of periodontal diseases, further revisions in the current classification system will be necessary.

THE 1989 CLASSIFICATION OF INFLAMMATORY PERIODONTAL DISEASES

The 1989 classification system (TABLE 4-1) included five types of periodontitis: (1) adult periodontitis, (2) early-onset periodontitis, (3) periodontitis associated with systemic disease, (4) necrotizing ulcerative gingivitis (NUG), and (5) refractory periodontitis [1]. The 1989 classification system emphasized the age of onset of disease—"adult periodontitis, early-onset periodontitis—and rates of disease progression—"rapidly progressing periodontitis." The main problems with the 1989 classification system were (1) unclear and overlapping disease categories, (2) inappropriate emphasis on the age of onset of disease and rates of progression, and (3) absence of a gingival disease classification [2].

TABLE 4-1.   1989 Classification of Inflammatory Periodontal Diseases
Adult Periodontitis (AP)
Early-Onset Periodontitis (EOP)
A. Prepubertal periodontitis (PPP)
B. Juvenile periodontitis (JP)
C. Rapidly progressive periodontitis (RPP)
Periodontitis Associated with Systemic Disease
Necrotizing Ulcerative Gingivitis (NUG)
Refractory Periodontitis (RP)

THE 1999 AAP CLASSIFICATION OF PERIODONTAL DISEASES AND CONDITIONS

The American Academy of Periodontology (AAP) initiated the currently accepted classification by organizing the International Workshop for a Classification of Periodontal Diseases and Conditions in 1999 [3]. The AAP Classification of Periodontal Diseases and Conditions attempts to correct some of the deficiencies of the 1989 classification system. The 1999 system is based on the concepts that plaque-induced periodontal diseases are bacterial infections and much of the destruction seen in these infections occurs as the result of the host response to the bacterial invaders. The 1999 classification includes eight main categories (TABLE 4-2).

TABLE 4-2.	Main Categories: AAP Classification of Periodontal Diseases and Conditions, 1999
Type I	**Gingival Diseases** Plaque-induced gingival diseases Non–plaque-induced gingival lesions
Type II	**Chronic Periodontitis** Localized Generalized
Type III	**Aggressive Periodontitis** Localized Generalized
Type IV	**Periodontitis as a Manifestation of Systemic Disease**
Type V	**Necrotizing Periodontal Disease**
Type VI	**Periodontitis Associated with Endodontic Lesions**
Type VII	**Developmental or Acquired Deformities and Conditions**
Type VIII	**Abscesses of the Periodontium**

COMPARING THE 1989 AND 1999 CLASSIFICATION SYSTEMS

Since the 1999 classification system has been in use for a relatively short period of time, much of the periodontal literature found in periodontal journals and textbooks is based on the earlier 1989 classification. For this reason, readers need to be somewhat familiar with both the 1989 and 1999 classification systems (TABLE 4-3).

TABLE 4-3.	Changes From 1989 to 1999 Classification
New Terminology	• *Chronic periodontitis* replaces the term *adult periodontitis* since epidemiological evidence suggests that chronic periodontitis is also seen in some adolescents. • *Aggressive periodontitis* replaces the term *early-onset periodontitis* because it is difficult to determine the age of onset of periodontitis in many cases. • *Necrotizing periodontal disease* replaces *necrotizing ulcerative gingivitis*
Additions	• Gingival disorders • Periodontitis as a manifestation of systemic disease • Periodontal abscess • Periodontitis in conjunction with endodontic lesions • Developmental or genetic conditions
Deletion	• The category of refractory periodontitis is eliminated. In the 1999 classification, the designation *refractory* can be applied to *all types* of periodontal disease that do not respond to treatment.

Section 3
AAP Classification System for Periodontal Diseases

Foundations of Periodontics for the Dental Hygienist uses the most recent, internationally accepted, consensus of the diseases and conditions affecting the periodontium, the AAP Classification of Periodontal Diseases and Conditions, 1999 (TABLE 4-4).

TABLE 4-4.   AAP Classification of Periodontal Diseases and Conditions

Type I

Gingival Diseases	I. Gingival Diseases
• **Plaque-Induced Gingival Diseases**	A. Dental plaque-induced gingival diseases[a]
○ Caused solely by plaque	1. Gingivitis associated with dental plaque biofilm only
○ Modified by systemic factors	a. Without other local contributing factors
	b. With local contributing factors
	2. Gingival diseases modified by systemic factors
	a. Associated with the endocrine system
	1) Puberty-associated gingivitis
	2) Menstrual cycle–associated gingivitis
	3) Pregnancy-associated
	a) Gingivitis
	b) Pyogenic granuloma
	4) Diabetes mellitus–associated gingivitis
	b. Associated with blood dyscrasias
	1) Leukemia-associated gingivitis
	2) Other
○ Modified by medications	3. Gingival diseases modified by medications
	a. Drug-influenced gingival diseases
	1) Drug-influenced gingival enlargements
	2) Drug-influenced gingivitis
	a) Oral contraceptive–associated gingivitis
	b) Other
○ Modified by malnutrition	4. Gingival diseases modified by malnutrition
	a. Ascorbic acid deficiency gingivitis
	b. Other
• **Non–Plaque-Induced Gingival Lesions**	B. Non–plaque-induced gingival lesions
○ Bacterial infections	1. Gingival diseases of specific bacterial origin
	a. *Neisseria gonorrhea*–associated lesions
	b. *Treponema pallidum*–associated lesions
	c. Streptococcal species–associated lesions
	d. Other

TABLE 4-4.	AAP Classification of Periodontal Diseases and Conditions (*Continued*)

Type I

- **Non–Plaque-Induced Gingival Lesions, continued**
  ○ Viral infections

  2. Gingival diseases of viral origin
     a. Herpes virus infections
        1) Primary herpetic gingivostomatitis
        2) Recurrent oral herpes
        3) Varicella zoster infections
     b. Other

  ○ Fungal infections

  3. Gingival diseases of fungal origin
     a. *Candida* species infections
        1) Generalized gingival candidosis
     b. Linear gingival erythema
     c. Histoplasmosis
     d. Other

  ○ Genetic origin

  4. Gingival lesions of genetic origin
     a. Hereditary gingival fibromatosis
     b. Other

  ○ Systemically related

  5. Gingival manifestations of systemic conditions
     a. Mucocutaneous disorders
        1) Lichen planus
        2) Pemphigoid
        3) Pemphigus vulgaris
        4) Erythema multiforme
        5) Lupus erythematosus
        6) Drug-induced
        7) Other
     b. Allergic reactions
        1) Dental restorative materials
           a) Mercury
           b) Nickel
           c) Acrylic
           d) Other
        2) Reactions attributable to
           a) Toothpastes/dentifrices
           b) Mouthrinses/mouthwashes
           c) Chewing gum additives
           d) Foods and additives
        3) Other

  ○ Trauma

  6. Traumatic lesions (factitious, iatrogenic, accidental)
     a. Chemical injury
     b. Physical injury
     c. Thermal injury

  ○ Reactions to foreign bodies
  ○ Other

  7. Foreign body reactions
  8. Not otherwise specified (NOS)

(continued)

TABLE 4-4. AAP Classification of Periodontal Diseases and Conditions (*Continued*)

Type II

Chronic Periodontitis (CP)	II. Chronic Periodontitis[b]
	   A. Localized
	   B. Generalized

Type III

Aggressive Periodontitis (AP)	III. Aggressive Periodontitis[b]
	   A. Localized
	   B. Generalized

Type IV

Periodontitis as Manifestation of Systemic Disease
   ○ Blood disorders
 	
   ○ Genetic factors
	IV. Periodontitis as a Manifestation of Systemic Diseases
	   A. Associated with hematological disorders
	      1. Acquired neutropenia
	      2. Leukemias
	      3. Other
	   B. Associated with genetic disorders
	      1. Familial and cyclic neutropenia
	      2. Down syndrome
	      3. Leukocyte adhesion deficiency syndromes
	      4. Papillon-Lefèvre syndrome
	      5. Chédiak-Higashi syndrome
	      6. Histiocytosis syndromes
	      7. Glycogen storage disease
	      8. Infantile genetic agranulocytosis
	      9. Cohen syndrome
	      10. Ehlers-Danlos syndrome (Types IV and VIII)
	      11. Hypophosphatasia
	      12. Other
	   C. Not otherwise specified (NOS)

Type V

Necrotizing Periodontal Diseases	V. Necrotizing Periodontal Disease
	   A. Necrotizing ulcerative gingivitis (NUG)
	   B. Necrotizing ulcerative periodontitis (NUP)

Type VI

Abscesses of the Periodontium	VI. Abscesses of the Periodontium
	   A. Gingival abscess
	   B. Periodontal abscess
	   C. Pericoronal abscess

TABLE 4-4. AAP Classification of Periodontal Diseases and Conditions (*Continued*)

Type VII

Periodontitis Associated with Endodontic Lesions

VII. Periodontitis Associated with Endodontic Lesions

    A. Combined periodontic-endodontic lesions

Type VIII

Deformities and Conditions

○ Tooth-related

VIII. Developmental or Acquired Deformities and Conditions

    A. Localized tooth-related factors that modify or predispose to plaque-induced gingival diseases or periodontitis

        1. Tooth anatomic factors

        2. Dental restorations/appliances

        3. Root fractures

        4. Cervical root resorption and cemental tears

○ Mucogingival conditions

    B. Mucogingival deformities and conditions around teeth

        1. Gingival/soft tissue recession

            a. Facial or lingual surfaces

            b. Interproximal (papillary)

        2. Lack of keratinized gingiva

        3. Decreased vestibular depth

        4. Aberrant frenum/muscle position

        5. Gingival excess

            a. Pseudopocket

            b. Inconsistent gingival margin

            c. Excessive gingival display

            d. Gingival enlargement

        6. Abnormal color

○ Mucogingival deformities

    C. Mucogingival deformities and conditions on edentulous ridges

        1. Vertical and/or horizontal ridge deficiency

        2. Lack of gingiva/keratinized tissue

        3. Gingival/soft tissue enlargement

        4. Aberrant frenum/muscle position

        5. Decreased vestibular depth

        6. Abnormal color

○ Occlusal trauma

    D. Occlusal trauma

        1. Primary occlusal trauma

        2. Secondary occlusal trauma

[a]Can occur on a periodontium with no attachment loss or on a periodontium with attachment loss that is not progressing.
[b]Can be further classified on the basis of extent and severity.
Data from Armitage GC. Development of a classification system for periodontal diseases and conditions. *Ann Periodontol.* 1999;4(1):1–6.

Section 4
Overview of Periodontal Diseases

GINGIVAL DISEASES

Gingival diseases usually involve inflammation of the gingival tissues, most often in response to bacterial plaque biofilm. Gingival diseases have been subdivided into two major categories: (1) dental plaque-induced gingival diseases and (2) non–plaque-induced gingival lesions.

1. **Dental Plaque-Induced Gingival Diseases**
   A. **Definition.** Plaque-induced gingival diseases are periodontal diseases involving inflammation of the gingiva in response to bacteria located at the gingival margin. Gingivitis associated with plaque biofilm formation is the *most common form* of gingival disease [4].
   B. **Subtypes.** There are four main subtypes of plaque-induced gingival diseases.
      1. Gingivitis associated with dental plaque biofilm only—the most common form is gingivitis resulting from dental plaque biofilm with no local or systemic complicating factors.
      2. Gingival diseases modified by systemic factors—gingival diseases with contributing systemic factors. Plaque biofilm formation still plays a central role in the etiology of gingival diseases modified by systemic factors. Systemic factors, however, play a contributing role. An example is pregnancy-associated gingivitis in which hormone fluctuations promote the growth of certain types of bacteria in the biofilm [5].
      3. Gingival diseases modified by medications—medication-induced gingival diseases. An example of this subcategory is medication-influenced gingival enlargement. Certain medications, such as phenytoin and cyclosporine, can promote enlargement of the gingival tissues in the presence of plaque biofilm formation.
      4. Gingival diseases modified by malnutrition—gingival diseases with malnutrition as a contributing factor. Severe malnutrition is seldom seen in well-developed countries. During early phases of experimental ascorbic acid deficiency, some increases in gingival inflammation and bleeding have been reported [6,7].
   C. **Disease Progression.** Gingivitis may persist for years without ever progressing to periodontitis.
2. **Non–plaque-induced gingival lesions.**
   A. **Less Common Type of Gingivitis.** A small percentage of gingival disease—termed non–plaque-induced gingival lesions—is not caused by bacterial plaque biofilm. Plaque biofilm does not have an etiologic role in non–plaque-induced gingival lesions.
   B. **Causes.** Non–plaque-induced gingival lesions can result from such varied causes as viral infections, fungal infections, dermatological (skin) diseases, allergic reactions, or mechanical trauma. Gingival inflammation in non–plaque-induced lesions might be caused by a specific bacterial, viral, or fungal infection [8,9].
      1. Gingival diseases of specific bacterial origin are becoming more common, especially those associated with sexually transmitted diseases such as *Neisseria gonorrhoeae* infection associated with gonorrhea.
      2. Herpes simplex virus types I and 2 and varicella zoster virus are two examples of viruses that can infect the gingiva [8].
      3. Fungal infections such as candidiasis can infect the gingiva [9]. Fungal infections are most common in immunocompromised individuals.

4. Gingival lesions are manifestations of some systemic diseases such a lichen planus, erythema multiforme, and psoriasis [10,11,12].
5. Allergic reactions to toothpastes and mouthrinses or even foods and chewing gum can result in gingival inflammation.

PERIODONTITIS

1. **Types of Periodontitis.** Periodontitis has been subdivided into seven major categories:
   A. Chronic periodontitis
   B. Aggressive periodontitis
   C. Periodontitis as a manifestation of systemic disease
   D. Necrotizing periodontal diseases
   E. Abscesses of the periodontium
   F. Periodontitis associated with endodontic lesions
   G. Developmental or acquired deformities and conditions
2. **Chronic Periodontitis (Most Common Form of Periodontitis)**
   A. **Definition.** Chronic periodontitis—the most common form of periodontitis—is a bacterial infection within the supporting tissues of the teeth.
      1. The disease is characterized by destruction of the periodontal ligament fibers and alveolar bone and by pocket formation and/or recession of gingival margin.
      2. This type of periodontitis was previously known as adult periodontitis because it was once believed to be primarily found in adults. Epidemiologic data, however, indicate that chronic periodontitis can be found in children and adolescents [13].
   B. **Clinical Features**
      1. Chronic periodontitis is initiated and sustained by plaque biofilms. The body's host response to the bacterial pathogens, however, is responsible for most of the tissue destruction seen in chronic periodontitis.
      2. Chronic periodontitis is most prevalent in adults but may occur in both the primary and adult dentitions.
      3. The disease usually progresses (worsens) at a slow to moderate rate, but there may be short periods of rapid disease progression [14–16]. Disease progression is characterized by loss of connective tissue and resorption of alveolar bone.
      4. Bacterial plaque biofilm and subgingival calculus are frequent findings. The amount of tissue destruction is consistent with the presence of local etiologic factors.
      5. The disease can be modified by and/or associated with systemic disease.
      6. Other factors, such as smoking, can be predisposing factors.
      7. Chronic periodontitis can be further classified on the basis of extent and severity.
3. **Aggressive Periodontitis (Highly Destructive Form of Periodontitis)**
   A. **Definition.** Aggressive periodontitis is bacterial infection characterized by a rapid loss of attachment and a less predictable response to periodontal therapy (than chronic periodontitis). The disease may be localized—localized aggressive periodontitis—or generalized—generalized aggressive periodontitis.
      1. Aggressive periodontitis was previously known as early-onset periodontitis.
      2. Localized aggressive periodontitis was formerly known as localized juvenile periodontitis.
      3. Generalized aggressive periodontitis was formerly known as rapidly progressing periodontitis.
   B. **Clinical Features**
      1. Aggressive periodontitis is much less common than chronic periodontitis and may occur in the primary and adult dentitions.

2. Aggressive periodontitis differs from chronic periodontitis in several characteristics:
   a. A rapid rate of disease progression that is seen in an otherwise healthy individual that results in rapid attachment loss and bone destruction.
   b. The amount of tissue destruction may be inconsistent with the presence of local etiologic factors. There are relatively small amounts of plaque biofilm or calculus deposits (as compared with those seen in chronic periodontitis).
   c. A family history of aggressive periodontitis. The disease can be modified by and/or associated with immune deficiencies and other genetic factors.

4. **Periodontitis as a Manifestation of Systemic Diseases.** The Periodontitis as a manifestation of systemic diseases category is a group of periodontal diseases that is associated with two general categories of systemic diseases: (1) hematological (blood) disorders, such as leukemia or acquired neutropenia, and (2) genetic disorders, such as Down syndrome or leukocyte adhesion deficiency syndrome.
   A. **Definition.** Periodontitis as a manifestation of systemic disease is the disease category used when the systemic condition is the major predisposing factor and the bacterial infection is considered a secondary feature of the systemic disease.
      1. This periodontal disease is associated with systemic conditions in which there is a significant reduction in the number of neutrophils or impairment in the ability of the neutrophils to fight infections.
      2. A severely decreased host resistance associated with a systemic condition is the major etiologic factor in the development of this category of periodontal disease.
   B. **Clinical Features.** The clinical manifestations of this category of periodontal disease occur at an early age.

5. **Necrotizing Periodontal Diseases** Necrotizing periodontal diseases are a unique type of periodontal disease that involves tissue necrosis (localized tissue death).
   A. **Definition**
      1. Necrotizing periodontal diseases include necrotizing ulcerative gingivitis and necrotizing ulcerative periodontitis.
         a. Necrotizing ulcerative gingivitis (NUG) is a type of periodontal disease that involves tissue necrosis that is limited to the gingival tissues with no clinical attachment loss.
         b. Necrotizing ulcerative periodontitis (NUP) is characterized by tissue necrosis of the gingival tissues combined with loss of attachment and alveolar bone loss.
      2. A diminished systemic resistance to bacterial infection of the periodontal tissues is a characteristic that is common to both NUG and NUP.
   B. **Clinical Features**
      1. Necrotic papillary and marginal gingiva covered by a yellowish or grayish coating
      2. Blunted or cratered papillae
      3. Spontaneous bleeding, fetid breath, and pain

6. **Abscesses of the Periodontium**
   A. **Definition**
      1. A periodontal abscess is a localized collection of pus that forms in a circumscribed area of the periodontal tissues.
         a. Bacteria in plaque biofilm attract high numbers of neutrophils from the soft tissue. Most of the time these neutrophils seep unnoticed from the periodontal pocket as exudate.

  b. If the drainage from the periodontal pocket is blocked, the neutrophil-rich exudate collects in the soft tissue wall of the pocket and forms a periodontal abscess.

 2. Periodontal abscesses are a common feature of moderate or advanced periodontitis.

B. Clinical Features

 1. Localized gingival swelling

 2. Drainage from the tissue (sinus tract)

 3. Pain on percussion (pressure with finger)

 4. Increased tooth mobility

7. Periodontitis Associated with Endodontic Lesions

A. Definition

 1. Periodontitis associated with endodontic lesions is a category of periodontal disease that involves infection or death of the tissues of the dental pulp.

 2. A tooth can be affected by both periodontal disease and pulpal disease at the same time. When periodontitis and pulpal disease affect the same tooth so severely that they become combined into one lesion, the condition usually is referred to as a combined periodontal-endodontic lesion.

  a. Periodontal Infection Leading to Infection of the Pulp. In some cases, periodontitis is so severe that it affects the apex of the tooth or one of the accessory openings into the pulp chamber that occur in some teeth. When this occurs, the bacterial infection of the periodontium can lead to infection of the dental pulp.

  b. Infection of Pulp Leading to Destruction of Periodontium. In advanced stages of pulpal disease, the pulpal disease can result in periodontal destruction by spreading of the infection from the dental pulp to the periodontal ligament and alveolar bone.

 3. A combined periodontal-endodontic lesion usually requires periodontal treatment and endodontic treatment (a root canal) to save the tooth.

B. Clinical Features

 1. Gingival inflammation

 2. Increased probing depths, loss of attachment

 3. Bleeding or pus evident on probing

8. Developmental or Acquired Deformities and Conditions. This category includes conditions that exist around the teeth that may predispose the periodontium to disease. This category is subdivided into localized tooth-related factors, mucogingival deformities and conditions, and occlusal trauma. Tooth-related factors include tooth position, root abnormalities, enamel pearls, defects in dental restorations, and occlusal trauma. Mucogingival deformities refer to defects in the normal shape of the gingiva and alveolar mucosa.

Chapter Summary Statement

The two basic diagnostic categories of periodontal disease are (1) gingivitis and (2) periodontitis. It is important to be thoroughly familiar with the terms periodontal disease, gingivitis, and periodontitis and the precise definition of each term.

 Classification systems provide a tool to study the etiology, pathogenesis, and treatment of periodontal diseases in an orderly manner. In addition, periodontal disease classifications assist the dental hygienist in communicating with other dental healthcare providers, patients, and dental insurance providers.

References

1. American Academy of Periodontology: Consensus report. Discussion section I, *Proceedings of the World Workshop in Clinical Periodontics*. Chicago, 1989. American Academy of Periodontology, 1999. p. I-23-I-32.
2. Armitage GC. Development of a classification system for periodontal diseases and conditions. *Ann Periodontol*. 1999;4(1):1–6.
3. Armitage GC. Classifying periodontal diseases—a long-standing dilemma. *Periodontol 2000*. 2002;30:9–23.
4. Aldred MJ, Bartold PM. Genetic disorders of the gingivae and periodontium. *Periodontol 2000*. 1998;18:7–20.
5. Amar S, Chung KM. Influence of hormonal variation on the periodontium in women. *Periodontol 2000*. 1994;6:79–87.
6. Mariotti A. Dental plaque-induced gingival diseases. *Ann Periodontol*. 1999;4(1):7–19.
7. Leggott PJ, Robertson PB, Rothman DL, et al. The effect of controlled ascorbic acid depletion and supplementation on periodontal health. *J Periodontol*. 1986;57(8):480–485.
8. Rivera-Hidalgo F, Stanford TW. Oral mucosal lesions caused by infective microorganisms. I. Viruses and bacteria. *Periodontol 2000*. 1999;21:106–124.
9. Stanford TW, Rivera-Hidalgo F. Oral mucosal lesions caused by infective microorganisms. II. Fungi and parasites. *Periodontol 2000*. 1999;21:125–144.
10. Gorsky M, Raviv M, Moskona D, et al. Clinical characteristics and treatment of patients with oral lichen planus in Israel. *Oral Surg Oral Med Oral Pathol Oral Radiol Endod*. 1996;82(6):644–649.
11. Farthing PM, Maragou P, Coates M, et al. Characteristics of the oral lesions in patients with cutaneous recurrent erythema multiforme. *J Oral Pathol Med*. 1995;24(1):9–13.
12. Yamada J, Amar S, Petrungaro P. Psoriasis-associated periodontitis: a case report. *J Periodontol*. 1992;63(10):854–857.
13. Papapanou PN. Periodontal diseases: epidemiology. *Ann Periodontol*. 1996;1(1):1–36.
14. Brown LJ, Loe H. Prevalence, extent, severity and progression of periodontal disease. *Periodontol 2000*. 1993;2:57–71.
15. Jeffcoat MK, Reddy MS. Progression of probing attachment loss in adult periodontitis. *J Periodontol*. 1991;62(3):185–189.
16. Papapanou PN, Wennstrom JL, Grondahl K. A 10-year retrospective study of periodontal disease progression. *J Clin Periodontol*. 1989;16(7):403–411.

Search for the Causes of Periodontal Disease

Learning Objectives

- Describe variables associated with periodontal disease that an epidemiologist might include in a research study.

- Define prevalence and incidence as measurements of disease within a population.

- Discuss historical and current theories associated with the progression of periodontal disease.

- Describe how clinical dental hygiene practice can be affected by epidemiological research.

Key Terms

Epidemiology
Incidence
Prevalence
Disease progression

Periodontal pathogens
Intermittent disease progression
Risk factors

Section 1
Epidemiology: Researching Periodontal Disease

Many generations of researchers have asked the question, "What causes periodontal disease?" while clinicians have asked, "What is the best care for my patients with periodontal disease?" This chapter discusses the study of disease in the population (epidemiology) and reviews historical and current perspectives on the causes and progression of periodontal disease.

1. **What is Epidemiology?**
    A. Epidemiology is the study of the health and disease within the total population (rather than an individual) and the risk factors that influence health and disease. An epidemiologist assesses how much disease, investigates possible causes, and applies results to treatment recommendations.
        1. Epidemiological research has three objectives: (1) to determine the amount and distribution of a disease in a population, (2) to investigate the causes of a disease, and (3) to apply this knowledge to the control of disease.
        2. Through research of population groups, epidemiologists strive to identify the risk factors associated with disease such as heredity, gender, physical environment, systemic factors, socioeconomic status, and personal behavior.
        3. An understanding of the risk factors associated with a certain disease can lead to theories of the cause of that disease and then to treatment standards for patient care.
    B. **Epidemiology of Periodontal Disease**
        1. A large percentage of the adult population has periodontal disease. Epidemiologists study periodontal disease to determine its occurrence in the population and to identify risk factors for periodontal disease. Some of the questions epidemiologists ask when researching periodontal disease are illustrated in Figure 5-1.
        2. Epidemiological research also provides current information to the clinical dental hygienist about methods and behaviors that are successful in the treatment and prevention of periodontal disease. Current research also may define the level of risk a patient may have for periodontal disease.
        3. Studies can be designed to look at the disparities or inequities of disease patterns. For instance, a study may explore why more periodontal disease

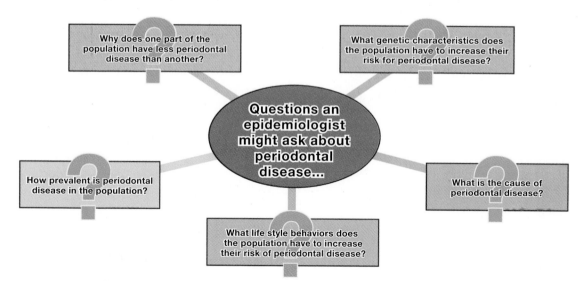

Figure 5.1. Researching Periodontal Disease. This diagram illustrates the types of questions asked by epidemiologists when studying periodontal disease.

is found in a specific segment of the population than in another group of people. Oral diseases occur disproportionately more among individuals with low socioeconomic status and with poor general health [1].

3. **Prevalence and Incidence of Disease**
   A. **Incidence and Prevalence**
      1. Prevalence refers to the number of all cases (both old and new) of a disease that can be identified within a specified population at a given point in time (FIG. 5-2). For example, in 2002 a study of 100 white adults, aged 35 to 45, was done with a prevalence of 50% of this population being recorded as having bleeding upon probing. The Gingival Bleeding Index (GBI) was used to record bleeding. This prevalence information does not indicate how long these adults have had gingival bleeding upon probing.
      2. Incidence is the number of **new disease cases** in a population that occur over a given period of time.
         For example, a follow-up study in 2003 of the same above adult population indicated an incidence of 10 additional cases recorded as bleeding upon probing. Now the new prevalence of bleeding upon probing with this population is 60%.

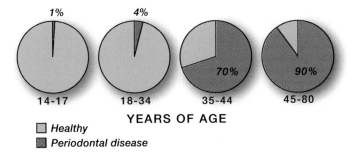

Figure 5.2. **Prevalence of Periodontal Disease**. Periodontal disease in various age groups. (Data from Oliver RC, Brown LJ, Loe H. Periodontal diseases in the United States population. *J Periodontol.* 1998;69(2):269–278.)

   B. **Variables Associated with the Prevalence of Disease.** Research findings show that variables associated with the prevalence of periodontal disease include a person's gender, race, socioeconomic status, and age.
      1. Gender
         a. Males have a greater prevalence and severity of periodontal disease than females.
         b. There has been some speculation that females have a tendency to practice better and more frequent self-care than males. These differences in self-care behaviors may lead to the greater prevalence of disease in males.
      2. Educational level and socioeconomic status
         a. Black and Hispanic males living in the United States have poorer periodontal health and a greater incidence of periodontal disease than White males.
         b. There is a greater incidence of periodontal disease in individuals with lower levels of education and income.
         c. Underdeveloped countries have a higher incidence of chronic periodontitis, possibly due to a lack of adequate information about disease prevention.
      3. Age
         a. Research studies have shown that the severity of periodontal disease increases with age; however, the exact role that age plays in periodontal disease is difficult to assess.

1) As an individual lives longer, the chances increase that he will be exposed to additional risk factors for periodontal disease. Such risk factors include systemic illness, medications, stress, and smoking.

2) The higher incidence of periodontal disease in the elderly, therefore, may not be due to age, but rather other risk factors to which an individual has been exposed during his or her long life.

b. Diminished dexterity is sometimes a problem in elderly individuals and can impact the individual's ability to perform self-care. Limited dexterity may also shorten the length of time that self-care is performed on a daily basis.

4. Access to dental care. Individuals who desire care or need care may not have access to dental care. Barriers to obtaining dental care include transportation—traveling long distances to a dental office—and the financial expense of dental care.

TABLE 5-1. Commonly Used Periodontal Indices

Index	Measurement
Community and Periodontal Index of Treatment Needs (CPITN)	Assesses probing depths and bleeding; developed to attain more uniform worldwide epidemiologic data; maybe used for measuring group periodontal needs
Eastman Interdental Bleeding Index (EIBI)	Assesses presence of inflammation and bleeding in the interdental area upon toothpick insertion
Gingival Bleeding Index (GBI)	Assesses presence of gingival inflammation by bleeding from interproximal sulcus within 10 seconds of flossing
Gingival Index (GI)	Assesses severity of gingivitis based on color, consistency, and bleeding on probing
Modified Gingival Index (MGI)	Similar to GI but assesses severity of gingivitis without probing; redefined scoring for mold/moderate inflammation
Periodontal Index (PI)	Assesses the severity of gingival inflammation without probing
Periodontal Disease Index (PDI)	Assesses the severity of gingival inflammation, pocket depth, and the level of gingival attachment
Periodontal Screening and Recording (PSR)	Assesses periodontal health in a rapid manner including probing depths, bleeding, and presence of hard deposits

C. **Measuring the Disease Prevalence**

1. The prevalence of periodontal disease in the U.S. adult population is determined by performing clinical examinations on cross sections of groups using indices. Indices measure the amount and severity of disease. Indices used to measure both gingivitis and periodontitis vary across epidemiological studies, as does the extent of disease present when a study begins. Refer to TABLE 5-1 for a list of indices commonly used to assess periodontal disease.

2. Prevalence is affected by new cases of disease (incidence), cures or deaths within a population, and the longer lives of subjects.

3. Historically, gingival indices have used criteria to measure variables of inflammation such as color changes, presence of edema, and bleeding upon probing. Clinical indices for measuring periodontitis include variables such as probing depth, clinical attachment level (CAL), and interpretation of radiographic bone levels (BLs). Many studies use sample groups numbering in the thousands. Several groups are then compared and statistically analyzed. Epidemiologists will have different approaches to research and will include different variables in studies. The selected population can be studied over time.

D. **Difficulties in Measurement of Periodontal Disease**

1. It is far easier to evaluate a population for prevalence and incidence of dental caries than for periodontal disease because caries lends itself for more objective measurement. The development and process of caries is well known and involves only tooth structure.

2. Periodontal disease, on the other hand, involves both hard and soft tissues and has multiple variables that must be considered. Determining the presence of gingivitis with or without the presence of periodontitis further complicates the assessment of disease. Assessment can include
   a. Soft tissue color changes (redness)
   b. Tissue swelling (edema)
   c. Loss of periodontal ligament fibers that support the teeth
   d. Loss of alveolar bone/ furcation involvement
   e. Bleeding upon probing/ spontaneous bleeding
   f. Probing depths

3. The multiple variables used to define periodontal disease make the numbers for prevalence and incidence of periodontal disease less specific, more of a range, and more subject to change.

E. **What the Research Shows.** Research on periodontal disease indicates that it is one of the most widespread diseases in adult Americans, with most individuals who have periodontal disease being unaware of its presence. Data on the dental health of the U.S. population come from the third National Health and Nutrition Examination Survey (NHANES III) [2].

1. Prevalence of gingivitis
   a. According to data from NHANES III, 54% of the noninstitutionalized civilian U.S. population aged 13 years and older had gingival bleeding in at least one gingival site [2].
   b. Adolescents have a higher prevalence of gingivitis than prepubertal children or adults [2].
   c. Males in all age groups are more likely to have gingivitis than females. The prevalence of gingivitis is especially high for males aged 13 to 17 years [2].

2. Prevalence of chronic periodontitis
   a. The presence of periodontal disease is measured clinically in several ways. One way is by calculation of the loss of periodontal attachment. Loss of attachment is the term used to describe the destruction of periodontal ligament fibers and alveolar bone that support the teeth. Figure 5-3 shows that attachment loss of 4 mm or more affects approximately half of adults aged 50 to 59 [2].
   b. By age 60 to 69, less than half of all adults in the United States have retained 21 teeth or more (FIG. 5-4) [2].

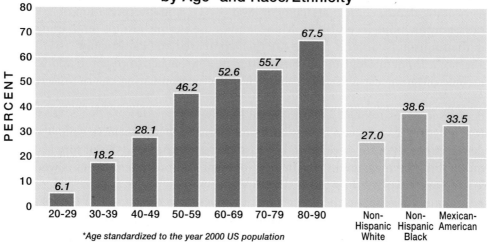

Figure 5.3. **Prevalence of Loss of Attachment.** Loss of attachment is the term used to describe the destruction of periodontal ligament fibers and alveolar bone that support the teeth. (Data source for graph: The Third National Health and Nutrition Examination Survey (NHANES III) 1988–1994, National Center for Health Statistics. Centers for Disease Control and Prevention.)

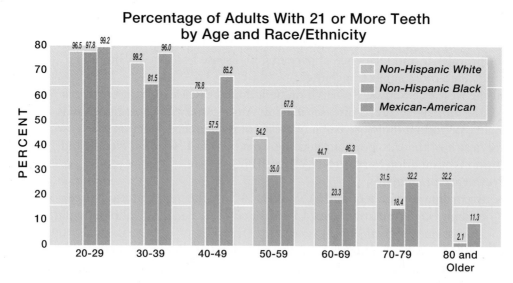

Figure 5.4. **Tooth Loss in Adults.** By age 60 to 69, less than half of all adults in the United States have retained 21 teeth or more. (Data source for graph: The Third National Health and Nutrition Examination Survey (NHANES III) 1988–1994, National Center for Health Statistics. Centers for Disease Control and Prevention.)

Section 2
Control and Progression of Periodontal Disease

CONTROL OF PERIODONTAL DISEASE

Over time, researchers have changed their ideas on the primary risk factors for periodontal disease. This chapter presents a brief historical review of how the understanding of disease risk factors has evolved over the years (TABLE 5-2). Awareness of past theories is helpful in understanding why recommendations for the prevention and treatment of periodontal disease have changed so much over the years. A 60-year-old patient who has received regular dental care over the years would have first visited a dental office in the 1950s (assuming that his of her first dental visit was by the age of 10).

TABLE 5-2. Theories on Disease Control of Periodontal Disease		
Theory	**Primary Risk Factors**	**Focus of Professional Care**
Calculus (Before 1960)	Calculus deposits	Removal of calculus deposits
Plaque Biofilm (1965–1985)	Bacterial plaque biofilm	Removal or disruption of bacterial plaque biofilm
Host–Bacterial Interaction (Current)	Many risk factors—a complex interaction of bacterial plaque biofilm, host response, and other risk factors	Identification and control of bacterial, host, local, and systemic risk factors

1. Historical Perspectives on Disease Control
   A. Calculus as Risk Factor—Before 1960
      1. Theory. Before 1960, clinicians believed that periodontal disease was caused solely by the presence of calculus deposits that act as a mechanical irritant to the tissue (FIG. 5-5).
      2. Treatment Before 1960
         a. Professional Care. Professional prophylaxis was scheduled every 6 months to remove accumulated calculus deposits.
         b. Patient Self-Care. Patients were advised to brush three times a day to remove food particles.

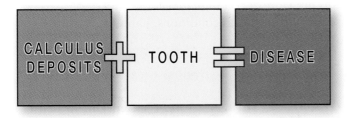

Figure 5.5. **Calculus Theory.** Before 1960, clinicians believed that periodontal disease was caused solely by the presence of calculus deposits.

   B. Bacterial Plaque Biofilm as Risk Factor—1965 to 1985
      1. Theory. Bacteria in dental plaque biofilm cause periodontal disease (FIG. 5-6).
         a. The classic research study by Löe et al. [3] demonstrated that an accumulation of bacterial plaque biofilm is important in the development of gingivitis.

b. In the years 1975 to 1985, research focused on the composition of plaque biofilm. Researchers hoped to determine which particular bacterial species were responsible for specific types of periodontal disease. Periodontal pathogens are bacteria that are capable of infecting the tissues of the periodontium.

c. During this time period, many clinicians believed that
   1) Daily plaque biofilm control efforts *alone* could prevent or control periodontal disease.
   2) If patients did not respond to treatment, they were at fault, probably due to infrequent or inadequate self-care.

2. Treatment 1965 to 1985
   a. Professional Care. Professional prophylaxis was scheduled two to three times a year.
   b. Patient Self-Care. The patient was instructed in self-care techniques and taught that prevention and control of periodontal disease depended on his or her daily plaque biofilm control efforts. If disease was not prevented or controlled, the patient was at fault for failing at plaque biofilm control.

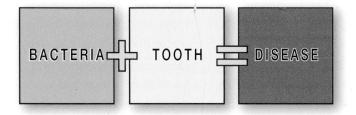

Figure 5.6. **Bacterial Theory.** During the years 1965 to 1985, most clinicians believed that the adequate daily plaque biofilm removal could prevent or control periodontal disease.

2. **Current Views on Disease Control.** In recent years, advances in research have led to a fundamental change in our understanding of periodontal disease and have led to the development of a new theory about the risk factors involved in periodontal disease. Researchers now believe that the presence of bacterial plaque biofilm, alone, is not enough to cause periodontal disease.
   A. **The Host–Bacterial Interaction as Risk Factor—Current.** It is the interaction of the host (patient) with the pathogenic bacteria that controls whether or not periodontal disease is present (FIG. 5-7).
      1. *A bacterial infection alone is insufficient to result in periodontal disease. The host response plays a critical role in the tissue destruction seen in periodontitis. Current research findings suggest that everyone is not equally susceptible to periodontal disease. Some individuals are more at risk than others.*
      2. Risk factors for periodontal disease include local oral conditions, habits, systemic disease, and genetic factors.

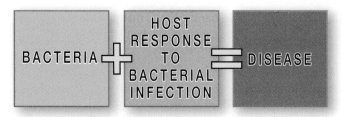

Figure 5.7. **Host-Bacterial Interaction Theory.** Current research has shown that it is the interaction of the patient with the dental plaque biofilm that controls whether or not periodontal disease is present.

3. **Current Views on Treatment**
   A. **Professional Care**
      1. Today, the treatment of periodontal disease is directed at managing the bacterial, local, and systemic etiologic factors for periodontal disease.

2. Periodontal maintenance appointments (recall appointments) should be scheduled as frequently as needed to assist the patient in controlling disease.
3. Treatment may involve not only the periodontal instrumentation of root surfaces but, when appropriate, includes control of local factors and referral to a physician for management of systemic disease or other risk factors.

B. **Patient Self-Care**
1. The patient is educated about the role of bacterial plaque biofilm in periodontal disease and in plaque biofilm control techniques.
2. If the disease continues to progress, the patient is not at fault for his or her failure to control the disease; instead, risk factors are identified and eliminated or controlled whenever possible. More frequent appointments for professional periodontal maintenance (recall visits) are recommended to assist the patient in controlling disease.

PROGRESSION OF PERIODONTAL DISEASE

For years, clinical researchers have been trying to find an answer to the question, "How does untreated periodontal disease progress?" In this context, disease progression means that the disease gets worse. Data from ongoing studies suggest that the pattern of disease progression may vary from (1) one individual to another, (2) one site to another in a person's mouth, and (3) one type of periodontal disease to another.

1. **Historical Perspective on Disease Progression**
   A. **Continuous Progression Theory (Historical View of Disease Progression: Prior to 1980).** The continuous disease progression theory states that periodontal disease progresses throughout the entire mouth in a slow and constant rate over the adult life of the patient (FIG. 5-8).
      1. This theory suggests that
         a. All cases of untreated gingivitis lead to periodontitis.
         b. All cases of periodontitis progress at a slow and steady rate of tissue destruction.
      2. Research studies conducted in the early 1980s indicated that periodontal disease neither progresses at a constant rate nor affects all areas of the mouth simultaneously. The continuous progression theory does not accurately reflect the complex nature of periodontal disease.

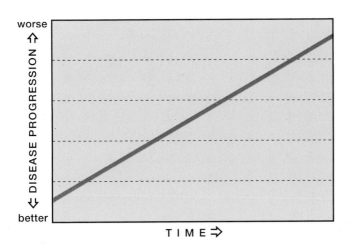

Figure 5.8. **The Continuous Disease Model of Disease Progression (Prior to 1980).** In the past, clinicians believed that periodontal disease progresses (worsens) throughout the entire mouth in a slow and constant rate over the life of the patient. It was believed that all cases of untreated gingivitis led to periodontitis.

2. **Current Theory of Disease Progression**
    A. **Intermittent Progression Theory (Current View).** Intermittent disease progression theory states that periodontal disease is characterized by periods of disease activity and inactivity (remission) (FIG. 5-9).
        1. Tissue destruction is sporadic, with short periods of tissue destruction alternating with periods of disease inactivity (no tissue destruction). The period of inactivity with no disease progression may last for months or for a much longer period of time.
        2. Tissue destruction progresses at different rates throughout the mouth. Destruction does not occur in all parts of the mouth at the same time. Instead, tissue destruction occurs in only a few specific sites (tooth surfaces) at a time.
        3. In the majority of cases, untreated gingivitis does not progress to periodontitis.
        4. Different forms of periodontitis progress at widely different rates.
        5. Susceptibility to periodontitis varies greatly from individual to individual and appears to be determined by the host response to periodontal pathogens.

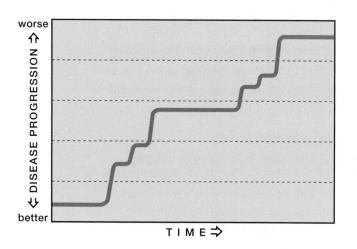

Figure 5.9. **Intermittent Disease Progression Theory.** Current research suggests that periodontal disease is characterized by periods of disease activity and inactivity. Furthermore, destruction does not occur in all parts of the mouth at the same time.

Section 3
Risk Factors for Periodontal Disease

Risk factors are factors that modify or amplify the likelihood of developing periodontal disease. The major established risk factors for periodontitis are specific bacterial pathogens, cigarette smoking, and diabetes mellitus.

1. **Local and Acquired Risk Factors**
   A. **Dental Plaque Biofilm**
      1. It has been known for years that periodontal disease is a bacterial infection. The presence of bacteria is necessary for periodontal disease to occur.
      2. Recent epidemiologic studies have investigated the specific role of specific bacteria as risk factors for periodontitis.
      3. The consensus report of the 1996 World Workshop in Periodontics identified three species, *Aggregatibacter actinomycetemcomitans*, *Porphyromonas gingivalis*, and *Tannerella forsythia* as causative factors for periodontitis.
      4. Only approximately 50% of the bacteria of the oral cavity are currently recognized [4]. Thus, these three species cannot be considered to be the only periodontal pathogens, but are the only ones for which sufficient data exists.
   B. **Local Oral Conditions**
      1. Local contributing factors for periodontal disease are oral conditions that increase an individual's susceptibility to periodontal infection in specific sites.
      2. Examples of local contributing factors include dental calculus and faulty restorations.
   C. **Cigarette Smoking**
      1. Numerous research studies established the association of smoking to poor periodontal health status [5–12].
      2. Data derived from the Third National Health and Nutrition Examination Survey (NHANES III) study suggest that as many as 42% of periodontitis cases in the United States can be attributed to current smoking, and another 11% to former smoking [12].
2. **Systemic Risk Factors.** Diabetes mellitus is a major risk factor for periodontitis [13–16]. There is good evidence to support an association between poorly controlled diabetes mellitus and periodontitis [17–19].

Chapter Summary Statement

Epidemiological research has three objectives: (1) to determine the amount and distribution of a disease in a population, (2) to investigate the causes of a disease, and (3) to apply this knowledge to the control of disease. Epidemiologists study periodontal disease to determine its occurrence in the population and to identify risk factors for periodontal disease. Epidemiological research also provides current information to the clinical dental hygienist about methods and behaviors that are successful in the treatment and prevention of periodontal disease. Current research also may define the level of risk a patient may have for periodontal disease. Advances in research have led to many changes in the understanding, prevention, and treatment of periodontal disease. In the future, ideas about causes and treatment will continue to be refined and changed as researchers delve further into the mysteries of periodontal disease.

Section 4
Focus on Patients

Case 1

You find a newspaper article that estimates that in your home state 73% of state residents have some form of periodontal disease. You would like to use this statistic in a paper you are writing. When you include this information in your paper, should you describe this statistic as incidence or prevalence of periodontitis?

Case 2

Two individuals who have exactly the same level of plaque biofilm control and exactly the same amount of plaque biofilm accumulation do not necessarily develop the same severity of periodontal disease. How do you explain this fact?

Case 3

Your dental team has a new patient who has gingivitis. The patient has poor plaque biofilm control, generalized calculus deposits, poorly controlled diabetes mellitus, a history of smoking cigarettes, and inadequate dietary intake of calcium. In your patient counseling, how would you characterize the likelihood that the patient will develop periodontitis in the future and what might you tell the patient about this?

References

1. United States Public Health Service. Office of the Surgeon General and National Institute of Dental and Craniofacial Research (U.S.), *Oral health in America a report of the Surgeon General.* 2000, Department of Health and Human Services, U.S. Public Health Service,: Rockville.

2. National Center for Health Statistics (U.S.), *National Health and Nutrition Examination Survey III, 1988–94.* 1998, U.S. Dept. of Health and Human Services, Centers for Disease Control and Prevention, National Center for Health Statistics,: Hyattsville

3. Loe H, Theilade E, Jensen SB. Experimental gingivitis in Man. *J Periodontol.* 1965;36:177–187.

4. Paster BJ, Boches SK, Galvin JL, et al. Bacterial diversity in human subgingival plaque. *J Bacteriol.* 2001;183(12):3770–3783.

5. Albandar JM, Streckfus CF, Adesanya MR, et al. Cigar, pipe, and cigarette smoking as risk factors for periodontal disease and tooth loss. *J Periodontol.* 2000;71(12):1874–1881.

6. Bergstrom J, Eliasson S, Dock J. A 10-year prospective study of tobacco smoking and periodontal health. *J Periodontol.* 2000;71(8):1338–1347.

7. Bergstrom J, Eliasson S, Dock J. Exposure to tobacco smoking and periodontal health. *J Clin Periodontol.* 2000;27(1):61–68.

8. Kocher T, Schwahn C, Gesch D, et al. Risk determinants of periodontal disease—an analysis of the Study of Health in Pomerania (SHIP 0). *J Clin Periodontol.* 2005;32(1):59–67.

9. Martinez-Canut P, Lorca A, Magan R. Smoking and periodontal disease severity. *J Clin Periodontol.* 1995;22(10):743–749.

10. Paulander J, Wennstrom JL, Axelsson P, et al. Some risk factors for periodontal bone loss in 50-year-old individuals. A 10-year cohort study. *J Clin Periodontol.* 2004;31(7):489–496.

11. Susin C, et al. Periodontal attachment loss attributable to cigarette smoking in an urban Brazilian population. *J Clin Periodontol.* 2004;31(11):951–958.

12. Tomar SL, Asma S. Smoking-attributable periodontitis in the United States: findings from NHANES III. National Health and Nutrition Examination Survey. *J Periodontol.* 2000;71(5):743–751.

13. Lalla E, Cheng B, Lal S, et al. Diabetes mellitus promotes periodontal destruction in children. *J Clin Periodontol.* 2007;34(4):294–298.

14. Lalla E, Lamster IB, Drury S, et al. Hyperglycemia, glycoxidation and receptor for advanced glycation endproducts: potential mechanisms underlying diabetic complications, including diabetes-associated periodontitis. *Periodontol 2000.* 2000;23:50–62.

15. Soskolne WA, Klinger A. The relationship between periodontal diseases and diabetes: an overview. *Ann Periodontol.* 2001;6(1):91–98.

16. Taylor GW. Bidirectional interrelationships between diabetes and periodontal diseases: an epidemiologic perspective. *Ann Periodontol.* 2001;6(1):99–112.

17. Grossi SG, Genco RJ. Periodontal disease and diabetes mellitus: a two-way relationship. *Ann Periodontol.* 1998;3(1):51–61.

18. Lalla E, Park DB, Papapanou PN, et al. Oral disease burden in Northern Manhattan patients with diabetes mellitus. *Am J Public Health.* 2004;94(5):755–758.

19. Taylor GW, Burt BA, Becker MP, et al. Glycemic control and alveolar bone loss progression in type 2 diabetes. *Ann Periodontol.* 1998;3(1):30–39.

Chapter 6

Oral Biofilms and Periodontal Infections

Learning Objectives

- Define the terms innocuous, pathogenic, virulent, Gram-positive, and Gram-negative.

- Recognize that not all bacteria are equally capable of causing periodontal disease.

- Define the term biofilm and explain the advantages to a bacterium of living in a biofilm.

- Name three everyday examples of biofilms in the environment.

- Name the three bacteria designated by The World Workshop in Periodontology as periodontal pathogens.

- Identify bacteria associated with health, gingival diseases, and periodontitis.

- Describe how the numbers of bacteria vary from health to disease in the periodontium.

- Name and describe the components of the biofilm structure.

- Given a drawing of a mature biofilm, label the following: bacterial microcolonies, fluid channels, extracellular slime layer, acquired pellicle, and tooth surface.

- Explain the significance of the extracellular slime layer to a bacterial microcolony.

- Explain the purpose of the fluid channels in a biofilm.

- Define coaggregation and explain its significance in bacterial colonization of the tooth surface.

- Explain why systemic antibiotics and antimicrobial agents are not effective in eliminating dental plaque biofilms.

- State the most effective ways to control dental plaque biofilms.

- Explain why frequent periodontal instrumentation is vital in the control of dental plaque biofilms located within periodontal pockets.

- Given a drawing of the subgingival plaque biofilm, label the zones of bacterial attachment.

- Explain to a patient how to prevent and delay the development of dental plaque biofilms.

Key Terms

Bacterium/bacteria
Innocuous
Pathogenic
Virulent
Cell membrane
Gram staining
Gram-positive bacteria
Gram-negative bacteria
Aerobic bacteria
Anaerobic bacteria
Facultative anaerobic bacteria
Biofilm
Extracellular slime layer
Nonmotile
Aggregatibacter actinomycetemcomitans
Tannerella forsythia
Porphyromonas gingivalis
Mixed infection
Transmission

Communicable
Acquired pellicle
Fimbriae
Bacteria blooms
Mushroom-shaped microcolonies
Extracellular slime layer
Fluid channels
Fluid forces
Coaggregation
Tooth-associated plaque biofilm
Tissue-associated plaque biofilm
Unattached bacteria
Virulence factors
Peptides
Exotoxin
Leukotoxin (LT)
Bacterial enzymes
Dormant bacteria

Section 1
Bacteria in the Oral Environment

One human mouth is home to more microorganisms than there are people on the planet Earth. More than 500 bacterial strains may be found in dental plaque biofilm [1]. These bacteria have evolved to survive in the environment of the tooth surface, gingival epithelium, and oral cavity. Since periodontal disease is a bacterial infection, understanding the role of bacteria in the initiation and progression of periodontal disease is critical to a dental hygienist's ability to prevent and treat periodontal diseases.

CHARACTERISTICS OF BACTERIA

1. **Characteristics of Bacteria**
   A. **Description**
      1. Bacterium (plural, bacteria). Bacteria are the simplest organisms and can be seen only through a microscope (FIG. 6-1).
      2. There are thousands of kinds of bacteria, most of which are harmless to humans.
         a. Innocuous—species of bacteria that are not harmful.
         b. Pathogenic—species of bacteria that are capable of causing disease. Another term for pathogenic bacteria is virulent bacteria. In the oral cavity, innocuous and pathogenic bacteria live together in a symbiotic relationship.
      3. Bacteria have existed on earth for longer than any other organisms and are still the most abundant type of cell.
      4. Bacteria can replicate quickly. This ability to divide quickly enables populations of bacteria to adapt rapidly to changes in their environment.
   B. **Structure of the Bacterial Cell Membrane.** A tough protective layer called a cell membrane encloses nearly all bacteria.
      1. The composition of the cell membrane is an important characteristic used in identifying and classifying bacteria.
      2. Gram staining is a laboratory method that reveals differences in the chemical and physical properties of bacterial cell membranes.
      3. Depending on their permeability, the bacterial cell membranes appear either purple or red in color under a microscope.
      4. Gram staining divides bacteria into Gram-positive (purple color) and Gram-negative (red color) bacterial cell membrane types (FIG. 6-1).
         a. Gram-positive bacteria (purple stain)
            1) Have a single, thick cell membrane
            2) Most of the bacteria associated with a healthy periodontium are Gram-positive
            3) Retain a purple color when stained with a dye known as crystal violet and so the bacterial cell membranes show a purple stain under the microscope
         b. Gram-negative bacteria (red stain)
            1) Have double cell membranes
            2) *Believed to play an important role in the tissue destruction seen in periodontitis*
            3) Do not stain purple with crystal violet and therefore, show a red stain under the microscope
            4) To remember that the membranes of Gram-negative bacteria stain red, it might be helpful to think "red = inflammation" (as these bacteria are believed to play an important role in inflammatory periodontitis)

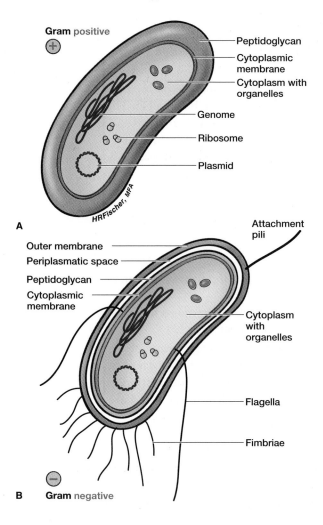

Gram positive
⊕

- Peptidoglycan
- Cytoplasmic membrane
- Cytoplasm with organelles
- Genome
- Ribosome
- Plasmid

HRFischer, MFA

A

Attachment pili

Outer membrane
Periplasmatic space
Peptidoglycan
Cytoplasmic membrane

Cytoplasm with organelles

Flagella

Fimbriae

⊖
B **Gram** negative

Figure 6.1. Structures of Gram-Positive and Gram-Negative Bacterial Cell Membranes. A: Gram-positive bacteria have a single cell membrane that retains a purple color when stained with crystal violet dye. **B:** Gram-negative bacteria have double cell membranes and show a red stain with the Gram staining technique. Gram-negative bacteria are believed to play an important role in periodontal disease.

2. **Where Bacteria Live.** Bacteria live almost everywhere, even in environments where other life forms cannot survive. Bacteria are always present on the skin and in the digestive and respiratory systems of humans.
   A. **Response to Gaseous Oxygen (O_2).** Most bacteria may be placed into one of three groups based on their response to O_2.
      1. Aerobic bacteria—require oxygen to live.
      2. Anaerobic bacteria—cannot live in the presence of oxygen.
      3. Facultative anaerobic bacteria—can exist either with or without oxygen.
   B. **Bacterial Lifestyles**
      1. Free-floating bacteria
         a. Bacteria may be free-floating. These free-floating bacteria are also known as planktonic bacteria.
         b. Until recently, most research done on bacteria was conducted on free-floating bacteria.
      2. Attached bacteria
         a. Bacteria can attach to surfaces and to one another. *Communities of bacteria that attach to each other and to a surface are described as living in a biofilm.*
         b. Once a bacterium attaches to a surface, it activates a whole different set of genes that give the bacterium different characteristics from those that it had as a free-floating organism.
         c. It has been estimated that more than 99% of all bacteria on earth live as attached bacteria.

BIOFILMS: BACTERIAL COMMUNITIES

Until recently, bacteria were studied as they grew on culture plates in a laboratory. Recent advances in research technology have allowed researchers to study bacteria in their natural environment. These studies have revealed that most bacteria live in complex communities called biofilms and that biofilms are found everywhere in nature.

In the oral cavity, dental plaque is a biofilm that adheres tenaciously to tooth surfaces, restorations, and prosthetic appliances. The dental plaque biofilm has the same complex structure as biofilms found elsewhere in nature: bacterial microcolonies, extracellular slime layer, and fluid channels.

1. **Biofilms and Where They Form**
    A. **Description**
        1. A biofilm is a living film—containing a well-organized community of bacteria—that grows on a surface.
        2. Usually, biofilms consist of many species of bacteria as well as other organisms and debris.
        3. Biofilms form rapidly on almost any surface that is wet.
    B. **Biofilm Environments**
        1. Biofilms are everywhere in nature (FIG. 6-2). "Biofilm" may seem like a new term, but everyone encounters biofilms on a regular basis. The plaque biofilm that forms on teeth (FIG. 6-3), the slime in fish tanks, and the slime deposit that clogs the sink drain are all examples of biofilms. The slimy rocks in a stream are biofilm-coated.
        2. *Biofilms can exist on any solid surface that is exposed to a bacteria-containing fluid.*
            a. Biofilms can be found on medical and dental implants, indwelling intravenous and urinary catheters, contact lenses, and prosthetic devices such as heart valves, biliary stents, pacemakers, and artificial joints.
            b. Legionnaires disease, which killed 29 people in 1976, was the result of a bacterial biofilm in the hotel's air conditioning system.

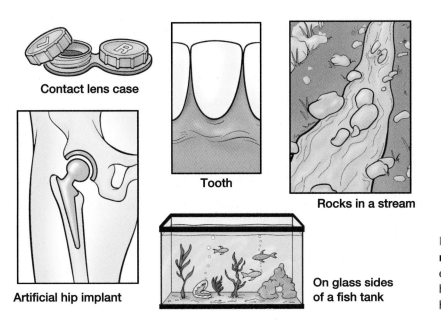

Contact lens case

Tooth

Rocks in a stream

Artificial hip implant

On glass sides of a fish tank

Figure 6.2. **Biofilm Environments.** Biofilms are found nearly everywhere in nature. They have a major impact on human health.

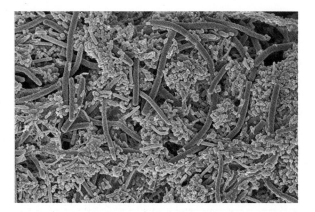

Figure 6.3. Dental Plaque Biofilm. Scanning electron micrograph (SEM) of dental plaque biofilm showing bacteria (red and yellow) and extracellular matrix (orange). (Courtesy of Getty Images.)

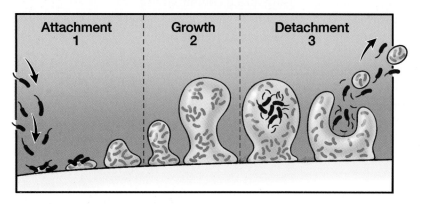

Figure 6.4. Biofilm Life Cycle. The three major stages in the life cycle of a biofilm: attachment, growth, and detachment in clumps.

    c. By some estimates 65% of all diseases maybe biofilm-induced. Biofilm-induced diseases include tuberculosis, cystic fibrosis, subacute bacterial endocarditis, and periodontal disease.

    3. Biofilms thrive in dental unit water and suction lines and have been shown to be the primary source of contaminated water delivered by dental units. Stagnant fluid flow allows free-floating bacteria to attach to the tubing walls in the dental unit and form intricate biofilms.

2. Life Cycle of a Biofilm. The biofilm life cycle has three stages: attachment, growth, and detachment (FIG. 6-4).

  A. Attachment. Bacteria attach to a surface.

  B. Growth

    1. The attached bacteria begin releasing substances that attract other free-floating bacteria to join the biofilm community (FIG. 6-8).

    2. The attached bacteria secrete a film known as the extracellular slime layer. This slimy film helps to keep the bacteria attached to the surface and acts as a protective shield for the bacteria.

    3. The bacteria multiply rapidly and grow away from the surface to form three-dimensional mushroom-shaped mature biofilms that attach to a surface at a narrow base.

    4. Movement of the fluid surrounding the mature biofilms results in extensions that stream from the main body of the biofilm.

  C. Detachment

    1. Clumps of the main biofilm break off and are carried away by the fluid surrounding the biofilm.

    2. These detached clumps can attach to other portions of a surface and form new bacterial colonies.

Section 2
Bacteria Associated with Periodontal Health and Disease

SPECIES CAPABLE OF COLONIZING THE MOUTH

Approximately 700 different species and subspecies are capable of colonizing the mouth. Figure 6-5 lists some of the cultivable species.

	Gram positive ⊕		Gram negative ⊖	
	Facultative anaerobes	**Obligate anaerobes**	**Facultative anaerobes**	**Obligate anaerobes**
Cocci 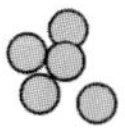	**Streptococcus** –*S. anginosus* (*S. milleri*) –*S. mutans* –*S. sanguis* • Ss –*S. oralis* –*S. mitis* –*S. intermedius*	**Peptostreptococcus** –*P. micros* • Pm **Peptococcus**	**Neisseria** **Branhamella**	**Veillonella** –*V. parvula*
Rods 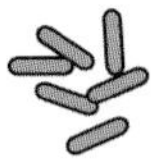	**Actinomyces** –*A. naeslundii* • An –*A. viscosus* • Av –*A. odontolyticus* –*A. israelii* **Propionibacterium** **Rothia** –*R. dentocariosa* **Lactobacillus** –*L. oris* –*L. acidophilus* –*L. salivarius* –*L. buccalis*	**Eubacterium** –*E. nodatum* • En –*E. saburreum* –*E. timidum* –*E. brachy* –*E. alactolyticum* **Bifidobacterium** –*B. dentium*	**Aggregatibacter** –*A. actinomycetem-comitans* • Aa **Capnocytophaga** –*C. ochracea* –*C. gingivalis* –*C. sputigena* **Campylobacter** –*C. rectus* • Cr –*C. curvus* –*C. showae* **Eikenella** –*E. corrodens* • Ec **Haemophilus** –*H. aphrophilus* –*H. segnis*	**Porphyromonas** –*P. gingivalis* • Pg –*P. endodontalis* **Prevotella** –*P. intermedia* • Pi –*P. nigrescens* –*P. denticola* –*P. loescheii* –*P. oris* –*P. oralis* **Tannerella** –*T. forsythia* • Tf **Fusobacterium** –*F. nucleatum* • Fn –*F. periodonticum* **Selenemonas** –*S. sputigena* –*S. noxia*
Spirochetes and mycoplasms 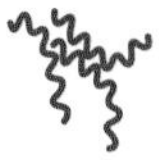	**Mycoplasm** –*M. orale* –*M. salivarium* –*M. hominis*		**Spirochetes of ANUG** **Treponema sp.** –*T. denticola* • Td –*T. socranskii* –*T. pectinovorum* –*T. vincentii*	
Eukaryotes	**Candida** –*C. albicans*	**Entamoeba**		**Trichomonas**

Figure 6.5. **Microorganisms Capable of Colonizing the Mouth.**

MICROORGANISMS ASSOCIATED WITH SPECIFIC PERIODONTAL STATES

Research studies clearly demonstrate that different bacterial groups are associated with periodontal health versus periodontal disease.

1. **Bacteria Associated with Health**
   A. In health, the number of bacteria that can be cultured from an individual healthy sulci is between 100 and 1,000 bacteria [1,2].
   B. About 75% of the bacteria found in periodontally healthy sites are Gram-positive facultative rods and cocci (FIG. 6-6). Gram-negative rods comprise about 13% of the bacteria found in healthy sites [3].
   C. Most of the bacteria in a healthy site are nonmotile—not capable of movement.
   D. The bacteria found in periodontal diseases are found in healthy sulci, but they make up a small proportion of the total bacteria in the site.

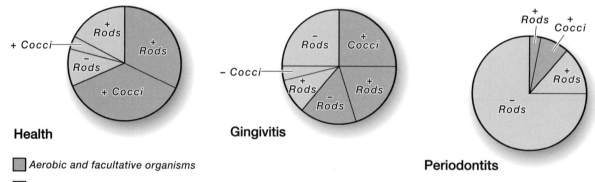

Figure 6.6. Proportions of Bacteria in Health Versus Disease. The relative proportions of facultative and anaerobic organisms found in subgingival samples in cases of periodontal health, gingivitis, and periodontitis.

2. **Bacteria Associated with Gingivitis**
   A. In gingivitis, the number of bacteria that can be cultured from an individual site ranges from 1,000 to 100,000 bacteria [2].
   B. *The bacteria found in chronic gingivitis consist of almost equal proportions of Gram-positive and Gram-negative bacteria.* Gram-negative rods comprise about 40% of the bacteria found in gingivitis (FIG. 6-6).
3. **Bacteria Associated with Periodontitis**
   A. Periodontitis is associated with an enormous number of Gram-negative bacteria.
      1. In periodontitis, the number of bacteria that can be cultured *from an individual tooth surface* ranges from 100,000 to 100,000,000 bacteria [2].
      2. Researchers have estimated the potential biofilm load in a patient with 28 teeth and generalized periodontitis. If the patient has 28 teeth and one considers the tooth roots to be circular with an average of 5 mm of biofilm on each tooth, the total mouth biofilm would cover an area about the size of the palm of an adult human hand [4].
      3. Gram-negative rods comprise about 74% of the bacteria associated with periodontitis (FIG. 6-6). *Chronic periodontitis is associated with high proportions of Gram-negative and motile bacteria.*
   B. The bacterial composition of periodontitis differs significantly from patient to patient and from site to site within the same mouth.

TABLE 6-1. Bacteria Strongly Associated with Chronic Periodontitis	
Bacteria	**Gram Stain/Motility**
Aggregatibacter actinomycetemcomitans	Gram-negative, nonmotile
Streptococcus intermedius	Gram-positive, nonmotile
Campylobacter rectus	Gram-negative, motile
Eubacterium nodatum	Gram-positive, nonmotile
Fusobacterium nucleatum	Gram-negative, nonmotile
Fusobacterium nucleatum, subspecies *polymorphum*	Gram-negative, nonmotile
Prevotella intermedia	Gram-negative, nonmotile
Peptostreptococcus micros	Gram-positive, nonmotile
Prevotella nigrescens	Gram-negative, nonmotile
Porphyromonas gingivalis	Gram-negative, nonmotile
Tannerella forsythia	Gram-negative, nonmotile
Treponema denticola	Not applicable, motile

Data from Socransky SS, Haffajee AD. Dental biofilms: difficult therapeutic targets. *Periodontol 2000*. 2002;28:12–55.

CURRENT SUSPECTED PERIODONTAL PATHOGENS

1. **Introduction to Periodontal Pathogens**
   A. Although more than 500 bacterial species have been isolated from periodontal pockets, it is likely that only a small percentage of these bacteria are periodontal pathogens.
   B. Several microorganisms have been strongly associated with chronic periodontitis [5]. Refer to TABLE 6-1 for a list of suspected periodontal pathogens. Future research will likely identify additional periodontal pathogens.
   C. In the future, dental healthcare providers may have diagnostic tests and treatments specifically directed at these periodontal pathogens.
2. **Periodontal Pathogens.** The World Workshop in Periodontology (Consensus Report, 1996) designated *A. actinomycetemcomitans*, *P. gingivalis*, and *T. forsythia* as periodontal pathogens (TABLE 6-2) [6].
   A. *Aggregatibacter actinomycetemcomitans*
      1. This species recently was renamed *Aggregatibacter actinomycetemcomitans* from its former name of *Actinobacillus actinomycetemcomitans* [7].
      2. This microorganism has been strongly associated with aggressive periodontitis [8–10].
      3. *Aggregatibacter actinomycetemcomitans* has also been implicated in chronic periodontitis cases, but less frequently and in lower numbers than from lesions in aggressive periodontitis [11,12].
      4. *Aggregatibacter actinomycetemcomitans is* capable of evading normal host immune response and of destroying gingival connective tissue and bone (FIG. 6-7).
   B. *Tannerella forsythia*
      1. This species was renamed *T. forsythia* from it former name *Bacteroides forsythus* [13].
      2. *The role of T. forsythia* in periodontal diseases has been clarified by numerous studies involving DNA probes or immunologic methods.

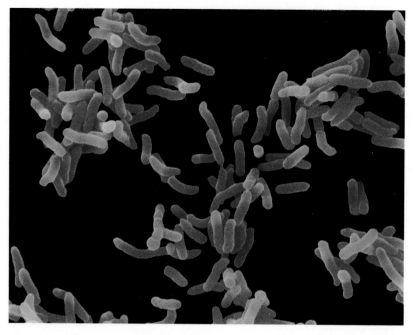

Figure 6.7. *Aggregatibacter actinomycetemcomitans.* A three dimensional image of *A. actinomycetemcomitans* taken with a scanning electron microscope (SEM). (Used with permission from Dennis Kunkel Microscopy, Inc.)

    3. Researcher S.G. Grossi and colleagues consider *T. forsythia* to be the most significant microbial risk factor that distinguishes subjects with periodontitis from those who are periodontally healthy [14,15].

    4. *T. forsythia* is the most common species detected on or in the epithelial cells recovered from periodontal pockets [16].

    5. The risk of periodontal attachment loss is higher in adolescents who are colonized by *T. forsythia* than in those in whom the species is not detected [17].

C. *Porphyromonas gingivalis*

    1. *P. gingivalis* can be found in low numbers in health or gingivitis but is more frequently detected in aggressive forms of periodontitis [18,19].

    2. The species is found in increased numbers in subjects exhibiting periodontal disease progression (worsening destruction of periodontium) [20].

    3. *P. gingivalis* commonly is seen in sites that exhibited recurrence of disease or persistence of deep periodontal pockets after periodontal therapy [20].

    4. *P. gingivalis* can inhibit migration of leukocytes across an epithelial barrier [21].

    5. The species has been shown to induce an elevated host response in subjects with various forms of periodontitis [22].

D. Periodontal Diseases are Mixed Infections

    1. *A. actinomycetemcomitans*, *P. gingivalis*, and *T. forsythia* have been extensively studied and strongly implicated etiologic risk factors for periodontitis. All periodontal infections, however, are associated with—caused by—multiple bacteria.

    2. Periodontal disease is a mixed infection. For this reason, if might be helpful to think of a bacterial soup of different bacteria within the plaque biofilm [2].

E. Transmission of Periodontal Pathogens

    1. Molecular epidemiology techniques that isolate DNA provide evidence that periodontal pathogens are transmissible. Transmission is the transfer of periodontal pathogens from the oral cavity of one person to another.

2. Transmission should not be confused with contagion. There is little or no evidence that periodontal infections are communicable. The term communicable refers to a disease that may be passed from one person to another by direct or indirect contact via substances such as inanimate objects.
3. Studies demonstrate that *A. actinomycetemcomitans* and *P. gingivalis* strains isolated from parents and children within the same family exhibited identical restriction endonuclease DNA fragment patterns [12,23–25].
4. Kissing is the primary means by which saliva and its bacterial contents are transmitted [25–27]. This means that the common contact of saliva in families puts children and couples at risk for contracting periodontal disease from another family member.

TABLE 6-2. Pronunciation Guide to Bacterial Tongue Twisters

Name	Pronunciation Guide
Aggregatibacter	ag-gre-gat-eee-bac-ter
actinomycetemcomitans	act-tin-oh-my-see-tem-comb-ah-tans
Tannerella	tann-er-ella
forsythia	fawr-sith-ee-uh
Fusobacterium	fuse-so-back-tier-EEE-um
nucleatum	nu-klee-ah-tum
Porphyromonas	pour-fy-roh-mo-nas
gingivalis	ging-jih-val-lis

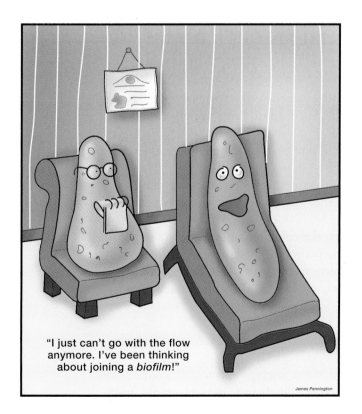

"I just can't go with the flow anymore. I've been thinking about joining a *biofilm*!"

James Pennington

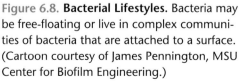

Figure 6.8. **Bacterial Lifestyles.** Bacteria may be free-floating or live in complex communities of bacteria that are attached to a surface. (Cartoon courtesy of James Pennington, MSU Center for Biofilm Engineering.)

Section 3
The Structure and Colonization of Plaque Biofilms

The pattern of dental plaque biofilm development can be divided into five phases:
(1) formation of acquired pellicle, (2) attachment of early bacterial colonizers,
(3) coaggregation of additional bacterial colonizers, and (4) formation of an
extracellular slime layer and microcolony formation. Phase 5 is a mature biofilm characterized by the bacterial microcolonies that form complex groups with
a primitive communication system and fluid channels (FIG. 6-9).

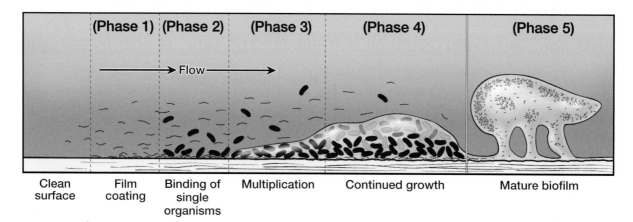

Figure 6.9. **Five Phases in the Formation of a Biofilm.** Phase 1, the acquired pellicle coats the tooth surface.
Phase 2, initial colonizers attach to the tooth surface. Additional bacteria coaggregate with the initial colonizers in
Phase 3. Phase 4 is signaled by the formation of the extracellular slime layer. Phase 5 is a mature biofilm.

THE COMPLEX STRUCTURE OF DENTAL PLAQUE BIOFILMS

1. Pattern of Plaque Biofilm Development
    A. Phase 1—Film Coating
        1. Within minutes after cleaning the tooth surface, a film forms over the tooth
           surface. This film, the acquired pellicle, is composed of a variety of salivary
           glycoproteins (mucins) and antibodies.
            a. The purpose of the acquired pellicle is to protect the enamel from acidic
               activity.
            b. Unfortunately, in addition to providing protection from acids, the
               acquired pellicle also alters the charge and energy of the tooth surface,
               facilitating bacterial adhesion.
            c. A helpful analogy in understanding the role of acquired pellicle in plaque
               biofilm formation is to think of the pellicle as "double-sided adhesive
               tape." The double-sided tape adheres to the tooth surface on one side and
               provides a sticky surface on the other side that facilitates attachment by
               bacteria to the tooth surface.
    B. Phase 2—Initial Attachment of Bacteria to Pellicle
        1. Within a few hours after pellicle formation, bacteria begin to attach to the
           outer surface of the pellicle.
        2. Some bacteria possess attachment structures, such as extracellular substances,
           and hundreds of hairlike structures that enable them to attach rapidly upon
           contact with the tooth surface. The hairlike structures are termed fimbriae.

C. **Phase 3—New Bacteria Join In.** Once bacteria stick to the tooth, they begin producing substances that stimulate other free-floating bacteria to join the community.

D. **Phase 4—Extracellular Slime Layer and Microcolony Formation**
  1. Production of an extracellular slime layer.
     a. It appears that the act of attaching to the tooth surface stimulates the bacteria to excrete a slimy, gluelike substance called the extracellular slime layer.
     b. This extracellular slime layer helps to anchor bacteria to the tooth surface and provides protection for the attached bacteria.
  2. Microcolony formation
     a. Once the surface of the tooth has been covered with attached bacteria, the biofilm grows primarily through cell division of the adherent bacteria (rather than through the attachment of new bacteria).
     b. Next, the proliferating bacteria begin to grow away from the tooth.
     c. Bacterial blooms are periods when specific species or groups of species grow at rapidly accelerated rates.

E. **Phase 5—Mature Biofilm: Mushroom-Shaped Microcolonies**
  1. The bacteria cluster together to form mushroom-shaped microcolonies that are attached to the tooth surface at a narrow base.
  2. The result is the formation of complex collections of different bacteria linked to one another.

2. **The Complex Structure of Mature Dental Plaque Biofilms**
  A. **Bacterial Microcolonies**
     1. The bacteria in a biofilm are not distributed evenly. As the bacteria attach to a surface and to each other, they cluster together to form mushroom-shaped microcolonies that are attached to the tooth surface at a narrow base (FIG. 6-10).
     2. Each microcolony is a tiny independent community containing thousands of compatible bacteria. Different microcolonies may contain different combinations of bacterial species.

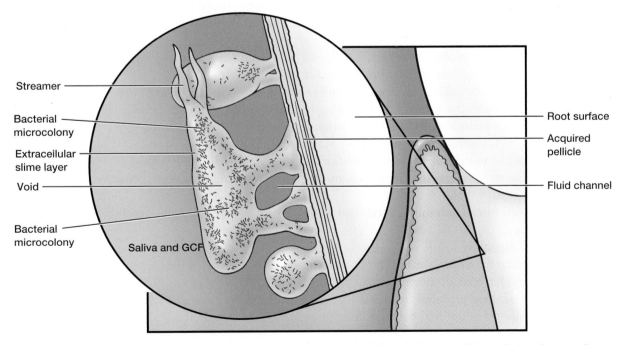

Figure 6.10. Structure of Plaque Biofilm. The complex structure of dental plaque biofilm includes clusters of bacterial microcolonies, streamers, and fluid channels. GCF, gingival crevicular fluid

    a. Environmental conditions within each microcolony of bacteria vary radically. The environmental conditions among several microcolonies may include differences in oxygen concentration, pH, and temperature.

    b. The differing environmental conditions within a biofilm mean that the bacterial population is very diverse—with each different bacterial species preferring a certain environment within the biofilm.

        1) This bacterial diversity helps to ensure the survivability of the plaque biofilm in widely varying oral conditions.

        2) If the plaque biofilm had only one species of bacteria, it would be much more likely that a toxic agent or condition would destroy the biofilm.

B. Extracellular Slime Layer

    1. The extracellular slime layer is a dense protective barrier that surrounds the bacterial microcolonies (FIG. 6-10).

    2. *The slime layer acts like a shield protecting the bacterial microcolonies from antibiotics, antimicrobials, and the body's immune system.*

C. Fluid Forces

    1. The fluid forces of the saliva surrounding the biofilm influence the shape of the plaque biofilm, as well as the spatial arrangement of the bacteria inside.

    2. These fluid forces result in the development of extensions from the main body of the biofilm. These biofilm extensions can break free and be swallowed, expectorated, or form new biofilm colonies in other areas of the mouth.

    3. Fluid forces also result in cell-to-cell collisions of the bacteria within the biofilm.

        a. Bacterial cell collisions lead to a more rapid spread of genes among the bacteria than there would be if there were no fluid forces acting on the biofilm.

        b. This rapid transfer of genes from bacterial cell to bacterial cell may result in enhanced bacterial virulence and antimicrobial resistance.

        c. *The continuous exchange of genetic information among bacteria means that the bacteria are constantly evolving.* This makes the bacterial biofilm very difficult to eradicate and helps to ensure the survivability of the biofilm.

D. Fluid Channels

    1. As the plaque biofilm develops, a series of fluid channels are formed that penetrate the extracellular slime layer (FIG. 6-10).

    2. These fluid channels direct fluids in and around the biofilm, bringing nutrients and oxygen to the bacteria and carrying bacterial waste products away.

    3. The fluids include everything from saliva to any beverages consumed.

E. Cell-to-Cell Communication System

    1. Direct cell-to-cell interaction occurs among the bacteria in the biofilm.

    2. The bacterial microcolonies use chemical signals to communicate with each other (FIG. 6-11).

    3. This cell-to-cell communication also results in the transfer of genes among bacteria.

F. Bacterial Signaling

    1. The bacteria within the biofilm produce hundreds of proteins that free-floating bacteria do not.

    2. Some of these proteins are signaling proteins that trigger events such as adhesion of additional bacteria and formation of the extracellular slime layer that surrounds the bacteria.

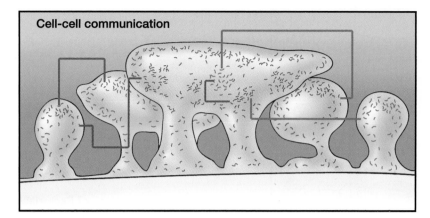

Figure 6.11. Cell-to-Cell Communication. Bacterial microcolonies use chemical signals to communicate with other microcolonies.

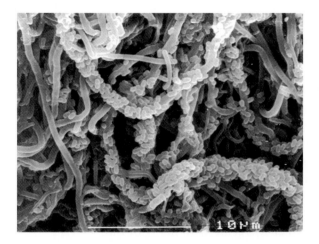

Figure 6.12. Bacterial Coaggregation. One example of coaggregation of bacteria has a corncob appearance that is created when a central rod-shaped bacterium becomes surrounded by many round cocci. (Courtesy of Ziedonis Skobe, PhD, Head, Biostructure Core Facility, The Forsyth Institute.)

BACTERIAL COLONIZATION AND SUCCESSION

1. Bacterial Colonization of the Tooth Surface
   A. **Layers and Layers of Bacteria.** The biofilm develops by stacking one bacterial species on top of another bacterial species. A mature dental biofilm does not consist of only one species of bacteria.
   B. **Coaggregation of Bacteria**
      1. *Coaggregation* is the cell-to-cell adherence of one oral bacterium to another (FIG. 6-12).
      2. *Coaggregation is not random; rather, each bacterial strain only has a limited set of bacteria to which they are able to adhere.*
      3. The ability to adhere and coaggregate is an important determinant in the development of the bacterial biofilm.
2. Sequence of Colonization
   A. **Early Bacterial Colonizers: Important to Bacterial Succession**
      1. The first bacteria to colonize the tooth surface are nonpathogenic (FIG. 6-13). The ability of these species to attach to the tooth surface lays the foundation for the growth of dental plaque biofilm (Box 6-1).

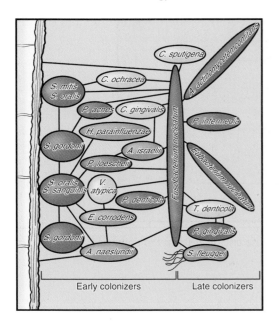

Figure 6.13. Coaggregation of Bacteria: Initial and Late Bacterial Colonizers. Early colonizers adhere to the acquired pellicle coating. Intermediate colonizers coaggregate with the early colonizers. The intermediate species coaggregate with the last colonizers including many periodontal pathogens. (Data from Kolenbrander PE, et al. Communication among oral bacteria. *Microbiol Mol Biol Rev.* 2002;66(3):486–505.)

a. Periodontal pathogens are unable to colonize the biofilm until the nonpathogenic species are attached to the tooth surface.

b. Periodontal pathogens remain freely floating in the oral cavity until signals from the early colonizers indicate that the conditions are favorable for the pathogenic species to join the biofilm.

2. Early bacterial colonizers of the tooth surface include many streptococcal species, such as *Streptococcus mitis* and *Streptococcus oralis* that have the ability to attach to the tooth pellicle, as well as, to each other [28,29]. Another early colonizer is *Actinomyces viscosus*.

3. The early bacterial colonizers release chemical signals that indicate to the next group of bacteria that conditions are favorable for them to join the biofilm.

4. The early streptococcal colonizers are able to coaggregate with many of the other early colonizing bacteria and intermediate species (FIG. 6-13). Many early and intermediate colonizing species are unable to attach to the tooth pellicle but have the ability to coaggregate with the streptococcal species.

5. Free-floating bacteria cannot join the biofilm until the conditions are favorable. The succession of bacteria joining the biofilm is comparable to elementary school students who are asked to line up in alphabetical order as their teacher calls out their names. Students whose last names start with the letter "O" cannot get in line until all the students whose last names start with "M and N" have taken their place in line.

B. **Intermediate and Late Colonizers**

1. As is the case with the early bacterial colonizers, the intermediate and late colonizers must join the biofilm in the proper sequence.

2. The intermediate species, such as *Fusobacterium nucleatum,* in turn coaggregate with the last colonizers. Many of the periodontal pathogens are late biofilm colonizers.

3. **Stages of Bacterial Colonization**

A. **Primary Colonization**

1. Within a short time after cleaning, Gram-positive cocci adhere and penetrate into the acquired pellicle film (FIG. 6-14A).

2. After 24 hours, plaque biofilm collected from the tooth surface consists mainly of streptococci with *Streptococcus sanguis* being the most dominant.

B. **Intermediate Coaggregation**
   1. In this stage, Gram-positive cocci and rods coaggregate and multiply.
   2. Gram-positive rods multiply and eventually outnumber the cocci.
C. **Gram-negative Organisms**
   1. Gram-negative bacteria, which have a poor ability to adhere to the tooth, coaggregate with Gram-positive cocci and rods.
   2. *F. nucleatum, Prevotella intermedia,* and other anaerobic Gram-negative bacteria adhere in this manner.
D. **Diverse Array of Gram-Negative Organisms**
   1. The numbers and diversity of the plaque biofilm increase and include large numbers of Gram-negative organisms.
   2. *P. gingivalis* and *Capnocytophaga gingivalis,* as well as large numbers of other Gram-negative organisms, thrive in the protective environment of the biofilm (Fig. 6-14D).
   3. A mature plaque biofilm is a very complex collection of multiple bacterial species. *The pathogenicity—disease-causing potential—of the bacteria combined in a biofilm is much greater than that of an individual pathogenic species.*

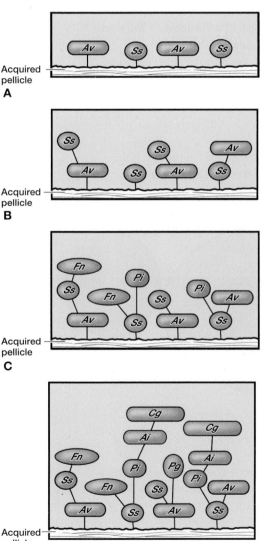

Figure 6.14. **Stages of Bacterial Colonization of the Tooth Surface.** A: Colonization of acquired pellicle. Early Gram-positive bacterial colonizers include *Actinomyces viscosus* (Av) and *Streptococcus sanguis* (Ss). *S. sanguis* is the most dominant. B: Intermediate coaggregation. Once an initial group of bacteria adhere to the pellicle, the bacteria begin to multiply. C: Coaggregation of Gram-negative organisms. Gram-negative bacteria join the biofilm, such as *Fusobacterium nucleatum* (Fn) and *Prevotella intermedia* (Pi). D: Diverse array of Gram-negative organisms. As the biofilm matures more Gram-negative anaerobic bacteria colonize the biofilm including *P. gingivalis* (Pg) and *Capnocytophaga gingivalis* (Cg). *Actinomyces israelii* (Ai) is a Gram-positive organism.

MICROBIAL COMPLEXES AND ATTACHMENT ZONES

1. **Microbial Complexes**
    A. **Internal Organization**
        1. The internal structure of plaque biofilm has been examined in a number of studies by light and electron microscopy [30–34].
        2. The organization of bacteria within biofilms is not random; rather there are specific associations among bacterial species [35]. The bacteria within a biofilm no longer work as single entities, but rather, act as a functioning system of interdependent parts.
    B. **Socransky's Microbial Complexes**
        1. Socransky grouped microorganisms into complexes and assigned each complex a color (FIG. 6-15) [35].
            a. The scheme for assigning colors to the microbial complexes is somewhat like the use of color designations for the Homeland Security Terror-Alert Status in the United States. In the terror-alert chart, the green color designates a low risk while the red color indicates a severe risk of terrorist attacks.
            b. Socransky assigned colors to each microbial complex based on the association with health or disease.
        2. The blue, purple, yellow and green complexes are early colonizers of the tooth surface and are thought to be compatible with gingival health.
        3. *The orange and red complexes are comprised of the species thought to be the major etiologic agents of periodontal disease.* The orange and red complexes become more dominant in the late stages of plaque biofilm development.

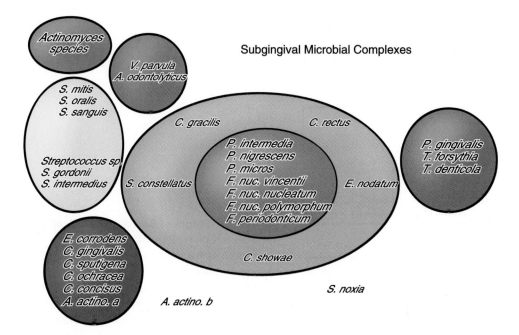

Figure 6.15. Socransky's Microbial Complexes. Bacteria in the plaque biofilm are organized in different complexes. Complexes on the left side of the diagram, green and yellow especially, are thought to be compatible with gingival health. The red and orange complexes are thought to be the most influential in causing periodontitis. The red complex is comprised of periodontal pathogens that are strongly associated with periodontitis. (Data from Socransky SS, et al. Microbial complexes in subgingival plaque. *J Clin Periodontol.* 1998;25(2):134–144.)

Box 6.1 The Importance of Early Colonizers in Biofilm Succession

1. Free-floating periodontal pathogens cannot cause periodontal disease.
2. Periodontal pathogens cannot colonize the biofilm until the nonpathogenic, early colonizers attach to the tooth surface.
3. If the biofilm is adequately disrupted by daily self-care and routine professional care, the biofilm will always be reforming. Every time the biofilm is disrupted, the entire process of bacterial succession starts over, beginning with the early colonizers.

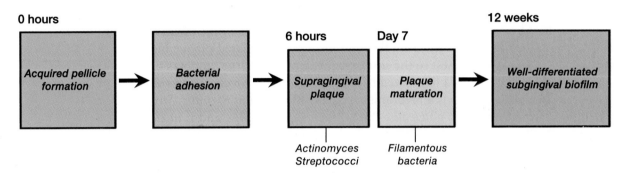

Figure 6.16. Sequence of Bacterial Attachment. Dental plaque biofilm development always begins supragingivally and progresses subgingivally.

2. **The Importance of Bacterial Attachment**
   A. **Free-Floating Pathogens Cannot Cause Periodontal Disease**
      1. Bacteria must be attached to a surface in order to cause periodontal disease.
      2. Free-floating bacteria—no matter how pathogenic—cannot cause periodontal disease.
      3. Bacteria attach to the tooth surface, pocket epithelium, or other bacteria that are attached to one of these surfaces.
      4. The most pathogenic bacteria attach to the pocket epithelium.
   B. **Sequence of Bacterial Attachment**
      1. Within minutes after cleaning the tooth surface, a film forms over the tooth surface.
      2. Within hours after pellicle formation, early colonizers begin to attach to the outer surface of the pellicle on the crown of the tooth (FIG. 6-16). Once bacteria attach to the tooth, they begin producing substances that stimulate other free-floating bacteria to join the community.
      3. Once the surface of the tooth has been covered, the proliferating bacteria begin to grow away from the tooth, forming a mature *supra*gingival biofilm. Biofilm development always begins *supra*gingivally (FIG. 6-16).
      4. Between 3 and 12 weeks after *supra*gingival plaque biofilm starts to form, the *sub*gingival biofilm is mature with predominantly Gram-negative anaerobic bacteria.

C. Bacterial Attachment Zones. The zones of *sub*gingival bacterial attachment (FIG. 6-17) are the tooth surface and the epithelial lining of the periodontal pocket. Bacteria also may attach to other bacteria that are attached to one of these surfaces.

1. Tooth-associated plaque biofilm—bacteria that are attached to the tooth surface.
   a. Bacteria attach to an area of the tooth surface that extends from the gingival margin almost to the junctional epithelium at the base of the pocket.
   b. Subgingival bacteria appear to have the ability to invade the dentinal tubules of the cementum.
   c. Filamentous microorganisms, cocci, and rods—including *S. mitis*, *S. sanguis*, and *A. viscosus*—dominate the tooth-associated plaque.

2. Tissue-associated plaque biofilm—bacteria that adhere to the epithelium.
   a. The bacteria that adhere loosely to the epithelium of the pocket wall are distinctly different from those of the tooth-associated plaque biofilm.
   b. The layers closest to the soft tissue wall contain large numbers of spirochetes and flagellated bacteria. Gram-negative cocci and rods also are present. There is a predominance of species such as *S. oralis, Streptococcus intermedius, P. gingivalis, P. intermedia, T. forsythia,* and *F. nucleatum.*
   c. Bacteria from the tissue-attached plaque biofilm can invade the gingival connective tissue and be found within the periodontal connective tissues and on the surface of the alveolar bone.
   d. *Research suggests that tissue-associated plaque biofilm is the most detrimental to the periodontal tissues.*

3. Unattached bacteria. In addition to the attached bacteria, the periodontal pocket also contains many free-floating bacteria that are not part of the biofilm.

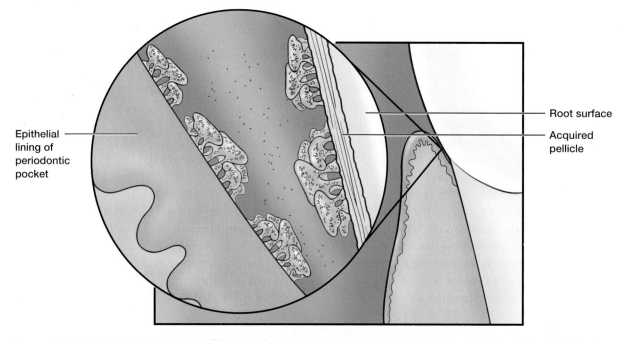

Epithelial lining of periodontic pocket

Root surface

Acquired pellicle

Figure 6.17. Subgingival Plaque Biofilm Attachment Zones. Within a periodontal pocket, bacteria attach to the tooth surface or the epithelial lining of the pocket.

Section 4
Mechanisms of Periodontal Destruction

1. **Host Response: The Primary Cause of Periodontal Destruction**
   A. **The Body's Inflammatory Response**
      1. Previously, investigators thought that bacteria were the primary cause of the tissue destruction seen in periodontitis. Perhaps bacterial virulence factors were inflaming the gingiva and destroying alveolar bone.
      2. *Current research shows that the body's immune response to plaque biofilm is the primary cause of the destruction seen in periodontitis.*
      3. The immune system is activated by the periodontal pathogens in the plaque biofilm.
      4. The inflammation that causes most of the damage in periodontitis is a continuous low-grade inflammation occurring 24 hours a day, month after month.
   B. **Bacteria and Host Response**
      1. Bacteria acting alone are not the cause of periodontal disease.
      2. Rather, it is the interplay between the bacteria and the host response that results in tissue destruction.

2. **Bacterial Virulence Factors: A Minor Cause of Periodontal Destruction.** The mechanisms that enable biofilm bacteria to colonize and invade the tissues of the periodontium are called virulence factors (TABLE 6-3). Virulence factors may be structural characteristics of the bacterium itself or substances produced and released into the environment by bacteria.
   A. **Bacterial Characteristics**
      1. Bacterial invasion factors
         a. Periodontal pathogens have the ability to actively penetrate the epithelium lining the pocket wall and invade the gingival connective tissue [36,37].
         b. Both Gram-positive and Gram-negative bacteria have been observed in the intercellular spaces of the gingival connective tissue and near the alveolar bone.
            1) Bacteria may invade the gingival connective tissue through ulcerations in the pocket epithelium.
            2) *A. actinomycetemcomitans, P. gingivalis, F. nucleatum,* and *Treponema denticola* have been demonstrated to directly invade host tissue cells.
            3) The ability to invade host tissue cells is believed to be a key factor that differentiates pathogenic from nonpathogenic Gram-negative bacteria [38].
            4) The presence of bacteria within the tissues makes periodontitis more resistant to treatment.
      2. Peptide proteins of bacterial cell membranes
         a. Previously, researchers thought that inflammation has something to do with lipopolysaccharide (LPS). Lipopolysaccharides make up the cell membranes of Gram-negative bacteria.
         b. Recently, researchers discovered a new class of proteins called peptides. Peptides are short chains of amino acids found in living bacterial cell membranes that control the transport of molecules in and out of the bacterial cell.
         c. T cells—a type of white blood cell—can identify the peptides on the cell membranes and lock into a peptide. Once locked into a peptide, the T cell alerts the rest of the immune system of the bacterial invasion.
         d. When a bacterium dies, the peptides unlink and become single amino acids again. There is nothing for the T cell to lock on to and the host immune response subsides.

B. **Bacterial Products**
   1. Exotoxin production
      a. Exotoxins are harmful proteins released from the bacterial cell that act on host cells at a distance.
      b. For example, *A. actinomycetemcomitans* produces leukotoxin (LT), an exotoxin that may enable these bacteria to destroy leukocytes in the sulcus or pocket.
   2. Bacterial enzyme production. Bacterial enzymes are agents that are harmful or destructive to host cells.
      a. A variety of enzymes produced by periodontal pathogens are important in tissue destruction [39,40].
      b. Enzymes function in a variety of ways to assist the bacteria in invading the tissues. Once released, bacterial enzymes have the ability to
         1) Increase permeability of the epithelial lining of the sulcus (allowing bacteria to penetrate sulcular epithelium more easily).
         2) Contribute to the breakdown of the collagen fibers in the gingival connective tissue.
         3) Promote apical migration of the junctional epithelium along the root surface.
         4) Cause widening of the intercellular spaces.
         5) Diminish the ability of immunoglobulins and other body proteins to defend the host.

TABLE 6-3. Bacterial Virulence Factors	
A. actinomycetemcomitans	Leukotoxin
	Endotoxin
	Enzymes
	Invades epithelial cells in vitro
	Invades buccal epithelial cells in vivo
P. gingivalis	Endotoxin
	Enzymes
	Bone resorption factor
	Invades epithelial cells in vitro
T. forsythia	Endotoxin
	Invades epithelial cells in vitro and in vivo

Section 5
Control of Plaque Biofilms

1. **Mechanisms of Bacterial Survival.** The biofilm provides the bacteria with an advantage that permits long-term survival within the sulcus or pocket environment. *The protective extracellular slime layer makes bacteria extremely resistant to antibiotics, antimicrobial agents, and the body's immune response.* It is likely that several mechanisms are responsible for biofilm resistance to systemic antibiotics, antimicrobial agents, and the immune system.
   A. **Resistance to Systemic Antibiotics and Antimicrobial Agents**
      1. Bacteria living in a biofilm are unusually resistant to systemic antibiotics (in dentistry, usually administered in pill form) and antimicrobials (placed locally in the oral cavity).
      2. *Antibiotic doses that kill free-floating bacteria, for example, need to be increased as much as 1,500 times to kill plaque biofilm bacteria* (and at these high doses, the antibiotic would kill the patient before the biofilm bacteria!) [41].
      3. Antimicrobial agents work best when used in conjunction with mechanical cleaning that removes or disrupts the dental plaque biofilm [42].
   B. **Protective Mechanisms of Biofilms**
      1. Extracellular slime layer
         a. The extracellular slime layer is very dense and may prevent the drugs from penetrating fully into the depth of the biofilm.
         b. The thick slime layer may protect the bacteria against leukocytes (defensive cells of the body's immune system).
         c. The dense slime layer may block substances released by leukocytes. As a result, the leukocyte substances end up causing more damage to the surrounding body tissue than to the biofilm bacteria.
      2. Enzymes. Some bacteria produce enzymes that degrade antibiotics faster than the drug can penetrate into the biofilm.
      3. Dormant Bacteria
         a. The biofilm is very thick and bacteria in the deepest layers become dormant—not dead—because they are cut off from the sources of nutrients. Dormant bacteria are in an inactive state in order to survive adverse environmental conditions.
         b. Antibiotics only work on bacteria that are active and reproducing.
         c. When the course of antibiotics is finished, the dormant inactive bacteria within the biofilm become reactivated.
2. **Physical Removal of Dental Plaque Biofilms is Essential**
   A. *Control of bacteria in dental plaque biofilms is best achieved by the physical disruption of plaque biofilm (such as brushing, flossing, and periodontal instrumentation).*
      1. The mature dental plaque biofilm is a very complex structure of bacterial microcolonies, extracellular slime layer, and fluid channels.
      2. It takes some time for the mature biofilm to form.
      3. Mechanical cleaning forces the bacteria to start over with initial attachment, initial colonization, secondary colonization and finally, to become a mature biofilm.
      4. In areas that are cleaned regularly, a mature biofilm will not be able to develop. The cleaner the tooth surface, the less complex the bacterial formation.
   B. Toothbrushes and floss cannot reach the subgingival plaque biofilm located within pockets. For this reason, frequent periodontal instrumentation of subgingival root surfaces by a dental hygienist or dentist is an essential component in the treatment of periodontitis.

Chapter Summary Statement

More than 500 bacterial strains have been identified in dental plaque biofilm. Experts agree that most forms of periodontal disease are caused by specific pathogens, particularly Gram-negative bacteria. The numbers of bacteria found at a site vary greatly in health, gingivitis, and periodontitis. Periodontitis is associated with large numbers of Gram-negative bacteria.

The recognition that dental plaque is a biofilm helps to explain why periodontal diseases have been so difficult to prevent and to treat. Periodontal pathogens within a biofilm environment behave very differently from free-floating bacteria. The protective extracellular slime matrix makes bacteria extremely resistant to systemic antibiotics, antimicrobial agents, and the body's immune system. Mechanical removal is the most effective treatment for the control of dental plaque biofilms.

Bacteria in dental plaque biofilms play a key role in the initiation and progression of periodontal disease. A bacterial infection alone, however, is insufficient to cause periodontal disease. The host response plays a critical role in the tissue destruction seen in periodontitis. Host response in periodontal disease is discussed in Chapter 9. Other contributing risk factors for periodontal disease include local oral conditions, habits, systemic disease, and genetic factors.

Section 6
Focus on Patients

Case 1

You have just completed a thorough cleaning of a tooth surface. Describe what deposits you might expect to form on the tooth surface over the next few days if the patient does absolutely no further cleaning of the tooth surface.

Case 2

Imagine that you are holding an "interview" of bacteria living in an oral biofilm. How might the bacteria respond to your question about advantages of living in a biofilm?

References

1. Kroes I, Lepp PW, Relman DA. Bacterial diversity within the human subgingival crevice. *Proc Natl Acad Sci USA*. 1999;96(25):14547–14552.

2. Darveau RP, Tanner A, Page RC. The microbial challenge in periodontitis. *Periodontol 2000*. 1997;14:12–32.

3. Roberts FA, Darveau RP. Beneficial bacteria of the periodontium. *Periodontol 2000*. 2002;30:40–50.

4. Page RC, Offenbacher S, Schroeder HE, et al. Advances in the pathogenesis of periodontitis: summary of developments, clinical implications and future directions. *Periodontol 2000*. 1997;14:216–248.

5. Socransky SS, Haffajee AD. Dental biofilms: difficult therapeutic targets. *Periodontol 2000*. 2002;28:12–55.

6. American Academy of Periodontology. *Annals of Periodontology*. Chicago: The Academy; 1996.

7. Norskov-Lauritsen N, Kilian M. Reclassification of *Actinobacillus actinomycetemcomitans*, *Haemophilus aphrophilus*, *Haemophilus paraphrophilus* and *Haemophilus segnis* as *Aggregatibacter actinomycetemcomitans* gen. nov., comb. nov., *Aggregatibacter aphrophilus* comb. nov. and *Aggregatibacter segnis* comb. nov., and emended description of *Aggregatibacter aphrophilus* to include V factor-dependent and V factor-independent isolates. *Int J Syst Evol Microbiol*. 2006;56(Pt 9):2135–2146.

8. Haffajee AD, Socransky SS, Ebersole JL, et al. Clinical, microbiological and immunological features associated with the treatment of active periodontosis lesions. *J Clin Periodontol*. 1984;11(9):600–618.

9. Haubek D, Ennibi OK, Poulsen K, et al. The highly leukotoxic JP2 clone of *Actinobacillus actinomycetemcomitans* and progression of periodontal attachment loss. *J Dent Res*. 2004;83(10):767–770.

10. Mandell RL. A longitudinal microbiological investigation of *Actinobacillus actinomycetemcomitans* and *Eikenella corrodens* in juvenile periodontitis. *Infect Immun*. 1984;45(3):778–780.

11. Rodenburg JP, van Winkelhoff AJ, Winkel EG, et al. Occurrence of *Bacteroides gingivalis*, *Bacteroides intermedius* and *Actinobacillus actinomycetemcomitans* in severe periodontitis in relation to age and treatment history. *J Clin Periodontol*. 1990;17(6):392–399.

12. Slots J, Feik D, Rams TE. *Actinobacillus actinomycetemcomitans* and *Bacteroides intermedius* in human periodontitis: age relationship and mutual association. *J Clin Periodontol*. 1990;17(9):659–662.

13. Sakamoto M, Suzuki M, Umeda M, et al. Reclassification of *Bacteroides forsythus* (Tanner et al. 1986) as *Tannerella forsythensis* corrig., gen. nov., comb. nov. *Int J Syst Evol Microbiol*. 2002;52(Pt 3):841–849.

14. Grossi SG, Genco RJ, Machtei EE, et al. Assessment of risk for periodontal disease. II. Risk indicators for alveolar bone loss. *J Periodontol*. 1995;66(1):23–29.

15. Grossi SG, Zambon JJ, Ho AW, et al. Assessment of risk for periodontal disease. I. Risk indicators for attachment loss. *J Periodontol*. 1994;65(3):260–267.

16. Dibart S, Skobe Z, Snapp KR, et al. Identification of bacterial species on or in crevicular epithelial cells from healthy and periodontally diseased patients using DNA-DNA hybridization. *Oral Microbiol Immunol*. 1998;13(1):30–35.

17. Hamlet S, Ellwood R, Cullinan M, et al. Persistent colonization with *Tannerella forsythensis* and loss of attachment in adolescents. *J Dent Res*. 2004;83(3):232–235.

18. Lau L, Sanz M, Herrera D, et al. Quantitative real-time polymerase chain reaction versus culture: a comparison between two methods for the detection and quantification of *Actinobacillus actinomycetemcomitans*, *Porphyromonas gingivalis* and *Tannerella forsythensis* in subgingival plaque samples. *J Clin Periodontol*. 2004;31(12):1061–1069.

19. Yang HW, Huang YF, Chou MY. Occurrence of *Porphyromonas gingivalis* and *Tannerella forsythensis* in periodontally diseased and healthy subjects. *J Periodontol*. 2004;75(8):1077–1083.

20. Bragd L, Dahlen G, Wikstrom M, et al. The capability of *Actinobacillus actinomycetemcomitans*, *Bacteroides gingivalis* and *Bacteroides intermedius* to indicate progressive periodontitis; a retrospective study. *J Clin Periodontol*. 1987;14(2):95–99.

21. Madianos PN, Papapanou PN, Sandros J. *Porphyromonas gingivalis* infection of oral epithelium inhibits neutrophil transepithelial migration. *Infect Immun*. 1997;65(10):3983–3990.

22. O'Brien-Simpson NM, Black CL, Bhogal PS, et al. Serum immunoglobulin G (IgG) and IgG subclass responses to the RgpA-Kgp proteinase-adhesin complex of *Porphyromonas gingivalis* in adult periodontitis. *Infect Immun.* 2000;68(5):2704–2712.

23. Alaluusua S, Saarela M, Jousimies-Somer H, et al. Ribotyping shows intrafamilial similarity in *Actinobacillus actinomycetemcomitans* isolates. *Oral Microbiol Immunol.* 1993;8(4):225–229.

24. DiRienzo JM, Slots J. Genetic approach to the study of epidemiology and pathogenesis of *Actinobacillus actinomycetemcomitans* in localized juvenile periodontitis. *Arch Oral Biol.* 1990;35 Suppl:79S–84S.

25. Petit MD, van Steenbergen TJ, Scholte LM, et al. Epidemiology and transmission of *Porphyromonas gingivalis* and *Actinobacillus actinomycetemcomitans* among children and their family members. A report of 4 surveys. *J Clin Periodontol.* 1993;20(9):641–650.

26. Petit MD, van Steenbergen TJ, Timmerman MF, et al. Prevalence of periodontitis and suspected periodontal pathogens in families of adult periodontitis patients. *J Clin Periodontol.* 1994;21(2):76–85.

27. Petit MD, van Winkelhoff AJ, van Steenbergen TJ, et al. *Porphyromonas endodontalis*: prevalence and distribution of restriction enzyme patterns in families. *Oral Microbiol Immunol.* 1993;8(4):219–224.

28. Bradshaw DJ, Bradshaw DJ, Marsh PD, et al. Role of *Fusobacterium nucleatum* and coaggregation in anaerobe survival in planktonic and biofilm oral microbial communities during aeration. *Infect Immun.* 1998;66(10):4729–4732.

29. Li J, Helmerhorst EJ, Leone CW, et al. Identification of early microbial colonizers in human dental biofilm. *J Appl Microbiol.* 2004;97(6):1311–1318.

30. Eastcott AD, Stallard RE. Sequential changes in developing human dental plaque as visualized by scanning electron microscopy. *J Periodontol.* 1973;44(4):218–224.

31. Lie T. Ultrastructural study of early dental plaque formation. *J Periodontal Res.* 1978;13(5):391–409.

32. Ronstrom A, Attstrom R, Egelberg J. Early formation of dental plaque on platic films. 1. Light microscopic observations. *J Periodontal Res.* 1975;10(1):28–35.

33. Saxton CA. Scanning electron microscope study of the formation of dental plaque. *Caries Res.* 1973;7(2):102–119.

34. Theilade E, Theilade J, Mikkelsen L. Microbiological studies on early dento-gingival plaque on teeth and Mylar strips in humans. *J Periodontal Res.* 1982;17(1):12–25.

35. Socransky SS, Haffajee SS, Cugini MA, et al. Microbial complexes in subgingival plaque. *J Clin Periodontol.* 1998;25(2):134–144.

36. Sandros J, Papapanou P, Dahlen G. *Porphyromonas gingivalis* invades oral epithelial cells in vitro. *J Periodontal Res.* 1993;28(3):219–226.

37. Sreenivasan PK, Meyer DH, Fives-Taylor PM. Requirements for invasion of epithelial cells by *Actinobacillus actinomycetemcomitans. Infect Immun.* 1993;61(4):1239–1245.

38. Loesche WJ. Bacterial mediators in periodontal disease. *Clin Infect Dis.* 1993;16 Suppl 4:S203–S210.

39. Curtis MA, et al. Molecular genetics and nomenclature of proteases of *Porphyromonas gingivalis. J Periodontal Res.* 1999;34(8):464–472.

40. Kuramitsu HK. Proteases of *Porphyromonas gingivalis*: what don't they do? *Oral Microbiol Immunol.* 1998;13(5):263–270.

41. Elder MJ, Stapleton F, Evans E, et al. Biofilm-related infections in ophthalmology. *Eye.* 1995;9(Pt 1):102–109.

42. Costerton JW, Lewandowski Z, Caldwell DE, et al. Microbial biofilms. *Annu Rev Microbiol.* 1995;49:711–745.

Chapter 7

Local Contributing Factors

Learning Objectives

- Define the terms pathogenicity and local contributing factors.

- Identify local etiologic factors that contribute to the retention and accumulation of microbial plaque biofilm.

- Explain the meaning of the phrase "pathogenicity of plaque biofilm."

- Identify and differentiate the location, composition, modes of attachment, mechanisms of mineralization, and pathologic potential of supragingival and subgingival calculus deposits.

- Describe four local contributing factors that can lead to direct damage to the periodontium.

- Describe the role of trauma from occlusion as a contributing factor in periodontal disease.

Key Terms

Local contributing factors
Disease site
Dental calculus
Pellicle
Morphology
Overhanging restoration
Palatogingival groove
Pathogenicity
Plaque biofilm pathogenicity
Food impaction
Tongue thrusting
Mouth breathing
Biologic width

Embrasure space
Encroaching on the embrasure space
Prosthesis
Removable prosthesis
Trauma from occlusion
Primary trauma from occlusion
Secondary trauma from occlusion
Functional occlusal forces
Parafunctional occlusal forces
Clenching
Bruxism
Occlusal adjustment

Section 1
Introduction to Local Contributing Factors

As discussed in Chapter 6, it is clear that both gingivitis and periodontitis have bacterial plaque biofilm as their primary etiology. There are, however, local contributing factors that can increase the risk of developing gingivitis or periodontitis or increase the risk of developing more severe disease when gingivitis or periodontitis is already established. Local contributing factors for periodontal disease are oral conditions or habits that increase an individual's susceptibility to periodontal infection. Local contributing factors do not actually initiate either gingivitis or periodontitis but only act to contribute to the disease process previously initiated by bacterial plaque biofilm.

It is critical for the dental team to recognize local contributing factors for periodontal disease during a periodontal assessment. The dental team should always eliminate or at least minimize the impact of local contributing factors during the nonsurgical periodontal treatment. The conditions discussed in this chapter refer to circumstances that favor periodontal breakdown and can contribute to gingivitis or periodontitis in individual sites in the mouth. In context of this discussion, a disease site is an individual tooth or specific surfaces of a tooth that are experiencing periodontal destruction. For instance, a local contributing factor might increase the susceptibility to periodontal infection on the distal surface of a maxillary premolar tooth. Examples of potential local contributing factors include dental calculus, faulty dental restorations, developmental defects in teeth, dental decay, certain patient habits, and trauma from occlusion.

MECHANISMS FOR INCREASED DISEASE RISK

Local contributing factors can increase the risk of developing gingivitis or periodontitis through several mechanisms or through combinations of these mechanisms. TABLE 7-1 summarizes mechanisms for increasing the disease risk in local sites, and each of these mechanisms is discussed in detail in the following sections of this chapter. There are three primary mechanisms by which local factors can increase the risk of developing periodontal disease or increase the severity of existing periodontal disease.
1. A local factor can increase plaque biofilm retention.
2. A local factor can increase plaque biofilm pathogenicity (disease-causing potential).
3. A local factor can cause direct damage to the periodontium.

TABLE 7-1. Mechanisms for Increasing Disease Risk in Local Sites	
Mechanism	**Clinical Example**
Local factor that increases plaque biofilm retention	Rough edge on a restoration harbors plaque biofilm and makes it difficult to remove plaque biofilm with a brush and floss
Local factor that increases plaque biofilm pathogenicity	Calculus which harbors plaque biofilm, allowing it to grow uninhibited for an extended period of time
Local factor that can inflict damage to the periodontium	Ill-fitting partial denture that puts excessive pressure on the gingiva

Section 2
Local Factors that Increase Plaque Biofilm Retention

This section presents local factors that can increase plaque biofilm retention. Most often these local contributing factors include rough or irregular surfaces that decrease the effectiveness of a patient's self-care and lead to the increased plaque biofilm retention.

1. **Dental Calculus.** Dental calculus is the most obvious example of a local contributing factor that can lead to increased plaque biofilm retention. Dental calculus is mineralized bacterial plaque biofilm, covered on its external surface by nonmineralized, living bacterial plaque biofilm. Mineralization of plaque biofilm can begin from 48 hours up to 2 weeks after plaque biofilm formation.
   A. **Effects of Calculus on the Periodontium**
      1. The surface of a calculus deposit at the microscopic level is quite irregular in contour and is always covered with disease-causing bacteria. Thus, even calculus that has not built up enough to result in a ledge or grossly altered tooth contour can lead to plaque biofilm retention at the site simply because of the rough nature of the calculus surface and its tendency to harbor bacteria.
      2. As dental calculus deposits build up, they can lead to even more irregular surfaces, ledges on the teeth, and other alterations of the contours of the teeth (FIG. 7-1). As calculus deposits accumulate, they create more and more areas of plaque biofilm retention that are difficult or impossible for a patient to clean.
   B. **Pathologic Potential**
      1. Since a layer of living bacterial plaque biofilm always covers a calculus deposit, dental calculus plays a significant role as a local contributing factor in periodontal disease.
      2. It is difficult to bring either gingivitis or periodontitis under control in the presence of dental calculus on affected teeth, and the importance of removing these deposits in patients with gingivitis and periodontitis cannot be overemphasized. The removal of dental calculus is discussed in Chapter 25.

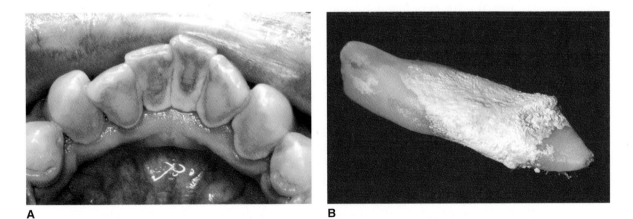

A **B**

Figure 7.1. Irregular Surface of Calculus Deposits. A: Heavy calculus deposits on the lingual surfaces of the mandibular anterior teeth. These deposits are so large that they interfere with the patient's self-care efforts. In addition, calculus deposits harbor living bacteria that can be in constant contact with the gingival tissue.
B: Calculus deposit on the crown and root surfaces of an extracted mandibular canine. (Photograph B courtesy of Dr Don Rolfs, Periodontal Foundations, Wenatchee, WA.)

C. **Composition of Dental Calculus.** Calculus is composed of an inorganic (or mineralized) component and an organic component.
   1. Inorganic portion of calculus
      a. The inorganic part of calculus makes up 70% to 90% of the overall composition of calculus.
      b. This inorganic part of dental calculus is primarily calcium phosphate, but the dental calculus also contains some calcium carbonate and magnesium phosphate.
      c. The inorganic part of calculus is similar to the inorganic components of bone.
   2. Organic portion of calculus
      a. The organic part of calculus makes up 10% to 30% of the overall composition of calculus.
      b. Components of the organic part include materials derived from plaque biofilm, derived from dead epithelial cells, and derived from dead white blood cells. It can also include living bacteria within the deposits of calculus.
D. **Types of Dental Calculus**
   1. Crystalline forms of dental calculus. As calculus ages on a tooth surface, the inorganic component changes through several different crystalline forms. It is interesting to note that some of these crystalline forms of calculus are quite similar to the crystal forms in the tooth itself.
      a. Newly formed calculus deposits appear as a crystalline form called brushite.
      b. In calculus deposits that are a bit more mature, but less than 6 months old, the crystalline form is primarily octocalcium phosphate.
      c. In mature deposits that are more than 6 months old, the crystalline form is primarily hydroxyapatite.
   2. Location of calculus deposits
      a. Supragingival calculus deposits are calculus deposits located coronal to (above) the gingival margin. Other terms that have been used to refer to deposits coronal to the gingival margin are supramarginal calculus and salivary calculus.
         1) Though supragingival calculus deposits can be found on any tooth surface, these usually are found in localized areas of the dentition, such as lingual surfaces of mandibular anterior teeth, facial surfaces of maxillary molars, and on teeth that are crowded or in malocclusion. It is interesting to note that supragingival calculus is frequently found in areas adjacent to large salivary ducts (such as the lingual surfaces of mandibular anterior teeth and the facial surfaces of maxillary posterior teeth).
         2) Though supragingival calculus can form in most any shape, these deposits most often are irregular, large deposits.
      b. Subgingival deposits are calculus deposits located apical to (below) the gingival margin. Other terms that have been used for deposits apical to the gingival margin are submarginal calculus and serumal calculus.
         1) The distribution of subgingival deposits may be localized in certain areas or generalized throughout the mouth.
         2) The shape of subgingival deposits is most often flattened. It is thought that the shape of the deposit may be guided by pressure of the pocket wall against the deposit.
E. **Modes of Attachment to Tooth Surfaces.** Dental calculus attaches to tooth surfaces through several different modes, and different attachment mechanisms can even exist in the same calculus deposit.

1. **Attachment by means of pellicle**
   a. Calculus can attach to the tooth surface by attaching to the pellicle on the surface. The pellicle is a thin, bacteria-free membrane that forms on the surface of the tooth during the late stages of eruption.
   b. This mode of attachment occurs most commonly on enamel surfaces.
   c. Calculus deposits attached via the pellicle are usually removed easily because this attachment is on the surface of the pellicle (and not actually locked into the tooth surface).

2. **Attachment to irregularities in the tooth surface**
   a. Calculus can also attach to irregularities in tooth surfaces. These irregularities include cracks in the teeth, tiny openings left where periodontal ligament fibers are detached, and grooves in cemental surfaces created as the result of faulty instrumentation during previous calculus removal procedures.
   b. Complete calculus removal in areas of irregularities in tooth surfaces is usually difficult since the deposits can be sheltered in these tooth defects.

3. **Attachment by direct contact of the calcified component and the tooth surface**
   a. Calculus can also attach to tooth surfaces by attaching directly to the calcified component of the tooth. In this mode of attachment, the matrix of the calculus deposit is interlocked with the inorganic crystals of the tooth.
   b. Deposits, firmly interlocked in the tooth surface, are usually difficult to remove.

2. **Tooth Morphology.** Morphology is the study of the anatomic surface features of the teeth. There are a variety of local contributing factors that relate to tooth morphology. Some of these variations in tooth morphology can occur when a tooth requires a restoration, and some of them occur simply because of variations in the way teeth form.
   A. **Poorly Contoured Restorations**
      1. When a dentist places a restoration, it is not always possible to contour the restoration perfectly smoothly with the existing tooth structure. When a restoration is not smoothly contoured with the tooth surfaces, this condition is referred to as an overhanging restoration or overhang (FIG. 7-2).
      2. Because of difficulty of access to tooth surfaces protected by an overhanging restoration, it is often impossible for a patient to remove plaque biofilm effectively from the tooth surface. This leads to plaque biofilm retention at the site and can subsequently lead to increased severity of either gingivitis or periodontitis at the site.

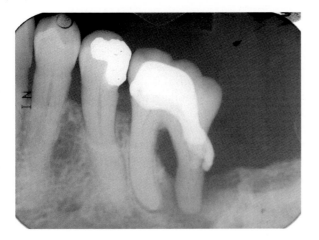

Figure 7.2. **Radiographic Evidence of Poorly Contoured Restorations.** Note that the restoration margins on the distal surface of the first molar and on the distal surface of the second premolar are not smoothly contoured with the actual tooth surfaces. This leads to increased plaque biofilm retention in both of the areas, thus making it impossible to control periodontitis in the presence of these poorly contoured restoration margins. (Courtesy of Dr Richard Foster, Guilford Technical Community College, Jamestown, NC.)

B. Dental Caries. Untreated tooth decay is another example of a local contributing factor that can increase plaque biofilm retention. Since tooth decay can result in defects in tooth structure (dental cavities), these defects (cavities) can also act as protected environments for bacteria that cause gingivitis and periodontitis to live and grow undisturbed (Fig. 7-3).

C. Tooth Grooves or Concavities

1. Naturally occurring developmental grooves and concavities in tooth surfaces frequently lead to difficulty in self-care at the site and can also be a local contributing factor for gingivitis and periodontitis because of the increased plaque biofilm retention at the site.

2. During the natural development of some incisor teeth, a groove forms on the palatal surface of the tooth. This groove is a developmental defect called a palatogingival groove and is most frequently seen on maxillary lateral incisors. Plaque biofilm retention is a common problem associated with a palatogingival groove since the groove is often difficult or impossible to clean effectively (Fig. 7-4).

3. Some tooth root surfaces have naturally occurring concavities or depressions that can lead to plaque biofilm retention (Fig. 7-5). The mesial surface of maxillary first premolar teeth often has a pronounced concavity in the surface. This concavity is a natural contour for that tooth, but if exposed in the oral cavity, can make it extremely difficult for a patient to maintain effective self-care at the site. Figure 7-6 illustrates how a tooth concavity can prevent thorough self-care even for a patient skilled in use of dental floss.

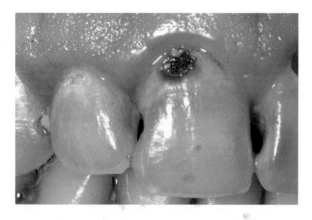

Figure 7.3. Untreated Decay. Note that this untreated tooth decay leaves an actual hole (cavity) in the tooth surface that can then harbor periodontal pathogens and can allow them to grow undisturbed by self-care efforts. (Courtesy of Dr Ralph Arnold, San Antonio, TX.)

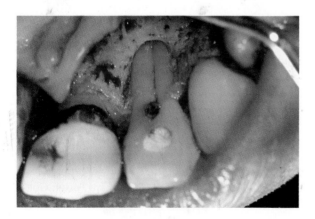

Figure 7.4. Palatogingival Groove. A palatogingival groove on the lingual surface of this maxillary lateral incisor is revealed during a periodontal surgical procedure. The gingiva has been lifted off the bone and tooth root. The palatal side of the root and the alveolar bone level are clearly visible. The palatogingival groove allowed plaque biofilm to mature undisturbed in the depth of the groove and has contributed to the extensive alveolar bone loss. (Courtesy of Dr Ralph Arnold, San Antonio, TX.)

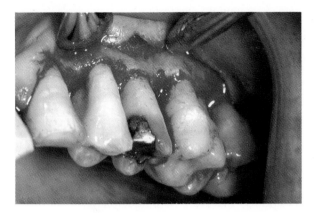

Figure 7.5. Root Concavity. The mesial root concavity on a maxillary first premolar. This photograph was taken during a periodontal surgical procedure designed to allow better visualization and treatment of the root concavity. (Courtesy of Dr Ralph Arnold, San Antonio, TX.)

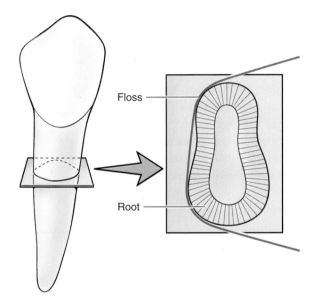

Floss

Root

Figure 7.6. Flossing a Tooth Surface with a Concavity. Note that even if floss is closely adapted to the tooth surfaces, the floss will not dislodge the plaque biofilm in the base of the concavity.

Section 3
Local Factors That Increase Plaque Biofilm Pathogenicity

Pathogenicity can be described as the ability of a disease-causing agent to actually produce the disease. In the dental context, pathogenicity can be thought of as the ability of the dental plaque biofilm to cause periodontal disease. Plaque biofilm pathogenicity relates to the character of the plaque biofilm rather than simply an increase in the amount of plaque biofilm.

1. **Undisturbed Plaque Biofilm Growth**
   A. **Plaque Biofilm Maturation**
      1. Plaque biofilm allowed to grow undisturbed is said to "mature." As plaque biofilm matures, it becomes colonized with larger and larger numbers of bacteria.
      2. Starting with a perfectly clean tooth surface, plaque biofilm bacteria accumulate in a predictable pattern on any tooth surface not being cleaned by the patient.
         a. Immediately after cleaning, salivary proteins attach to the tooth surface and form the pellicle.
         b. Within the first 2 days, the pellicle becomes colonized with Gram-positive aerobic cocci and rods. These bacteria can cause gingivitis but do not cause periodontitis.
         c. Over the next week, other bacteria enter the plaque biofilm. These new bacteria include those that can cause periodontitis.
            1) The bacteria in this stage of plaque biofilm development include some Gram-negative anaerobic cocci and Gram-negative rods.
            2) In addition, at this stage specific periodontal pathogens can colonize the plaque biofilm including Fusobacterium species and *Prevotella intermedia*.
         d. Later, other bacteria including *Porphyromonas gingivalis* colonize the plaque biofilm. Some of these other bacteria are also associated with periodontitis.
   B. **Increased Plaque Biofilm Pathogenicity**
      1. The concept of plaque biofilm pathogenicity refers to the ability of the bacteria in the dental plaque biofilm to produce periodontal disease.
         a. It is important to understand that all plaque biofilm that is left undisturbed and allowed to mature (i.e., age) on a tooth surface is eventually colonized by bacteria known to cause periodontitis.
         b. As plaque biofilm matures into a true plaque biofilm, it becomes more pathogenic than the plaque biofilm that first developed on the tooth surface since it includes more of the bacteria that are the causative agents in periodontitis (FIG. 7-7).
      2. Increased plaque biofilm pathogenicity is closely related to some plaque biofilm retention factors. Plaque biofilm retention factors not only allow an increase in the amount of plaque biofilm at the site, but they can also allow plaque biofilm to mature and increase in pathogenicity.

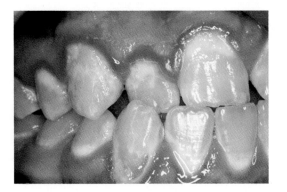

Figure 7.7. Mature Dental Plaque Biofilm. Note the thick dental plaque biofilm at the gingival margin of the teeth in this photograph. This plaque biofilm has been present for several weeks and is more pathogenic than a less mature plaque biofilm because it now harbors periodontal pathogens. (Courtesy of Dr Richard Foster, Guilford Technical Community College, Jamestown, NC.)

Section 4
Local Factors That Cause Direct Damage

The fourth section discusses a few of the local contributing factors that may actually cause direct damage to the periodontium. These factors also may alter the progress of periodontitis at individual sites. Some local contributing factors that can directly damage the periodontium include food impaction, patient habits, and faulty restorations or appliances.

1. **Direct Damage Due to Food Impaction**
    A. **Definition.** Food impaction refers to forcing food (such as pieces of tough meat) between teeth during chewing, trapping the food in the interdental area.
    B. **Effect of Food Impaction**
        1. Food forced into a tooth sulcus can strip the gingival tissues away from the tooth surface and contribute to periodontal breakdown in addition to the more obvious danger of serving as nutrients for tooth decay causing bacteria.
        2. Food impaction not only damages the gingival tissues directly but can also lead to alterations in the gingival contour that result in interdental areas that are difficult for patients to clean (FIG. 7-8).
2. **Direct Damage from Patient Habits.** In some patients, habits such as tongue thrusting, mouth breathing, or the improper use of toothbrushes, toothpicks, and other dental cleaning aids can also cause direct damage to the periodontium.
    A. **Improper Use of Plaque Biofilm Control Aids.** Improper use of plaque biofilm control aids can result in direct damage to the gingival tissues, causing alteration of the natural contours of the tissues (FIG. 7-9).

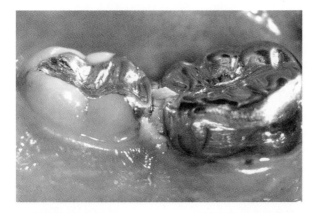

Figure 7.8. **Food Impaction.** Note the food impaction between the two molar teeth. As this patient chews food, the food is forced between these teeth and produces direct damage to the periodontium. (Courtesy of Dr Don Rolfs, Periodontal Foundations, Wenatchee, WA.)

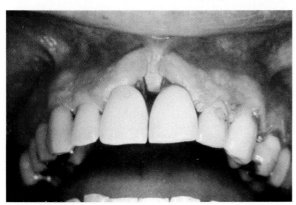

Figure 7.9. **Misuse of Toothpick.** The interdental papilla between the two central incisors has been destroyed by the patient's habit of repeatedly forcing a toothpick between the teeth. This damage to the papillae is an example of direct damage to the periodontium.

B. Tongue Thrusting. Tongue thrusting is the application of forceful pressure against the anterior teeth with the tongue.
1. Tongue thrusting is often the result of an abnormal tongue positioning during the initial stage of swallowing.
2. This oral habit exerts excessive lateral pressure against the teeth and may be traumatic to the periodontium (FIG. 7-10).

C. Mouth Breathing. Mouth breathing is the process of inhaling and exhaling air primarily through the mouth, rather than the nose, and often occurs while the patient is sleeping. Mouth breathing has a tendency to dry out the gingival tissues in the anterior region of the mouth.

3. Direct Damage Due to Faulty Restorations and Appliances

A. Inappropriate Crown Placement. A crown is a metal, ceramic, or ceramic-bonded-to-metal covering for a badly damaged tooth. Placing a crown on a damaged tooth is a common mechanism used to preserve a badly damaged tooth.
1. Crowns can sometimes be placed inappropriately when the tooth structure is minimal. There can be direct damage to the periodontium when the edges of a crown (called margins) are placed below the gingival margin and too near the alveolar bone.
2. A crown margin that is closer than 2 mm to the crest of the alveolar bone can result in resorption of alveolar bone (FIG. 7-11).

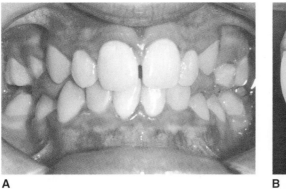
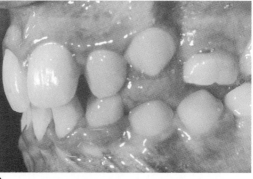

A   B

Figure 7.10. Tongue Thrust. A: Facial view of a patient with a tongue thrust. As this patient swallows, the patient applies lateral pressure with her tongue against the teeth. **B:** Side view of the tongue thrust. The tongue is visible in the canine region of the mouth as the patient presses her tongue forward when swallowing. (Courtesy of Dr Don Rolfs, Periodontal Foundations, Wenatchee, WA.)

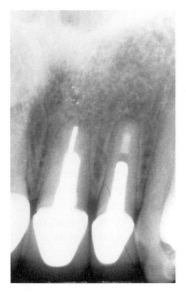

Figure 7.11. Direct Damage to the Periodontium. This radiograph reveals a crown with a margin that is approximately 1 mm from the alveolar bone. This distance is too close to the bone to allow for normal soft tissue attachment to the tooth.

3. Biologic width refers to the space on the tooth surface occupied by the junctional epithelium and the connective tissue attachment fibers immediately apical to (below) the junctional epithelium (FIG. 7-12). This biologic width can be "violated" or damaged by restoration margins. The series of drawings in FIG. 7-13 shows the biologic width and its relationship to a properly placed margin and a restoration margin that violates or damages the biologic width.

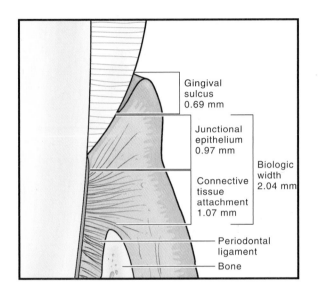

Figure 7.12. **Biologic Width in Health.** Illustration showing the biologic width in health with average dimensions that have been reported in the literature.

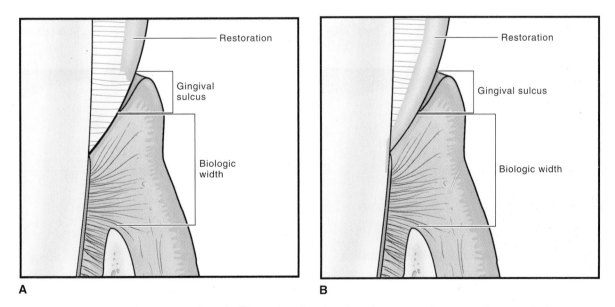

Figure 7.13. **Margins of a Restoration. A:** Illustration showing the placement of a restoration margin in a position that leaves the biologic width undamaged by the restoration. **B:** Illustration showing the placement of a restoration margin in a position that violates or damages the biologic width.

B. **Improperly Contoured Restorations**
1. Bulky or overcontoured crowns or restorations can result in inadequate space between the teeth to accommodate the natural form of the interdental papilla.
2. The open space apical to the contact area of two adjacent teeth is referred to as an embrasure space. In health, the embrasure space is filled by an interdental papilla.
3. Bulky crowns reduce the size of the embrasure space so that inadequate space exists between the teeth to accommodate the interdental papilla. In this situation, the bulky crowns are described as encroaching upon the embrasure space (FIG. 7-14).

C. **Faulty Removable Prosthesis**
1. A prosthesis is an appliance used to replace missing teeth.
   a. A removable prosthesis is one that the patient can remove for cleaning and before going to bed. A removable prosthesis that replaces a few teeth is commonly called a removable partial denture.
   b. A removable prosthesis should be differentiated from a fixed prosthesis. A fixed prosthesis is a prosthesis that is cemented to the teeth (also known as a fixed bridge).
2. A damaged or poorly fitting removable prosthesis can impinge on gingival tissue and favor plaque biofilm accumulation and thus hasten the progress of periodontitis (FIG. 7-15).

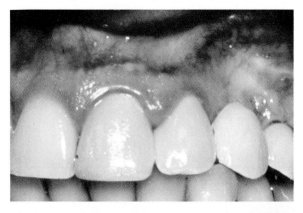

Figure 7.14. **Bulky Crown Encroaching on Interdental Space.** The crowns shown here are so bulky in contour on their proximal surfaces that they fill the embrasure space leaving no room for the natural form of the papilla. Note that the papilla between the central and lateral incisor appears enlarged because it is being pushed from between the teeth.

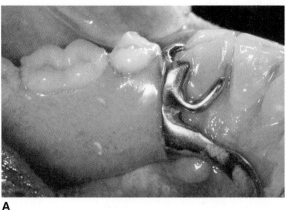

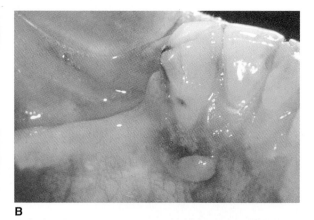

A   B

Figure 7.15. **Tissue Damage by a Poorly Fitting Removable Prosthesis.** A: Clinical photograph showing a removable prosthesis (lower partial denture) that replaces extracted posterior teeth. B: With the prosthesis removed, the tissue damage to the mandibular canine is revealed. Recession of gingival margin on the canine is due in part to the clasp of the faulty prosthesis impinging upon the gingival tissue. (Courtesy of Dr Don Rolfs, Periodontal Foundations, Wenatchee, WA.)

4. **Direct Damage from Occlusal Forces**
   A. **Trauma from Occlusion**
      1. Direct damage to the periodontium can result from excessive occlusal (or biting) forces on the teeth.
      2. When excessive occlusal forces cause damage to the periodontium, this is referred to as trauma from occlusion.
         a. When trauma from occlusion occurs, some alveolar bone resorption can result simply because of increased pressure placed on the surrounding alveolar bone.
         b. When there is loss of some alveolar bone due to pressures from trauma from occlusion, there can be a more rapid destruction by any existing periodontitis.
      3. A thorough clinical exam and a thorough radiographic exam can frequently reveal signs of trauma from occlusion.
         a. Some of the clinical signs of trauma from occlusion that have been reported include the following.
            1) Tooth mobility
            2) Sensitivity to pressure
            3) Migration of teeth
         b. Some of the radiographic signs of trauma from occlusion that have been reported include the following:
            1) Enlarged, funnel-shaped periodontal ligament space
            2) Alveolar bone resorption. Figure 7-16 shows a radiograph of a tooth that has been subjected to excessive occlusal forces (trauma from occlusion).
      4. Trauma from occlusion has been classified in the dental literature for many years as either primary trauma from occlusion or secondary trauma from occlusion.
         a. Primary trauma from occlusion is defined as excessive occlusal forces on a sound periodontium.
            1) Examples of causes of primary trauma from occlusion include accidental placement of a high restoration or insertion of a fixed bridge or partial denture that places excessive force on the abutment teeth.
            2) The changes seen in primary occlusal trauma include a wider periodontal ligament space, tooth mobility, and even tooth and jaw pain. These changes are reversible if the trauma is removed.

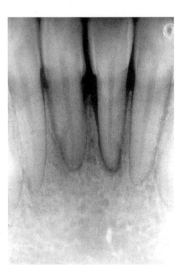

Figure 7.16. Radiographic Evidence of Trauma from Occlusion. Note the dramatic widening of the periodontal ligament space along the lateral root surfaces on the mandibular right central incisor (center tooth on radiograph). The alveolar bone has been destroyed because of the pressures resulting from trauma from occlusion.

TABLE 7-2. Terms Associated with Trauma from Occlusion	
Term	**Definition**
Trauma from occlusion	Injury to the periodontium resulting from excessive occlusal forces
Primary trauma from occlusion	Injury to the periodontium resulting from excessive occlusal forces
Secondary trauma from occlusion	Injury from normal occlusal forces applied to a periodontium previously damaged by periodontitis

b. **Secondary trauma from occlusion** is defined as normal occlusal forces on an unhealthy periodontium previously weakened by periodontitis.
   1) Secondary trauma from occlusion occurs to a tooth in which the surrounding periodontium has experienced apical migration of the junctional epithelium, loss of connective tissue attachment, and loss of alveolar bone. In this type of trauma, the periodontium was unhealthy prior to experiencing excessive occlusal forces. TABLE 7-2 summarizes definitions of some terms used to describe trauma from occlusion.
   2) A tooth with an unhealthy, inflamed periodontium that is subjected to excessive occlusal forces is thought to be subject to more rapid bone loss and pocket formation.
   3) Teeth can be tipped laterally easily when subjected to lateral occlusal forces. These tipping forces frequently accompany trauma from occlusion and can create areas of pressure and tension within the PDL that are transmitted to the bone. Figure 7-17 illustrates how this tipping can occur. As alveolar bone loss progresses, this lateral tipping becomes even more likely because of the longer lever arm created by the part of the tooth out of the bone compared to the part of the tooth encased in the bone.
   4) Teeth with reduced alveolar bone support can have additional damage to the periodontium because of the tipping action of lateral forces placed on the teeth. Figure 7-18 shows a series of drawings that illustrate this concept.

B. **Parafunctional Occlusal Forces**
   1. A series of other terms are used to describe excessive occlusal forces. Two of these terms are functional and parafunctional occlusal forces.
      a. **Functional occlusal forces** are the normal forces produced during the act of chewing food.
      b. **Parafunctional occlusal forces** result from tooth-to-tooth contact made when not in the act of eating.
         1) Examples of these parafunctional habits are clenching of the teeth together as a release of nervous tension or grinding the teeth together for the same release.
            a) **Clenching** is the continuous or intermittent forceful closure of the maxillary teeth against the mandibular teeth.
            b) **Bruxism** is forceful grinding of the teeth.
            c) These parafunctional habits can occur without the person having conscious knowledge of the habit. Some individuals exhibit these habits while asleep.
         2) Parafunctional habits can exert excessive force on the teeth and to the periodontium.

2. There are several clinical therapies that can be used by a dentist to help control the damage from trauma from occlusion.
   a. When the trauma is a result of a faulty bite (referred to as a faulty occlusion), the dentist can make minor adjustments in the bite to minimize the damaging forces. This procedure is called an occlusal adjustment.
   b. When the trauma is a result of bruxism, the dentist can fabricate an acrylic appliance sometimes referred to as a night guard appliance that can protect the teeth during part of each day.

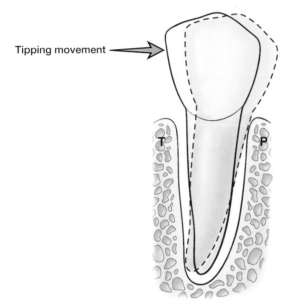

Tipping movement

Figure 7.17. Tipping Movement from Lateral Occlusal Forces. Tipping of a tooth within the socket due to lateral occlusal forces often accompanies trauma from occlusion. This tipping can result in areas of pressure and tension within the PDL. In this illustration, "T" indicates an area of tension. The letter "P" indicates an area of pressure in the PDL and alveolar bone.

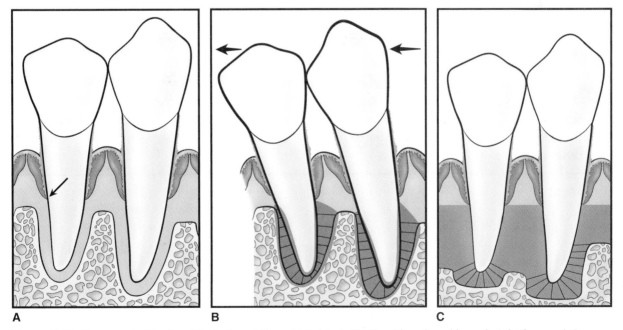

A   B   C

Figure 7.18. Damage to Teeth with Reduced Bone Height. A: Teeth with reduced bone height from existing periodontitis. **B:** Teeth being subjected to lateral forces and being moved laterally by those forces. **C:** Additional bone loss to the periodontium as a result of pressure on bone from the lateral tooth movement. This additional bone loss can be additive to the bone loss already occurring in a periodontitis patient.

Chapter Summary Statement

Local contributing factors can increase the risk of developing gingivitis or periodontitis or increase the risk of developing more severe disease when gingivitis or periodontitis is already established. The three mechanisms in which local factors can increase the risk of periodontal disease are by (1) increasing plaque biofilm retention, (2) increasing plaque biofilm pathogenicity, and (3) causing direct damage to the periodontium. As discussed in Chapter 19, the dental team must identify these local contributing factors during a clinical assessment so that any local contributing factors can be eliminated or minimized during the nonsurgical periodontal treatment.

Section 5
Focus on Patients

Case 1

Examination of a patient reveals gingivitis. In addition, the patient has generalized calculus deposits and numerous restorations with overhangs. What steps might be necessary to bring the gingivitis under control in this patient?

Case 2

In a dental hygiene journal, you find an article that refers to mature dental plaque biofilm. Explain what the author means by this term mature dental plaque.

Case 3

Examination of a patient reveals periodontitis. The patient also has a severe tooth clenching habit. Explain how the tooth clenching habit could be related to the progress of the periodontitis.

Basic Concepts of Immunity and Inflammation

Learning Objectives

- Define the term immune system and name its primary function.

- Define the term inflammation and name two events that can trigger the inflammatory response.

- Name the five classic symptoms of acute inflammation and explain what events in the tissues result in these classic symptoms.

- Give an example of a type of injury or infection that would result in inflammation in an individual's arm. Describe the symptoms of inflammation that the individual would experience.

- Compare and contrast acute inflammation and chronic inflammation.

- Define the term phagocytosis and describe the steps in this process.

- Describe the role of polymorphonuclear leukocytes in the immune system.

- Describe the role of macrophages in the immune system.

- Contrast the terms macrophage and monocyte.

- Describe the role of B lymphocytes in the immune system.

- Describe the role of T lymphocytes in the immune system.

- Describe the three ways that antibodies participate in the host defense.

- Define the term inflammatory mediator.

- Define complement system and explain its principle functions in the immune response.

Key Terms

Immune system

Host

Host response

Leukocyte

Polymorphonuclear leukocytes (PMNs)

Neutrophil

Chemotaxis

Lysosome

Neutropenia

Macrophage

Monocyte

Lymphocyte

B Lymphocyte

Antibody

Immunoglobulin

T lymphocyte

Cytokine

Complement system

Membrane attack complex

Opsonization

Endothelium

Transendothelial migration

Phagocytosis

Phagosome

Phagolysosome

Inflammation

Inflammatory biochemical mediator

Chemokines

Acute Inflammation

C-reactive protein (CRP)

Chronic Inflammation

Section 1
The Body's Defense System

Humans are surrounded by millions of microorganisms, many of which may prove to be deadly. Our hands, alone, harbor up to 2 million microorganisms. The only reason that the human body survives is that it has a protective defense system that is remarkably effective in recognizing and fighting disease-causing microorganisms. The immune system is a complex system that is responsible for defending the body against millions of bacteria, viruses, fungi, toxins, and parasites.

INTRODUCTION TO THE IMMUNE SYSTEM

1. Description
   A. **A Complex System of Responses**
      1. The immune system is a collection of responses that protects the body against infections by bacteria, viruses, fungi, toxins, and parasites (FIG. 8-1).
      2. Bacteria, viruses, and other disease-causing microorganisms attack the human body over 100 million times a day. For this reason, the human immune system attempts to control quickly the spread of invading microorganisms.
   B. **Self Versus Nonself.** When the immune system encounters cells or molecules, it must determine whether these are *self* (part of the body) or foreign substances. Molecules might be harmless substances, such as pollen, or constitute part of a microorganism. Microorganisms, in turn, might be innocuous or pathogenic.
2. Function
   A. **Prime Purpose**
      1. The prime purpose of the human immune system is to defend the life of the individual (host) by identifying the foreign substances in the body (bacteria, viruses, fungi or parasites) and develop a defense against them [1,2].
      2. The body recognizes bacteria, viruses, fungi, and parasites as something foreign to itself and *responds by (1) sending certain types of cells to the infection site and (2) producing biochemical substances to counteract the foreign invaders*.
   B. The way that an individual's body responds to an infection is known as the host response.
3. **Consequences of Loss of Immune Function.** Loss of immune function is deadly to the body. An example is the human immunodeficiency virus (HIV), the virus that causes acquired immune deficiency syndrome (AIDS). HIV disables a specific group of immune system cells responsible for coordinating immune responses. People infected with HIV often develop infections from microorganisms that rarely cause infection in individuals with normal, healthy immune systems.
4. **Consequences of an Overzealous Immune Response.** The immune system can sometimes become confused or so intense in its response *that it begins to harm the body that it is trying to protect*. Rheumatic heart disease is an example of a confused immune response to infection. The problem begins as an infection of the skin or pharynx with streptococcal bacteria. Unfortunately, there are similarities between certain molecules of the streptococcal bacteria and molecules of human heart tissue. As a result of this molecular similarity, immune responses against the streptococcal bacteria also attack and damage the heart tissue of the infected individual.

Infectious organisms taking advantage
of breaches in the body's barriers

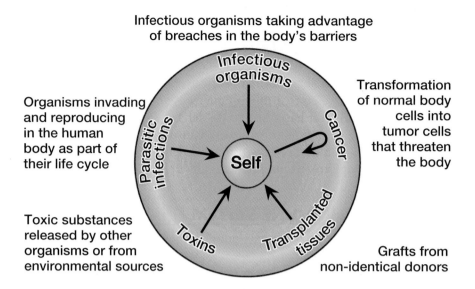

Transformation
of normal body
cells into
tumor cells
that threaten
the body

Organisms invading
and reproducing
in the human
body as part of
their life cycle

Toxic substances
released by other
organisms or from
environmental sources

Grafts from
non-identical donors

Figure 8.1. The Immune Defense System. The immune system defends the body against invading microorganisms, as well as toxins in the environment. Basically, the immune system recognizes body cells as "self" and tries to protect these cells. This includes protection against infectious organisms, parasitic infections, toxins, and cancerous cells. Unfortunately, cells of transplanted tissues are recognized as "nonself" or invaders. For this reason, strong drugs are needed to keep the body's immune system from rejecting a transplant.

COMPONENTS OF THE IMMUNE SYSTEM

Components of the immune system that play an important role in combating periodontal disease are the (1) cellular defenders (phagocytes, lymphocytes) and (2) the complement system (Fig. 8-2 and Table 8-1) [1,2].

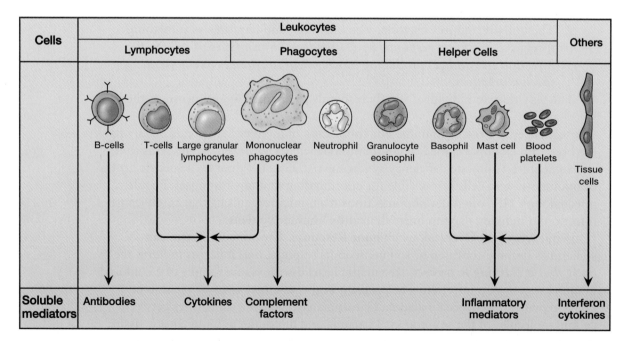

Figure 8.2. Components of the Immune System. Components of the immune system include cells and chemical mediators. The cells and the chemical mediators are closely related since the cells produce most of the mediators.

CELLS OF THE IMMUNE SYSTEM

1. **Leukocytes.** Leukocytes are white blood cells that act much like independent single-cell organisms able to move and capture microorganisms on their own.
   A. **Polymorphonuclear leukocytes.** Polymorphonuclear leukocytes (PMNs) are phagocytes that play a vital role in combating the pathogenic bacteria responsible for periodontal disease (FIG. 8-3).
      1. PMNs, also known as neutrophils, are phagocytic cells that actively engulf and destroy microorganisms.
      2. These cells are the *rapid responders* and provide the first line of defense against many common microorganisms and are essential for the control of bacterial infections.
      3. Once in the blood stream, PMNs can move through capillary walls and into the tissue. PMNs are attracted to bacteria by a process called chemotaxis.
      4. The cytoplasm of a PMN contains many granules filled with strong bactericidal and digestive enzymes. These granules (called lysosomes) can kill and digest bacterial cells after phagocytosis.
      5. PMNs are *short-lived cells* that die when they become engorged with the bacteria they phagocytize. The pus formed at sites of inflammation contains many dead and dying PMNs. PMNs have a short life span, generally less than 1 day.
      6. The bacteria associated with periodontal disease are most effectively phagocytized by PMNs.
      7. Normally, each milliliter of blood contains between 3,000 and 6,000 PMNs. A PMN count of less than 1,000 cells/mL is called neutropenia and indicates an increased risk of infection.
   B. **Monocytes/Macrophages.** Macrophages are large phagocytes with one kidney-shaped nucleus and some granules (FIG. 8-4).
      1. These leukocytes are called monocytes when found in the bloodstream and macrophages when they are located in the tissues.
      2. Macrophages are highly phagocytic cells that actively engulf and destroy microorganisms (FIG. 8-5). Macrophages contain a few lysosomes that are filled with bactericidal and digestive enzymes.
      3. Macrophages are slower to arrive at the infection site than PMNs. The *slower, long-lived* macrophages are often the most numerous cells in chronic inflammation.
      4. Macrophages present antigen to T cells. Together macrophages and T lymphocytes play an important role in chronic inflammation.

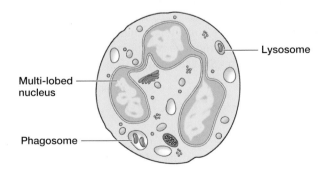

Multi-lobed nucleus

Lysosome

Phagosome

Figure 8.3. Morphology of a Polymorphonuclear Leukocyte. PMNs contain granules called lysosomes that are used to digest bacteria.

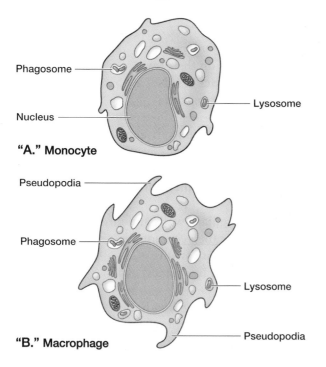

"A." Monocyte

Phagosome

Nucleus

Lysosome

"B." Macrophage

Pseudopodia

Phagosome

Lysosome

Pseudopodia

Figure 8.4. Morphology of a Monocyte and a Macrophage. These phagocytic leukocytes are called monocytes (A) when found in the bloodstream, and macrophages (B) when they are located in the tissues. Of the blood cells, macrophages are the largest—thus, the name "macro." Macrophages are five- to tenfold larger than monocytes and contain more lysosomes.

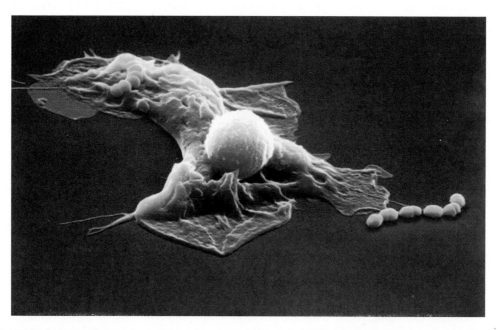

Figure 8.5. SEM of Macrophage. A scanning electron micrograph (SEM) of a human macrophage (*gray*) approaches a chain of Streptococcus pyogenes (*orange*). Riding atop the macrophage is a spherical lymphocyte. Both macrophages and lymphocytes are important in eliminating infection. (SEM courtesy of Cells Alive.)

2. **Lymphocytes.** Lymphocytes are small white blood cells that play an important role in recognizing and controlling foreign invaders. The two main types of lymphocytes that are important in the defense against periodontal pathogens are B lymphocytes (B cells) and T lymphocytes (T cells).

  A. **B Lymphocytes**

    1. **Description**

      a. B lymphocytes are small leukocytes that help in the defense against bacteria, viruses, and fungi.

      b. B lymphocytes can further differentiate into one of the two types of B cells: plasma B cells and memory B cells.

      c. The principal functions of B lymphocytes are to **make antibodies**. Once a B cell has been activated, it manufactures millions of antibodies and pours them into the bloodstream (FIG. 8-6).

    2. **Antibodies**

      a. Antibodies are Y-shaped proteins. One end of the Y binds to the outside of the B cell. The other end binds to a microorganism and helps to kill it.

      b. Antibodies are known collectively as immunoglobulins. The five major classes of immunoglobulin are immunoglobulin M (IgM), immunoglobulin D (IgD), immunoglobulin G (IgG), immunoglobulin A (IgA), and immunoglobulin E (IgE).

      c. Antibodies participate in host defense in three main ways:

        1) Neutralize bacteria or bacterial toxins to prevent bacteria from destroying host cells.

        2) Coat bacteria making them more susceptible to phagocytosis.

        3) Activate the complement system.

  B. **T Lymphocytes**

    1. T lymphocytes are small leukocytes whose main function is to intensify the response of other immune cells—such as B lymphocytes and macrophages—to the bacterial invasion.

    2. T cells can produce substances called cytokines, such as the interleukins (ILs), that further stimulate the immune response. Cytokine is a general name for any protein that is secreted by cells and affects the behavior of nearby cells. Cytokines that play an important role in periodontitis include interleukin-1 (IL-1), interleukin-6 (IL-6), interleukin-8 (IL-8), and tumor necrosis factor-alpha (TNF-alpha).

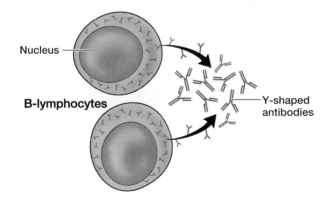

Nucleus

B-lymphocytes

Y-shaped antibodies

Figure 8.6. B-Lymphocytes. Diagram of a B cell showing the Y-shaped antibody protein attached to the cell wall.

THE COMPLEMENT SYSTEM

In addition to the cellular defenders, the other major component of the immune response is the complement system. The cellular defenders only respond after they encounter a microorganism. Pathogens, however, can evade contact with the immune cells. If this happens, the complement system provides a second means of defense.

1. **Definition.** The Complement System is a complex series of proteins circulating in the blood that works to facilitate phagocytosis or kill bacteria directly by puncturing bacterial cell membranes. The complement proteins are activated by and work with (complement) the antibodies, hence the name.

2. **Four Principal Functions of Complement.** After activation, the complement proteins interact, in a highly regulated cascade, to carry out a number of defensive functions (FIG. 8-7):
   A. **Destruction of Pathogens.** Components of complement can destroy certain microorganisms directly by forming pores in their cell membranes.
   To accomplish this task, the complement system creates a protein unit called the membrane attack complex that is capable of puncturing the cell membranes of certain bacteria (lysis).
   B. **Opsonization of Pathogens.** The complement system facilitates the engulfment and destruction of microorganisms by phagocytes. This process, known as opsonization of pathogens, is the most important action of the complement system. Complement components coat the surface of the bacterium allowing the phagocytes to recognize, engulf, and destroy the bacterium.
   C. **Recruitment of Phagocytes.** The complement system recruits additional phagocytic cells to the site of the infection.
   D. **Immune Clearance.** Finally, the complement system performs a "housekeeping" function, the removal of immune complexes from circulation.

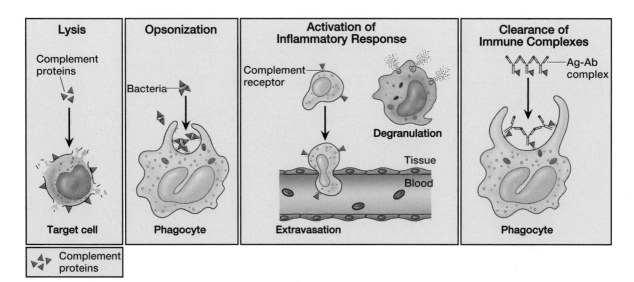

Figure 8.7. **Activities of the Complement System.** In this diagram, complement proteins are represented by small red triangles. Complement proteins facilitate a number of immune activities: puncturing the cell membranes of certain bacteria (lysis), phagocytosis of bacteria (opsonization), further activation of the inflammatory response by recruitment of additional phagocytic cells to the infection site, and clearance of immune complexes from circulation.

TABLE 8-1. Summary: Components of the Immune System

Component	Function
Polymorphonuclear leukocyte (PMN)  **A**	• Phagocytosis • Release of lysosomes • Release of powerful regulatory proteins (cytokines) that signal the immune system to send additional phagocytic cells to the site of an infection
Macrophage  **B**	• Phagocytosis • Release of lysosomes • Release of powerful regulatory proteins (cytokines) that signal the immune system to send additional phagocytic cells to the site of an infection
B-lymphocyte/ Plasma cell 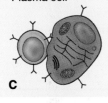 **C**	• Production of immunoglobulins
T-lymphocytes 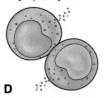 **D**	• Further stimulate the immune response
Immunoglobulins IgG, IgM, IgA, IgD, IgE **E**	• Neutralize bacteria or bacterial toxins • Coat bacteria to facilitate phagocytosis • Activate the complement system
Complement System 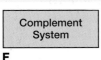 **F**	• Lysis of cell membranes of certain bacteria • Phagocytosis • Recruitment of additional phagocytic cells to the infection site and clearance of immune complexes from circulation

Section 2
Leukocyte Migration, Chemotaxis, and Phagocytosis

1. **Leukocyte Migration from the Blood Vessels**
    A. **Transendothelial Migration**
        1. In order to fight an infection, the cells of the immune system travel through the bloodstream and into the tissues (FIG. 8-9).
            a. Near the infection site, the immune cells push their way between the endothelial cells lining the blood vessels (extravasation) and enter the connective tissue [3].
            b. The thin layer of epithelial cells that line the interior surface of the blood vessels is called the endothelium. For this reason, the process of immune cells exiting the vessels and entering the tissues is called transendothelial migration.
        2. Defects in transendothelial migration are associated with aggressive periodontitis underscoring the importance of this process in the defense against periodontal pathogens.
    B. **Leukocyte Migration to the Infection Site**
        1. Once the leukocytes enter the connective tissue, the cells must migrate to the site of the infection.
        2. Chemotaxis is the process whereby leukocytes are attracted to the infection site in response to biochemical compounds released by the invading microorganisms.

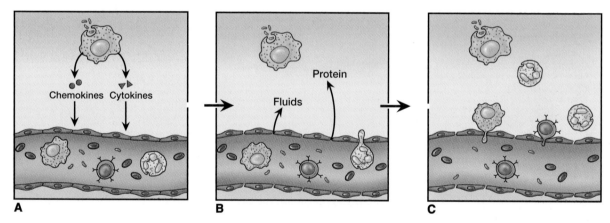

Figure 8.9. Leukocyte Migration To Connective Tissue. A: Leukocytes travel through the blood stream to the site of infection. **B:** Leukocytes squeeze between the cells of the blood vessel wall. **C:** Leukocytes enter the connective tissue and are attracted to the invading bacteria.

2. **Phagocytosis**
    A. **Description.** Phagocytosis is the process by which leukocytes engulf and digest microorganisms [4].
        1. Steps in phagocytosis
            a. First, the external cell wall of a phagocytic cell (such as a neutrophil or macrophage) adheres to the bacterium (FIG. 8-10). The phagocytic cell extends fingerlike projections (pseudopodia) that surround the bacterium.
            b. Next, a phagocytic vesicle called a phagosome surrounds the bacterium.
            c. Lysosome granules fuse with the vesicle to form a phagolysosome.
            d. The bacterium is digested within the phagolysosome.

   e. Finally, the phagocytic cell discharges the contents of the phagolysosome into the surrounding tissue.

2. **Local tissue destruction from phagocytosis**

   a. Lysosomal enzymes and other microbial products are released from a leukocyte after phagocytosis or when the leukocyte dies.

   b. Once released, the lysosomal enzymes cause damage to tissue cells in the same manner that they destroy bacteria.

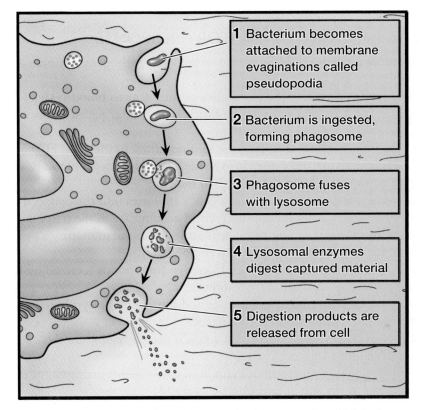

1 Bacterium becomes attached to membrane evaginations called pseudopodia

2 Bacterium is ingested, forming phagosome

3 Phagosome fuses with lysosome

4 Lysosomal enzymes digest captured material

5 Digestion products are released from cell

Figure 8.10. **Phagocytosis**. The steps involved in phagocytosis, the process by which leukocytes engulf and digest microorganisms.

Section 3
The Inflammatory Process

Inflammation is the body's reaction to injury or invasion by disease-producing organisms. The inflammatory response focuses host defense components at the site of the infection to eliminate microorganisms and heal damaged tissue. Inflammation is part of the immune response. It is a process that depends both on the physical actions of leukocytes and the biochemical compounds that these cells produce [1,2].

MAJOR EVENTS IN THE INFLAMMATORY RESPONSE

1. The inflammatory response is triggered by the invasion of pathogens or tissue injury.
2. Immediately, mast cells (located in the connective tissues near to blood vessels) release chemicals that dilate the capillaries and increase vascular permeability (FIG. 8-11).
3. Minutes after tissue injury, there is an increase in blood flow to the area. Higher blood volume heats the tissue and causes it to redden. This increased blood flow is needed to deliver immune "cellular defenders" to the site.
4. Within hours, leukocytes pass through the walls of capillaries into the connective tissue. Plasma proteins leak from the capillaries and accumulate in the tissues.
5. The leukocytes phagocytose invading pathogens and release inflammatory mediators that contribute to the inflammatory response.
   A. **Inflammatory biochemical mediators** are bioactive compounds secreted by cells that activate the body's inflammatory response.
   B. Inflammatory mediators of importance in periodontitis are the cytokines, prostaglandins, and matrix metalloproteinases.
      1. Leukocytes secrete cytokines that play a major role in regulating the behavior of immune cells.
      2. Chemokines, a major subgroup of cytokines, cause additional immune cells to be attracted to the site of infection or injury [5].

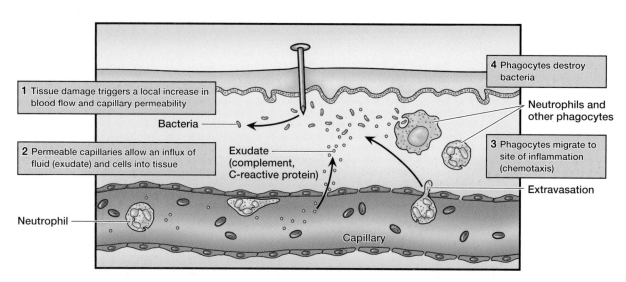

Figure 8.11. Inflammatory Response. In this illustration, bacteria have entered the body through a wound created by a nail puncture. The entry of bacteria initiates an inflammatory response that begins with the release of chemical substances that attract phagocytic cells to the site of the bacterial invasion.

TWO STAGES OF INFLAMMATION

1. **Acute Inflammation**
    A. **Description**
        1. Acute inflammation is a short-term, **normal** process that protects and heals the body following physical injury or infection (FIG. 8-12).
        2. In the absence of inflammation, wounds and infections would never heal and the progressive tissue destruction would threaten the life of the individual.
        3. The acute inflammatory process is achieved by the increased movement of plasma and leukocytes from the blood into the injured tissues.

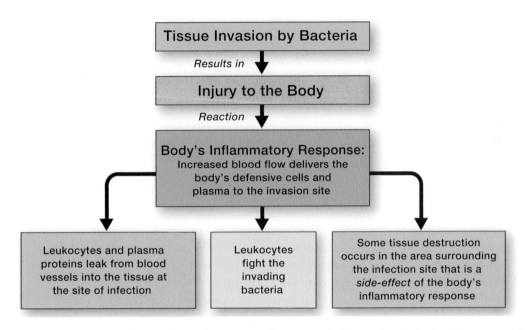

Figure 8.12. **Major Events in the Body's Inflammatory Response.** Inflammation is the body's response to injury or invasion by disease-producing organisms. This response focuses the body's defense mechanisms at the site of an injury or infection.

    B. **Five Classic Symptoms of Acute Inflammation.** To inflame means "to set on fire," which makes us think of red, heat, and pain. Clinically, there are five classic symptoms of acute inflammation (Box 8-1) at the site of infection or injury:
        1. **Heat**—a localized rise in temperature due to an increased amount of blood at the site.
        2. **Redness**—the result of increased blood in the area.
        3. **Swelling**—the result of the accumulation of fluid at the site. The leukocytes and plasma that collect at the site cause the swelling (edema) associated with inflammation.
        4. **Pain**—the result of pressure from edema in the tissue. The excess fluid in the tissues puts pressure on sensitive nerve endings, causing pain.
        5. **Loss of function**—the result of swelling and pain. For example, inflammation of a finger (swelling and pain) would cause you to favor that finger and not use it in a normal manner.

Box 8.1 Everyday Example of Acute Inflammation

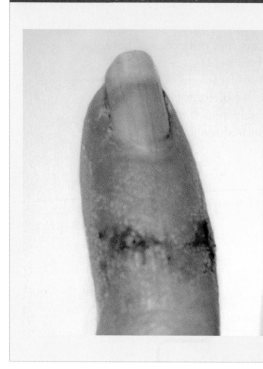

Callie L. sustained a deep cut to her little finger. She applied an antiseptic cream and covered the wound with an adhesive bandage. A few hours later, the injured finger is quite painful. When Callie applies pressure to the area near the wound, it feels warm and the pressure of her touch is quite painful. The finger looks red and swollen.

What is the source of the redness?
The redness is due to increased blood flow at the injury site.

What is the primary source of the swelling?
The primary source of the swelling is caused by the entry of fluid into the connective tissue. Cells entering the connective tissue also contribute to the swelling.

What is the cause of the warmth?
The warmth of an inflamed area results from increased blood flow to the area that brings with it the warmth.

C. The Acute Inflammatory Process
  1. **Description.** The process of acute inflammation is initiated by the blood vessels near the injured tissue, which alter to allow the release of plasma proteins and leukocytes into the surrounding tissue.
  2. PMNs are the first leukocytes to arrive at the injured site.
     a. These cells phagocytose and kill invading microorganisms through the release of nonspecific toxins. These nonspecific toxins kill pathogens as well as adjacent host cells, sick and healthy alike.
     b. The PMNs release cytokines, including IL and tumor necrosis factor (TNF).
     c. Such inflammatory cytokines in turn induce the liver to synthesize various plasma proteins called acute phase reactant proteins.
        1) The liver produces C-reactive protein (CRP), a type of acute phase protein, during episodes of acute inflammation. The levels of CRP increase up to 50,000-fold in acute inflammation.
        2) Recent research indicates that patients with elevated levels of CRP are at increased risk for diabetes, hypertension, and cardiovascular disease.
        3) *A study published in the Journal of Periodontology reports that the inflammatory effects from periodontal disease cause oral bacterial by-products to enter the bloodstream. These bacterial by-products trigger the liver to make CRP that inflames the arteries and promotes blood clot formation* [6].
  3. PMNs are short lived and so are primarily involved in the early stages of inflammation.
  4. If the body succeeds in eliminating all microorganisms, the tissue will heal and the inflammation will cease.
  5. Inflammation is the body's first line of defense against injury and infection, but it is a double-edged sword. If the acute inflammatory responses are not effective in controlling the invading microorganisms, the inflammatory response becomes chronic (FIG. 8-14).

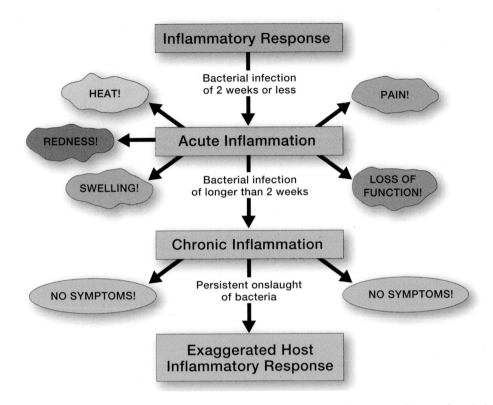

Figure 8.14. Two Stages of Inflammation. Acute inflammation is of short duration, whereas chronic inflammation is a long-lived inflammatory response.

2. **Chronic inflammation**
   A. **Description**
      1. Chronic inflammation is a long-lived, **out-of-control** inflammatory response that continues for more than a few weeks.
         a. It is a pathological condition characterized by active inflammation, tissue destruction, and attempts at repair.
         b. *The warning signs of acute inflammation are absent in chronic inflammation—such as periodontitis—and the problem may go unnoticed by the host (patient). Clinically, pain often is absent.*
      2. The inflammatory response has one all-important goal: respond immediately to destroy infectious microorganisms in the damaged tissue before they can spread to other areas of the body.
         a. Chronic inflammation occurs when the body is unable to eliminate the infection. In this stage, the invading microorganisms are persistent and stimulate an exaggerated response by the host's immune system.
         b. In its zeal to protect the body, the inflammatory response will destroy as much tissue as necessary to accomplish this goal.
         c. *In cases where inflammation becomes chronic, the inflammation can become so intense that it inflicts permanent damage to the body tissues.* This is the case in periodontitis.
   B. **The Chronic Inflammatory Process**
      1. The accumulation of macrophages characterizes chronic inflammation.
      2. Macrophages engulf and digest microorganisms.
      3. Leukocytes release several different inflammatory mediators, including IL-1, TNF-alpha, and prostaglandins that perpetuate the inflammatory response (FIG. 8-15).

a. One of the principle cytokines secreted by macrophages is TNF-alpha [7]. Evidence indicates that TNF-alpha contributes to the tissue destruction that characterizes chronic inflammation (TABLE 8-2).

b. In fact, ***tissue damage is the hallmark of chronic inflammation.***

4. If the infection persists, inflammation can last months or even years.

5. Chronic inflammation is abnormal and does not benefit the body. ***Chronic inflammation is an out-of-control response that can destroy healthy tissue and cause more damage than the original problem.***

a. Left unchecked, a hyperactive inflammatory response can even start attacking healthy tissue.

b. Chronic inflammation is associated with a number of disease states, including asthma, rheumatoid arthritis, diabetes, atherosclerosis, gingivitis, and periodontitis.

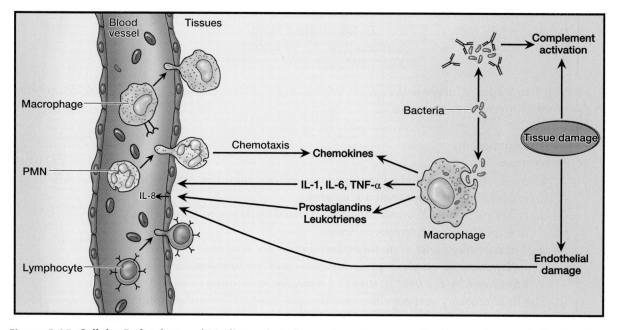

Figure 8.15. Cellular Defenders and Mediators in Inflammatory Response. The three primary cells involved in the inflammatory response are the Polymorphonuclear leukocytes (PMNs), macrophages, and lymphocytes. The first of these cells to migrate into the tissues are the PMNs, followed by macrophages, and then the lymphocytes. In addition, this illustration shows some of the many chemical mediators that play a part in the inflammatory response. These include chemokines, IL-1, IL-6, TNF-alpha, prostaglandins, and leukotrienes.

TABLE 8-2. Inflammatory Biochemical Mediators

Name	Effects
IL-1	Increased vascular permeability
	T-cell and B-cell activation
	Fever
	Synthesis of proteins, such as C-reactive protein, by liver
IL-6	Increased vascular permeability
	T-cell and B-cell activation
	Increased immunoglobulin synthesis
	Fever
	Synthesis of proteins, such as C-reactive protein, by liver
IL-8	Attraction of PMNs to the infection site
Leukotrienes	Allow leukocytes to exit the blood vessel and move into the connective tissue
Prostaglandins	Cause vasodilatation, fever, and pain
TNF-alpha	Increased vascular permeability
	Chemotaxis
	T-cell and B-cell activation
	Fever
	Synthesis of proteins, such as C-reactive protein, by liver
	Systemic effects of inflammation such as loss of appetite and increased heart rate

Chapter Summary Statement

The immune system is a collection of responses that is responsible for defending the body against millions of bacteria, viruses, fungi, toxins, and parasites. The prime purpose of the human immune system is to defend the life of the individual (host) by identifying foreign substances and developing a defense against them. The way that an individual's body responds to infection is known as the host response. Without an effective immune system, human beings would not survive.

Components of the immune system that play an important role in combating periodontal disease are the cellular defenders and the complement system. In order to fight an infection, immune cells travel through the blood stream and into the tissues (transendothelial migration). The process whereby leukocytes are attracted to the infection site in response to the invading microorganisms is known as chemotaxis. Phagocytosis is the process by which leukocytes engulf and digest microorganisms.

Inflammation is the body's reaction to injury or invasion by disease-producing organisms. The inflammatory response focuses host immune components at the site of an infection to eliminate microorganisms and heal damaged tissue. It relies on both the physical actions of leukocytes and the biochemical compounds that these cells produce. Acute inflammation is a short-term, normal process that protects and heals the body. Chronic inflammation is a long-lived, out-of-control response that continues for more than a few weeks. In chronic inflammation, the immune system response can sometimes become so intense that it begins to harm the body that it is trying to protect. Tissue damage is the hallmark of chronic inflammation.

Periodontal disease is a bacterial infection that induces an inflammatory response in the periodontal tissues. Chapter 9 focuses on the host immune response to periodontal pathogens.

Section 4
Focus on Patients

Case 1

You suddenly injure your arm by accidentally stabbing it with an ice pick. Within minutes following the injury, you note some changes in the tissues in the area of the injury. What changes in the tissues should you expect if your body responds with a typical inflammatory response?

References

1. Janeway C, Murphy KP, Travers P, et al. *Janeway's Immunobiology*. 7th ed. New York: Garland Science; 2008:887, xxi.

2. Paul WE. *Fundamental Immunology*. 6th ed. Philadelphia: Wolters Kluwer Health/Lippincott Williams & Wilkins; 2008:1603, xviii.

3. Marshall D, Haskard DO. Clinical overview of leukocyte adhesion and migration: where are we now? *Semin Immunol*. 2002;14(2):133–140.

4. Greenberg S, Grinstein S. Phagocytosis and innate immunity. *Curr Opin Immunol*. 2002;14(1):136–145.

5. Van Haastert PJ, Devreotes PN. Chemotaxis: signalling the way forward. *Nat Rev Mol Cell Biol*. 2004;5(8):626–634.

6. Noack B, Genco RJ, Trevisan M, et al. Periodontal infections contribute to elevated systemic C-reactive protein level. *J Periodontol*. 2001;72(9):1221–1227.

7. Tieri P, Valensin S, Latora V, et al. Quantifying the relevance of different mediators in the human immune cell network. *Bioinformatics*. 2005;21(8):1639–1643.

Host Immune Response to Periodontal Pathogens

Learning Objectives

- Define the term immune system and name its primary function.

- Examine the periodontium of a patient with gingivitis and point out the signs of inflammation that are visible in the tissues.

- Define the term biochemical mediator and name three types of mediators.

- Describe the tissue destruction that can be initiated by the biochemical mediators secreted by immune cells.

- Describe the sequential development of periodontal disease.

- Describe the role of the host response in the severity and tissue destruction seen in periodontitis.

- Explain immunologic interactions of the host in periodontal diseases.

- Describe and differentiate the mechanisms of tissue destruction in periodontal disease.

- Describe and discuss current knowledge of the immunopathology of periodontal disease.

Key Terms

Host response
Host
Biochemical mediators
Cytokines

Prostaglandins
Prostaglandins of the E series (PGE)
Matrix metalloproteinases (MMPs)

Section 1
The Role of Host Response in Periodontal Disease

Periodontal disease is a bacterial infection that induces an inflammatory response in the periodontal tissues [1]. For the progression from gingivitis to periodontitis, pathogenic bacteria must be present. For many years, it was assumed that pathogenic bacteria were the sole cause of the tissue destruction seen in periodontal disease. *Research findings indicate that although bacteria are essential for disease to occur, the presence of periodontal pathogens alone is insufficient to cause the tissue destruction seen in periodontitis. Rather, it is the body's response to the periodontal pathogens that is the cause of nearly all the destruction seen in periodontal disease* [2–6].

The way that the body responds to periodontal pathogens is known as the host response. The prime purpose of the human immune system is to defend the life of the individual (host). In the instance of periodontal disease, the immune system strives to defend the body against periodontal pathogens. The body's defenses are employed with the purpose of saving the life of the host, not to preserve the tooth or its supporting periodontal tissues. This chapter focuses on the host immune response to periodontal pathogens and the tissue destruction that ensues when periodontal pathogens elicit a chronic inflammatory response in the host.

INFLAMMATORY BIOCHEMICAL MEDIATORS

When pathogenic bacteria successfully infect the periodontium, the body responds by mobilizing defensive immune cells and releasing a series of biochemical mediators to combat them. Immune cells secrete biologically active compounds—called biochemical mediators—that activate the body's inflammatory response. Biochemical mediators are the "middlemen" sent by the host cells to activate the inflammatory response. Inflammatory mediators of importance in periodontitis are the cytokines, prostaglandins, and matrix metalloproteinases (TABLE 9-1).

1. **Cytokines.** Cytokines are powerful regulatory proteins released by immune cells that influence the behavior of other cells. The cytokine (literally "cell protein") is a molecule that transmits information or signals from one cell to another. When released by host cells, cytokines signal the immune system to send additional phagocytic cells to the site of an infection.
   A. **Sources of Cytokines.** Many different cells including PMNs, macrophages, B lymphocytes, epithelial cells, gingival fibroblasts, and osteoblasts produce cytokines in response to microorganisms or tissue injury.
   B. **Functions of Cytokines**
      1. Recruit cells such as PMNs and macrophages to the infection site.
      2. Increase vascular permeability allowing immune cells and complement to move into the tissues at the infection site.
      3. *Have the potential to initiate tissue destruction and bone loss in chronic inflammatory diseases, such as periodontitis.*
      4. Cytokines that play an important role in periodontitis include interleukin-1 (IL-1), interleukin-6 (IL-6), interleukin-8 (IL-8), and tumor necrosis factor-α (TNF-α) [7].
2. **Prostaglandins.** Prostaglandins are a series of powerful biochemical mediators, of which prostaglandins D, E, F, G, H, and I are the most important biologically. Prostaglandins of the E series (PGE) play an important role in the bone destruction seen in periodontitis.

A. **Sources of Prostaglandins.** Most cells can produce prostaglandins, but PMNs and macrophages are particularly important sources. The major source of PGE in inflamed periodontal tissues is the macrophage, although PMNs and gingival fibroblasts also produce them.

B. **Functions of Prostaglandins**

1. Increase the permeability and dilation of the blood vessels, leading to redness and edema of the connective tissue.
2. Trigger osteoclasts—bone-consuming cells—to destroy the alveolar bone.
3. Promote the overproduction of destructive MMP enzymes.
4. *Prostaglandins initiate most of the alveolar bone destruction in periodontitis.*

3. **Matrix Metalloproteinases.** Matrix metalloproteinases (MMPs) are a family of at least 12 different enzymes produced by various cells of the body. These enzymes can act together to break down the connective tissue matrix.

A. **Sources of MMPs.** PMNs, macrophages, gingival fibroblasts, and junctional epithelial cells produce MMPs. PMNs and gingival fibroblasts are the major source of MMPs in periodontitis.

B. **Functions of MMPs.**

1. MMPs' effects in health. Under normal, healthy conditions, MMPs facilitate the normal turnover of the periodontal connective tissue matrix.
2. MMPs' effects in chronic infection and inflammation
   a. In the presence of chronic bacterial infection, large amounts of MMPs are released in an attempt to kill the invading bacteria.
   b. This overproduction of MMPs results in the breakdown of the connective tissue of the periodontium.
   c. *In the presence of increased MMP levels, extensive collagen destruction occurs in the periodontal tissues.* Collagen provides the structural framework of all periodontal tissues. Without collagen, the tissues of the gingiva, periodontal ligament, and supporting alveolar bone degrade, resulting in recession of gingival margin, pocket formation, and tooth mobility.

TABLE 9-1. Tissue Destruction by Biochemical Mediators in Periodontitis

Mediators	Local Effects
Cytokine IL-1	Stimulates osteoclast activity, resulting in bone resorption [8–10]
	Induces breakdown of collagen matrix in the gingiva, periodontal ligament, and alveolar bone [10,11]
Cytokine IL-6	Stimulates bone resorption [12]
	Inhibits bone formation [13]
Cytokine IL-8	Stimulates connective tissue destruction [14]
	Stimulates bone resorption [8,9,15,16]
Cytokine TNF-α	Stimulates bone resorption [9]
	Induces breakdown of collagen matrix in the gingiva, periodontal ligament, and alveolar bone [9]
Prostaglandin E_2	Stimulates MMP secretion [4,17]
	Stimulates bone resorption [9,18–20]
MMP enzymes	Induce breakdown of collagen matrix in the gingiva, periodontal ligament, and alveolar bone [11,21]

Section 2
Pathogenesis of Inflammatory Periodontal Disease

Marked changes occur in the periodontium as the result of the body's inflammatory response to bacterial invasion of the junctional epithelium and gingival connective tissue. R.C. Page and H.E. Schroeder [4,5] described the distinct stages in histologic development of gingivitis and periodontitis: (1) early plaque biofilm accumulation phase, (2) early gingivitis, (3) established gingivitis, and (4) periodontitis.

EARLY BACTERIAL ACCUMULATION PHASE (FIG. 9-1)

1. **Initial Bacterial Colonization.** Bacteria colonize the tooth surface near the gingival margin.

2. **Initiation of Host Response.** The presence of Gram-negative bacteria and their metabolic products initiates the host immune response.
   A. In response to the bacterial pathogens, the junctional epithelial cells release various biochemical mediators, including *cytokines, PGE$_2$, MMPs, and TNF-α.*
   B. These mediators stimulate the immune response, recruiting polymorphonuclear leukocytes (PMNs) to the site.
   C. PMNs pass from blood vessels into the gingival connective tissue.
      1. The PMNs need to reach the sulcus in order to fight the bacterial infection located there and so must travel through the gingival connective tissue toward the junctional epithelium and the gingival sulcus.
      2. As they pass into the gingival connective tissue, the PMNs release cytokines. *Cytokines released by the PMNs destroy healthy gingival connective tissue, creating a pathway that allows the PMNs to move quickly through the tissue.*
      3. The goal of the PMNs is to reach the bacteria in the sulcus and destroy them. The damage to the healthy connective tissue is not a concern. In a healthy body, this tissue destruction will be repaired after the bacterial infection is brought under control.
   D. PMNs migrate into sulcus and phagocytize bacteria.

3. **Activation of Complement System.** The presence of Gram-negative bacteria activates the complement system.

4. **Outcome of Host Response**
   A. The host response is successful if all the periodontal pathogens are destroyed.
   B. Initiation of good patient self-care can disrupt the plaque biofilm and result in a return to health. If the bacterial infection is brought under control—through the efforts of the immune system and effective plaque biofilm control—the body is able to repair the destruction caused by the immune response.
   C. If the bacterial pathogens are not controlled, however, early gingivitis develops.

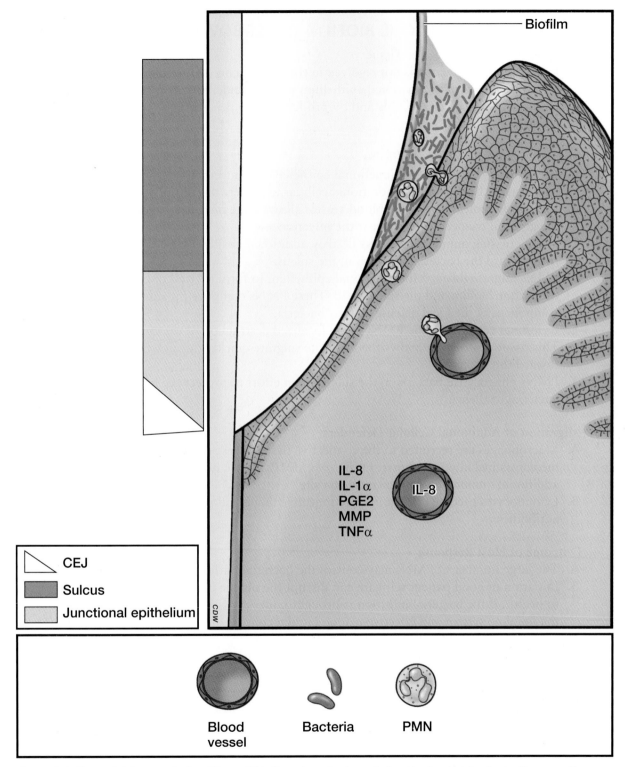

IL-8
IL-1α
PGE2
MMP
TNFα

CEJ
Sulcus
Junctional epithelium

Blood vessel

Bacteria

PMN

Biofilm

Figure 9.1. Bacterial Accumulation Phase. This first phase is characterized by bacterial colonization near the gingival margin.

EARLY GINGIVITIS: PLAQUE BIOFILM OVERGROWTH PHASE (FIG. 9-2)

1. **Pathogens Invade Connective Tissue**
   A. If the bacterial infection is not resolved in the early accumulation phase, the bacteria penetrate through the junctional epithelium into the underlying connective tissue.
   B. Unfortunately, bacterial toxins and by-products easily penetrate the junctional epithelium.

2. **Migration and Chemotaxis of PMNs**
   A. *Cytokines*—released by the junctional epithelial cells in response to the increased bacterial challenge—attract additional cellular defenders to the site.
   B. Increased permeability of the blood vessels allows large numbers of PMNs to rush into the gingival connective tissue near the infection site.
   C. The increasing numbers of PMNs destroy additional healthy gingival connective as they rush toward the bacterial invaders in the sulcus.
   D. PMNs migrate through the junctional epithelium to form a "wall of cells" between the plaque biofilm and the sulcus wall. These PMNs comprise the most important component of the local defense against bacteria.
   E. *Cytokines* released by the PMNs cause localized destruction of the connective tissue. This tissue destruction allows the PMNs to migrate quickly through the connective tissue toward the sulcus.
   F. PMNs phagocytize bacteria in the sulcus in an effort to protect the host tissues from the bacterial challenge.

3. **Migration of Additional Cellular Defenders**
   A. Macrophages are recruited to the connective tissue. These cells release many biochemical mediators including *cytokines, PGE_2, and MMPs*. These biochemical mediators recruit additional immune cells to the infection site.
   B. Lymphocytes become evident in the connective tissue and produce *cytokines* and antibodies.

4. **Outcome of Host Response**
   A. The large number of PMNs may control the bacterial pathogens.
   B. Initiation of good patient self-care can disrupt the plaque biofilm and result in a return to health. If the bacterial infection is brought under control—through the efforts of the immune system and effective plaque biofilm control—the body is able to repair the destruction caused by the immune response.
   C. If bacterial pathogens continue to proliferate, this early gingivitis will become established gingivitis—the next phase of disease progression.

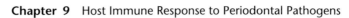

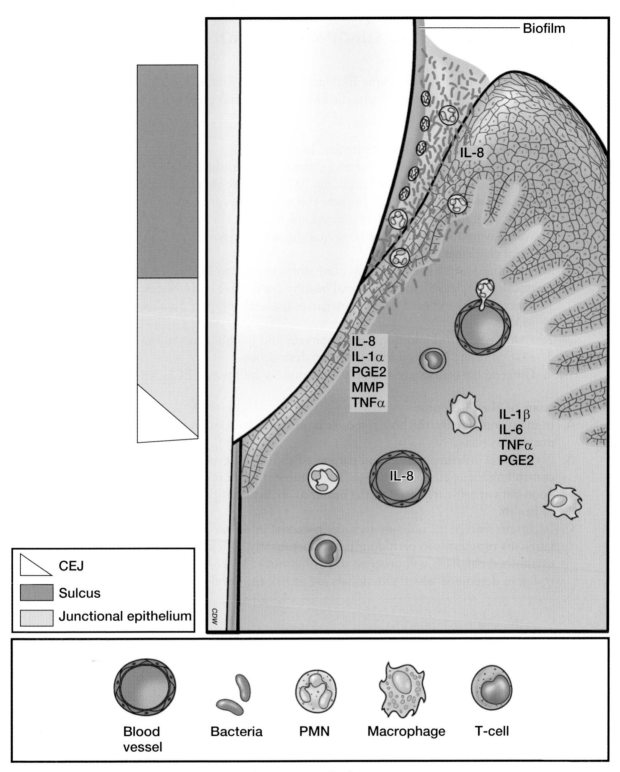

Figure 9.2. **Early Gingivitis: The Plaque Biofilm Overgrowth Phase.**

ESTABLISHED GINGIVITIS: SUBGINGIVAL PLAQUE BIOFILM PHASE (FIG. 9-3)

1. **Establishment of Subgingival Plaque Biofilm.** The plaque biofilm extends subgingivally into the gingival sulcus, disrupting the attachment of the coronal-most portion of the junctional epithelium from the tooth surface.

2. **Migration of Additional Cellular Defenders to Site**
    A. Large numbers of subgingival bacteria stimulate the epithelial cells to secrete *cytokines*, resulting in the recruitment of additional PMNs, macrophages, and lymphocytes.
    B. Macrophages and lymphocytes become the most numerous cells in the tissue. PMNs, however, continue to fight bacteria in the sulcus.
    C. Activated lymphocytes produce large quantities of antibodies to assist in controlling the bacterial challenge.
    D. The immune system keeps sending more immune cells to fight the bacteria. More toxic chemicals are released and additional healthy connective tissue is destroyed.
        1. Macrophages exposed to Gram-negative bacteria produce *cytokines, PGE_2*, and *MMPs*.
        2. *Cytokines* recruit additional macrophages and lymphocytes to the area.
        3. *PGE_2* and the *MMPs* initiate collagen destruction.
        4. Gingival fibroblasts are stimulated to produce additional *PGE_2* and *MMPs*.

3. **Outcome of Host Response**
    A. In many individuals, the host response is adequate to contain the bacterial challenge during this phase.
    B. Periodontal instrumentation and patient education, at this point, can be helpful in controlling the bacterial challenge. The combination of professional treatment and good patient self-care can stop the bacterial challenge and return the periodontium to health.
    C. In certain susceptible individuals if the bacterial infection is not controlled, established gingivitis progresses to periodontitis. Unfortunately, no one can predict when and if established gingivitis will progress to periodontitis. Much current research is directed to trying to determine which individuals are at risk for developing periodontitis.

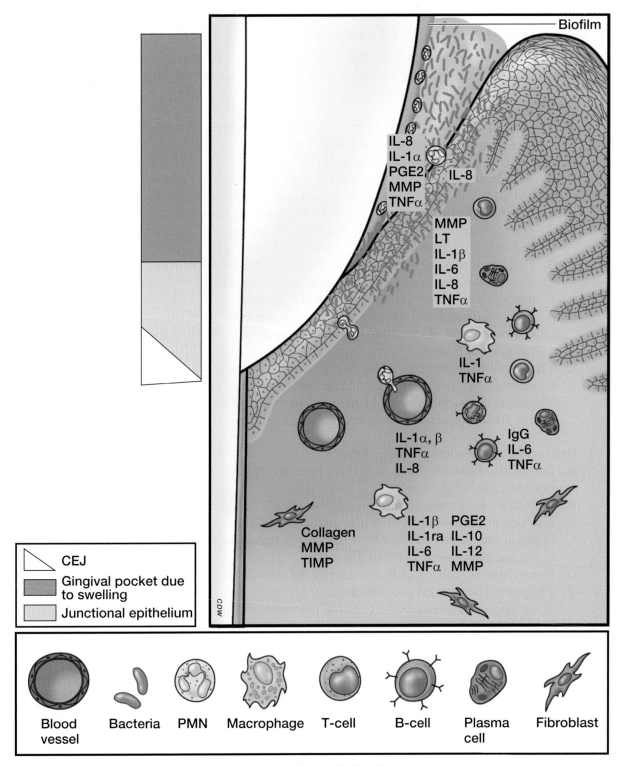

Figure 9.3. **Established Gingivitis: The Subgingival Plaque Biofilm Phase.**

PERIODONTITIS: TISSUE DESTRUCTION PHASE (FIG. 9-4)

1. **Bacterial Pathogens Flourish in Biofilm.** The plaque biofilm grows laterally and apically along the root surface and the transition from gingivitis to periodontitis is initiated.

2. **Host Response Intensifies**
   A. The bacterial infection becomes chronic, leading to chronic inflammation. *The immune response becomes so intense that it begins to harm the periodontium that it is trying to protect from the bacterial pathogens* [21,22].
   B. Cellular defenders intensify their defense against the bacterial pathogens.
      1. PMNs, macrophages, and epithelial cells produce *cytokines* that cause the *destruction of the gingival connective tissue and periodontal ligament fibers* [11].
      2. Macrophages produce high concentrations of *cytokines, PGE$_2$, and MMPs* that result in *destruction of connective tissue and alveolar bone* [9,21].
      3. High levels of *MMPs* are present in the tissues. MMPs mediate destruction of the extracellular matrix of the gingiva, attached collagen fibers at the apical edge of the junctional epithelium, and the periodontal ligament.
      4. *PGE$_2$* mediates bone destruction by stimulating large numbers of osteoclasts to resorb the crest of the alveolar bone. The gingival pocket progresses to become a periodontal pocket.
   C. The immune system keeps trying to eliminate the bacteria but the bacteria are not eliminated. As more and more immune cells rush to the site, more tissue is damaged. *The tissue destruction caused by the immune response now overwhelms any tissue repair. Tissue destruction becomes the main outcome of the immune system response.*

3. **Destruction of Periodontal Tissues Ensues**
   A. Basal cells of the junctional epithelium begin to replicate and extend epithelial ridges into the connective tissue.
   B. Cells of the junctional epithelium migrate apically and attach to the root surface, resulting in the development of a periodontal pocket.
   C. Gingival fibroblasts shift to a state that favors the *destruction of the gingival connective tissue and periodontal ligament fibers* (FIG. 9-5).
   D. Osteoclasts, stimulated by PGE$_2$, *destroy the crest of the alveolar bone* (FIG. 9-5).
   E. The periodontal pocket provides an ideal protected environment for continued growth of subgingival bacteria. These bacterial pathogens present a chronic, repeated challenge to the host.

4. **Outcome of Host Response**
   A. Chronic infection by the periodontal pathogens induces a chronic inflammatory response. *This chronic inflammation is an out-of-control response that destroys periodontal tissues and causes more damage to the periodontium than the bacterial infection. Tissue damage is the hallmark of periodontitis.*
   B. Factors influencing the host's failure to control the bacterial challenge may include
      1. Abnormal PMN function
      2. Persistence and virulence of bacteria in the biofilm
      3. Acquired and environmental factors such as smoking and stress
      4. Systemic factors such as uncontrolled diabetes mellitus or genetic factors

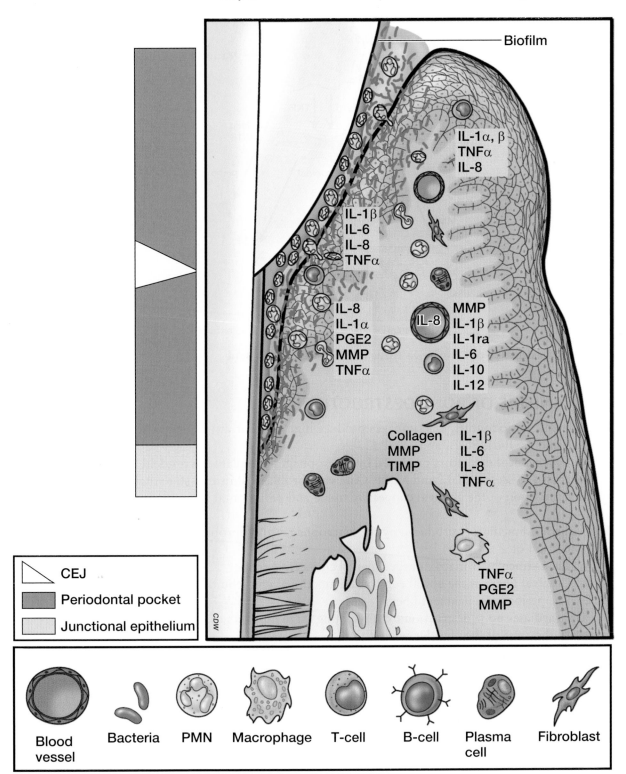

Figure 9.4. **Periodontitis: The Tissue Destruction Phase.**

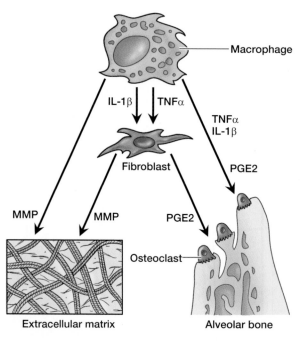

Figure 9.5. Destruction of Connective Tissue Matrix and Alveolar Bone.

MECHANISMS OF BONE DESTRUCTION

1. In chronic periodontitis, macrophages produce high concentrations of cytokines (IL-L and TNF-α), PGE$_2$, and MMP [23].
2. The biochemical mediators produced by macrophages stimulate the resident fibroblasts also to secrete PGE$_2$ and MMP. Gingival fibroblasts shift to a state that favors the destruction of the gingival connective tissue and periodontal ligament fibers [24].
3. Biochemical mediators produced by the macrophages and fibroblasts result in destruction of
   A. The extracellular matrix of the gingival connective tissue
   B. Gingival fibers at the apical edge of the junctional epithelium
   C. The periodontal ligament fibers.
4. PGE$_2$ mediates bone destruction by stimulating large numbers of osteoclasts to resorb the crest of the alveolar bone [9].

Chapter Summary Statement

The immune system provides the body with a strong defense against invading periodontal pathogens. In many cases, PMNs attracted to the site are able to contain the bacterial challenge and no tissue damage occurs. If the bacterial challenge is not contained, the plaque biofilm extends subgingivally and develops into a highly organized biofilm. In many cases, the host response still is able to contain the bacterial pathogens. In some individuals, however, the host resistance is insufficient to contain the bacterial challenge. Biochemical mediators produced by immune cells are largely responsible for the tissue destruction seen in periodontitis. High levels of cytokines, MMPs, and PGE_2 characterize periodontitis. The unrelenting, chronic bacterial infection triggers immune responses that (1) destroy the connective tissue of the gingiva and periodontal ligament and (2) resorb the alveolar bone.

Page and Schroeder described the distinct stages in histologic development of gingivitis and periodontitis: (1) early plaque biofilm accumulation phase, (2) early gingivitis, (3) established gingivitis, and (4) periodontitis.

Section 3
Focus on Patients

Case 1

In reading a dental journal you find an article that describes a new medication that is reported to stop collagen destruction by one of the matrix metalloproteinases (MMPs). If this new medication does indeed block such collagen destruction, what effect might this medication have on a patient with periodontitis?

Case 2

Mrs. Smith is a new patient in the dental office. Mrs. Smith is 45 years of age and works as an accountant. Mrs. Smith had not received regular dental care in the past; however, her new employer provides dental insurance for his employees. Mrs. Smith has chronic periodontitis. How will you explain inflammatory periodontal disease to Mrs. Smith?

References

1. Darveau RP, Tanner A, Page RC. The microbial challenge in periodontitis. *Periodontol 2000.* 1997;14:12–32.
2. Van Dyke TE, Serhan CN. Resolution of inflammation: a new paradigm for the pathogenesis of periodontal diseases. *J Dent Res.* 2003;82(2):82–90.
3. Kornman KS, Page RC, Tonetti MS. The host response to the microbial challenge in periodontitis: assembling the players. *Periodontol 2000.* 1997;14:33–53.
4. Page RC, Offenbacher S, Schroeder HE, et al. Advances in the pathogenesis of periodontitis: summary of developments, clinical implications and future directions. *Periodontol 2000.* 1997;14:216–248.
5. Page RC, Schroeder HE. Pathogenesis of inflammatory periodontal disease. A summary of current work. *Lab Invest.* 1976;34(3):235–249.
6. Oringer RJ. Modulation of the host response in periodontal therapy. *J Periodontol.* 2002;73(4):460–470.
7. Page RC. The role of inflammatory mediators in the pathogenesis of periodontal disease. *J Periodontal Res.* 1991;26(3 Pt 2):230–242.
8. Qwarnstrom EE, MacFarlane SA, Page RC. Effects of interleukin-1 on fibroblast extracellular matrix, using a 3-dimensional culture system. *J Cell Physiol.* 1989;139(3):501–508.
9. Schwartz Z, Goultschin J, Dean DD, et al. Mechanisms of alveolar bone destruction in periodontitis. *Periodontol 2000.* 1997;14:158–172.
10. McDevitt MJ, Wang HY, Knobelman C, et al. Interleukin-1 genetic association with periodontitis in clinical practice. *J Periodontol.* 2000;71(2):156–163.
11. Reynolds JJ, Meikle MC. Mechanisms of connective tissue matrix destruction in periodontitis. *Periodontol 2000.* 1997;14:144–157.
12. Roodman GD. Interleukin-6: an osteotropic factor? *J Bone Miner Res.* 1992;7(5):475–478.
13. Hughes FJ, Howells GL. Interleukin-6 inhibits bone formation in vitro. *Bone Miner.* 1993;21(1):21–28.
14. Meikle MC, Atkinson SJ, Ward RV, et al. Gingival fibroblasts degrade type I collagen films when stimulated with tumor necrosis factor and interleukin 1: evidence that breakdown is mediated by metalloproteinases. *J Periodontal Res.* 1989;24(3):207–213.
15. Bertolini DR, Nedwin GE, Bringman TS, et al. Stimulation of bone resorption and inhibition of bone formation in vitro by human tumour necrosis factors. *Nature.* 1986;319(6053):516–518.
16. Thomson BM, Mundy GR, Chambers TJ. Tumor necrosis factors alpha and beta induce osteoblastic cells to stimulate osteoclastic bone resorption. *J Immunol.* 1987;138(3):775–779.
17. Gemmell E, Marshall RI, Seymour GJ. Cytokines and prostaglandins in immune homeostasis and tissue destruction in periodontal disease. *Periodontol 2000.* 1997;14:112–143.
18. Dietrich JW, Goodson JM, Raisz LG. Stimulation of bone resorption by various prostaglandins in organ culture. *Prostaglandins.* 1975;10(2):231–240.
19. Offenbacher S, Farr DH, Goodson JM. Measurement of prostaglandin E in crevicular fluid. *J Clin Periodontol.* 1981;8(4):359–367.
20. Zubery Y, Dunstan CR, Story BM, et al. Bone resorption caused by three periodontal pathogens in vivo in mice is mediated in part by prostaglandin. *Infect Immun.* 1998;66(9):4158–4162.
21. Giannobile WV. Host-response therapeutics for periodontal diseases. *J Periodontol.* 2008; 79(8 Suppl):1592–1600.
22. Graves DT. The potential role of chemokines and inflammatory cytokines in periodontal disease progression. *Clin Infect Dis.* 1999;28(3):482–490.
23. McCauley LK, Nohutcu RM. Mediators of periodontal osseous destruction and remodeling: principles and implications for diagnosis and therapy. *J Periodontol.* 2002;73(11):1377–1391.
24. Dongari-Bagtzoglou AI, Ebersole JL. Gingival fibroblast cytokine profiles in *Actinobacillus actinomycetemcomitans*-associated periodontitis. *J Periodontol.* 1996;67(9):871–878.

Chapter 10

Systemic Factors Associated with Periodontal Disease

Learning Objectives

- Describe systemic factors that may modify or amplify the host response to periodontal pathogens.

- In the clinical setting, for a patient in your care with periodontitis, explain to your clinical instructor the risk factors that may have contributed to your patient's periodontitis.

- Define the terms Type I diabetes, Type II diabetes, and gestational diabetes.

- Discuss the implications of diabetes on the periodontium.

- Define the term osteoporosis and discuss the link between skeletal osteoporosis and alveolar bone loss in the jaw.

- Discuss how hormone alterations may affect the periodontium.

- Define the term pregnancy-associated pyogenic granuloma.

- Explain how abnormalities of polymorphonuclear leukocytes may affect the body's response to periodontal pathogens.

- Describe the genetic and physical characteristics of Down syndrome.

- Discuss the implications of Down syndrome on the periodontium.

- Define the term drug-influenced gingival enlargement.

- Name three medications that can cause gingival enlargement.

Key Terms

Systemic risk factors
Diabetes mellitus
Type I diabetes mellitus
Type II diabetes mellitus
Gestational diabetes
Well-controlled diabetes
Leukemia
Acquired immunodeficiency syndrome (AIDS)
Linear gingival erythema (LGE)
Osteoporosis

Osteopenia
Postmenopausal osteoporosis
Pregnancy gingivitis
Pregnancy-associated pyogenic granuloma
Menopausal gingivostomatitis
Drug-influenced gingival enlargement
Phenytoin
Cyclosporine
Nifedipine

Section 1
Systemic Risk Factors for Periodontitis

Additional factors, other than the presence of bacteria, play a significant role in determining why some individuals are more susceptible to periodontal disease than others.

Susceptibility to periodontitis may be increased by systemic risk factors that modify or amplify the host response to the bacterial infection. Systemic risk factors are conditions or diseases that increase an individual's susceptibility to periodontal infection by modifying or amplifying the host response to the bacterial infection.

Proven systemic risk factors include diabetes mellitus, osteoporosis, hormone alteration, medications, tobacco use, and genetic influences. *Tobacco use as a risk factor for periodontal disease is discussed in Chapter 11.*

DIABETES MELLITUS

1. **Introduction to Diabetes Mellitus.** Diabetes mellitus is a disease in which the body does not produce or properly use insulin. Insulin is a hormone that is needed to convert sugar, starches, and other food into energy that the body uses to sustain life.
   A. **Types of Diabetes Mellitus**
      1. Type I Diabetes Mellitus (previously called insulin-dependent diabetes mellitus or juvenile-onset diabetes)
         a. Type I diabetes mellitus (type 1 DM) is caused by destruction of the insulin-producing cells of the pancreas. The pancreas is an organ (located near the stomach) that produces insulin. Insulin is a hormone that allows the body cells to take in the glucose that they need. Without insulin, the glucose stays in the bloodstream instead of going into the cells. The glucose builds up in the blood, resulting in diabetes.
         b. This type accounts for approximately 10% of all diagnosed cases of diabetes mellitus.
         c. Treatment of type 1 diabetes includes a carefully calculated diet, exercise, home blood glucose testing several times a day, and multiple daily insulin injections to replace the insulin hormone that the pancreas no longer makes.
      2. Type II Diabetes Mellitus (previously called non–insulin-dependent diabetes mellitus [NIDDM] or adult-onset diabetes)
         a. Type II diabetes mellitus (type 2 DM) occurs when (1) the body does not make enough insulin hormone and/or (2) the body cells ignore the insulin and fail to use it to help bring glucose into the cells.
         b. This type is the most common form of diabetes. The onset of symptoms in type 2 DM is more gradual and less severe, usually presenting after the age 40 years.
         c. Treatment of type 2 diabetes includes diet control, exercise, home glucose testing, oral medication, and/or insulin. Approximately 40% of people with type 2 diabetes require insulin injections.
      3. Gestational Diabetes
         a. Gestational diabetes is a form of diabetes that occurs during pregnancy in women who have never had diabetes before pregnancy. Gestational diabetes starts when a woman's body is not able to make and use all the insulin it needs for pregnancy. This type of diabetes usually disappears when the pregnancy is over.
         b. This type affects about 4% of all pregnant women, about 135,000 cases in the United States each year.

    c. Persons at risk for gestational diabetes include women who are 25 years or older; were overweight before becoming pregnant; have a family history of diabetes; and are Hispanics, African Americans, Native Americans, Asian Americans, or Pacific Islanders.

  B. Children and Adolescents with Diabetes

    1. Researchers at Columbia University reported on the largest study, to date, of 6- to 18-year-old individuals with diabetes and 350 individuals in the same age group without diabetes.

    2. The children and adolescents with diabetes showed significantly more periodontal disease than those without diabetes. Children and adolescents with diabetes had greater attachment loss than those without diabetes.

    3. Based on these findings, children with diabetes should be examined for signs of periodontal disease and receive early intervention and prevention [1].

2. Diabetes Mellitus and Risk of Periodontitis.

  A. Incidence of Periodontitis

    1. Patients with well-controlled diabetes have no more periodontal disease than persons without diabetes.

      a. Diabetes is well-controlled if the blood glucose levels are stabilized within the recommended range.

      b. The short-term nonsurgical periodontal treatment response of individuals with controlled diabetes is similar to that of nondiabetic controls, with similar trends in improved probing depth and attachment gain [2].

    2. Individuals with *undiagnosed or poorly controlled diabetes* are at greater risk for severe periodontitis than are persons with controlled diabetes and nondiabetic individuals.

      a. There is good evidence to support an association between poorly controlled diabetes mellitus and periodontitis. Periodontal disease is considered a complication of uncontrolled diabetes.

      b. Periodontal attachment loss (connective tissue destruction and bone loss) occurs more frequently in individuals with poorly controlled diabetes, of both type 1 and type 2 DM, than in individuals with well-controlled diabetes [3].

    3. An unfavorable treatment outcome may occur in long-term maintenance therapy of individuals with poorly controlled diabetes [4].

  B. Effects of Increased Glucose Blood Levels on the Periodontium. An individual with uncontrolled or poorly controlled blood glucose levels has an increased risk for developing acute periodontal abscesses, more extensive attachment loss, and a much greater risk of progressive bone loss.

    1. Hyperglycemia (high blood sugar) in uncontrolled diabetics results in increased glucose in the gingival crevicular fluid and blood. Since many bacteria thrive on sugars, this glucose-rich crevicular fluid may result in altered bacterial composition within the plaque biofilm microcolonies and influence the development of periodontal disease [5].

    2. Reduced PMN function and defective chemotaxis in uncontrolled diabetics can contribute to impaired host defenses (FIG. 10-1). Since PMNs are the first line of defense against periodontal pathogens, reduced PMN function allows the bacteria to increase greatly in number [6].

    3. Individuals who have both diabetes and periodontitis have significantly higher levels of IL-1β and PGE2 in the gingival crevicular fluid compared to nondiabetic controls with a similar degree of periodontal disease [7].

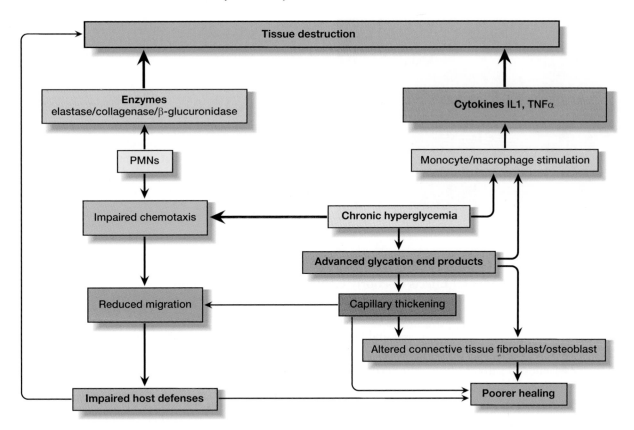

Figure 10.1. **Effects of Uncontrolled Diabetes Mellitus on the Host Response.**

   4. Hyperglycemia can affect the synthesis, maturation, and maintenance of collagen and extracellular matrix.
   a. The hyperglycemic state results in the excessive formation of accumulated glycation end-products (AGE). AGE are derived from the reaction of glucose and proteins. These substances are involved in biological processes relating to collagen turnover. Excessive accumulation of AGE is believed to contribute to the chronic health complications associated with diabetes. AGE may play a significant role in the progression of periodontal disease, as well, in uncontrolled diabetes.
   b. Collagen is cross-linked by AGE formation, making it less likely to be normally repaired or newly synthesized. Collagen in the gingival tissues of individuals with uncontrolled diabetes is aged and more susceptible to breakdown.
C. Implications of Diabetes for the Periodontium
   1. The rate of development of periodontal disease in subjects with poorly controlled diabetes is two to three times greater than that observed in nondiabetic patients (Fig. 10-2).
   2. The response of well-controlled diabetics to nonsurgical periodontal therapy, including periodontal debridement of tooth surfaces, appears to be similar to that of nondiabetic individuals.
   3. Patients with poorly controlled diabetes have a poorer response to nonsurgical and surgical periodontal therapies, more rapid recurrence of deep pockets, and a less favorable long-term response to treatment.
   4. A diabetic who smokes, and who is age 45 or older, is 20 times more likely than a nondiabetic, nonsmoking individual to experience severe periodontitis.

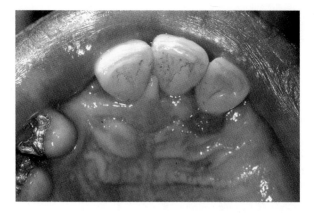

Figure 10.2. Inflammatory Reaction. Note the localized inflammatory swelling of the gingiva on the palatal surface of the maxillary lateral incisor. The patient has uncontrolled diabetes mellitus. This intense inflammatory reaction is typical for individuals with uncontrolled diabetes. (Courtesy of Dr Ralph Arnold, San Antonio, TX.)

D. **Oral and Periodontal Effects of Poorly Controlled Diabetes Mellitus**
  1. Reduced salivary flow and burning mouth or tongue are common complaints of patients with uncontrolled diabetes. Dental healthcare professionals should suspect undiagnosed diabetes as a likely cause of burning tongue and refer the patient to a physician for follow-up care.
  2. Reduced salivary flow and xerostomia can encourage the growth of *Candida albicans* and the development of oral candidiasis [6].
  3. Individuals with undiagnosed or poorly controlled diabetes frequently present with multiple periodontal abscesses, leading to rapid destruction of periodontal bone support.
E. **Implications for the Dental Hygienist**
  1. The level of diabetic control and the health status should be carefully monitored for all individuals with diabetes.
  2. The dental hygienist should emphasize the importance of careful self-care at home and frequent professional care visits.

LEUKEMIA

1. **Introduction to Leukemia**
  A. **Characteristics**
    1. Leukemia is cancer that begins in blood cells. In people with leukemia, the bone marrow produces a large number of abnormal white blood cells that do not function properly. At first, leukemia cells function almost normally. In time, they may crowd out normal white blood cells, red blood cells, and platelets. This makes it hard for the blood to do its work.
    2. The National Cancer Institute estimates that there were 44,270 new cases and 21,710 deaths from leukemia in the United States in 2008. Leukemia is a disease of both children and adults and is more common in men and boys than girls and women.
  B. **Types of Leukemia**
    1. Leukemia is classified on the duration (acute or chronic) and the type of cell involved (myeloid or lymphoid).
    2. Leukemia is either *chronic* (gets worse slowly) of *acute* (gets worse quickly).
    3. Leukemia that affects the lymphoid cells is called *lymphocytic*. Leukemia that affects the myeloid cells is called *myelogenous* leukemia.

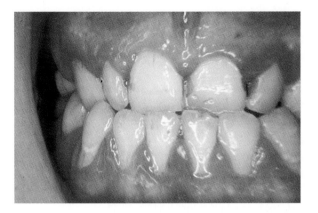

Figure 10.3. Leukemia-Associated Gingivitis. Note the swollen, red gingival tissues in this patient with leukemia. (Courtesy of Dr Ralph Arnold, San Antonio, TX.)

2. **Leukemia-Associated Gingivitis**
   A. **Inflammation of the Gingiva.** Signs of inflammation in the gingiva include swollen, glazed, and spongy tissues that are red to deep purple in appearance (FIG. 10-3). Gingival bleeding is also a common sign [8].
   B. **Gingival Enlargement.** Gingival enlargement has also been reposted, initially beginning at the interdental papilla followed by marginal and attached gingiva.

ACQUIRED IMMUNODEFICIENCY SYNDROME

1. **Characteristics of AIDS.** Acquired immunodeficiency syndrome (AIDS) is a communicable disease caused by human immunodeficiency virus (HIV). People with acquired immunodeficiency syndrome are at an increased risk for developing certain cancers and for infections that usually occur only in individuals with a weak immune system.
2. **Linear Gingival Erythema**
   A. **Characteristics of LGE**
      1. In the gingiva, manifestations of HIV infection were formerly known as HIV-associated gingivitis but currently are designated as linear gingival erythema. Linear gingival erythema (LGE) is characterized by a 2- to 3-mm marginal band of intense erythema (redness) in the free gingiva [9] (FIG. 10-4).
      2. The band of gingival erythema may extend into the attached gingiva and/or extend beyond the mucogingival line into the alveolar mucosa [9].

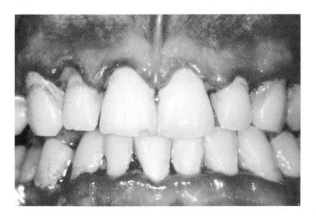

Figure 10.4. Linear Gingival Erythema. Gingival changes associated with LGE. Note the marginal band of intense erythema in the free gingiva.

3. LGE may be localized to one or two teeth but is more commonly a generalized gingival condition.

4. LGE does not respond to conventional plaque biofilm control and periodontal instrumentation [9–11].

5. *With the advent of antiretroviral therapy for HIV-positive patients, the prevalence of HIV-specific lesions has been dramatically reduced* [12].

B. Etiology of LGE

1. The etiology of LGE is not well understood.

2. Research indicates that organisms not generally associated with gingivitis, such as *Candida* species, are associated with LGE [13].

3. In addition, LGE lesions have reduced proportions of T cells and macrophages and an increased number of IgG plasma cells and PMNs [14].

4. These host cell responses and unusual organisms associated with LGE may be responsible for the nonresponsive nature of LGE to plaque biofilm control and periodontal instrumentation.

OSTEOPOROSIS

1. **Characteristics of Osteoporosis**

   A. **Definitions**

   1. Osteoporosis is a reduction in bone mass that causes an increased susceptibility to fractures. Osteoporosis occurs most frequently in postmenopausal women, in sedentary or bedridden individuals, and in patients receiving long-term steroid therapy.

   2. Osteopenia is a condition in which there is a decrease in bone density but not necessarily an increase in the risk or incidence of fracture. Osteopenia is commonly seen in people over the age of 50 who have lower than average bone density but do not have osteoporosis.

   3. Postmenopausal osteoporosis is a disorder caused by the cessation of estrogen production and is characterized by bone fractures.

   B. **Incidence.** Osteoporosis affects more than 20 million men and women in the United States and results in nearly 2 million bone fractures per year.

2. **Osteoporosis and the Risk of Periodontitis**

   A. **Link Between Osteoporosis and Alveolar Bone Loss**

   1. There may be a link between skeletal osteoporosis and alveolar bone loss in the jaw. Preliminary studies report significant correlations between mandibular bone mineral density and hip bone mineral density [15].

   2. In and of itself, osteoporosis does not initiate periodontitis. Loss of density of the alveolar bone, however, may exacerbate the bone resorption seen in preexisting periodontitis.

   B. **Postmenopausal Osteoporosis and Alveolar Bone Loss**

   1. Postmenopausal women with osteoporosis and low educational levels have a greater chance of having periodontal disease than do those without osteoporosis [16,17].

   2. Deficient absorption of dietary calcium and increased excretion of calcium due to diminished estrogen levels in postmenopausal women can account for some bone changes, usually involving the mandible more than the maxilla [18].

   3. Hormone replacement therapy (HRT) is associated with reduced gingival inflammation and a reduced frequency of clinical attachment loss in osteopenic/osteoporotic women in early menopause [19].

HORMONAL VARIATIONS

Levels of sex hormones vary during various periods of life, most strikingly during puberty, pregnancy, and menopause. Some studies indicate that changes in hormone levels may have an effect on the periodontium, particularly in the presence of preexisting, plaque-induced gingival inflammation.

1. **Puberty, Pregnancy, and Menopause**
   A. **Puberty.** During puberty there are increased levels of estradiol in females and testosterone in males.
      1. Increased levels of sex hormones during puberty cause increased blood circulation to the gingival tissues and may cause an increased sensitivity to local irritants, such as bacterial plaque biofilm, resulting in pubertal gingivitis.
      2. An association between (1) the serum levels of testosterone, estrogen and progesterone and (2) in the proportions of *Prevotella intermedia, P. nigrescens* and *Capnocytophaga* species have been seen in puberty gingivitis. These organisms have been implicated in the increased bleeding tendency and gingival inflammation observed during puberty [20–22].
      3. Pubertal gingivitis occurs equally in girls and boys. The tendency for plaque-induced gingivitis decreases as the young person progresses through puberty.
      4. The dental hygienist should explain the importance of thorough plaque biofilm control and its role in the prevention of plaque-induced gingivitis during puberty.
      5. The American Dental Association (ADA) recommends the use of antimicrobial mouth rinses, antibiotic therapy, and aggressive periodontal therapy for any *severe* cases of puberty gingivitis.
   B. **Menstruation**
      1. Usually, the menstrual cycle does not cause any changes in the gingiva.
      2. Women with *preexisting gingivitis* experience increased inflammation and crevicular fluid exudate during menstruation when compared to controls with a healthy periodontium [23].
      3. Gingival inflammation seems to be exacerbated by an imbalance or increase in sex hormones. Numerous studies have demonstrated that sex hormones modify the actions of the cells of the immune system.
      4. When the progesterone level is highest before menstruation, intraoral aphthous ulcers, herpes lesions, and candidiasis occur in some women as a cyclic pattern [24].
   C. **Pregnancy**
      1. Inflammation of the gingiva increases in pregnant women in the presence of small amounts of bacterial plaque biofilm. Gingival inflammation initiated by plaque biofilm and exacerbated by hormonal changes in the second and third trimesters of pregnancy, is referred to as pregnancy gingivitis.
      2. Probing depths, bleeding on probing, and crevicular fluid flow are increased in pregnancy gingivitis.
      3. The likelihood of gingival inflammation increases in the second month when the circulating hormones related to pregnancy rise in the blood, increasing sensitivity to bacterial plaque biofilm and other local irritants. Pregnant women, near or at term, produce large quantities of estradiol, estriol, and progesterone. The incidence of gingival inflammation is highest in the eighth month when the levels of circulating hormones are at their peak.

4. Effects on Subgingival Plaque Biofilm Composition
   a. There is an increase in the selective growth of periodontal pathogens in subgingival plaque biofilm during the onset of pregnancy gingivitis at the third to fourth month of pregnancy. Gestational hormones act as growth factors for bacteria [25].
   b. A 55-fold increase in the proportion of *P. intermedia* has been demonstrated in pregnant women compared with nonpregnant controls [26].
5. Effects on Tissues and Host Response
   a. The increase in severity of gingivitis during pregnancy may be related to the increased circulatory levels of progesterone and its effects on the capillary vessels [27].
   b. Elevated progesterone levels in pregnancy enhance capillary permeability and dilation, resulting in increased gingival exudate.
   c. High levels of progesterone and estrogen associated with pregnancy have been shown to suppress the immune response to dental plaque biofilm [28].
   d. PMN chemotaxis and phagocytosis have been reported to be depressed in response to high levels of gestational hormones [29].
6. Oral Manifestations of Inflammation of the Periodontium
   a. The gingival tissue may be edematous and dark red, with bulbous interdental papillae (FIG. 10-5).
   b. In some cases, a gingival papilla can react so strongly to bacterial plaque biofilm that a large, localized overgrowth of gingival tissue called a pregnancy-associated pyogenic granuloma (pregnancy tumor) may form on the interdental gingiva or on the gingival margin (FIG. 10-6).

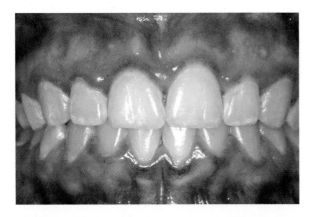

Figure 10.5. Pregnancy Gingivitis. Clinical appearance of reddened, swollen tissues of pregnancy gingivitis. (Courtesy of Dr Richard Foster, Guilford Technical Community College, Jamestown, NC.)

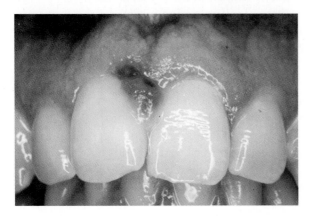

Figure 10.6. Pregnancy-Associated Pyogenic granuloma. The clinical appearance of a pyogenic granuloma (pregnancy tumor).

> **1)** These growths are benign and are generally not painful.
>
> **2)** If the growth persists after delivery, it can be surgically removed.

> c. Dental hygienists should educate pregnant women on the effects of pregnancy on the gingival tissues and stress the importance of thorough self-care for plaque biofilm control and professional care.

D. **Menopause and Postmenopause**

1. Menopausal gingival problems affect only a small percentage of women. If menopause does affect the gingiva, it is called menopausal gingivostomatitis.
2. During menopause there is a decline in hormonal levels. Decreased levels of circulating hormones in women who are menopausal or postmenopausal may result in oral changes, such as thinning of the oral mucosa, dry mouth, burning sensations, altered taste, recession of the gingival margin, and alveolar bone loss.
3. Menopausal and postmenopausal women taking hormone replacement therapy (HRT) may experience pregnancy-like symptoms of gingivitis.
4. Postmenopausal women may experience osteopenia or osteoporosis. The possible link between skeletal osteoporosis and alveolar bone loss in the jaw is discussed under the topic of "Osteoporosis" in this chapter.

2. **Oral Contraceptives**

A. **Synthetic Hormones**

1. Oral contraceptive agents are one of the most widely used classes of drugs in the world.
2. Clinical studies in the 1960s and 1970s demonstrated that women using oral contraceptives had a higher incidence of gingival inflammation than women who did not use these agents. All studies prior to the 1980s recording changes to the gingival tissues by oral contraceptives were completed when hormone concentrations were at much higher levels than are currently available.
3. A recent clinical study evaluating the effects of low-dose oral contraceptives found no effect of oral contraceptives on gingival inflammation in young women [30].
4. Cross-sectional data from the Third National Health and Nutrition Examination Survey (NHANES III) failed to show a relationship between low-dose oral contraceptive use and increased levels of gingivitis [31].
5. From these data it appears that current low-dose oral contraceptives probably are not as harmful to the periodontium as the early formulations.

B. **Oral Contraceptives and Aggressive Periodontitis.** A recent research study looked at oral contraceptives to see if the newer lower-dose pills influenced aggressive periodontitis [32]. Researchers evaluated 50 women aged 20 to 35 years *who were diagnosed with aggressive periodontitis.*

1. Of the 50 women, only 8 had never taken oral contraceptives.
2. Those taking oral contraceptives had deeper pockets and more attachment loss than women not taking the pill.
3. The average attachment loss was 1 mm greater in those taking oral contraceptives compared to those not taking the pill.
4. The researchers concluded that women at risk of generalized aggressive periodontitis should be advised that oral contraceptive use might lead to more advanced disease.

C. **Patient Education.** For patients taking oral contraceptives, dental hygienist should stress the importance of thorough plaque biofilm control and its role in the prevention of plaque-induced gingivitis.

Section 2
Genetic Risk Factors For Periodontitis

Periodontitis is widely recognized as a complex disease. As discussed in other sections of this textbook, it is clear that fundamentally periodontitis is a bacterial infection; numerous studies have even identified the specific bacteria that are associated with the development of the various types of periodontitis. For many years, however, clinical observations that severe periodontitis can occur in successive generations of some families led to speculation about the potential role of genetic factors in periodontitis. Research has begun to clarify the true role of genetics as a risk factor in this complex disease.

1. The Role of Genetics in Periodontitis
   A. Genetics and General Health
      1. Many diseases arise as a result of a combination of both environmental factors and genetic factors.
      2. For periodontitis, "environmental factors" can mean the presence of periodontal pathogenic bacteria in plaque biofilm on a tooth surface and "genetic factors" refer to inherited characteristics such as certain genes in cells.
      3. Genes can have a dramatic effect on an organism by determining the specific characteristics of proteins that are needed for cells to live and function normally.
      4. It is common knowledge today that genes within cell nuclei have a huge influence on most of our characteristics.
      5. Mutations or variations within these genes can lead to specific diseases, and sometimes these diseases can even affect the periodontium.
   B. Rare Genetic Syndromes Associated with Periodontitis
      1. There are several rare genetic disorders that in addition to creating multiple medical problems for patients can also lead to very unusual forms of periodontitis.
      2. Examples of some of these rare disorders include conditions such as Chédiak-Higashi syndrome, Down syndrome, leukocyte adhesion deficiency syndrome, Job syndrome, Papillon-Lefèvre syndrome, Crohn disease, acute monocytic leukemia, and cyclic and chronic neutropenia.
         a. Many of these rare disorders are accompanied by a PMN malfunction that makes patients more susceptible to infections such as periodontitis.
         b. Heredity abnormalities in PMN function can lead to overwhelming systemic bacterial infections and are often associated with increased susceptibility to severe periodontal destruction.
         c. Dental hygienists are unlikely to encounter patients with most of these severe genetic disorders outside a hospital dentistry setting.
      3. These rare genetic syndromes have been studied to help clarify the role of genetics and periodontal diseases, but most of these studies are not very helpful to a clinician in understanding the relationship between genetics and the more common forms of periodontal disease such as chronic or aggressive periodontitis.
   C. Genetics and Chronic Periodontitis
      1. Chronic periodontitis is the most common form of periodontitis, and genetic studies related to chronic periodontitis have focused mainly on studies of twins.
      2. The studies are difficult to interpret, but from these studies of twins it appears that approximately 50% of chronic periodontitis susceptibility may indeed be due to genetic factors.

3. The genetic risk factor for chronic periodontitis appears quite complex, and there does not appear to be a specific gene mutation associated with this disease.

4. It is probable that the genetic risk of developing chronic periodontitis lies in the additive effect of multiple genes.

D. **Genetics and Aggressive Periodontitis Not Associated with Specific Syndromes**

1. Aggressive periodontitis is a relatively rare condition, and genetic studies of this condition have been difficult to conduct because of its rarity.

2. Genetic studies related to aggressive periodontitis do indicate that there are likely to be different genetic forms of aggressive periodontitis, but specific genes have not yet been identified for these diseases.

2. **Down Syndrome and Periodontitis.** Though most of these rare genetic syndromes are unlikely to be encountered by the dental hygienist outside a hospital setting, persons with Down syndrome are frequently treated by members of the dental team in general and periodontal dental offices. Down syndrome is one of the most common birth defects. Usually, children born with this condition have some degree of mental retardation, as well as characteristic physical features. Many of these children also have other health problems.

A. **Genetic Changes in Down Syndrome**

1. Normally, the nucleus of each cell contains 46 chromosomes. In Down syndrome, however, the nucleus contains 47 chromosomes. Most cases of Down syndrome occur because there are three copies of the 21st chromosome. For this reason, Down syndrome is also referred to as trisomy 21.

2. More than 350,000 people in the United States have Down syndrome.

3. Due to advances in medical treatment, 80% of adults with Down syndrome reach age 55 and many live longer. As the mortality rate associated with Down syndrome decreases, the prevalence of adults with Down syndrome in our society will increase. More and more dental healthcare providers will interact with individuals with this condition, increasing the need for education and acceptance.

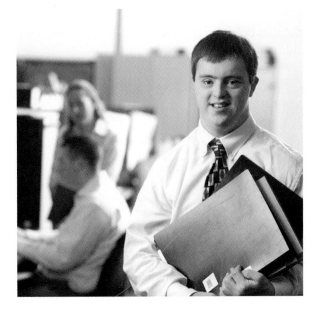

Figure 10.7. Individuals with Down Syndrome in the Workforce. With appropriate training and support people with Down syndrome can and do make a huge contribution to their workplace. (Courtesy of Getty Images.)

B. **Physical Characteristics of Patients with Down Syndrome.** Among the most common physical traits of infants with Down syndrome are
   1. Flat facial profile with a small nose with a depressed nasal bridge
   2. Upward slant to the eyes and small skin folds on the inner corners of the eyes
   3. Protruding tongue and an open mouth

C. **Medical and Developmental Problems of Patients with Down Syndrome**
   1. Children with Down syndrome are at increased risk for congenital heart defects, increased susceptibility to infection, respiratory problems, gastrointestinal abnormalities, and childhood leukemia.
   2. Abnormal PMN function is seen in about half of all patients with Down syndrome.
   3. Most individuals with Down syndrome have some level of mental retardation, with IQs in the mild to moderate range of mental retardation. Those who receive good medical care and experience a supportive social environment can attend school, hold jobs, and participate in decisions that affect them. Some live with family or friends, and some live independently (FIG. 10-7).

D. **Implications of Down Syndrome for the Periodontium**
   1. It is widely known that individuals with Down syndrome often develop severe, aggressive periodontitis. The prevalence of periodontal disease ranges from 58% to 96% of young adults under 35 years of age with Down syndrome [33].
   2. The prevalence of periodontal disease cannot simply be attributed to poor oral hygiene. The etiology of periodontal disease in persons with Down syndrome is complex. In recent years, much focus has been placed on the altered immune response resulting from the underlying genetic disorder [33].
      a. Impaired PMN chemotaxis and phagocytosis most likely explain the high prevalence and increased severity of periodontitis associated with Down syndrome [34,35].
      b. Impaired cellular motility of gingival fibroblasts that prevents wound healing and regeneration of periodontal tissues may be involved in the etiology of Down syndrome periodontitis [36].
   3. Substantial plaque biofilm formation, deep periodontal pockets, and extensive gingival inflammation characterize periodontal disease in Down syndrome (FIG. 10-8) [37].
   4. Studies indicate that various periodontal pathogens colonize the gingival tissues in the very early childhood years of children with Down syndrome [38].

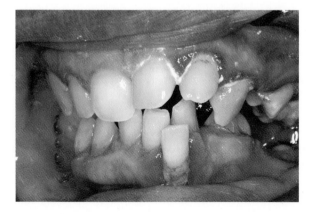

Figure 10.8. Periodontitis and Down Syndrome. Severe periodontal destruction in a 25-year-old patient with Down syndrome. (Courtesy of Dr Richard Foster, Guilford Technical Community College, Jamestown, NC.)

3. **Tests for Genetic Susceptibility to Periodontitis.** Genetic tests for chronic periodontitis are difficult to develop, since it appears that there is no single gene that is responsible for the susceptibility to this condition.
   A. **Genetic Tests for Gene Mutations**
      1. Genetic tests for gene mutations that lead to some of the syndrome forms of periodontitis such as Chédiak-Higashi syndrome and Papillon-Lefèvre syndrome have already been used.
      2. It is important to realize that gene mutations for these rare conditions do not appear to be of value when attempting to assess the risk for the more common forms of periodontitis such as chronic periodontitis and aggressive periodontitis.
   B. **Genetic Tests for Gene Variations**
      1. Gene variations (or polymorphisms) have been investigated for possible association with chronic periodontitis; the most promising of these include several interleukin (IL) genes.
      2. Currently a genetic test is being marketed in the United States for testing for polymorphisms of IL genes.
         a. When two variations or polymorphisms of two of the IL-1 genes are found together, there appears to be an increased risk of developing severe periodontitis. This relationship, however, has only been demonstrated in nonsmokers.
         b. Testing for variations of certain IL-1 genes is the basis for this genetic test.
         c. Though this test does underscore relationships between periodontitis and genetics, further research is needed to clarify the clinical usefulness of this type of testing.

Section 3
Systemic Medications with Periodontal Side Effects

A number of medications used to treat systemic diseases can cause oral complications. Effects of medications can modify oral hygiene habits, plaque biofilm composition, size of gingival tissues, level of bone, and salivary flow. Educating patients about potential oral side effects is critical to reducing the medication-related risks of periodontal disease. Commonly prescribed medications that can affect the periodontium are summarized in TABLE 10-1.

TABLE 10-1. Effects of Commonly Prescribed Medications on Periodontium		
Medication Class	**Generic Name (Brand Name)**	**Effect on Periodontium**
Antibiotic	Tetracycline (Achromycin)	Inhibits alveolar bone loss
Anticonvulsant	Phenytoin (Dilantin)	Gingival overgrowth
Antianxiety agents	Alprazolam (Xanax)	Increased plaque biofilm formation
Antihypertensive	Enalapril (Vasotec)	Increased gingival inflammation
Calcium channel blocker	Nifedipine (Procardia)	Gingival overgrowth
Immunosuppressive	Cyclosporine (Sandimmune)	Gingival overgrowth
Nonsteroidal anti-inflammatory	Ibuprofen (Advil, Midol, Nuprin)	Inhibits alveolar bone loss

1. **Medications that Alter Plaque Biofilm Composition, pH, or Salivary Flow**
   A. **Plaque Biofilm Composition or pH**
      1. Many oral medications alter plaque biofilm composition and pH in ways that are harmful to the periodontium.
      2. Medications Containing Sugar
         a. Sugar is a major component of some cough drops, liquid medications, cough syrups, tonics, chewable vitamins, antacid tablets, and other medications. Medications that contain sugar add significantly to the alteration of plaque biofilm pH and composition.
         b. Sugar-containing liquid or chewable medications are sometimes used in the treatment of children with chronic medical problems. Parents should be made aware of the oral health consequences of such medications. Giving the medications at mealtimes instead of between meals is helpful.
         c. Sugar is metabolized by bacteria to form acid, causing the enamel to demineralize. The demineralized areas are rough and act as attachment sites for bacteria, keeping bacterial plaque biofilm against tissues and eventually resulting in inflammation of the gingiva.
      3. Medications that Lower pH
         a. Some over-the-counter (OTC) preparations contain sugar and vitamin C. This combination of sugar and vitamin C causes an acid pH.

    b. Examples of products containing sugar and vitamin C include chewable vitamin C tablets, certain cough drops, and certain liquid cough preparations.

    c. Products that alter the plaque biofilm pH significantly can cause root-surface caries in older adults and have an effect on the metabolism of periodontal pathogens [39,40].

B. Salivary Flow and pH

  1. Adequate saliva flow is necessary for the maintenance of healthy oral tissues. The ability of saliva to limit the growth of pathogens is a major determinant of systemic and oral health.

    a. The physical flow of the saliva helps to dislodge microbes from the teeth and mucosa surfaces. Saliva can also cause bacteria to clump together so that they can be swallowed before they become firmly attached.

    b. Saliva is rich in antimicrobial components. Certain molecules in saliva can directly kill or inhibit a variety of microbes.

  2. Patients with xerostomia suffer from an increase in the incidence of oral candidiasis, coronal and root-surface caries, as well as excess plaque biofilm formation.

  3. More than 400 over-the-counter and prescription drugs have xerostomia as a possible side effect [41,42].

  4. Some of the more common groups of medications that cause xerostomia are cardiovascular medications (blood pressure, diuretics, calcium channel blockers); antidepressants; sedatives; centrally acting analgesics; antiparkinsonism medications; allergy medications; and antacids [43].

3. Drug-Influenced Gingival Enlargement

A. Introduction

  1. Drug-influenced gingival enlargement is an esthetically disfiguring overgrowth of the gingiva that is a side effect associated with certain medications.

  2. Drugs associated with gingival enlargement can be broadly divided into three categories: anticonvulsants, calcium channel blockers, and immunosuppressants (TABLE 10-2). These three classes of medications influence gingival fibroblasts to overproduce collagen matrix when stimulated by gingival inflammation [44].

    a. More than 20 medications have been shown to have the potential to induce gingival enlargement.

    b. Among the old and relatively newer pharmacologic agents involved in gingival enlargement, overall, the anticonvulsant phenytoin still has the highest prevalence rate (approximately 50%), with calcium channel blockers and immunosuppressant-associated enlargements about half as prevalent [44].

  3. The clinical characteristics of drug-influenced gingival enlargement include enlargement of the gingiva, tendency to occur more often in the anterior gingiva, prevalence in younger age groups, and onset within 3 months of use [45–47].

  4. Current studies on the mechanism of drug-associated enlargement are focusing on the direct and indirect effects of these drugs on gingival fibroblast metabolism.

  5. If possible, treatment is generally targeted on drug substitution and effective control of local inflammatory factors such as plaque biofilm and calculus. When these measures fail to cause resolution of the enlargement, surgical intervention is recommended.

TABLE 10-2. Estimated Prevalence of Drug-Associated Gingival Enlargement			
Category	Pharmacologic Agent	Trade Name	Prevalence
Anticonvulsants	Phenytoin	Dilantin	50% [48,49]
	Sodium valproate	Depakene, Depacon, Epilim, Valpro	Rare [49–51]
	Phenobarbitone	Phenobarbital, Donnatal	>5% [52]
	Vigabatrin	Sabril	Rare [53]
	Carbamazepine	Tegretol	None reported
Immunosuppressants	Cyclosporin	Neoral, Sandimmune	Adults 25% to 30% [54–56] Children >70% [57]
Calcium channel blockers	Nifedipine	Adalat, Nifecard, Procardia, Tenif	6% to 15% [58–60]
	Diltiazem	Cardizem, Dilacor, Diltiamax, Tiazac	5% to 20% [61]
	Verapamil	Calan, Covera, Isoptin, Tarka, Verelan	<5% [62]
	Felodipine	Agon, Felodur, Lexxel, Plendil	Rare [50, 59]
	Amlodipine	Lotrel, Norvasc	Rare [50, 59]
	Isradipine	DynaCirc	None reported

B. **Anticonvulsants**
1. Phenytoin (FEN-i-toyn) is one of the most commonly used anticonvulsant medications to control convulsions or seizures in the treatment of epilepsy. It remains the drug of choice for treatment of grand mal, temporal lobe, and psychomotor seizures [50]. Phenytoin is marketed under various trade names including Dilantin 4, Dilantin Kapseals 4, and Phenytoin. Phenytoin is among the 20 most-prescribed drugs in the world.
2. Overgrowth of the gingiva is one of the most common side effects of phenytoin. It has been estimated that 40% to 50% of the millions of individuals who take phenytoin will develop gingival overgrowth to some extent. Overgrowths appear to be more common in children and young adults.
3. Gingival overgrowth begins with enlargement of the interdental papillae.
   a. The interdental papillae overgrow, forming firm triangular tissue masses that protrude from the interdental area.
   b. Gradually, the enlarged papillae may fuse mesially and distally and partially cover the anatomical crown with the marginal gingiva (FIG. 10-9). Overgrowths are most commonly seen on the facial aspect of the anterior teeth.

c. In the presence of good plaque biofilm control, the enlarged tissue is pink in color and firm and rubbery in consistency. In the presence of poor plaque biofilm control, the tissue appears red, edematous, and spongy.

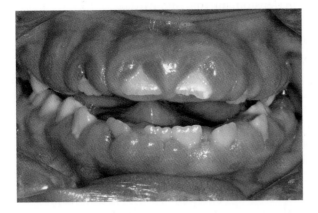

Figure 10.9. Phenytoin-Influenced Gingival Overgrowth. Severe enlargement of the gingiva associated with phenytoin (Dilantin) medication in an individual with epilepsy. (Courtesy of Dr Ralph Arnold, San Antonio, TX.)

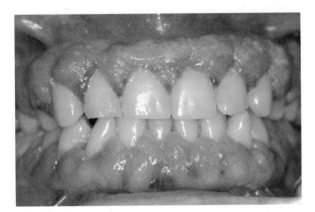

Figure 10.10. Cyclosporine-Influenced Gingival Overgrowth. The clinical appearance of cyclosporine-associated gingival overgrowth resembles that of phenytoin-associated gingival enlargement. (Courtesy of Dr Ralph Arnold, San Antonio, Texas.)

C. **Immunosuppressants**
1. Cyclosporine (SIGH-kloe-spor-een) belongs to the group of medicines known as immunosuppressive agents used for prevention of transplant rejection as well as for management of a number of autoimmune conditions such as rheumatoid arthritis. When a patient receives an organ transplant, the body will try to reject the transplanted organ. Cyclosporine works by preventing this response.
2. The incidence of cyclosporine-associated gingival overgrowth affects approximately 25% of patients taking the medication.
3. The clinical appearance of cyclosporine-associated gingival overgrowth resembles that of phenytoin-associated gingival enlargement (FIG. 10-10).
4. Patients receiving cyclosporine are usually medically compromised, requiring close consultation with the patient's physician to assure safe management of the patient's periodontal condition.

D. Calcium Channel Blockers

1. Antihypertensive drugs in the calcium channel blocker group are used extensively in elderly patients who have angina or peripheral vascular disease [50,63].

2. Nifedipine (nye-FED-I-peen), one type of calcium channel blocker, is used as a coronary vasodilator in the treatment of hypertension, angina, and cardiac arrhythmias. Calcium channel blockers are a class of drugs that block the influx of calcium ions through cardiac and vascular smooth muscle cell membranes. This results in the dilation of the main coronary and systemic arteries.

   a. Approximately 38% of patients taking nifedipine experience gingival enlargement.

   b. The clinical appearance of nifedipine-associated gingival overgrowth resembles that of phenytoin-associated gingival enlargement (FIG. 10-11).

3. Various other calcium channel blocking medications, such as diltiazem, felodipine, nitrendipine, and verapamil also may induce gingival enlargement (FIG. 10-12).

4. Surgical elimination of the tissue overgrowth is often required. Unfortunately, the gingival overgrowth is likely to recur within 1 to 2 years even in the presence of good plaque biofilm control, especially if the patient is younger than age 25. If plaque biofilm control is inadequate, the regrowth will occur rapidly. The patient should be advised of the likelihood of the recurrence of the gingival overgrowth following surgery.

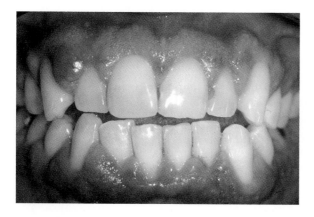

Figure 10.11. Nifedipine-Associated Enlargement. Gingival overgrowth in a patient who takes nifedipine for the treatment of cardiac arrhythmia. (Courtesy of Dr Ralph Arnold, San Antonio, TX.)

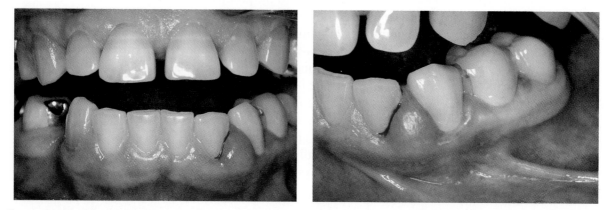

Figure 10.12. Gingival Enlargement Associated with Calcium Channel Blocking Drugs. Gingival enlargement of the papilla between the lateral incisor and canine induced by the calcium channel blocking medication Norvasc. (Courtesy of Dr Richard Foster, Guilford Technical Community College, Jamestown, NC.)

Section 4
Focus on Patients

Case 1

A patient, who has been previously treated for chronic periodontitis and has been followed by your dental team for several years, calls your dental office with a concern. She is scheduled to undergo a liver transplant and has been warned by her physician that the medications she will need will make her more susceptible to infections. She asks if these medications might have an effect on her continuing treatment for periodontitis. How might you respond to her concern?

Case 2

The parents of a young patient currently being treated by your dental team inform you that following a lengthy illness, their daughter has recently been diagnosed by her physician with a neutrophil defect. Neutrophils are also known as polymorphonuclear leukocytes. They inquire about any dental implications of this diagnosis. How might you respond to this inquiry?

References

1. Lalla E, Cheng B, Lal S, et al. Diabetes mellitus promotes periodontal destruction in children. *J Clin Periodontol.* 2007;34(4):294–298.
2. Christgau M, Palitzsch KD, Schmalz G, et al. Healing response to non-surgical periodontal therapy in patients with diabetes mellitus: clinical, microbiological, and immunologic results. *J Clin Periodontol.* 1998;25(2):112–124.
3. Westfelt E, Rylander H, Blohme G, et al. The effect of periodontal therapy in diabetics. Results after 5 years. *J Clin Periodontol.* 1996;23(2):92–100.
4. Tervonen T, Karjalainen K. Periodontal disease related to diabetic status. A pilot study of the response to periodontal therapy in type 1 diabetes. *J Clin Periodontol.* 1997;24(7):505–510.
5. Gugliucci A. Glycation as the glucose link to diabetic complications. *J Am Osteopath Assoc.* 2000;100(10):621–634.
6. Ueta E, Osaki T, Yoneda K, et al. Prevalence of diabetes mellitus in odontogenic infections and oral candidiasis: an analysis of neutrophil suppression. *J Oral Pathol Med.* 1993;22(4):168–174.
7. Salvi GE, Yalda B, Collins JG, et al. Inflammatory mediator response as a potential risk marker for periodontal diseases in insulin-dependent diabetes mellitus patients. *J Periodontol.* 1997;68(2):127–135.
8. Dreizen S, McCredie KB, Keating MJ. Chemotherapy-associated oral hemorrhages in adults with acute leukemia. *Oral Surg Oral Med Oral Pathol.* 1984;57(5):494–498.
9. Winkler JR, Grassi M, Murray PA. Clinical description and etiology of HIV-associated periodontal diseases. In: *Robertson: Perspectives on oral manifestations of AIDS: diagnosis and management of HIV-associated infections: proceedings of a symposium held January 18–20, 1988 in San Diego, California.* Littleton: PSG Publishing Co.; 1988.
10. Winkler JR, Murray PA. Periodontal disease. A potential intraoral expression of AIDS may be rapidly progressive periodontitis. *CDA J.* 1987;15(1):20–24.
11. Winkler JR, Murray PA, Grassi M, et al. Diagnosis and management of HIV-associated periodontal lesions. *J Am Dent Assoc.* 1989;(Suppl):25S–34S.
12. Kroidl A, Schaeben A, Oette M, et al. Prevalence of oral lesions and periodontal diseases in HIV-infected patients on antiretroviral therapy. *Eur J Med Res.* 2005;10(10):448–453.
13. Lamster IB, Grbic JT, Mitchell-Lewis DA, et al. New concepts regarding the pathogenesis of periodontal disease in HIV infection. *Ann Periodontol.* 1998;3(1):62–75.
14. Gomez RS, da Costa JE, Loyola AM, et al. Immunohistochemical study of linear gingival erythema from HIV-positive patients. *J Periodontal Res.* 1995;30(5):355–359.
15. Jeffcoat M. The association between osteoporosis and oral bone loss. *J Periodontol.* 2005;76(11 Suppl):2125–2132.
16. Gomes-Filho IS, Passos-Jde S, Cruz SS, et al. The association between postmenopausal osteoporosis and periodontal disease. *J Periodontol.* 2007;78(9):1731–1740.
17. Wactawski-Wende J, Hausmann E, Hovey K, et al. The association between osteoporosis and alveolar crestal height in postmenopausal women. *J Periodontol.* 2005;76(11 Suppl):2116–2124.
18. Shapiro S, Bomberg TJ, Benson BW, et al. Postmenopausal osteoporosis: dental patients at risk. *Gerodontics.* 1985;1(5):220–225.
19. Reinhardt RA, Payne JB, Maze CA, et al. Influence of estrogen and osteopenia/osteoporosis on clinical periodontitis in postmenopausal women. *J Periodontol.* 1999;70(8):823–828.
20. Gusberti FA, Mombelli A, Lang NP, et al. Changes in subgingival microbiota during puberty. A 4-year longitudinal study. *J Clin Periodontol.* 1990;17(10):685–692.
21. Mombelli A, Rutar A, Lang NP. Correlation of the periodontal status 6 years after puberty with clinical and microbiological conditions during puberty. *J Clin Periodontol.* 1995;22(4):300–305.
22. Nakagawa S, Fujii H, Machida Y, et al. A longitudinal study from prepuberty to puberty of gingivitis. Correlation between the occurrence of Prevotella intermedia and sex hormones. *J Clin Periodontol.* 1994;21(10):658–665.
23. Holm-Pedersen P, Loe H. Flow of gingival exudate as related to menstruation and pregnancy. *J Periodontal Res.* 1967;2(1):13–20.
24. Ferguson MM, Carter J, Boyle P. An epidemiological study of factors associated with recurrent aphthae in women. *J Oral Med.* 1984;39(4):212–217.
25. Di Placido G, Tumini V, D'Archivio D, et al. Gingival hyperplasia in pregnancy. II. Etiopathogenic factors and mechanisms. *Minerva Stomatol.* 1998;47(5):223–229.
26. Jensen J, Liljemark W, Bloomquist C. The effect of female sex hormones on subgingival plaque. *J Periodontol.* 1981;52(10):599–602.

27. Lundgren D, Magnusson B, Lindhe J. Connective tissue alterations in gingivae of rats treated with estrogen and progesterone. A histologic and autoradiographic study. *Odontol Revy*. 1973;24(1):49–58.

28. Sooriyamoorthy M, Gower DB. Hormonal influences on gingival tissue: relationship to periodontal disease. *J Clin Periodontol*. 1989;16(4):201–208.

29. Raber-Durlacher JE, Leene W, Palmer-Bouva CC, et al. Experimental gingivitis during pregnancy and post-partum: immunohistochemical aspects. *J Periodontol*. 1993;64(3):211–218.

30. Preshaw PM, Knutsen MA, Mariotti A. Experimental gingivitis in women using oral contraceptives. *J Dent Res*. 2001;80(11):2011–2015.

31. Taichman LS, Eklund SA. Oral contraceptives and periodontal diseases: rethinking the association based upon analysis of National Health and Nutrition Examination Survey data. *J Periodontol*. 2005;76(8):1374–1385.

32. Mullally BH, Coulter WA, Hutchinson JD, et al. Current oral contraceptive status and periodontitis in young adults. *J Periodontol*. 2007;78(6):1031–106.

33. Morgan J. Why is periodontal disease more prevalent and more severe in people with Down syndrome? *Spec Care Dentist*. 2007;27(5):196–201.

34. Cutler CW, Wasfy MO, Ghaffar K, et al. Impaired bactericidal activity of PMN from two brothers with necrotizing ulcerative gingivo-periodontitis. *J Periodontol*. 1994;65(4): 357–363.

35. Izumi Y, Sugiyama S, Shinozuka O, et al. Defective neutrophil chemotaxis in Down's syndrome patients and its relationship to periodontal destruction. *J Periodontol*. 1989;60(5):238–242.

36. Murakami J, Kato T, Kawai S, et al. Cellular motility of Down syndrome gingival fibroblasts is susceptible to impairment by *Porphyromonas gingivalis* invasion. *J Periodontol*. 2008;79(4): 721–727.

37. Barr-Agholme M, Dahllof G, Modeer T, et al. Periodontal conditions and salivary immuno-globulins in individuals with Down syndrome. *J Periodontol*. 1998;69(10):1119–1123.

38. Amano A, Kishima T, Kimura S, et al. Periodontopathic bacteria in children with Down syndrome. *J Periodontol*. 2000;71(2):249–255.

39. Touger-Decker R, van Loveren C. Sugars and dental caries. *Am J Clin Nutr*. 2003;78(4): 881S–892S.

40. Steele JG, Sheiham A, Marcenes W, et al. Clinical and behavioural risk indicators for root caries in older people. *Gerodontology*. 2001;18(2):95–101.

41. Ciancio SG. Medications' impact on oral health. *J Am Dent Assoc*. 2004;135(10):1440–1448; quiz 1468–1469.

42. Sreebny LM, Schwartz SS. A reference guide to drugs and dry mouth—2nd edition. *Gerodontology*. 1997;14(1):33–47.

43. Guggenheimer J, Moore PA. Xerostomia: etiology, recognition and treatment. *J Am Dent Assoc*. 2003;134(1):61–69; quiz 118–119.

44. Dongari-Bagtzoglou A. Drug-associated gingival enlargement. *J Periodontol*. 2004;75(10): 1424–1431.

45. Hassell TM, Hefti AF. Drug-induced gingival overgrowth: old problem, new problem. *Crit Rev Oral Biol Med*. 1991;2(1):103–137.

46. Hefti AF, Eshenaur AE, Hassell TM, et al. Gingival overgrowth in cyclosporine A treated multiple sclerosis patients. *J Periodontol*. 1994;65(8):744–749.

47. Mariotti A. Dental plaque-induced gingival diseases. *Ann Periodontol*. 1999;4(1):7–19.

48. Casetta I, Granieri E, Desidera M, et al. Phenytoin-induced gingival overgrowth: a community-based cross-sectional study in Ferrara, Italy. *Neuroepidemiology*. 1997;16(6):296–303.

49. Ciancio SG, Bartz NW Jr, Lauciello FR. Cyclosporine-induced gingival hyperplasia and chlorhexidine: a case report. *Int J Periodontics Restorative Dent*. 1991;11(3):241–245.

50. Marshall RI, Bartold PM. A clinical review of drug-induced gingival overgrowths. *Aust Dent J*. 1999;44(4):219–232.

51. Seymour RA, Heasman PA, Macgregor IDM. *Drugs, Diseases, and the Periodontium. Oxford Medical Publications*. Oxford; New York: Oxford University Press; 1992: 206; xiii.

52. Gregoriou AP, Schneider PE, Shaw PR. Phenobarbital-induced gingival overgrowth? Report of two cases and complications in management. *ASDC J Dent Child*. 1996;63(6):408–413.

53. Katz J, Givol N, Chaushu G. et al. Vigabatrin-induced gingival overgrowth. *J Clin Periodontol*. 1997;24(3):180–182.

54. Boltchi FE, Rees TD, Iacopino AM. Cyclosporine A-induced gingival overgrowth: a comprehensive review. *Quintessence Int*. 1999;30(11):775–783.

55. Fu E, Nieh S, Hsiao CT, et al. Nifedipine-induced gingival overgrowth in rats: brief review and experimental study. *J Periodontol.* 1998;69(7):765–771.

56. Myers BD, Newton L. Cyclosporine-induced chronic nephropathy: an obliterative microvascular renal injury. *J Am Soc Nephrol.* 1991;2(2 Suppl 1):S45–S52.

57. Kilpatrick NM, et al. Gingival overgrowth in pediatric heart and heart-lung transplant recipients. *J Heart Lung Transplant.* 1997;16(12):1231–1237.

58. Barak S, Engelberg IS, Hiss J. Gingival hyperplasia caused by nifedipine. Histopathologic findings. *J Periodontol.* 1987;58(9):639–642.

59. Ellis JS, Seymour RA, Steele JG, et al. Prevalence of gingival overgrowth induced by calcium channel blockers: a community-based study. *J Periodontol.* 1999;70(1):63–67.

60. Fattore L, Stablein M, Bredfeldt G, et al. Gingival hyperplasia: a side effect of nifedipine and diltiazem. *Spec Care Dentist.* 1991;11(3):107–109.

61. Andriani F, Margulis A, Lin N, et al. Analysis of microenvironmental factors contributing to basement membrane assembly and normalized epidermal phenotype. *J Invest Dermatol.* 2003;120(6):923–931.

62. Meller AT, Rumjanek VM, Sansone C, et al. Oral mucosa alterations induced by cyclosporin in mice: morphological features. *J Periodontal Res.* 2002;37(6):412–415.

63. Hallmon WW, Rossmann JA. The role of drugs in the pathogenesis of gingival overgrowth. A collective review of current concepts. *Periodontol 2000.* 1999;21:176–196.

Chapter 11

Smoking and Periodontal Disease

Learning Objectives

- Discuss the implications of smoking on periodontal health status.
- Discuss the implications of smoking on the host response to periodontal disease.
- Discuss the effects of smoking on periodontal treatment outcomes.
- Discuss current theories as to why smokers have more periodontal disease than nonsmokers.
- Explain why tobacco cessation counseling is a valuable part of patient care in the dental setting.
- Value the importance of providing tobacco cessation counseling as a routine part of periodontal treatment.

Key Term

Ask. Advise. Refer. Model for tobacco cessation counseling

Section 1
Introduction to Smoking and Periodontal Disease

Epidemiological studies, clinical trials, and animal research consistently indicate that periodontal disease has a multifactorial etiology. Specific risk factors alter the susceptibility of the host to periodontal infection and affect disease severity. In the past 30 years, there is increasing awareness of the role of tobacco use in the severity of periodontal diseases. *It appears that smoking may be one of the most significant risk factors in the development and progression of periodontal disease.* (FIG. 11-1).

In the United States approximately 25% of the adult population smoke cigarettes. In the Canadian Tobacco Use Monitoring Survey for 2001, 22% of the population aged 15 years and older identified themselves as smokers.

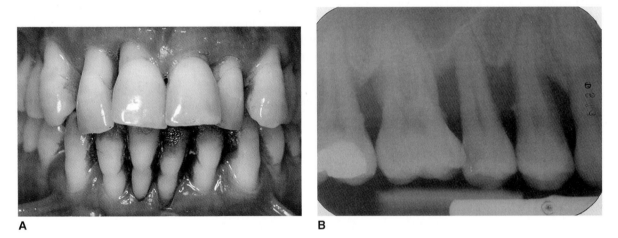

A   **B**

Figure 11.1. **Periodontitis Associated with Smoking.** A: Clinical and B: radiographic evidence shows advanced periodontitis with horizontal and vertical bone loss in this 37-year-old male, cigarette smoker, with 20 pack years of smoking.

1. **Smoking Increases the Risk for Severe Periodontal Disease**
   A. **Increased Risk for Periodontal Disease**
      1. A substantial number of large-scale studies establish that smoking increases the risk for severe periodontal disease by 2.6 to 6 times [1–14].
      2. In the United States adult population, 41.9% of periodontitis cases are attributable to current cigarette smoking and 10.9% to former smoking.
      3. With more than half of the periodontitis cases among adults in the United States associated with smoking, it is important to understand its impact on disease initiation and progression in patients who smoke.
      4. A large proportion of chronic periodontitis may be preventable through prevention and cessation of cigarette smoking.
   B. **Effects of Smoking on the Periodontium**
      1. A large number of studies establish that in comparing smokers and nonsmokers with periodontitis, smokers have
         a. More attachment loss and more recession of the gingival margin [9,15,16]
         b. More alveolar bone loss [6,8,18–21]
         c. Deeper probing depths and a greater number of deep pockets [6,8,17–20]
         d. More teeth with furcation involvement [23,24]
         e. More tooth loss [25,26]

2. The more cigarettes smoked and the longer an individual has smoked, the more severe the attachment loss (FIGS. 11-1 and 11-2) [9].

3. Smoking is strongly associated with aggressive periodontal destruction in young adults. Tobacco smoking may play an important role in the development of forms of periodontitis that do not respond to treatment despite excellent patient compliance and appropriate periodontal therapy [27].

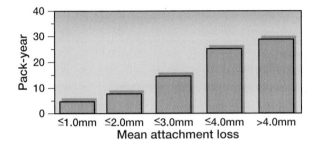

Figure 11.2. Effect of Cigarette Smoking and Severity of Attachment Loss. For every 10 pack-year increment, there is a 1-mm increase in mean attachment loss. (Data from Grossi SG, Zamgon JJ, Ho AW, et al. Assessment of risk for periodontal disease. I. Risk indicators for attachment loss. *J Periodontol.* 1994;65:260–267.)

2. **Impact of Tobacco Products on the Periodontium**
   A. **Cigarette, Cigar, and Pipe Smoking.** Most of the evidence supporting tobacco use as a risk factor for periodontal disease is from cigarette smoking; however, cigar and pipe use also are significant risk factors for attachment loss [1–14,28].
      1. Tobacco products contain nicotine that enters the bloodstream through the lungs, skin, or mucous membranes.
      2. In smokers, the periodontal tissues are continuously exposed to nicotine and its metabolites due to deposition of nicotine on the root surface and its release via saliva and gingival crevicular fluid. Local and systemic effects of nicotine also are believed to have an impact on periodontal tissues.
   B. **Smokeless Tobacco**
      1. The use of smokeless tobacco worldwide is increasing since more people tend to stay away from smoked tobacco as a consequence of public pressure.
      2. The use of smokeless tobacco has been shown to result in an increased inflammatory response in the gingival tissues. Increased inflammatory responses contribute to an accelerated periodontal breakdown and subsequent attachment loss at the site of placement.
      3. Additional mechanical trauma resulting from the abrasive nature of the smokeless tobacco being held in close proximity to thin gingival tissues could also be contributory to recession of gingival margin.

Section 2
Mechanisms of Periodontal Disease Progression in Smokers

There are several theories as to why smokers have more periodontal disease than nonsmokers. These theories involve effects on bacteria in the plaque biofilm, host response, healing, and response to treatment (Fig. 11-3) [29–31].

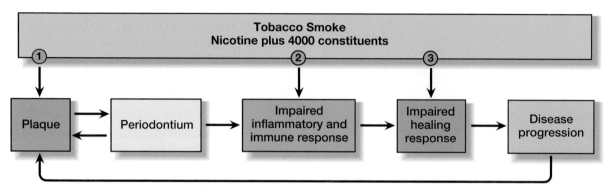

Figure 11.3. **Why Smokers Have More Periodontal Disease.** Mechanisms of periodontal disease in smokers may involve effects on (*1*) plaque biofilm bacteria, (*2*) host response, and (*3*) healing response.

1. **Effects on Bacteria in the Plaque Biofilm**
    A. **Microbial Species Hypothesis.** One hypothesis regarding the role of tobacco smoking in the development of periodontal diseases is that when compared to nonsmokers, smokers harbor different types of bacteria in the plaque biofilm.
        1. Several studies have shown that smokers harbor more microbial species that are associated with periodontitis than nonsmokers.
            a. One large study showed that smokers harbored significantly higher levels of *Tannerella forsythia* (formerly *Bacteroides forsythus*), *Aggregatibacter actinomycetemcomitans*, and *Porphyromonas gingivalis* [32].
            b. Another study showed that smoking is a determining factor for the composition of the subgingival microflora in adult patients with periodontitis and may select for a specific cluster of periodontal pathogens, notably *Tannerella forsythia* (formerly *Bacteroides forsythus*), *Peptostreptococcus micros* and *Fusobacterium nucleatum* and *Campylobacter rectus* [33].
            c. A third study showed that *Staphylococcus aureus, Peptostreptococcus micros, Campylobacter concisus, Escherichia coli, Tannerella forsythia, Porphyromonas gingivalis, Candida albicans*, and *Aspergillus fumigatus* are found in significantly higher numbers and more frequently in smokers [34].
            d. Smoking may cause changes in the pocket environment that could result in different microflora in smokers. Cigarette smoking may decrease the oxygen tension in periodontal pockets and may lead to a different selection of the pathogenic bacteria [35,36].
        2. **No Difference in Microbial Species.** In contrast, several studies have failed to show differences in bacterial species between smokers and nonsmokers [37–40]. More research is needed to clarify the effects of smoking on the plaque biofilm.

2. **Effects on Host Response**
   A. **Diminished Inflammation**
      1. *The development of inflammation is suppressed in smokers with fewer sites exhibiting redness or bleeding on probing* [41].
      2. Smokers exhibit less gingivitis with less inflamed marginal tissue [7,15,41,42]. The typical clinical appearance of the smoker's gingival tissue exhibits relatively little gingival inflammation and a tendency to a more fibrotic appearance with little edema. Despite the clinical appearance, deep pockets, attachment loss, and bone loss are common.
      3. Reduced bleeding is most likely due to decreased vascularization. Histological comparisons of inflammatory lesions from smokers and nonsmokers show fewer blood vessels in the inflammatory lesions of smokers [43].
         a. In nonsmokers, vascularization of the periodontal tissues is very pronounced. Typical signs of inflammation, such as changes in gingival redness, swelling of the gingiva, an increase of gingival crevicular fluid flow as well as bleeding on probing (BOP) are caused by alterations of the vascular system.
         b. In smokers, however, the clinical signs of inflammation including BOP are suppressed (FIG. 11-4). For this reason, great care should be taken in performing periodontal screening and examination of smokers. *In smokers, the lack of bleeding on probing does not indicate healthy tissue as it does in nonsmokers.*
      4. Gingival bleeding on probing increases within 4 to 6 weeks of quitting smoking [44]. The resumption of bleeding on probing provides further evidence that tobacco smoking affects the inflammatory response and that these changes are reversible on quitting.

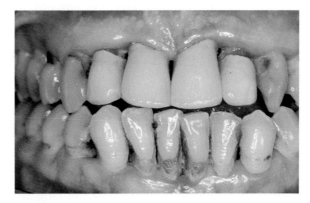

Figure 11.4. Diminished Clinical Signs of Inflammation in a Smoker. A 58-year-old female, cigarette smoker of 20 pack years with advanced periodontitis. Note that clinical signs of inflammation, such as marginal redness, are minimal. The teeth are discolored due to nicotine deposits.

   B. **Impairment of Normal Host Response**
      1. It is well documented that tobacco smoke and its constituents can inhibit neutrophil (PMN) and monocyte-macrophage defensive functions [44–52].
      2. The PMN is the first line of defense in the periodontal tissue.
         a. The normal passage of the PMN from a vessel to the periodontal tissues involves a series of steps including capture, rolling, adhesion, and transmigration through the vessel wall into the connective tissue.
         b. In smokers, a minor defect in adhesion and function compromises the leukocyte in defending the periodontal tissue [53,54].

3. Components in tobacco also may modify the production of cytokines or inflammatory mediators. Nicotine has been shown to increase the release of interleukin-6 by osteoblasts. Smokers have been reported to have increased levels of TNF-alpha in the crevicular fluid [55].

3. **Effects on Healing and Treatment Response**
   A. *Smoking impairs healing in all aspects of periodontal treatment* including nonsurgical treatment, basic periodontal surgery, regenerative periodontal surgery, mucogingival plastic periodontal surgery, and dental implant surgery [56–65].
   B. In nonsurgical treatment, smoking is associated with less probing depth reduction and less attachment gain [57,58,60,63,66–68].
   C. Tobacco smoking is a major risk factor for biologic complications around oral implants, including peri-implantitis, and the risk increases in a time- and dose-dependent manner.
      1. Some studies have shown that implant success rates are reduced in smokers [69–71].
      2. Other retrospective data, however, did not identify smoking as a variable associated with implant failure [72,73].

Section 3
Smoking Cessation

1. **Effects of Smoking Cessation on the Periodontium.** There have been few publications in the periodontal literature to specifically address the impact of smoking cessation on the periodontium, most probably because of the common challenges in motivating patients to quit smoking. Most investigations on the impact of smoking cessation on the periodontium have been either cross-sectional studies of periodontal status in current smokers, former smokers, and never smokers, or have been prospective cohort studies.
   A. The Effect of Smoking Cessation on Periodontal Status
      1. *Current smokers usually have significantly worse periodontal conditions (greater probing depths, more attachment loss, and alveolar bone loss) than either never smokers or former smokers.*
      2. In general, the periodontal health status of former smokers is not as good as that of never smokers but is better than that of current smokers [10,74,75].
      3. These findings suggest that while the past effects of smoking on the periodontium cannot be reversed, smoking cessation is beneficial to periodontal health [76].
      4. *The American Academy of Periodontology strongly recommends inclusion of tobacco cessation counseling is an integral part of periodontal therapy.*
   B. The Effect of Smoking Cessation on Periodontal Treatment Outcomes
      1. Studies have confirmed that treatment outcomes in former smokers are generally similar to those that can be expected in never smokers, but are usually better than those that can be expected in current smokers [77].
      2. The benefits of smoking cessation on the periodontium likely result from (1) a reduction in pathogenic bacteria in the subgingival plaque biofilm, (2) improved circulation in the gingiva, and (3) improvements in the host's immune-inflammatory response.

2. **Smoking Cessation Counseling**
   A. **Smoking Cessation and the Prevention of Periodontal Disease**
      1. Smoking may be responsible for more than half the cases of periodontal disease among adults in the United States.
      2. The knowledge that smoking is a significant risk factor suggests that *in smokers*, smoking cessation might prevent more periodontal disease than daily plaque biofilm control self-care. All patients should be assessed for smoking status and smokers should be given smoking cessation counseling. Examples of counseling sessions are presented in Boxes 11-1 to 11-3.
   B. **A User-Friendly Model for Cessation Counseling**
      1. The American Dental Hygienists' Association (ADHA) has developed a "user-friendly" model for tobacco cessation counseling. Ask. Advise. Refer. (AAR) is the ADHA's national Smoking Cessation Initiative designed to promote cessation intervention by dental hygienists.
      2. As part of the "Ask. Advise. Refer." campaign, dental hygienists refer their patients who use tobacco to quitlines as well as to web-based and local cessation programs.
      3. The "Ask. Advise. Refer." program is designed as a program that dental hygienists can easily integrate into their tobacco cessation efforts. Detailed information is available on the American Dental Hygienists' Association's website at www.askadviserefer.org (Boxes 11-1–11-3).

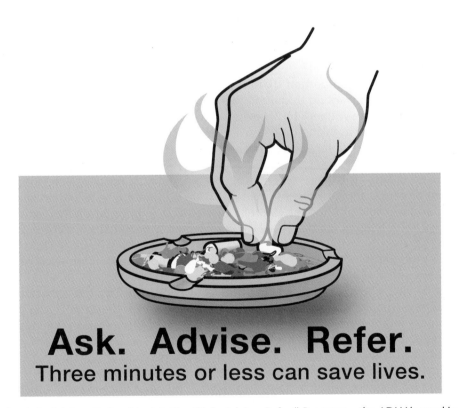

Ask. Advise. Refer.
Three minutes or less can save lives.

Figure 11.5. The Ask. Advise. Refer. Model. The "Ask. Advise. Refer." Program—the ADHA's smoking cessation initiative—is an easy to use three-step tobacco use cessation program.

Box 11.1 Sample Cessation Counseling Dialog #1

Ms. W is a 22-year-old radiology technician who has come to the dental office for her biannual exam. There are no significant findings on Ms. W's health history. The periodontal assessment reveals chronic periodontitis. Ms. W began smoking at age 12 and has smoked ¾ to 1 pack a day for almost 10 years. She is very excited because she has just become engaged but admits that her fiancé will not set a wedding date until she has quit smoking.

Clinician: Your oral exam shows evidence of damage from smoking. How do you feel about quitting?

Ms W: I want to quit. My fiancé hates that I am smoking. Every day I tell myself not to smoke but I just cannot seem to quit.

Clinician: What is the most difficult part about quitting? What is your biggest barrier?

Ms W: I feel like cigarettes are my best friends! The only time I relax is when I smoke—or when I am out drinking and smoking with my friends. Almost all my friends smoke.

Clinician: Have you ever tried to quit?

Ms W: Every day!! But nothing works! And then my fiancé yells at me so I feel worse and end up smoking more. I feel so guilty and so embarrassed!

Clinician: It sounds like you are in a vicious circle that is probably making it harder to quit. Let's put this in perspective. Of all addictions, it is harder to take control over the nicotine addiction than any other. It is also harder for women to quit than for men. But the good news is that there are more things available to help smokers quit than ever before. And quitting at your young age will be so beneficial in every way—including your oral health! The longer we do anything, the harder it is to stop. So stopping now would be the best thing you will ever do for yourself and while it will be very difficult, it will definitely be easier than if you continue to smoke for another 20 years.

Ms W: What is the best way to quit?

Clinician: Probably the most important thing is for you to do is make the decision to quit. That is even more important than wanting to quit. Rather than telling yourself "today I am not going to smoke," set a firm quit date within 1 to 2 weeks of this appointment and make plans on how not to smoke. Think of quitting as taking on a new job. With all the other responsibilities you have, quitting has to be your priority for about 3 months. And get help—the more support you have the better.

Ms W: What kind of help? My fiancé tells me to just stop—that if I really wanted to quit I could.

Clinician: A lot of people think smokers should just stop. But that is like telling an alcoholic to just stop drinking and we wouldn't do that. We tell other addicts to get quit therapy and that's what smokers should do! It is about learning how to quit. We rarely get what we want in life unless we work at it.

Ms W: I never thought of it that way. I thought I couldn't stop because I am weak or just don't have any will power.

Clinician: Not at all. I would suggest calling 1 800 QUIT NOW. This is a free service that provides counseling on how to quit. This quit line can also tell you about programs near you if you are interested in more intensive treatment. There are also excellent programs on the internet such as www.quitnet.com. And as your dental healthcare provider I will assist you in any way I can—including educate you about the medications that help people quit.

Ms W: Thank you. I will call the quit line and let you know what I decide to do.

Clinician: Good for you. You will miss your "best friend" but your life will be so much better once you have made the break!

Box 11.2 Sample Cessation Counseling Dialog #2

Ms. G is a 50-year-old grant writer who has come to the dental office for follow-up care. Ms. G has type 2 diabetes, COPD (chronic bronchitis), and severe enough periodontal disease that several of her teeth have been extracted in the past few years. Ms. G began smoking at age 13 and has smoked a pack a day for most of her life. About a year ago she decreased her daily consumption to half a pack.

Clinician: Congratulations on being able to cut down on your smoking! Have you thought about quitting completely? We might be able to save your remaining teeth if you are able to quit.

Ms G: I know I should quit but I really love my cigarettes.

Clinician: Has it been hard for you to cut down?

Ms G: Actually it's been horrible.

Clinician: What has been the most difficult part for you?

Ms G: I can't stop thinking about my next cigarette. I find myself thinking about when I can get the next cigarette in as soon as I put one out!

Clinician: It almost sounds like the cigarettes have become even more important to you since you cut down! While quitting is the most difficult thing you might ever do, it might in fact make your life easier to not have to worry about when you can get in your next cigarette.

Ms G: That's true—it would be so nice to not to have to think about them any more.

Clinician: So you still love your cigarettes but don't love that you are smoking!

Ms G: Yes that is exactly it. I hate that I am still smoking. I know it is so bad for my health. I feel that I must quit but I have tried to quit before and the longest I have ever gone without a cigarette has only been 4 hours! Cigarettes are the only things that calm me down.

Clinician: How soon do you smoke when you first get up in the morning and do you ever smoke if you wake during the night?

Ms G: I smoke before my feet hit the ground every morning and I often take a couple of drags if I wake up during the night.

Clinician: It sounds like you have a strong physical addiction as well as a significant psychological addiction. Have you considered using medication to help you quit? You would be a good candidate for pharmacotherapy.

Ms G: No. I take insulin for my diabetes and I don't want to take anything that would interfere with that.

Clinician: Actually, smoking interferes with controlling your diabetes much more than a quit-smoking medication. And were you aware that with every cigarette your blood sugar goes up? So your diabetes would be much easier to control if you quit.

Ms G: I had no idea that was the case.

Clinician: One suggestion would be to look at quitting the same way you look at having diabetes. A nicotine addiction is a chronic condition just as diabetes is. You do whatever you can to control your blood sugar with diet, exercise, and medication in order to enhance your quality of life and decrease risks—even though you may not want to do all those things. Try to look at quitting that way. Even though you love cigarettes, you will benefit by taking control! Look at quitting as something you are doing for yourself rather than to yourself. That approach may make it easier to let go of smoking.

Ms G: I like that. It puts me in control of the situation—rather than letting the cigarettes control me! Maybe I will consider trying a medication to help me.

Box 11.3 Sample Smoking Cessation Counseling Dialog #3

Mr. R is a 48-year-old attorney who has come to the dental office for his care. Mr. R has hypertension and high cholesterol. His periodontal assessment reveals aggressive periodontitis. Mr. R. began smoking at age 17 and has smoked 2 packs a day for 30 years.

Clinician: As you know, your oral exam shows significant damage from smoking and your blood pressure is elevated today. Have you tried to quit since our last visit?

Mr. R: Not really. And I don't want to talk about it. Everyone is on me. My doctors, my wife, my kids, and now I suppose you are going to give me a hard time too.

Clinician: I don't want to give you a hard time. But I do want you to encourage you to at least try and quit. The more times you try, the more chance you have of success. I am not going to tell you how dangerous it is to smoke. But I am going to remind you that by quitting you can reverse so much of the damage cigarettes have caused in you.

Mr. R: Look I really don't want to quit. I exercise and I watch what I eat. I'll keep coming to you for my teeth and take medicine for my heart problems and hope for the best.

Clinician: You are such a "take charge" person in every other aspect of your life. How about taking control over this addiction rather than hoping for the best?

Mr. R: I will quit when I am ready. I know myself. When I decide to do something, it gets done.

Clinician: Take advantage of that! Consider what is available to help you quit now. It is possible to quit even if you don't want to quit or don't feel ready.

Mr. R: It would get people off my back anyway. My kids nag me every day.

Clinician: People in your life are concerned about you. But you cannot quit for them. You can use the fact that you will have a longer, better quality life with your kids as a motivation though the decision to quit is yours. No one, nothing, can make you quit but there are plenty of us who can help you quit.

Mr. R: If I do this, I am doing it on my own.

Clinician: I understand your wanting to take that approach. However, it would be so much easier if you use a medication. You have been smoking for a long time and a medication would increase your chance of permanent success.

Mr. R: Is it ok to take something with all my heart problems?.

Clinician: Absolutely. In fact the newest medications have high success rates. It should be started one to two weeks prior to quitting and once there is a therapeutic dose in your system, you should notice a significant decrease in your desire to smoke. I can provide you with more information and arrange for a prescription.

Mr. R: I have heard that some people get depressed when they try to quit smoking.

Clinician: Feeling depressed is very common with quitting! I will show you a list of the most common withdrawal symptoms so you will be aware of what to expect. And also give you information on the other 6 FDA-approved medications so you will have all the options. Think about setting a quit date within a couple of weeks and let me know how I can best assist you through the process. I will keep working with you until you are able to quit.

Mr. R: OK I will try but this is just between you and me.

Clinician: I understand and will respect that. At some point people in your life will be aware that you are trying to quit and it might help you to let them know what they can do to help you— including NOT nag you! I am very proud of you for making the attempt. You will not regret it!

Chapter Summary Statement

Tobacco use is a major risk factor for the onset and progression of periodontal disease. There are several theories as to why smokers have more periodontal disease than nonsmokers, involving effects on (1) bacteria in plaque biofilm, (2) host response, (3) healing, and (4) response to treatment. There is sufficient evidence for the benefits of smoking cessation on a wide variety of oral health outcomes, including periodontal treatment. Advice and assistance on smoking cessation is, therefore, an integral part in the management of all patients seeking periodontal care.

Section 4
Focus on Patients

Case 1

A new patient with severe chronic periodontitis has a history of smoking one to two packs of cigarettes each day. The patient informs you that he will do "anything" to save his teeth, but that he cannot quit smoking. What counsel would you provide this patient about the effect of the smoking habit on the likelihood of long-term control of his periodontitis?

References

1. Albandar JM, et al. Cigar, pipe, and cigarette smoking as risk factors for periodontal disease and tooth loss. *J Periodontol.* 2000;71(12):1874–1881.
2. Anerud A, Loe H, Boysen H. The natural history and clinical course of calculus formation in man. *J Clin Periodontol.* 1991;18(3):160–170.
3. Beck JD, Koch GG, Offenbacher S. Incidence of attachment loss over 3 years in older adults— new and progressing lesions. *Community Dent Oral Epidemiol.* 1995;23(5):291–296.
4. Beck JD, et al. Prevalence and risk indicators for periodontal attachment loss in a population of older community-dwelling blacks and whites. *J Periodontol.* 1990;61(8):521–528.
5. Dolan TA, et al. Behavioral risk indicators of attachment loss in adult Floridians. *J Clin Periodontol.* 1997;24(4):223–232.
6. Feldman RS, Alman JE, Chauncey HH. Periodontal disease indexes and tobacco smoking in healthy aging men. *Gerodontics.* 1987;3(1):43–46.
7. Feldman RS, Bravacos JS, Rose CL. Association between smoking different tobacco products and periodontal disease indexes. *J Periodontol.* 1983;54(8):481–487.
8. Grossi SG, et al. Assessment of risk for periodontal disease. II. Risk indicators for alveolar bone loss. *J Periodontol.* 1995;66(1):23–29.
9. Grossi SG, et al. Assessment of risk for periodontal disease. I. Risk indicators for attachment loss. *J Periodontol.* 1994;65(3):260–267.
10. Haber J, Kent RL. Cigarette smoking in a periodontal practice. *J Periodontol.* 1992; 63(2):100–106.
11. Krall EA, Garvey AJ, Garcia RI. Alveolar bone loss and tooth loss in male cigar and pipe smokers. *J Am Dent Assoc.* 1999;130(1):57–64.
12. Machtei EE, et al. Longitudinal study of prognostic factors in established periodontitis patients. *J Clin Periodontol.* 1997;24(2):102–109.
13. Martinez-Canut P, Lorca A, Magan R. Smoking and periodontal disease severity. *J Clin Periodontol.* 1995;22(10):743–749.

14. Tomar SL, Asma S. Smoking-attributable periodontitis in the United States: findings from NHANES III. National Health and Nutrition Examination Survey. *J Periodontol.* 2000;71(5):743–751.

15. Haffajee AD, Socransky SS. Relationship of cigarette smoking to attachment level profiles. *J Clin Periodontol.* 2001;28(4):283–295.

16. Linden GJ, Mullally BH. Cigarette smoking and periodontal destruction in young adults. *J Periodontol.* 1994;65(7):718–723.

17. Bergstrom J, Eliasson S. Cigarette smoking and alveolar bone height in subjects with a high standard of oral hygiene. *J Clin Periodontol.* 1987;14(8):466–469.

18. Bergstrom J, Eliasson S, Dock J. Exposure to tobacco smoking and periodontal health. *J Clin Periodontol.* 2000;27(1):61–68.

19. Bergstrom J, Eliasson S, Preber H. Cigarette smoking and periodontal bone loss. *J Periodontol.* 1991;62(4):242–246.

20. Bergstrom J, Floderus-Myrhed B. Co-twin control study of the relationship between smoking and some periodontal disease factors. *Commun Dent Oral Epidemiol.* 1983;11(2):113–116.

21. Bergstrom J, Eliasson S. Noxious effect of cigarette smoking on periodontal health. *J Periodontal Res.* 1987;22(6):513–517.

22. Bergstrom J, Eliasson S, Dock J. A 10-year prospective study of tobacco smoking and periodontal health. *J Periodontol.* 2000;71(8):1338–1347.

23. Axelsson P, Paulander J, Lindhe J. Relationship between smoking and dental status in 35-, 50-, 65-, and 75-year-old individuals. *J Clin Periodontol.* 1998;25(4):297–305.

24. Mullally BH, Linden GJ. Molar furcation involvement associated with cigarette smoking in periodontal referrals. *J Clin Periodontol.* 1996;23(7):658–661.

25. Krall EA, Dawson-Hughes B, Garvey AJ, Garcia RI. Smoking, smoking cessation, and tooth loss. *J Dent Res,* 1997;76(10):1653–1659.

26. Osterberg T, Mellstrom D. Tobacco smoking: a major risk factor for loss of teeth in three 70-year-old cohorts. *Commun Dent Oral Epidemiol.* 1986;14(6):367–370.

27. MacFarlane GD, Herzberg MC, Wolff LF, Hardie NA. Refractory periodontitis associated with abnormal polymorphonuclear leukocyte phagocytosis and cigarette smoking. *J Periodontol.* 1992;63(11):908–913.

28. Haber J, Wattles J, Crowley M, et al. Evidence for cigarette smoking as a major risk factor for periodontitis. *J Periodontol.* 1993;64(1):16–23.

29. American Academy of Periodontology. Position paper: tobacco use and the periodontal patient. Research, Science and Therapy Committee of the American Academy of Periodontology. *J Periodontol.* 1999;70(11):1419–1427.

30. Barbour SE, Nakashima K, Zhang JB, et al. Tobacco and smoking: environmental factors that modify the host response (immune system) and have an impact on periodontal health. *Crit Rev Oral Biol Med.* 1997;8(4):437–460.

31. Palmer RM, Wilson RF, Hasan AS, Scott DA. Mechanisms of action of environmental factors—tobacco smoking. *J Clin Periodontol.* 2005;32 Suppl 6:180–195.

32. Zambon JJ, Grossi SG, Machtei EE, et al. Cigarette smoking increases the risk for subgingival infection with periodontal pathogens. *J Periodontol.* 1996;67(10 Suppl):1050–1054.

33. van Winkelhoff AJ, Bosch-Tijhof CJ, Winkel EG, van der Reijden WA. Smoking affects the subgingival microflora in periodontitis. *J Periodontol.* 2001;72(5):666–671.

34. Kamma JJ, Nakou M, Baehni PC. Clinical and microbiological characteristics of smokers with early onset periodontitis. *J Periodontal Res.* 1999;34(1):25–33.

35. Loesche WJ, Gusberti F, Mettraux G, et al. Relationship between oxygen tension and subgingival bacterial flora in untreated human periodontal pockets. *Infect Immun.* 1983;42(2):659–667.

36. Mettraux GR, Gusberti FA, Graf H. Oxygen tension (pO2) in untreated human periodontal pockets. *J Periodontol.* 1984;55(9):516–521.

37. Bostrom L, Bergstrom J, Dahlen G, Linder LE. Smoking and subgingival microflora in periodontal disease. *J Clin Periodontol.* 2001;28(3):212–219.

38. Darby IB, Hodge PJ, Riggio MP, Kinane DF. Microbial comparison of smoker and non-smoker adult and early-onset periodontitis patients by polymerase chain reaction. *J Clin Periodontol.* 2000;27(6):417–424.

39. Preber H, Bergstrom J. Occurrence of gingival bleeding in smoker and non-smoker patients. *Acta Odontol Scand.* 1985;43(5):315–320.

40. Van der Velden U, Varoufaki A, Hutter JW, et al. Effect of smoking and periodontal treatment on the subgingival microflora. *J Clin Periodontol.* 2003;30(7):603–610.

41. Bergstrom J, Preber H. The influence of cigarette smoking on the development of experimental gingivitis. *J Periodontal Res*. 1986;21(6):668–676.
42. Preber H, Bergstrom J, Linder LE. Occurrence of periopathogens in smoker and non-smoker patients. *J Clin Periodontol*. 1992;19(9 Pt 1):667–671.
43. Nair P, Sutherland G, Palmer RM, et al. Gingival bleeding on probing increases after quitting smoking. *J Clin Periodontol*. 2003;30(5):435–437.
44. Kenney EB, Kraal JH, Saxe SR, Jones J. The effect of cigarette smoke on human oral polymorphonuclear leukocytes. *J Periodontal Res*. 1977;12(4):227–234.
45. Codd EE, Swim AT, Bridges RB. Tobacco smokers' neutrophils are desensitized to chemotactic peptide-stimulated oxygen uptake. *J Lab Clin Med*. 1987;110(5):648–652.
46. Eichel B, Shahrik HA. Tobacco smoke toxicity: loss of human oral leukocyte function and fluid-cell metabolism. *Science*. 1969;166(911):1424–1428.
47. Lannan S, McLean A, Drost E, et al. Changes in neutrophil morphology and morphometry following exposure to cigarette smoke. *Int J Exp Pathol*. 1992;73(2):183–191.
48. Nowak D, Ruta U, Piasecka G. Nicotine increases human polymorphonuclear leukocytes chemotactic response—a possible additional mechanism of lung injury in cigarette smokers. *Exp Pathol*. 1990;39(1):37–43.
49. Pabst MJ, Pabst KM, Collier JA, Coleman TC, Lemons-Prince ML, Godat MS, Waring MB, Babu JP. Inhibition of neutrophil and monocyte defensive functions by nicotine. *J Periodontol*. 1995;66(12):1047–1055.
50. Ryder MI, Fujitaki R, Johnson G, Hyun W. Alterations of neutrophil oxidative burst by in vitro smoke exposure: implications for oral and systemic diseases. *Ann Periodontol*. 1998;3(1):76–87.
51. Selby C, Drost E, Brown D, Howie S, MacNee W. Inhibition of neutrophil adherence and movement by acute cigarette smoke exposure. *Exp Lung Res*. 1992;18(6):813–827.
52. Totti N III, McCusker KT, Campbell EJ, et al. Nicotine is chemotactic for neutrophils and enhances neutrophil responsiveness to chemotactic peptides. *Science*. 1984;223(4632): 169–171.
53. Koundouros E, Odell E, Coward P, et al. Soluble adhesion molecules in serum of smokers and non-smokers, with and without periodontitis. *J Periodontal Res*. 1996;31(8):596–599.
54. Palmer RM, Scott DA, Meekin TN, et al. Potential mechanisms of susceptibility to periodontitis in tobacco smokers. *J Periodontal Res*. 1999;34(7):363–369.
55. Bostrom L, Linder LE, Bergstrom J. Clinical expression of TNF-alpha in smoking-associated periodontal disease. *J Clin Periodontol*. 1998;25(10):767–773.
56. Bostrom L, Linder LE, Bergstrom J. Influence of smoking on the outcome of periodontal surgery. A 5-year follow-up. *J Clin Periodontol*. 1998;25(3):194–201.
57. Grossi SG, Skrepcinski FB, DeCaro T, et al. Response to periodontal therapy in diabetics and smokers. *J Periodontol*. 1996;67(10 Suppl):1094–1102.
58. Grossi SG, Zambon J, Machtei EE, et al. Effects of smoking and smoking cessation on healing after mechanical periodontal therapy. *J Am Dent Assoc*. 1997;128(5):599–607.
59. Heasman L, Stacey F, Preshaw PM, et al. The effect of smoking on periodontal treatment response: a review of clinical evidence. *J Clin Periodontol*. 2006;33(4):241–253.
60. Kaldahl WB, Johnson GK, Patil KD, Kalkwarf KL. Levels of cigarette consumption and response to periodontal therapy. *J Periodontol*. 1996;67(7):675–681.
61. Kinane DF, Chestnutt IG. Smoking and periodontal disease. *Crit Rev Oral Biol Med*. 2000;11(3):356–365.
62. Miller PD, Jr. Root coverage with the free gingival graft. Factors associated with incomplete coverage. *J Periodontol*. 1987;58(10):674–681.
63. Preber H, Bergstrom J. The effect of non-surgical treatment on periodontal pockets in smokers and non-smokers. *J Clin Periodontol*. 1986;13(4):319–323.
64. Tonetti MS. Cigarette smoking and periodontal diseases: etiology and management of disease. *Ann Periodontol*. 1998;3(1):88–101.
65. Tonetti MS, Pini-Prato G, Cortellini P. Effect of cigarette smoking on periodontal healing following GTR in infrabony defects. A preliminary retrospective study. *J Clin Periodontol*. 1995;22(3):229–234.
66. Ah MK, Johnson GK, Kaldahl WB, et al. The effect of smoking on the response to periodontal therapy. *J Clin Periodontol*. 1994;21(2):91–97.
67. Haffajee AD, Cugini MA, Dibart S, et al. The effect of SRP on the clinical and microbiological parameters of periodontal diseases. *J Clin Periodontol*. 1997;24(5):324–334.

68. Renvert S, Dahlen G, Wikstrom M. The clinical and microbiological effects of non-surgical periodontal therapy in smokers and non-smokers. *J Clin Periodontol*. 1998;25(2):153–157.

69. Bain CA, Moy PK. The association between the failure of dental implants and cigarette smoking. *Int J Oral Maxillofac Implants*. 1993;8(6):609–615.

70. Gorman LM, Lambert PM, Morris HF, et al. The effect of smoking on implant survival at second-stage surgery: DICRG Interim Report No. 5. Dental Implant CLinical Research Group. *Implant Dent*. 1994;3(3):165–168.

71. Jones JK, Triplett RG. The relationship of cigarette smoking to impaired intraoral wound healing: a review of evidence and implications for patient care. *J Oral Maxillofac Surg*. 1992;50(3):237–239; discussion 9–40.

72. Minsk L, Polson AM, Weisgold A, et al. Outcome failures of endosseous implants from a clinical training center. *Compend Contin Educ Dent*. 1996;17(9):848–850, 52–54, 56 passim.

73. Weyant RJ. Characteristics associated with the loss and peri-implant tissue health of endosseous dental implants. *Int J Oral Maxillofac Implants*. 1994;9(1):95–102.

74. Bolin A, Eklund G, Frithiof L, Lavstedt S. The effect of changed smoking habits on marginal alveolar bone loss. A longitudinal study. *Swed Dent J*. 1993;17(5):211–216.

75. Haber J, Wattles J, Crowley M, et al. Evidence for cigarette smoking as a major risk factor for periodontitis. *J Periodontol*. 1993;64(1):16–23.

76. Preshaw PM, Heasman L, Stacey F, et al. The effect of quitting smoking on chronic periodontitis. *J Clin Periodontol*. 2005;32(8):869–879.

76. Ramseier CA. Potential impact of subject-based risk factor control on periodontitis. *J Clin Periodontol*. 2005;32(Suppl 6):283–290.

77. Preshaw PM, Heasman L, Stacey F, et al. The effect of quitting smoking on chronic periodontitis. *J Clin Periodontol*. 2005;32(8):869–879.

Chapter 12

Etiologic Factors: Risk for Periodontitis

Learning Objectives

- Define the term biologic equilibrium and discuss factors that can disrupt the balance between health and disease in the periodontium.

- Define and give examples of the term contributing risk factors.

- In the clinical setting, for a patient with periodontitis, explain to your clinical instructor the factors that may have contributed to your patient's disease.

Key Terms

Multifactorial etiology
Biologic equilibrium
Disease-promoting factors

Health-promoting factors
Risk assessment

Section 1
Risk Factors for Periodontal Disease

Research studies have clearly demonstrated that periodontal disease is a bacterial infection of the periodontium and that bacteria are the primary etiologic agents in periodontal disease. The presence of pathogenic bacteria, however, does not necessarily mean that an individual will experience periodontitis.

Periodontitis has a multifactorial etiology, that is, periodontitis is a disease that results from the interaction of many factors (FIG. 12-1). Some persons with abundant bacterial plaque biofilm exhibit only mild disease, while others with light dental plaque biofilm suffer severe disease. Untreated gingivitis does not always lead to periodontitis and everyone infected with periodontal pathogens does not experience periodontitis.

These findings suggest that additional factors, other than the presence of bacteria, must play a significant role in determining why some individuals are more susceptible to periodontal disease than others. Many contributing factors help to determine the initiation and progression of periodontal disease (TABLE 12-1). Contributing etiologic factors negatively influence the periodontium as well as the host immune response. It is critical for the dental team to recognize contributing factors for periodontal disease during a periodontal assessment. Whenever possible, the dental team should eliminate or minimize the impact of contributing factors during the nonsurgical periodontal treatment (TABLE 12-2).

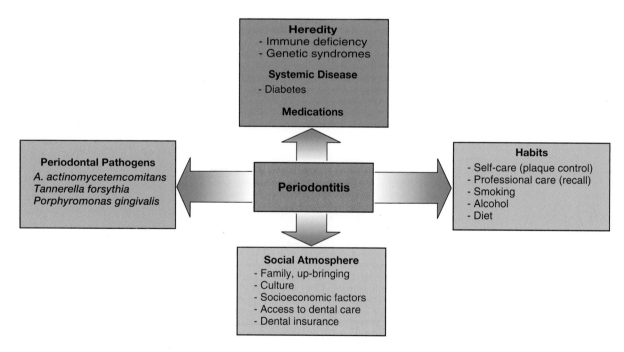

Figure 12.1. Risk Factors for Periodontal Disease. Periodontitis has a multifactorial etiology. Additional factors—other than the presence of bacteria—play a significant role in determining why some individuals are more susceptible to periodontal disease than others.

TABLE 12-1. Risk Factors for Periodontal Disease

Poor self care
- Plaque biofilm
- Calculus deposits

Faulty dentistry
- Overhangs
- Subgingival margins

Smoking/tobacco
- Frequency
- Current history
- Past history

Nutrition
- Poor nutritional habits

Medications
- Dilantin
- Calcium channel blockers
- Cyclosporin
- Drugs known to cause xerostomia

Diabetes
- Duration
- Poor glycemic control

Hormonal variations
- Puberty
- Pregnancy
- Menopause

Heredity
- Family history
- Genetic testing

Immunocompromised
- Neutropenia
- Human immunodeficiency virus

TABLE 12-2. Risk Management for Periodontal Disease

Poor self-care
- Improved plaque biofilm control
- Frequent professional care

Faulty dentistry
- Corrective dentistry

Smoking/tobacco
- Cessation counseling
- Smoking quit lines
- Chemotherapeutics

Nutrition
- Supplements

Medications
- Change medications
- Work with physician
- Good plaque biofilm control
- Frequent professional care

Diabetes
- Good glycemic control
- Work with physician
- Good plaque biofilm control
- Frequent professional care

Hormonal variations
- Good plaque biofilm control
- Frequent professional care
- Chemotherapeutics

Heredity
- Chemotherapeutics
- Frequent professional care

Immunocompromised
- Consult with physician
- Chemotherapeutics

Section 2
Balance Between Periodontal Health and Disease

BIOLOGIC EQUILIBRIUM

1. **Biologic Equilibrium.** The human body is continually working to maintain a state of balance in the internal environment of the body, known as biologic equilibrium.
   A. **Periodontal Health**
      1. In the oral cavity, most of the time, things are in a state of balance between the bacterial plaque biofilm and the host.
      2. For the periodontium to remain healthy, the bacterial challenge must be contained at a level that can be tolerated by the host.
      3. The situation can be thought of as a balance scale, with the disease-promoting factors on one side of the scale and the health-promoting factors on the other (FIG. 12-2). As long as the two sides of the scale are in balance, there will be no disease progression.
   B. **Periodontal Disease**
      1. The intermittent pattern of disease activity seen in periodontitis is believed to result from the changing balance between the pathogenic bacteria and the host's inflammatory and immune responses.
      2. This balance also can be affected by other risk factors, such as local or systemic variables.

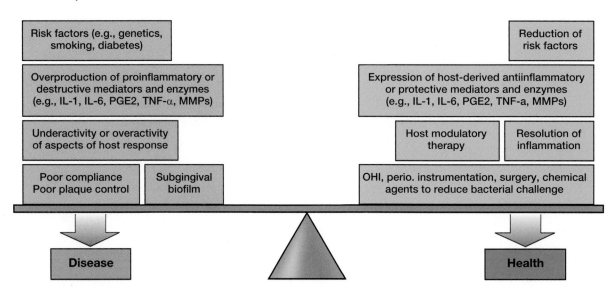

Figure 12.2. Periodontal Equilibrium. The balance between periodontal health and disease is tipped toward disease by risk factors. OHI, oral hygiene instructions.

2. **The Delicate Balance Between Health and Disease.** When active periodontal disease sites are present in the mouth, the goal is to return the oral cavity to a state of biologic equilibrium.
   A. **Periodontal Equilibrium and Dental Plaque Biofilm**
      1. Experienced dental hygienists will attest to the fact that major differences exist in the way that individuals respond to the plaque biofilm.
         a. Many patients return to the dental office year after year with generalized bacterial plaque biofilm. These patients exhibit gingivitis and yet, year after year, show no clinical signs of progression to periodontitis. For some reason, gingivitis never progresses to periodontitis in these individuals. Perhaps these individuals have no systemic or acquired factors that add

stress to the biologic equilibrium. Basically, if an individual's immune system can effectively deal with a mouthful of periodontal pathogens, there will be no destructive periodontal disease (FIG. 12-3).

b. In a few individuals, gingivitis progresses to periodontitis. It is theorized that such individuals may possess systemic risk factors (such as genetic variables or systemic disease) that significantly increase their susceptibility to periodontitis (FIG. 12-4).

2. There are many patients who are unable or unwilling to perform the self-care necessary to control bacterial plaque biofilm. For these patients, it is necessary to increase the frequency of professional care to compensate for the inadequate level of patient self-care. A professional care at frequent intervals can be effective in restoring the balance between health and disease (FIG. 12-5).

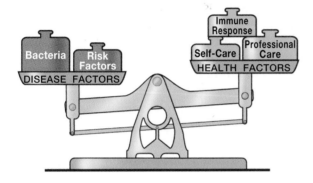

Figure 12.3. **Gingivitis in the Presence of Plaque Biofilms**. In individuals with a low susceptibility to periodontitis, gingivitis may never progress to periodontitis.

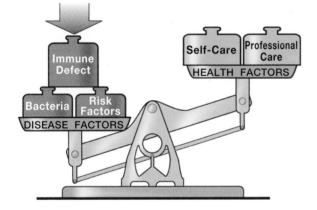

Figure 12.4. **Periodontitis in the Presence of Plaque Biofilm**. In susceptible individuals, gingivitis processes to periodontitis.

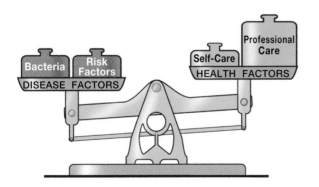

Figure 12.5. **Frequent Professional Care**. An individual who is unwilling or unable to obtain adequate plaque biofilm control on a daily basis. More frequent periodontal instrumentation can help to control the development of mature plaque biofilms.

B. Local Contributing Factors

1. It is possible to totally eliminate a local risk factor in many cases. A faulty restoration is a good example of a local factor that can be corrected, restoring the balance between local disease-promoting and health-promoting factors at the site.

2. In other cases, it is possible to compensate for a local risk factor by improving the patient's self-care and/or increasing the frequency of professional care. For example, the patient may need to use tufted dental floss to clean around the abutment teeth of a fixed bridge. This situation can be compared to adding more weight on the health-side of the balance scale to equal or exceed the weight on the disease-side of the scale.

C. Systemic or Genetic Contributing Factors

1. Certain systemic or acquired risk factors are possible to control or eliminate if the patient is willing to do so. For example, the individual can work with a physician to keep diabetes well controlled. A smoker may decide to stop smoking. In both cases the individual has made a change that is health promoting, both systemically and for the periodontium (FIG. 12-6).

2. In the case of a contributing risk factor that cannot be controlled, it is necessary to add weight to the health-side of the scale. For example, some individuals have a genetic risk factor—such as abnormal PMN function—that causes them to be susceptible to severe periodontitis. At the present time, we are unable to eliminate or control genetic risk factors. It is possible, however, to assist the patient in maintaining health by increasing the extent of professional care. Frequent professional care will increase the weight on the health-side of the scale (FIG. 12-7).

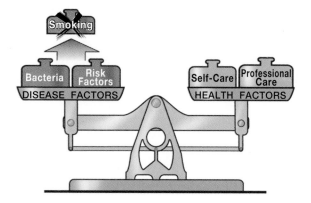

Figure 12.6. Eliminating a Systemic Risk Factor. Smoking cessation, combined with adequate self-care and professional care, restores the balance.

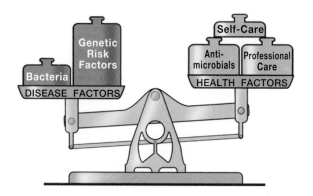

Figure 12.7. Management of a Genetic Risk Factor. At the present time, there are some risk factors that cannot be eliminated or controlled. Professional care can help slow disease progression.

PERIODONTAL RISK ASSESSMENT

Dental healthcare providers are interested not only in diagnosing periodontal disease, but also in predicting which individuals are more likely to develop periodontitis. The process of identifying risk factors that increase an individual's probability of disease is called risk assessment. It is becoming possible to consider an individual's risk factors for periodontal disease (systemic disease, genetic information, personal habits, and characteristics) and to classify patients into high- or low-risk groups. For example, individuals who smoke have a higher risk of periodontitis than nonsmokers. Clinicians also use the risk assessment process to prevent disease. For example, identifying smokers and offering smoking cessation counseling.

Information concerning individual risk for developing periodontal disease is obtained through careful evaluation of the individual's demographic data, medical history, dental history, and comprehensive periodontal clinical examination (TABLE 12-3).

Risk assessment questionnaires are practical tools that can be helpful in identifying individuals who are at a high-risk for periodontal disease. Figures 12-8A and B are examples of a two-page periodontal risk questionnaire that can be used to elicit the presence of common periodontal risk factors. Dental hygienists can use risk questionnaires to initiate discussion with patients about periodontal risk factors.

TABLE 12-3.   Clinical Risk Assessment for Periodontal Disease

Demographic data

    Age

    Duration of exposure to contributing risk factors

    Self-care (plaque biofilm control)

    Frequency of professional care

    Male gender

    Dental awareness

    Socioeconomic status

Medical history

    Tobacco use

    Diabetes

    Osteoporosis

    Certain medications

    Genetic predisposition to aggressive disease

Dental history

    Frequency of professional care

    Family history of early tooth loss

    Previous history of periodontal disease

Clinical examination

    Plaque biofilm accumulation

    Calculus deposits

    Bleeding on probing

    Loss of attachment

    Plaque biofilm retentive areas

    Anatomic contributing factors

    Restorative contributing factors

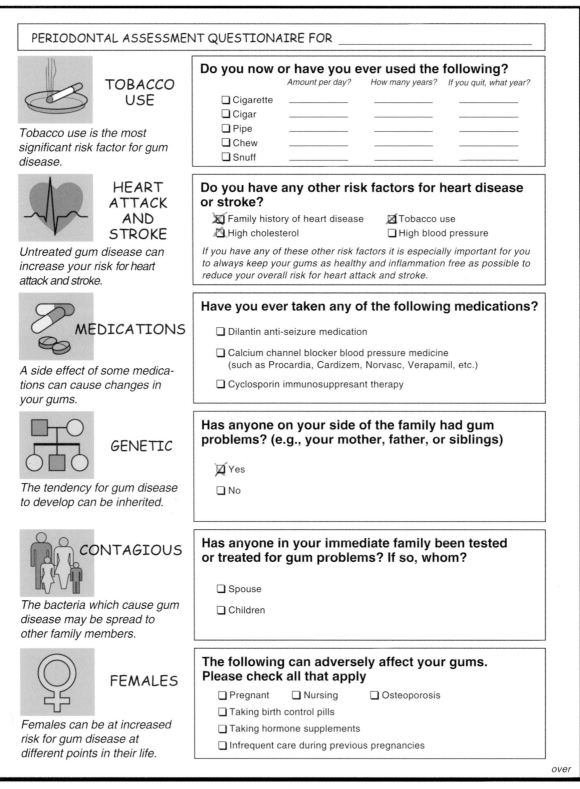

PERIODONTAL ASSESSMENT QUESTIONAIRE FOR _____

TOBACCO USE

Tobacco use is the most significant risk factor for gum disease.

Do you now or have you ever used the following?

	Amount per day?	How many years?	If you quit, what year?
☐ Cigarette	_____	_____	_____
☐ Cigar	_____	_____	_____
☐ Pipe	_____	_____	_____
☐ Chew	_____	_____	_____
☐ Snuff	_____	_____	_____

HEART ATTACK AND STROKE

Untreated gum disease can increase your risk for heart attack and stroke.

Do you have any other risk factors for heart disease or stroke?

☒ Family history of heart disease   ☒ Tobacco use
☒ High cholesterol   ☐ High blood pressure

If you have any of these other risk factors it is especially important for you to always keep your gums as healthy and inflammation free as possible to reduce your overall risk for heart attack and stroke.

MEDICATIONS

A side effect of some medications can cause changes in your gums.

Have you ever taken any of the following medications?

☐ Dilantin anti-seizure medication

☐ Calcium channel blocker blood pressure medicine (such as Procardia, Cardizem, Norvasc, Verapamil, etc.)

☐ Cyclosporin immunosuppresant therapy

GENETIC

The tendency for gum disease to develop can be inherited.

Has anyone on your side of the family had gum problems? (e.g., your mother, father, or siblings)

☒ Yes

☐ No

CONTAGIOUS

The bacteria which cause gum disease may be spread to other family members.

Has anyone in your immediate family been tested or treated for gum problems? If so, whom?

☐ Spouse

☐ Children

FEMALES

Females can be at increased risk for gum disease at different points in their life.

The following can adversely affect your gums. Please check all that apply

☐ Pregnant   ☐ Nursing   ☐ Osteoporosis
☐ Taking birth control pills
☐ Taking hormone supplements
☐ Infrequent care during previous pregnancies

over

A

Figure 12.8A. Side 1 of Periodontal Risk Questionnaire. Risk assessment questionnaires are practical tools that can be helpful in identifying individuals who have a high susceptibility to periodontitis. Side one of a risk assessment questionnaire is shown here. See Figure 12-8B for side two of this questionnaire. (Used with permission of Timothy G. Donley, DDS, MSD, Bowling Green, KY.)

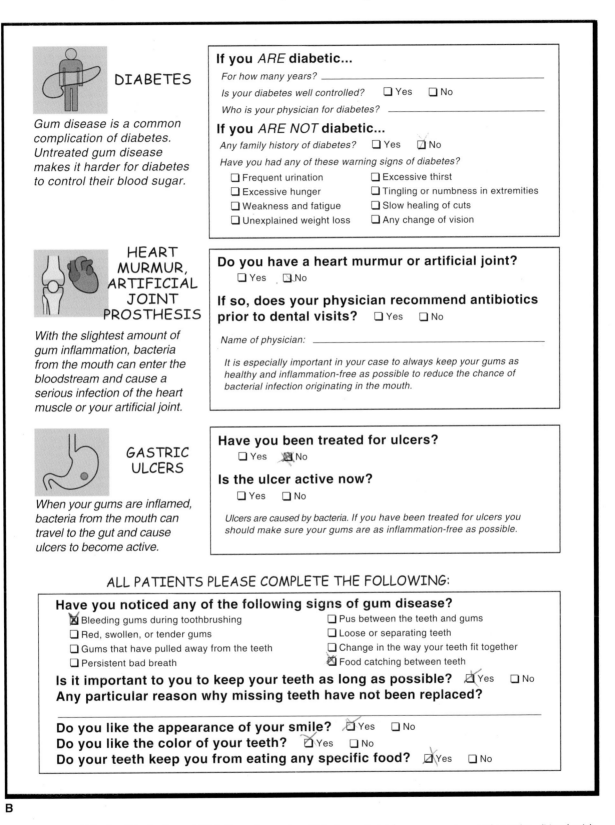

DIABETES

Gum disease is a common complication of diabetes. Untreated gum disease makes it harder for diabetes to control their blood sugar.

If you *ARE* diabetic...

For how many years? _____

Is your diabetes well controlled?   ☐ Yes   ☐ No

Who is your physician for diabetes? _____

If you *ARE NOT* diabetic...

Any family history of diabetes?   ☐ Yes   ☒ No

Have you had any of these warning signs of diabetes?

☐ Frequent urination   ☐ Excessive thirst
☐ Excessive hunger   ☐ Tingling or numbness in extremities
☐ Weakness and fatigue   ☐ Slow healing of cuts
☐ Unexplained weight loss   ☐ Any change of vision

HEART MURMUR, ARTIFICIAL JOINT PROSTHESIS

With the slightest amount of gum inflammation, bacteria from the mouth can enter the bloodstream and cause a serious infection of the heart muscle or your artificial joint.

Do you have a heart murmur or artificial joint?
☐ Yes   ☒ No

If so, does your physician recommend antibiotics prior to dental visits?   ☐ Yes   ☐ No

Name of physician: _____

It is especially important in your case to always keep your gums as healthy and inflammation-free as possible to reduce the chance of bacterial infection originating in the mouth.

GASTRIC ULCERS

When your gums are inflamed, bacteria from the mouth can travel to the gut and cause ulcers to become active.

Have you been treated for ulcers?
☐ Yes   ☒ No

Is the ulcer active now?
☐ Yes   ☐ No

Ulcers are caused by bacteria. If you have been treated for ulcers you should make sure your gums are as inflammation-free as possible.

ALL PATIENTS PLEASE COMPLETE THE FOLLOWING:

Have you noticed any of the following signs of gum disease?

☒ Bleeding gums during toothbrushing   ☐ Pus between the teeth and gums
☐ Red, swollen, or tender gums   ☐ Loose or separating teeth
☐ Gums that have pulled away from the teeth   ☐ Change in the way your teeth fit together
☐ Persistent bad breath   ☒ Food catching between teeth

Is it important to you to keep your teeth as long as possible?   ☒ Yes   ☐ No
Any particular reason why missing teeth have not been replaced?

_____

Do you like the appearance of your smile?   ☒ Yes   ☐ No
Do you like the color of your teeth?   ☒ Yes   ☐ No
Do your teeth keep you from eating any specific food?   ☒ Yes   ☐ No

B

Figure 12.8B. Side 2 of Periodontal Risk Questionnaire. Side two of a risk assessment questionnaire. (Used with permission of Timothy G. Donley, DDS, MSD, Bowling Green, KY.)

Chapter Summary Statement

In the oral cavity, most of the time, things are in a state of balance between the bacterial plaque biofilm and the host.

- For the periodontium to remain healthy, the bacterial challenge must be contained at a level that can be tolerated by the host.
- The situation can be thought of as a balance scale, with the disease-promoting factors on one side of the scale and the health-promoting factors on the other.
- As long as the two sides of the scale are in balance, there will be no disease progression.
- The intermittent pattern of disease activity seen in periodontitis is believed to result from the changing balance between the pathogenic bacteria and the host's inflammatory and immune responses.

Periodontal disease is a bacterial infection of the periodontium. The presence of pathogenic bacteria, however, does not necessarily mean that an individual will experience periodontitis.

- Additional factors play a role in determining why some individuals are more susceptible to periodontitis than others.
- Contributing factors are factors that increase an individual's susceptibility to periodontitis by modifying the host response to bacterial infection.
- Contributing factors such as systemic disease, smoking, and genetic factors can play a significant role in determining the onset and progression of periodontitis.

Daily plaque biofilm control by the patient and routine professional care are the best methods for prevention of periodontal disease. Other risk factors must be evaluated, however, to develop the best treatment plan for each individual. In addition, dental healthcare providers should provide tobacco cessation and other health promotion programs that contribute to both overall and periodontal health.

Section 3
Focus on Patients

Case 1

Mr. Archie Newcomer is a new patient in your dental office. Mr. Newcomer is 35 years of age and reports that this is his first dental check-up in 5 or 6 years. Mr. Newcomer's completed Periodontal Assessment Questionnaire is shown in Figures 12-9A and B on the next two pages of this module. Review Mr. Newcomer's questionnaire, make a list of periodontal risk factors and suggest strategies for managing these risk factors.

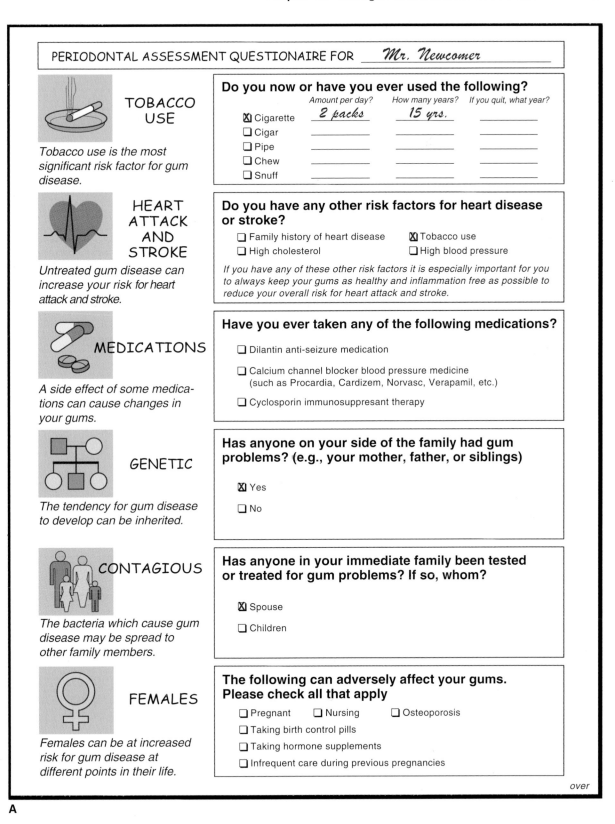

PERIODONTAL ASSESSMENT QUESTIONAIRE FOR ___*Mr. Newcomer*___

TOBACCO USE

Tobacco use is the most significant risk factor for gum disease.

Do you now or have you ever used the following?

	Amount per day?	How many years?	If you quit, what year?
☒ Cigarette	*2 packs*	*15 yrs.*	
☐ Cigar			
☐ Pipe			
☐ Chew			
☐ Snuff			

HEART ATTACK AND STROKE

Untreated gum disease can increase your risk for heart attack and stroke.

Do you have any other risk factors for heart disease or stroke?

☐ Family history of heart disease   ☒ Tobacco use
☐ High cholesterol   ☐ High blood pressure

If you have any of these other risk factors it is especially important for you to always keep your gums as healthy and inflammation free as possible to reduce your overall risk for heart attack and stroke.

MEDICATIONS

A side effect of some medications can cause changes in your gums.

Have you ever taken any of the following medications?

☐ Dilantin anti-seizure medication

☐ Calcium channel blocker blood pressure medicine
   (such as Procardia, Cardizem, Norvasc, Verapamil, etc.)

☐ Cyclosporin immunosuppresant therapy

GENETIC

The tendency for gum disease to develop can be inherited.

Has anyone on your side of the family had gum problems? (e.g., your mother, father, or siblings)

☒ Yes

☐ No

CONTAGIOUS

The bacteria which cause gum disease may be spread to other family members.

Has anyone in your immediate family been tested or treated for gum problems? If so, whom?

☒ Spouse

☐ Children

FEMALES

Females can be at increased risk for gum disease at different points in their life.

The following can adversely affect your gums. Please check all that apply

☐ Pregnant   ☐ Nursing   ☐ Osteoporosis
☐ Taking birth control pills
☐ Taking hormone supplements
☐ Infrequent care during previous pregnancies

over

A

Figure 12.9A. Page 1 of Mr. Newcomer's Risk Questionnaire.

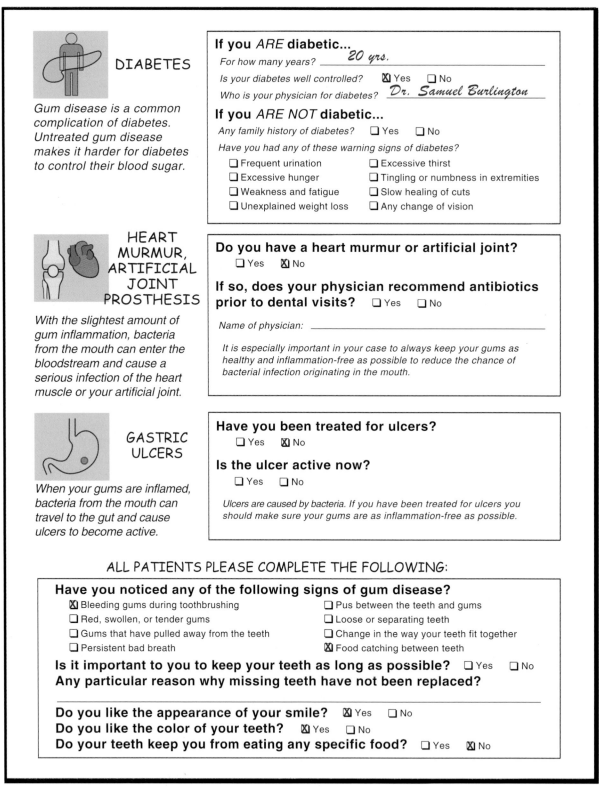

DIABETES

Gum disease is a common complication of diabetes. Untreated gum disease makes it harder for diabetes to control their blood sugar.

If you *ARE* diabetic...

For how many years? _____ 20 yrs. _____

Is your diabetes well controlled? ☒ Yes ☐ No

Who is your physician for diabetes? _Dr. Samuel Burlington_

If you *ARE NOT* diabetic...

Any family history of diabetes? ☐ Yes ☐ No

Have you had any of these warning signs of diabetes?

☐ Frequent urination   ☐ Excessive thirst
☐ Excessive hunger   ☐ Tingling or numbness in extremities
☐ Weakness and fatigue   ☐ Slow healing of cuts
☐ Unexplained weight loss   ☐ Any change of vision

HEART MURMUR, ARTIFICIAL JOINT PROSTHESIS

With the slightest amount of gum inflammation, bacteria from the mouth can enter the bloodstream and cause a serious infection of the heart muscle or your artificial joint.

Do you have a heart murmur or artificial joint?
☐ Yes ☒ No

If so, does your physician recommend antibiotics prior to dental visits? ☐ Yes ☐ No

Name of physician: _____

It is especially important in your case to always keep your gums as healthy and inflammation-free as possible to reduce the chance of bacterial infection originating in the mouth.

GASTRIC ULCERS

When your gums are inflamed, bacteria from the mouth can travel to the gut and cause ulcers to become active.

Have you been treated for ulcers?
☐ Yes ☒ No

Is the ulcer active now?
☐ Yes ☐ No

Ulcers are caused by bacteria. If you have been treated for ulcers you should make sure your gums are as inflammation-free as possible.

ALL PATIENTS PLEASE COMPLETE THE FOLLOWING:

Have you noticed any of the following signs of gum disease?

☒ Bleeding gums during toothbrushing   ☐ Pus between the teeth and gums
☐ Red, swollen, or tender gums   ☐ Loose or separating teeth
☐ Gums that have pulled away from the teeth ☐ Change in the way your teeth fit together
☐ Persistent bad breath   ☒ Food catching between teeth

Is it important to you to keep your teeth as long as possible? ☐ Yes ☐ No

Any particular reason why missing teeth have not been replaced?

_____

Do you like the appearance of your smile? ☒ Yes ☐ No
Do you like the color of your teeth? ☒ Yes ☐ No
Do your teeth keep you from eating any specific food? ☐ Yes ☒ No

B

Figure 12.9B. Page 2 of Mr. Newcomer's Risk Questionnaire.

Suggested Readings

American Academy of Periodontology statement on risk assessment. *J Periodontol.* 2008;79(2):202.

Douglass CW. Risk assessment and management of periodontal disease. *J Am Dent Assoc.* 2006;137 Suppl:27S–32S.

Page RC, Martin J, Krall EA, et al. Longitudinal validation of a risk calculator for periodontal disease. *J Clin Periodontol.* 2003;30(9):819–827.

Chapter 13

Clinical Features of the Gingiva

Learning Objectives

- Describe characteristics of the gingiva in health.
- List clinical signs of gingival inflammation.
- Compare and contrast clinical features of healthy and inflamed gingival tissue.
- Explain the difference in color between acute and chronic inflammation.
- Differentiate between bulbous, blunted, and cratered papilla.

Key Terms

Stippling
Inflammation
Gingivitis
Bulbous papilla
Blunted papilla
Cratered papilla
Extent of inflammation

Distribution of inflammation
Localized inflammation
Generalized inflammation
Papillary inflammation
Marginal inflammation
Diffuse inflammation

Section 1
Clinical Features of Healthy Gingiva

It is important for clinicians to recognize the appearance of healthy gingiva and to recognize all of its variations in health. In addition, clinicians must be able to describe gingiva accurately when documenting the findings from a periodontal assessment.

1. **Tissue Color and Contour in Health**
   A. **Tissue Color**
      1. Healthy gingival tissue has a uniform, pink color. The shade of pink depends on the number and size of blood vessels and the density of the gingival epithelium.
      2. The shade of pink usually is lighter in blondes with fair complexions and darker in brunettes with dark complexions (FIG. 13-1).
      3. The coral pink of the gingiva is easily distinguished from the darker alveolar mucosa.
      4. Healthy tissue also can be pigmented. The pigmented areas of the attached gingiva may range from light brown to black.
   B. **Tissue Contour (Size and Shape)**
      1. In health, the gingival tissue lies snugly around the tooth and firmly against the alveolar bone (FIG. 13-2).
      2. The gingival margin is smoothly scalloped in an arched form as the gingiva margin flows across the tooth surface from papilla to papilla.
      3. The gingival margin meets the tooth with a tapered (knife-edge), flat, or slightly rounded edge.
      4. Papillae come to a point and fill the space between teeth (FIG. 13-2).
      5. Teeth with a diastema—no contact between adjacent teeth—or large spaces between teeth will have flat papillae.
2. **Tissue Consistency and Texture in Health**
   A. **Tissue Consistency**
      1. The attached gingiva is firmly connected to the underlying cementum and alveolar bone.
      2. The tissue is resilient (elastic). If gentle pressure is applied to the gingiva with the side of a probe, the tissue resists compression and springs back almost immediately.
      3. The attached gingiva will not pull away from the tooth when air is blown into the sulcus.

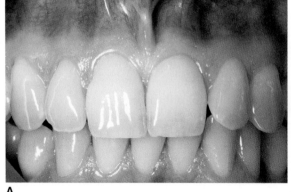

A

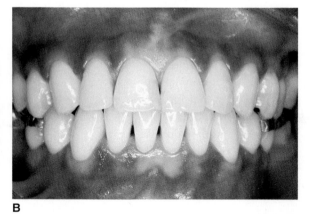

B

Figure 13.1. Tissue Color in Health. A: Periodontal health showing coral pink gingiva. Note the distinct difference in appearance between the keratinized gingiva and the nonkeratinized alveolar mucosa. **B:** Pigmentation of the gingiva showing how the gingiva can vary in color in some patients.

B. Surface Texture of the Tissue
   1. In health, the surface of the attached gingiva is firm and may have a dimpled appearance similar to the skin of an orange peel (FIG. 13-3).
   2. This dimpled appearance is known as stippling. The presence of stippling is best viewed by drying the tissue with compressed air.
   3. Healthy tissue may or may not exhibit a stippled appearance as the presence of stippling varies greatly from individual to individual.
3. **Position of Gingival Margin in Health.** The gingival margin is slightly coronal to the cementoenamel junction (FIG. 13-4).
4. **Absence of Bleeding in Health.** Healthy tissue does not bleed when disturbed by clinical procedures such as gentle probing of the sulcus.

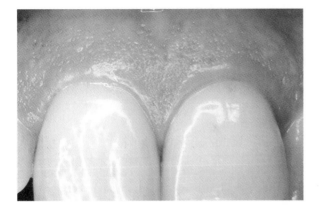

Figure 13.2. Contours of Healthy Gingiva. This tissue on the facial aspect of the maxillary anteriors exhibits all the characteristics of health, including a smoothly scalloped gingival margin, a tapered margin slightly coronal to the CEJ, and pointed papillae that completely fill the space between the teeth. (Courtesy of Dr Don Rolfs, Wenachee, WA.)

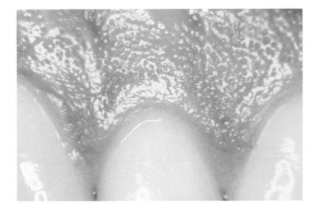

Figure 13.3. Stippling of Gingival Tissue. Healthy gingival tissue showing a stippled appearance. Stippling varies greatly from individual to individual and in some patients healthy tissue may not exhibit a stippled appearance.

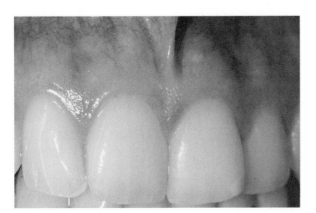

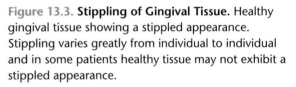

Figure 13.4. Position of the Margin in Health. In health, the gingival margin is slightly coronal to the cementoenamel junction.

Section 2
Clinical Features of Gingival Inflammation

Gingival inflammation is the body's reaction to the bacterial infection of the gingival tissues by periodontal pathogens. The inflammatory response to this bacterial infection results in clinical changes in the gingival tissue involving the free and attached gingiva, as well as the papillae. A clinician with a trained eye can discern subtle differences in color, contour, and consistency even in gingival tissues that appear relatively healthy at first glance. The phrase "tissue talks" is good to remember when assessing the gingival tissue. TABLE 13-1 contrasts of the characteristics of healthy versus inflamed gingival tissue.

TABLE 13-1.	Characteristics of Healthy Versus Inflamed Gingival Tissue	
	Healthy Tissue	**Gingivitis**
Color	Uniform pink color Pigmentation may be present	Acute: bright red Chronic: bluish red to purplish red

Contour	Marginal gingiva:
	  Meets the tooth in a tapered or slightly rounded edge
	Interdental papillae:
	  Pointed papilla fills the space between the teeth
		Marginal gingiva:
		  Meets the tooth in a rolled, thickened edge
		
		Interdental papillae:
		  Bulbous, blunted, cratered

Consistency	Firm Resilient under compression	Spongy, flaccid Indents easily when pressed lightly Compressed air deflects the tissue
Texture	Smooth and/or stippled	Tissue shiny Stretched appearance
Margin	Slightly coronal to the CEJ	Coronal to the CEJ
Bleeding	No bleeding upon probing	Bleeding upon probing

1. Characteristics of Gingivitis
   A. Tissue Color in Gingivitis
      1. Gingivitis is an inflammation of the gingiva often causing the tissue to become red and swollen, to bleed easily, and sometimes to become slightly tender.
      2. Inflammation results in increased blood flow to the gingiva causing the tissue to appear bright red. Figures 13-5 and 13-6 show examples of common clinical presentations of gingivitis.

B. Tissue Contour (Size and Shape) in Gingivitis

1. An increase of fluid in the inflamed gingival tissue causes enlargement of the tissues. The normal scalloped appearance of the gingiva is lost if the gingival papillae are swollen.
2. Examples of types of changes in the appearance of the papillae are listed below.
   a. Bulbous papilla—a papilla that is enlarged and appears to bulge out of the interproximal space (FIG. 13-7).
   b. Blunted papilla—a papilla is flat and does not fill the interproximal space (FIG. 13-8).
   c. Cratered papillae—a papilla that appears to have been "scooped out" leaving a concave depression in the mid-proximal area. Cratered papillae are associated with necrotizing ulcerative gingivitis (FIG. 13-9).

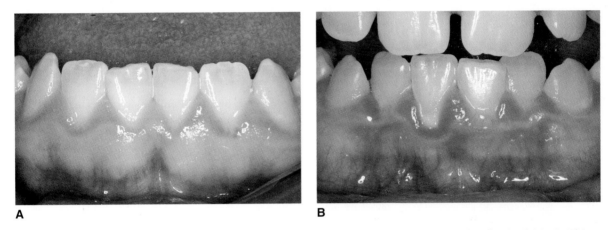

A   **B**

Figure 13.5. Color Changes in Gingivitis. A: Slight marginal redness is a clinical sign of early gingivitis. **B:** This gingival tissue shows more inflammation than seen in photograph **A.** The marginal and papillary gingival tissues are bright red in color. Note, also, the swelling of the marginal gingival and papillae in this example. (Courtesy of Dr Richard Foster, Guilford Technical Community College, Jamestown, NC.)

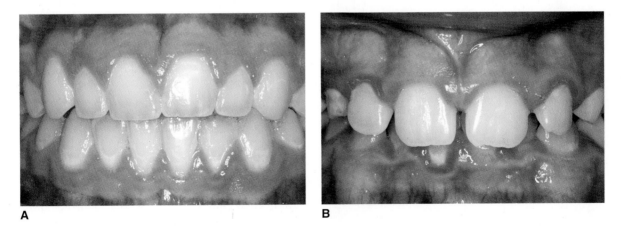

A   **B**

Figure 13.6. Color Changes in Gingivitis. A: This example shows subtle color changes in the marginal and papillary gingival tissues. **B:** In this example, the color changes are pronounced with fiery red marginal gingiva and papillae. (Courtesy of Dr Richard Foster, Guilford Technical Community College, Jamestown, NC.)

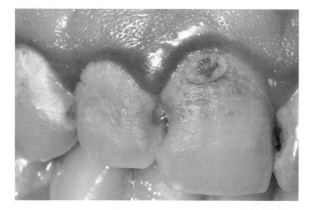

Figure 13.7. Bulbous Papillae. In gingivitis, the papillae may be enlarged and appear to bulge out of the interproximal space as seen in the papilla between the central and lateral incisors in this clinical photograph. (Courtesy of Dr Ralph Arnold, San Antonio, TX.)

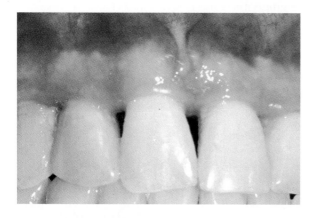

Figure 13.8. Blunted Papillae. In gingivitis, the papillae may be blunted and missing as seen in the papillae between the central and lateral incisors. (Courtesy of Dr Don Rolfs, Wenachee, WA.)

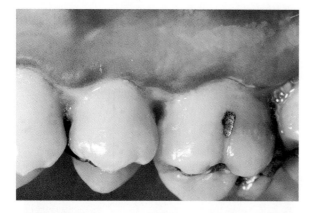

Figure 13.9. Cratered Papillae. The papillae may have a concave appearance in the midproximal area as seen in the papillae between second premolar and molar in this clinical photo. (Courtesy of Dr Don Rolfs, Wenachee, WA.)

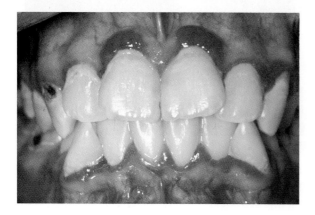

Figure 13.10. Soft, Spongy Tissue. Inflamed gingival tissue may be soft and spongy. The inflammatory fluids can cause the gingival tissues to feel somewhat like a moist sponge. (Courtesy of Dr Ralph Arnold, San Antonio, TX.)

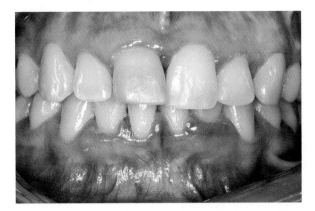

Figure 13.11. Smooth, Shiny Tissue. In gingivitis, fluid in the tissue can cause the tissue to appear smooth and shiny with a stretched appearance. (Courtesy of Dr Richard Foster, Guilford Technical Community College, Jamestown, NC.)

2. **Tissue Consistency and Texture in Gingivitis**
   A. **Tissue Consistency in Gingivitis**
      1. Increased fluid in the inflamed tissue also may cause the gingiva to be soft, spongy, and nonelastic (FIG. 13-10).
      2. When pressure is applied to the inflamed gingiva with the side of a probe, the tissue is easily compressed and can retain an imprint of the probe for several seconds.
      3. Inflamed gingival tissue loses its firm consistency becoming flaccid (soft, movable). When compressed air is directed into the sulcus, it readily deflects the gingival margin and papillae away from the neck of the tooth.
   B. **Surface Texture in Gingivitis**
      1. The increase in fluid due to the inflammatory response can cause the gingival tissues to appear smooth and very shiny (FIG. 13-11).
      2. The tissue almost has a "stretched" appearance that resembles plastic wrap that has been pulled tightly.
3. **Position of Margin in Gingivitis**
   A. In gingivitis, the position of the gingival margin may move more coronally (further above the CEJ).
   B. This change in the position of the gingival margin is due to tissue swelling and enlargement (FIG. 13-12).
4. **Presence of Bleeding in Gingivitis**
   A. Bleeding upon gentle probing is seen clinically before changes in color are clinically detectible (FIG. 13-13).
   B. In gingivitis, the sulcus lining becomes ulcerated and the blood vessels become engorged. The tissues bleed easily during probing or instrumentation.
   C. There is a direct relationship between inflammation and bleeding: the more severe the inflammation, the heavier the bleeding.

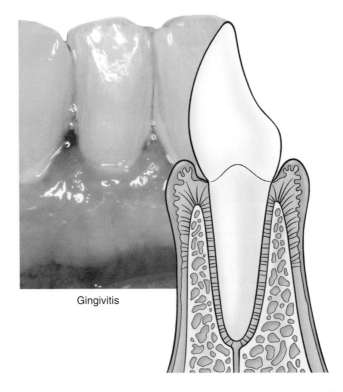

Gingivitis

Figure 13.12. Tissue Margin in Gingivitis. The tissue swelling in gingivitis may cause the position of the gingival margin to move coronally—further above the CEJ—than in health. There is no destruction of periodontal ligament fibers or alveolar bone in gingivitis.

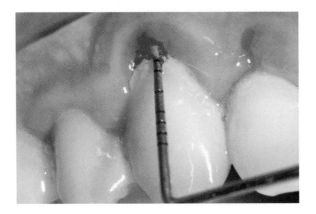

Figure 13.13. Bleeding on Probing. Inflammation causes the gingival tissues to bleed easily during gentle probing. The inflammation results in ulceration of the pocket wall exposing delicate blood vessels. Bleeding is an important clinical indicator of inflammation.

Section 3
Extent and Distribution of Inflammation

In documenting inflammation of the gingival tissues it is useful to note both the extent and distribution of the inflammation.

1. **Gingival Inflammation**
   A. **Extent of Inflammation.** The extent of inflammation is the area of tissue that is affected by inflammation. The extent of inflammation is described as localized or generalized in the mouth.
      1. Localized inflammation is confined to the gingival tissue of a single tooth—such as the maxillary right first molar—or to a group of teeth—such as the mandibular anterior sextant.
      2. Generalized inflammation involves all or most of the tissue in the mouth.
   B. **Distribution of Inflammation.** The distribution of inflammation describes the area where the gingival tissue is inflamed.
      1. The inflammation may affect only the interdental papilla, the gingival margin and the papilla, or the gingival margin, papilla, and the attached gingiva.
      2. TABLE 13-2 summarizes how to describe the extent and distribution of inflammation of the gingival tissue. Figures 13-14 to 13-18 illustrate the use of this descriptive terminology.

TABLE 13-2. Gingival Inflammation	
Extent	• Localized—inflammation confined to the tissue of a single tooth or a group of teeth • Generalized—inflammation of the gingival tissue of all or most of the mouth
Distribution	• Papillary—inflammation of the interdental papilla only • Marginal—inflammation of the gingival margin and papilla • Diffuse—inflammation of the gingival margin, papilla, and attached gingiva
Descriptions	Descriptive terms may be combined to create a verbal picture of the inflammation, such as: • "Localized marginal inflammation in the mandibular anterior sextant" • "Localized papillary inflammation on the maxillary right canine" • "Generalized marginal inflammation" • "Generalized diffuse inflammation"

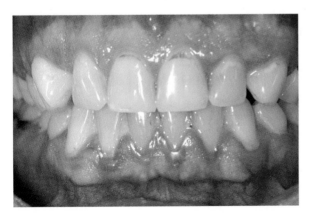

Figure 13.14. **Localized Marginal Inflammation.** Note the redness and swelling of the marginal and papillary gingival tissues that is localized to the mandibular anterior sextant. (Courtesy of Dr Ralph Arnold, San Antonio, TX.)

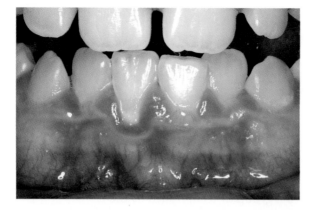

Figure 13.15. Localized Diffuse Inflammation. Redness and edema of the gingival margin, papillae, and attached gingiva in the mandibular anterior sextant. (Courtesy of Dr Richard Foster, Guilford Technical Community College, Jamestown, NC.)

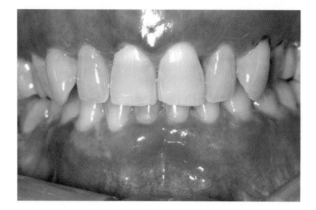

Figure 13.16. Generalized Diffuse Inflammation. Diffuse inflammation of the gingival margin, papillae, and attached gingiva throughout the entire mouth. (Courtesy of Dr Ralph Arnold, San Antonio, TX.)

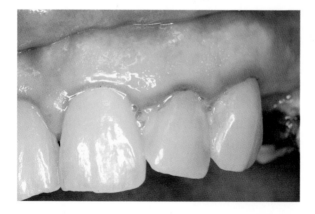

Figure 13.17. Localized Marginal Inflammation. Note the reddened tissue color along the gingival margin, extending down into the papillae on these maxillary anterior teeth. (Courtesy of Dr Richard Foster, Guilford Technical Community College, Jamestown, NC.)

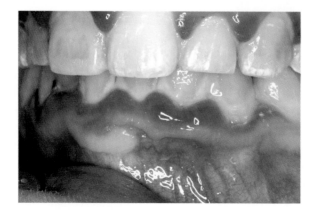

Figure 13.18. Localized Diffuse Inflammation. Inflammation involving the gingival margin, papillae, and attached gingiva of the mandibular anterior sextant. (Courtesy of Dr Richard Foster, Guilford Technical Community College, Jamestown, NC.)

Chapter Summary Statement

Clinicians must have a clear mental image of gingival health to recognize the signs of gingival inflammation when it occurs. Inflammation in the gingiva causes changes in the color, contour, and consistency of the gingiva that can be recognized even in the earliest stages by the trained clinician.

Section 4
Focus on Patients

Case 1

A patient new to your dental team has been appointed with you for a dental prophylaxis. The patient has just relocated to your town. The patient tells you that he saw a dentist just before moving who told him that he has gingivitis. During your discussion with the patient, he asks if there is some way he can tell at home if he has gingivitis. How might you reply to this patient's question?

Chapter 14

Diseases of the Gingiva

Learning Objectives

- Name and define the two major subdivisions of gingival disease as established by the American Academy of Periodontology.

- Compare and contrast dental plaque-induced gingival diseases and non–plaque-induced gingival lesions.

- Describe the clinical signs of inflammation you would expect to find in a patient with moderate plaque-induced gingivitis.

- List systemic factors that may modify gingival disease.

- Name three types of medications that may cause gingival enlargement.

- Explain how the use of certain medications and malnutrition can modify gingival disease.

- Develop a list of suggestions for managing patients with primary herpetic gingivostomatitis.

Key Terms

Gingival diseases
Dental plaque-induced gingival diseases
Acute gingivitis
Chronic gingivitis

Gingival diseases with modifying
 factors
Pregnancy-associated pyogenic granuloma
Non–plaque-induced gingival lesions

Section 1
Classification of Gingival Diseases

Gingival diseases usually involve inflammation of the gingival tissues, most often in response to bacterial plaque biofilm. Certain characteristics must be present for a periodontal disease to be classified as a gingival disease (Box 14-1). The 1999 AAP Classification of Periodontal Diseases and Conditions subdivides gingival diseases into two major categories: (1) dental plaque-induced gingival diseases and (2) non–plaque-induced gingival lesions. Each of these major categories has two or more subcategories (Fig. 14-1).

Box 14-1. Characteristics Common to Gingival Diseases

1. Signs or symptoms of inflammation are confined to the gingiva.

2. No loss of attachment (no destruction of periodontal ligament fibers or alveolar bone) is associated with the inflammation of the gingival tissues.

3. The presence of dental plaque biofilm initiates and/or aggravates the inflammation.

4. Clinical signs of inflammation include changes such as enlarged gingival contours, color transition to a red and/or bluish-red hue, bleeding upon stimulation, increased crevicular fluid flow).

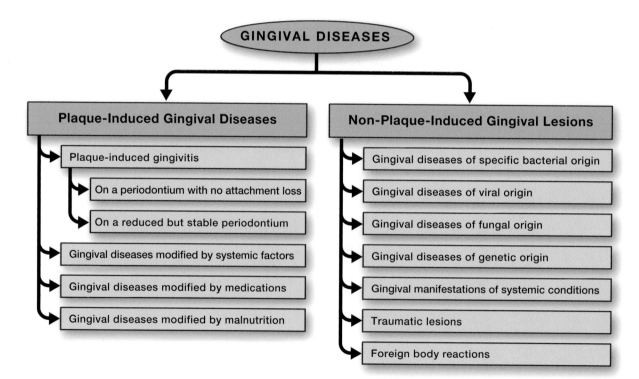

Figure 14.1. Two Major Subdivisions of Gingival Diseases. The two major subdivisions of gingival diseases are (1) dental plaque-induced gingival diseases and (2) non–plaque-induced gingival lesions. These two major subdivisions are further subdivided into types.

Section 2
Dental Plaque-Induced Gingival Diseases

Dental plaque-induced gingival diseases are periodontal diseases involving inflammation of the gingiva in response to dental plaque biofilm. Ineffective plaque biofilm control triggers the body's immune response. As long as bacteria remain in contact with the gingival tissue, inflammation continues. Certain species of bacteria that are elevated during times of gingival inflammation are listed in TABLE 14-1.

TABLE 14-1. Bacteria Associated with Health and Gingivitis		
	Bacterial Species Associated With Health	**Bacterial Species Elevated in Gingivitis**
Gram-positive rods	Actinomyces israelii Actinomyces naeslundii Actinomyces odontolyticus Rothia dentocariosa Actinomyces gerencseriae	Actinomyces naeslundii III
Gram-positive cocci	Streptococcus mitis Streptococcus oralis Peptostreptococcus micros Streptococcus sanguis Streptococcus gordonii	Streptococcus anginosis Streptococcus sanguis
Gram-negative rods	Selenomonas sputigena Capnocytophaga gingivalis Prevotella intermedia Fusobacterium nucleatum	Campylobacter concisus

1. **Gingivitis Associated with Dental Plaque Biofilm Only**
   A. **Characteristics**
      1. Gingivitis associated with dental plaque biofilm is by far the most common type of periodontal disease.
      2. The clinical signs of gingivitis may vary between individuals and also within the dentition of an individual.
         a. Inflammation is not as intense in children versus young adults with the same quantity of plaque biofilm [1]. A possible explanation for this variation is that children may have fewer pathogenic bacteria in their plaque biofilm, a thicker junctional epithelium, and a less developed immune response [2].
         b. Gingival inflammation in senior adults is more pronounced even when similar amounts of dental plaque biofilms are present. The reason for pronounced inflammation in senior adults may be the result of age-related differences in cellular inflammatory response to plaque biofilm [3,4].
      3. Local factors—such as dental restorations, appliances, root fractures, and tooth anatomy—act as a site for bacterial plaque biofilm retention and may contribute to the disease.

B. **Clinical Signs of Gingivitis Associated with Dental Plaque Biofilm Only**
1. Clinical signs of gingival inflammation include changes in gingival contour, color, and consistency. Common clinical signs include erythema (redness), swelling, bleeding, and tenderness (Box 14-2).
2. The disease process begins at the gingival margin and is characterized clinically by red, swollen, tender gums that bleed easily.

C. **Duration of Gingivitis**
1. Acute gingivitis—gingivitis of a short duration, after which professional care and patient self-care returns the gingiva to a healthy state.
2. Chronic gingivitis—long-lasting gingivitis; gingivitis may exist for years without ever progressing to periodontitis.

Box 14.2 Gingivitis Associated with Dental Plaque Biofilm Only

- Most common form of periodontal disease
- Plaque biofilm present at the gingival margin
- Gingival redness; tenderness
- Increase in sulcular temperature
- Bleeding upon probing
- Stable attachment levels
- Condition reversible with plaque biofilm removal

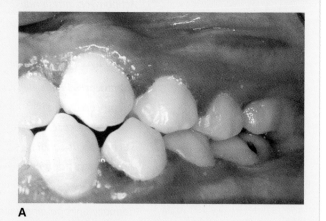

A

Figure 14.2A. **Plaque-Induced Gingivitis.** Plaque-induced gingivitis in this patient has resulted in rolled gingival margins and enlarged papillae.

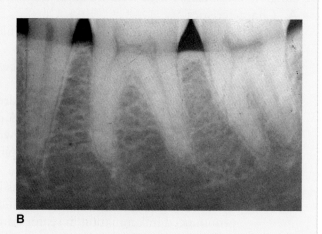

Figure 14.2B. **Radiograph Reveals No Bone Loss.** The dental radiographs of an individual with plaque-induced gingivitis do not reveal any changes in either the alveolar bone height or the character of the alveolar bone.

B

2. **Plaque-Associated Gingival Diseases with Modifying Factors.** The category gingival diseases with modifying factors includes the less common types of plaque-induced gingivitis. There are three main subcategories of gingival diseases with modifying factors: (1) gingival diseases modified by systemic factors, (2) gingival diseases modified by medications, and (3) gingival diseases modified by malnutrition.

  A. **Gingival Diseases Modified by Systemic Factors.** In this form of gingival disease, plaque biofilm initiates the disease; then, specific systemic factors found in the host will modify the disease process.

    1. *Gingival diseases associated with the endocrine system and fluctuations in sex hormones.* In this subcategory, changes in the endocrine system or levels of sex hormones result in an exaggerated response to the presence of bacterial plaque biofilm. Gingival tissues may appear bright red, soft, friable, smooth and exhibit bleeding from slight provocation.

      a. *Puberty-associated gingivitis* is an exaggerated inflammatory response of the gingiva to a relatively small amount of dental plaque biofilm and hormones during puberty.

        1) Although severity is directly related to the amount of plaque biofilm, puberty-associated gingivitis will manifest with a very small amount of plaque biofilm.

        2) Puberty-associated gingivitis is found in both male and female adolescents.

        3) Clinical features are inflamed gingiva with prominent bulbous papillae on the facial aspect (FIG. 14-3). Bulbous papillae rarely are seen on the lingual gingival tissue.

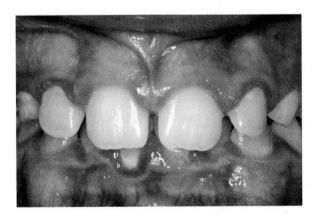

Figure 14.3. Puberty-Associated Gingivitis. Puberty-associated gingivitis is an exaggerated inflammatory response of the gingiva to a relatively small amount of dental plaque biofilm. The exaggerated response is modulated by hormones released during puberty. (Courtesy of Dr Richard Foster, Guilford Technical Community College, Jamestown, NC.)

      b. *Menstrual cycle-associated gingivitis* is an exaggerated inflammatory response of the gingiva to dental plaque biofilm and hormones before ovulation.

      c. *Oral contraceptive-associated gingivitis* is an exaggerated inflammatory response of the gingiva to dental plaque biofilm and **high-dose** oral contraceptives.

        1) Usually seen in patients taking *high-dose* oral contraceptives. A recent study evaluating the effects of *low-dose* oral contraceptives found no effect on gingival inflammation in young women [5].

        2) Gingival enlargement is reversed with discontinuation of high-dose oral contraceptives.

        3) Long term use of high-dose oral contraceptives may affect periodontal attachment levels.

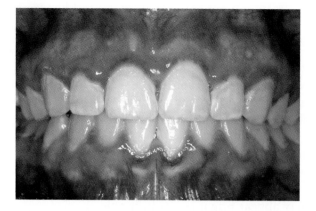

Figure 14.4. **Pregnancy-Associated Gingivitis.** Note the red gingiva and bulbous interdental papilla on this patient with pregnancy-associated gingivitis. (Courtesy of Dr Richard Foster, Guilford Technical Community College, Jamestown, NC.)

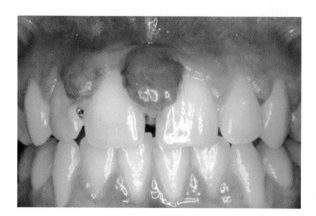

Figure 14.5. **Pregnancy-Associated Pyogenic Granuloma.** This mushroom-like mass of the gingiva bleeds easily if disturbed.

d. *Pregnancy-associated gingivitis* is an exaggerated inflammatory response of the gingiva to dental plaque biofilm and hormone changes usually occurring during the second and third trimesters of pregnancy.

   1) Pregnancy-associated gingivitis can manifest in response to even small amounts of plaque biofilms.
   2) The gingival tissue may be edematous and dark red, with bulbous interdental papillae (FIG. 14-4).
   3) In some cases, a gingival papilla can react so strongly to bacterial plaque biofilm that a large, localized overgrowth of gingival tissue called a pregnancy-associated pyogenic granuloma (pregnancy tumor), may form on the interdental gingiva or on the gingival margin.

e. *Pregnancy-associated pyogenic granuloma ("pregnancy tumor")* is a localized, mushroom-shaped gingival mass projecting from the gingival margin or more commonly from a gingival papilla during pregnancy.

   1) An exaggerated tissue response to plaque biofilm or other irritants that usually occurs after the first trimester of pregnancy.
   2) Characterized by a mushroom-like tissue mass that most commonly occurs in the maxilla and interproximally (FIG. 14-5).
   3) The tissue mass is painless and noncancerous.
   4) The tissue mass bleeds easily if disturbed and may appear to be covered with dark red pinpoint markings.
   5) The growth usually resolves after childbirth.

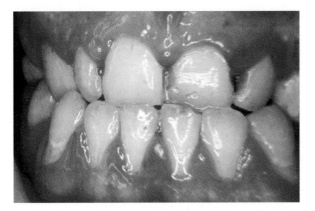

Figure 14.6. Leukemia-Associated Gingivitis. Note the red, swollen appearance of the gingiva in this patient with leukemia. (Courtesy of Dr Ralph Arnold, San Antonio, TX.)

  f. *Diabetes-associated gingivitis* is an inflammatory response of the gingiva to dental plaque biofilm that is aggravated by poorly controlled blood glucose levels.

   1) Often seen in children with poorly controlled Type I diabetes mellitus.

   2) Reduction in gingival inflammation in adults with diabetes may reduce the amount of insulin needed to control blood glucose levels [6]. Diabetes mellitus is discussed in more detail in Chapter 10.

 2. *Gingival diseases associated with blood dyscrasias.*

  a. *Leukemia-associated gingivitis* is an exaggerated inflammatory response of the gingiva to plaque biofilm resulting in increased bleeding and tissue enlargement. Oral lesions are usually the first clinical signs of leukemia; therefore, dental healthcare providers are quite often the first to suspect that a patient may have leukemia.

   1) Gingival tissues appear swollen, spongy, shiny, red to deep purple in appearance (Fig. 14-6).

   2) Tissues are very friable (tear easily) and have a tendency to hemorrhage with slight provocation.

   3) Plaque biofilm is not a prerequisite for gingivitis in patients with leukemia.

   4) Gingivitis begins in the papillae and spreads to the marginal and then, the attached gingiva.

  b. *Blood dyscrasias-associated gingivitis* is gingivitis associated with abnormal function or number of blood cells.

3. Plaque-Associated Gingival Diseases Modified by Medications

 A. *Drug-influenced gingivitis* is an exaggerated inflammatory response of the gingiva to dental plaque biofilm and a systemic medication.

 B. *Drug-influenced gingival enlargement* is an increase in size of the gingiva resulting from systemic medications, most commonly anticonvulsants, calcium channel blockers, and immunosuppressants. Plaque biofilm accumulation is not necessary for the initiation of gingival enlargement but it will exacerbate the gingival disease. Meticulous plaque biofilm control can reduce but will not eliminate gingival overgrowth.

  1. Medications associated with gingival enlargement

   a. Anticonvulsants (e.g., Phenytoin, Celontin, Zerontin, Paganone, sodium valproate). Anticonvulsants are a diverse group of pharmaceuticals used in the treatment of epileptic seizures. In addition, anticonvulsants are now used in the treatment of bipolar disorder.

   b. Immunosuppressants (e.g., cyclosporine). Immunosuppressant drugs suppress the natural immune responses. Immunosuppressants are given to transplant patients to prevent organ rejection or to patients with autoimmune diseases. The immunosuppressant stimulates fibroblast proliferation with excessive extracellular matrix accumulation in gingival tissues.

   c. Calcium channel blocking agents (e.g., amlodipine, nifedipine, verapamil). Calcium channel blocking agents relax the blood vessels and increase the supply of blood and oxygen to the heart while reducing its workload. Some of the calcium channel blocking agents are used to relieve and control angina pectoris (chest pain). Some are also used to treat high blood pressure (hypertension). These drugs affect gingival connective tissues by stimulating an increase of fibroblasts and increasing the production of connective tissue matrix.

  2. Clinical appearance of gingival enlargement

   a. Tissue enlargement is an exaggerated inflammatory response in relation to the amount of plaque biofilm present.

   b. Onset within 3 months of taking medication.

   c. The pattern of tissue enlargement is irregular, first observed in papillae. Begins as a painless area of enlargement on the papilla and then proceeds to the marginal gingiva.

   d. Gingiva in anterior sextants is most commonly affected, however, can occur in posterior sextants (Figs. 14-7 and 14-8).

   e. Severity of overgrowth is directly affected by level of self-care; scrupulous homecare can reduce the severity of the overgrowth.

   f. Appears more frequently in the maxillary and mandibular anterior sextants.

   g. Characterized by increased flow of crevicular fluid, bleeding upon probing with no attachment loss.

   h. More commonly seen in children.

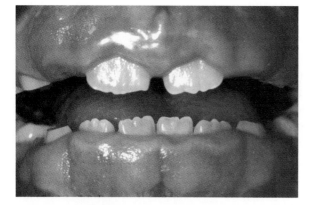

Figure 14.7. Phenytoin-Induced Gingival Enlargement. Massive-tissue overgrowth may be seen in phenytoin-induced gingival enlargement.

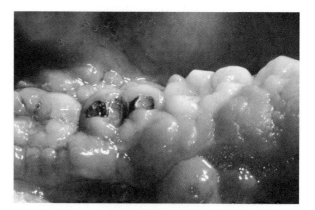

Figure 14.8. Cyclosporine-Induced Gingival Enlargement. Gingival changes seen in cyclosporine-induced gingival enlargement.

4. **Plaque-Associated Gingival Diseases Modified by Malnutrition.** Even with our adequate food supply in North America, infants, institutionalized elderly, and alcoholics are all at risk for vitamin deficiencies.

   A. *Ascorbic acid-deficiency gingivitis* is an inflammatory response of the gingiva to dental plaque biofilm aggravated by chronically low ascorbic acid (vitamin C) levels. Ascorbic acid-deficiency gingivitis manifests as bright red, swollen, ulcerated gingival tissue that bleeds with the slightest provocation (FIG. 14-9).

   B. **Other.** Specific nutrient deficiencies can exacerbate the response of gingival tissues to plaque biofilm. In animal studies, a deficiency in vitamin A, B-complex vitamins, and starvation have all had an effect on gingival tissues. Vitamin A helps maintain healthy sulcular epithelium. B-complex vitamins help maintain healthy mucosal tissues. Starvation eliminates all nutrients necessary for healthy periodontium.

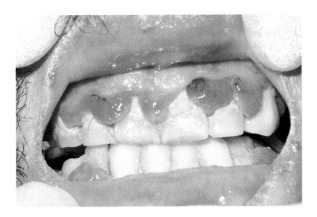

Figure 14.9. Ascorbic Acid-deficiency Gingivitis. A photograph of a patient with scurvy. Scurvy is the clinical state arising from dietary deficiency of vitamin C (ascorbic acid). Note the bright red, swollen, and ulcerated gingival tissue. (Courtesy of Mediscan Company.)

Section 3
Non–Plaque-Induced Gingival Lesions

A small percentage of gingival diseases—non–plaque-induced gingival lesions—are not caused by bacterial plaque biofilm and do not disappear after plaque biofilm removal. *It should be emphasized, however, that the presence of dental plaque biofilm could increase the severity of the gingival inflammation in non–plaque-induced lesions.*

Non–plaque-induced gingivitis can result from such varied causes as: bacterial, viral, or fungal infections, genetic origin, dermatological (skin) diseases, allergic reactions, and mechanical trauma.

- Specific bacteria can infect the gingival tissues and cause a form of gingivitis [7].
- Some types of gingivitis can be caused by an infection with a specific virus [8–10].
- Although rare in otherwise healthy individuals, gingival lesions can be caused by fungal infections [8,11].
- There are some gingival lesions that are not infections at all, but rather have a genetic etiology [12].
- There are a wide variety of gingival lesions that occur as manifestations of systemic conditions such as mucocutaneous disorders or allergic reactions [8].

This section presents some examples of this small percentage of gingival disease in which dental plaque biofilm does not have an etiologic role. Of the non–plaque-induced gingival lesions, the two most commonly seen in the dental office are primary herpetic gingivostomatitis and allergic reactions.

1. **Gingival Diseases of Specific Bacterial Origin**
   A. **Definition.** Gingival diseases in this category are characterized by a bacterial infection of the gingiva by a specific bacterium that is *not a common component* of the bacterial plaque biofilm.
   B. **Characteristics of Gingival Diseases of Specific Bacterial Origin**
      1. Gingival diseases of specific bacterial origin that occur on rare occasions when a bacterial infection overwhelms the host resistance. In these cases, the gingivitis is due to an infection by a specific bacterium that is usually not considered a periodontal pathogen. Examples include infections with *Neisseria gonorrhea*, *Treponema pallidum*, and streptococcal species [13–15].
      2. The gingival lesions manifest as painful ulcerations, chancres or mucous patches, or atypical highly inflamed gingivitis (FIG. 14-10).
      3. Lesions may not be present elsewhere on the body.

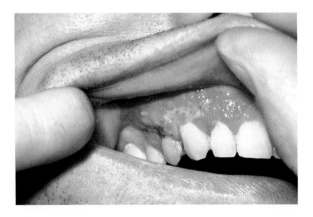

Figure 14.10. Atypical Mycobacterial Infection. This patient has an atypical bacterial infection of the gingiva. The fingers shown in this photograph are the patient's own. (Courtesy of Mediscan Company.)

2. Primary Herpetic Gingivostomatitis (PHG) is a severe reaction to the initial infection with—first exposure of an individual to—the herpes simplex virus type-1 (HSV-1).

   A. Disease Characteristics

      1. By the time individuals reach middle age, about 70% have been infected with HSV-1.

         a. In most cases, the virus never causes symptoms during this primary HSV-1 infection. This is known as a subclinical—symptom free—infection.

         b. In some individuals, however, this initial infection presents with intensely painful gingivitis and multiple vesicles that easily rupture to form painful ulcers. This severe reaction to the initial HSV-1 infection is known as primary herpetic gingivostomatitis (FIG. 14-11).

         c. Once infected, most individuals develop immunity to the virus. In certain individuals, the HSV-1 can remain latent in the trigeminal ganglion and is responsible for recurrent oral herpetic lesions (cold sores).

      2. The initial infection with the HSV-1 usually affects young children—with heightened incidence from 1 to 3 years of age—but may affect adolescents and adults.

         a. Of children with primary infections, 99% are symptom free or the symptoms are attributed to teething.

         b. The remaining 1% develop significant gingival inflammation and ulceration of the lips and mucous membranes [16].

      3. The infection is contagious during the vesicular stage as the virus is contained in the clear fluid in the vesicles. The virus may be easily spread through close personal contact.

      4. PHG is associated with severe pain that makes eating and drinking difficult.

      5. Associated symptoms of PHG are headache, swollen lymph nodes, and sore throat. Because this condition is a viral infection, there may be a low-grade fever usually not above 101°F.

      6. Regresses spontaneously within 10 to 20 days without scarring.

   B. Clinical Manifestations of PHG. PHG may occur anywhere on the free or the attached gingiva or in the alveolar mucosa.

      1. PHG is characterized by widespread inflammation of the marginal and attached gingiva.

      2. The gingiva will demonstrate intense gingivitis and pain.

      3. Small clusters of vesicles rapidly erupt throughout the mouth.

      4. Later, these vesicles burst, forming yellowish ulcers that are surrounded by a red halo. Ulcers may occur on the lips, tongue, palate, and buccal mucosa (FIG. 14-12).

      5. Headache, fever, swollen lymph nodes, and sore throat usually are present.

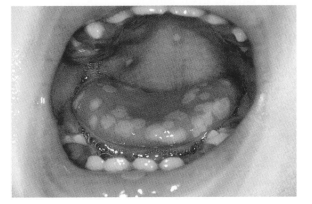

Figure 14.11. **Primary Herpetic Gingivostomatitis.** This photograph shows an initial HSV-1 infection in a young child. (Courtesy of Mediscan Company.)

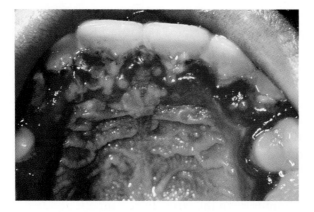

Figure 14.12. Primary Herpetic Gingivostomatitis. Primary herpetic gingivostomatitis is seen on the palate of this patient. Note the fiery red gingival margins and ulcers surrounded by red halos.

C. **Treatment for Primary Herpetic Gingivostomatitis**
  1. Encourage the intake of fluids to prevent dehydration that can result from fever. Athletic drinks, such as Gator Aid, can be consumed to replenish electrolytes lost due to dehydration.
  2. A dietary replacement drink, such as PedaSure or Ensure, can be a good source of nutrition since eating will be difficult. The patient may be able to eat foods processed in a blender.
  3. Counsel the patient that adequate intake of fluids is important. Since eating and drinking are painful, dehydration is a major concern with these individuals.
  4. An antimicrobial mouthwash like Listerine or Peridex should be recommended to prevent a secondary infection.
  5. Precautions should be taken to prevent the spread of the virus to the patient's eyes or from the infected individual to other persons. The infected patient should wash with soap and water frequently. Wash toys that an infected child puts in his or her mouth before and after play time. Do not let an infected child share contaminated items, such as eating utensils with another person.
3. **Linear Gingival Erythema (LGE)**
  A. **Disease Characteristics**
    1. LGE is a gingival manifestation of immunosuppression.
    2. It is characterized by inflammation that is exaggerated for the amount of plaque biofilm present.
    3. LGE does not respond well to improved oral self-care or professional therapy.
    4. For a diagnosis of LGE, the condition must persist after removal of plaque biofilm [17].
  B. **Clinical Manifestations of LGE**
    1. LGE is characterized by a distinct red band that is limited to the free gingiva (Fig. 14-13).
    2. There is no evidence of attachment loss in LGE.
    3. A key feature of LGE is a lack of bleeding on probing [18].
    4. LGE is often associated with HIV infection.
    5. LGE usually does not respond well to therapy.

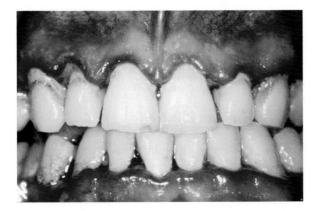

Figure 14.13. **Linear Gingival Erythema**. This patient has linear gingival erythema associated with HIV infection. Note the distinct red band along the free gingiva.

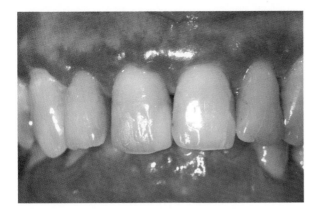

Figure 14.14. **Oral Lichen Planus**. Oral lichen planus of the maxillary gingiva. The gingival tissues are erythematous, ulcerated, and painful. (Courtesy of Dr Ralph Arnold, San Antonio, TX.)

4. **Lichen Planus**
   A. **Disease Characteristics**
      1. Lichen planus is a disease of the skin and mucous membranes in which there is an itchy, swollen rash on the skin or in the mouth. Both the skin and mucous membranes may be affected, however, oral involvement or skin involvement alone is common. The exact cause of lichen planus is unknown. However, it is likely to be related to an allergic or immune reaction.
      2. Lichen planus is the most common mucocutaneous disease affecting the gingiva.
      3. Oral lichen planus may affect persons of any age although it is rarely seen in children [19].
      4. An initial episode of oral lichen planus may last for weeks or months. Unfortunately, oral lichen planus is usually a chronic condition and can last for many years.
   B. **Clinical Manifestations**
      1. Oral manifestations include intense erythema of the gingiva (FIG. 14-14).
      2. Ulcerations of the gingiva may be present and are associated with pain.
      3. Interlacing white lines (Wickham striae) may be present on the buccal mucosa and gingiva.
      4. Raised white lesions may be present as individual papules or in plaque–like configurations.

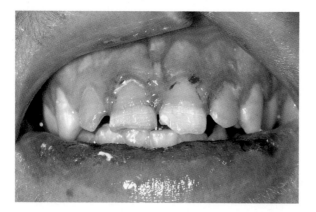

Figure 14.15. **Erythema Multiforme**. Erythema multiforme with ulcerations of the gingiva and crust formation of the lower lip. (Courtesy of Dr Ralph Arnold, San Antonio, TX.)

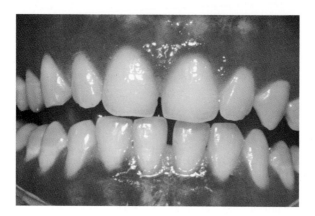

Figure 14.16. **Allergic Reaction**. Clinical signs of allergic reactions in the gingival tissues include redness extending from the gingival margin to the mucogingival junction.

5. **Erythema Multiforme**
   A. **Disease Characteristics**
      1. Erythema multiforme is a disorder of the skin and mucous membranes due to an allergic reaction or infection. Large, symmetrical red blotches, resembling a target, appear all over the skin in a circular pattern.
      2. On mucous membranes, it begins as blisters and progresses to ulcers. Oral involvement occurs in as many as 25% to 60% of cases and is sometimes the only involved site [20].
      3. The exact cause is unknown, though may involve a hypersensitivity reaction.
   B. **Clinical Manifestations**
      1. Oral manifestations include swollen lips often with extensive crust formation.
      2. Lesions on the gingiva involve bullae that rupture and leave ulcers (Fig. 14-15).
6. **Allergic Reactions.** Allergic reactions can occur to ingredients in toothpastes, mouthwashes, or chewing gum [21]. These reactions are usually the result of a flavor additive or preservatives in the product. Flavor additives known to cause gingival reactions are cinnamon and carvone [22].
   A. **Occurrence of Allergic Reactions**
      1. Allergic reactions occur most commonly in patients who have a history of allergic conditions such as hay fever, allergic skin rashes, or asthma.

2. Allergic patients seem to be particularly sensitive to the flavoring agent. The most secret part of the formulation of toothpastes and mouthwashes is the flavoring agent, and this is usually the most allergenic component.

B. Clinical Manifestations. The clinical manifestations of allergy are a diffuse fiery red gingivitis sometimes with ulcerations (FIG. 14-16).

C. Recognition and Treatment of Allergic Reaction

1. The hygienist might suspect this problem in a patient with good plaque biofilm control who previously has had healthy gingiva (especially if the patient has a history of allergies). Inquire if the patient is using a new toothpaste or mouthwash or chewing gum.

2. Advise the patient to change brands of toothpaste or mouthwash. Cessation of the allergen-containing toothpaste or mouthwash should result in a resolution of the gingivitis.

3. If necessary, the diagnosis of allergic response can be confirmed by a biopsy with a diagnosis of plasma cell gingivitis.

4. When the manufacturer becomes aware of allergic reactions, the flavoring agent or additive causing the problem is usually altered. For this reason, the patient sometimes can switch back to the original product (after 6 to 12 months) and use it without problem.

Chapter Summary Statement

Gingival diseases are the mildest form of periodontal disease. Plaque-induced gingivitis is the most common of the periodontal diseases. Clinically, plaque-induced gingivitis is characterized by gingiva that is red, swollen, bleeds easily, and is slightly tender. Plaque-induced gingivitis may be modified by systemic factors, medications, or malnutrition.

Non–plaque-induced gingival lesions are a group of uncommon gingival lesions that are not caused by bacterial plaque biofilm. Non–plaque-induced gingivitis can result from such diverse causes as infection, skin diseases, allergic reactions, or trauma.

Section 4
Focus on Patients

Case 1

You are scheduled to do a dental prophylaxis on a patient with a diagnosis of localized severe plaque-induced gingivitis. At the time of the appointment the patient informs you that she has just received notice that lab results indicate that she is pregnant. How might this pregnancy alter the periodontal diagnosis?

Case 2

A patient who has been cared for by your dental team suddenly exhibits poor self-care with quite a bit of plaque biofilm accumulation. This is unusual for this patient. Discussions reveal that the patient is having difficulty with brushing and flossing due to soreness of the mouth. Examination reveals numerous small mucosal ulcers. Further discussions reveal that the patient has been experiencing this soreness since she began using tartar control toothpaste. How might your dental team manage this patient's diminished effectiveness of self-care?

Case 3

Your patient is a 12-year-old male, who in spite of good oral hygiene practices, presents with generalized marginal redness and bleeding upon probing. His demonstration of tooth brushing and flossing indicates high dexterity and ability to remove bacterial plaque biofilm and in talking with his mother, she confirms that he practices daily oral hygiene. How would you explain the presence of gingival disease to this patient and what would you recommend to improve his gingival health?

References

1. Matsson L, Goldberg P. Gingival inflammatory reaction in children at different ages. *J Clin Periodontol.* 1985;12(2):98–103.
2. Bimstein E, Matsson L. Growth and development considerations in the diagnosis of gingivitis and periodontitis in children. *Pediatr Dent.* 1999;21(3):186–191.
3. Fransson C, Berglundh T, Lindhe J. The effect of age on the development of gingivitis. Clinical, microbiological and histological findings. *J Clin Periodontol.* 1996;23(4):379–385.
4. Fransson C, Mooney J, Kinane DF, et al. Differences in the inflammatory response in young and old human subjects during the course of experimental gingivitis. *J Clin Periodontol.* 1999;26(7):453–460.
5. Taichman LS, Eklund SA. Oral contraceptives and periodontal diseases: rethinking the association based upon analysis of National Health and Nutrition Examination Survey data. *J Periodontol.* 2005;76(8):1374–1385.
6. Mealey BL, Oates TW. Diabetes mellitus and periodontal diseases. *J Periodontol.* 2006;77(8):1289–1303.
7. Siegel MA. Syphilis and gonorrhea. *Dent Clin North Am.* 1996;40(2):369–383.
8. Holmstrup P. Non-plaque-induced gingival lesions. *Ann Periodontol.* 1999;4(1):20–31.
9. Miller CS, Redding SW. Diagnosis and management of orofacial herpes simplex virus infections. *Dent Clin North Am.* 1992;36(4):879–895.
10. Scully C, Epstein J, Porter S, et al. Viruses and chronic disorders involving the human oral mucosa. *Oral Surg Oral Med Oral Pathol.* 1991;2(5):537–544.
11. Loh FC, Yeo JF, Tan WC, et al. Histoplasmosis presenting as hyperplastic gingival lesion. *J Oral Pathol Med.* 1989;18(9):533–536.
12. Hart TC, Zhang Y, Gorry MC, et al. A mutation in the SOS1 gene causes hereditary gingival fibromatosis type 1. *Am J Hum Genet.* 2002;70(4):943–954.
13. Littner MM, Dayan D, Kaffe I, et al. Acute streptococcal gingivostomatitis. Report of five cases and review of the literature. *Oral Surg Oral Med Oral Pathol.* 1982;53(2):144–147.
14. Ramirez-Amador V, Madero JG, Pedraza LE, et al. Oral secondary syphilis in a patient with human immunodeficiency virus infection. *Oral Surg Oral Med Oral Pathol Oral Radiol Endod.* 1996;81(6):652–654.
15. Rivera-Hidalgo F, Stanford TW. Oral mucosal lesions caused by infective microorganisms. I. Viruses and bacteria. *Periodontol 2000.* 1999;21:106–124.
16. King DL, Steinhauer W, Garcia-Godoy F, et al. Herpetic gingivostomatitis and teething difficulty in infants. *Pediatr Dent.* 1992;14(2):82–85.
17. Umadevi M, Adeyemi O, Patel M, et al. (B2) Periodontal diseases and other bacterial infections. *Adv Dent Res.* 2006;19(1):139–145.
18. Robinson PG, Winkler JR, Palmer G, et al. The diagnosis of periodontal conditions associated with HIV infection. *J Periodontol.* 1994;65(3):236–243.
19. Scully C, de Almeida OP, Welbury R. Oral lichen planus in childhood. *Br J Dermatol.* 1994;130(1):131–133.
20. Huff JC, Weston WL, Tonnesen MG. Erythema multiforme: a critical review of characteristics, diagnostic criteria, and causes. *J Am Acad Dermatol.* 1983;8(6):763–775.
21. Skaare A, Kjaerheim V, Barkvoll P, et al. Skin reactions and irritation potential of four commercial toothpastes. *Acta Odontol Scand.* 1997;55(2):133–136.
22. Drake TE, Maibach HI. Allergic contact dermatitis and stomatitis caused by a cinnamic aldehyde-flavored toothpaste. *Arch Dermatol.* 1976;112(2):202–203.

Chronic Periodontitis

Learning Objectives

- Name and define the three major categories of periodontitis.

- Recognize and describe clinical and radiographic features of chronic periodontitis.

- Define the term clinical attachment loss.

- In the clinical setting, explain to your patient the signs and symptoms of chronic periodontal disease.

- In a clinical setting for a patient with chronic periodontitis, describe to your clinical instructor the clinical signs of disease present in the patient's mouth.

- List systemic factors that may be contributing factors to periodontitis.

- Define recurrent chronic periodontitis.

- Define refractory chronic periodontitis.

Key Terms

Periodontitis
Chronic periodontitis
Clinical attachment loss
Peri-implantitis
Extent
Localized chronic periodontitis
Generalized chronic periodontitis
Disease progression

Site-specific
Severity
Slight (mild) periodontitis
Moderate periodontitis
Severe periodontitis
Recurrent disease
Refractory disease
Refractory chronic periodontitis

Section 1
Classification of Periodontitis

Periodontitis is a bacterial infection that affects all parts of the periodontium including the gingiva, periodontal ligament, bone, and cementum. It is the result of a complex interaction between the plaque biofilm that accumulates on tooth surfaces and the body's efforts to fight this infection. Periodontitis is the number one cause of tooth loss in adults and is particularly prevalent in smokers and those with modifying factors such as undiagnosed or poorly controlled diabetes mellitus. There are also some individuals who are genetically predisposed to developing periodontitis.

The 1999 AAP Classification of Periodontal Diseases and Conditions subdivides periodontitis into three major categories: (1) chronic periodontitis, (2) aggressive periodontitis, and (3) less common types of periodontitis. Each major category has two or more subcategories (FIG. 15-1).

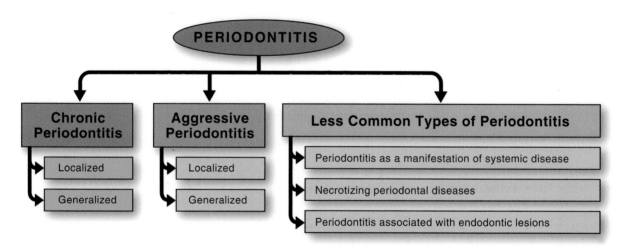

Figure 15.1. **Three Major Categories of Periodontitis.** The 1999 AAP Classification of Periodontal Diseases and Conditions subdivides periodontitis into three major categories of periodontitis. Each of the three major categories has two or more subcategories.

Section 2
Chronic Periodontitis—The Most Common Form

Chronic periodontitis is a bacterial infection resulting in inflammation within the supporting tissues of the teeth, progressive destruction of the periodontal ligament, and loss of supporting alveolar bone. Chronic periodontitis begins as plaque-induced gingivitis. Plaque-induced gingivitis is a reversible condition that if left untreated may develop into chronic periodontitis. *Chronic periodontitis involves irreversible loss of attachment and bone and is the most frequently occurring form of periodontitis.*

GENERAL CHARACTERISTICS OF CHRONIC PERIODONTITIS

1. **Alternative Terminology.** Chronic periodontitis was previously known as adult periodontitis. The name adult periodontitis, however, is misleading as this type of periodontitis can occur in individuals of any age: children, adolescents, and adults.
2. **Signs and Symptoms of Chronic Periodontitis**
   A. **Alterations in Color, Texture, and Size of the Marginal Gingiva**
      1. Red or purplish tissue. In chronic periodontitis, the gingival tissue may appear bright red or purplish.
         a. In such cases, the clinical signs of chronic periodontitis are very evident at the initial examination of the oral cavity. The gingiva appears swollen with the color ranging from pale red to magenta. Alterations in contour and form are evident such as rolled gingival margins, blunted or flattened papillae.
         b. An example of chronic periodontitis exhibiting this type of appearance is shown in Box 15-1.
      2. Pale pink tissue. In chronic periodontitis, the gingival tissue may be pale pink and have an almost normal-looking appearance.
         a. *The clinical appearance of the tissues is not a reliable indicator of the presence or severity of chronic periodontitis.*
         b. In many patients, the changes in color, contour, and consistency may not be visible on inspection. At first glance, an inexperienced clinician may mistake the clinical appearance of chronic periodontitis for one of health. Closer examination will reveal firm, rigid (fibrotic) tissue, the presence of pocketing, and bleeding upon probing. Chronic periodontitis exhibiting this type of appearance is shown in Box 15-1.
   B. **Bleeding, Crevicular Fluid, and Exudate**
      1. Gingival bleeding is common, either spontaneous bleeding or bleeding in response to probing.
      2. Increased flow of gingival crevicular fluid or suppuration (pus) from periodontal pockets is common.
   C. **laque Biofilm and Calculus Deposits**
      1. Chronic periodontitis is characterized by mature supragingival and subgingival plaque biofilms and calculus deposits.
      2. Although chronic periodontitis is initiated and sustained by plaque biofilms, host factors determine the pathogenesis and rate of progression of the disease.

Box 15.1 Chronic Periodontitis

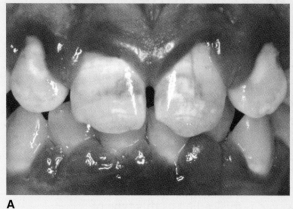

A

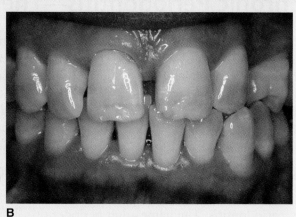

B

Figure 15.2A. Highly Visible Changes in the Gingiva. Chronic periodontitis may exhibit many clinically visible signs, such as, changes in the contour of the tissue.

Figure 15.2B. Minimal Visible Changes in Gingiva. In this example of chronic periodontitis, there are minimal visible tissue changes. Since periodontitis is a disease affecting the deeper tissues of the periodontium, the appearance of the surface tissue often is not a reliable indicator of disease severity.

Characteristics of Chronic Periodontitis

- Most commonly seen in adults over 35 years of age, but can occur in children and adolescents
- Initiated and continued by dental plaque but the host response plays an essential role in its pathogenesis
- Signs and symptoms include swelling, redness, gingival bleeding, periodontal pockets, bone loss, tooth mobility, suppuration (pus), plaque biofilm, dental calculus
- Bone loss may be evident on radiographs
- Disease progresses at a slow to moderate rate
- Attachment loss may occur in one area of a tooth's attachment, on several teeth, or the entire dentition
- It can be modified by other factors, especially cigarette smoking

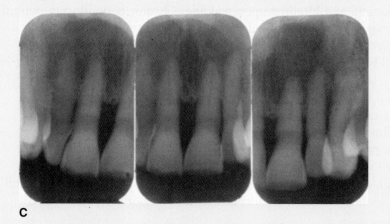

C

Figure 15.2C. Radiographic Evidence of Chronic Periodontitis. Dental radiographs of patients with chronic periodontitis usually reveal horizontal patterns of alveolar bone loss.

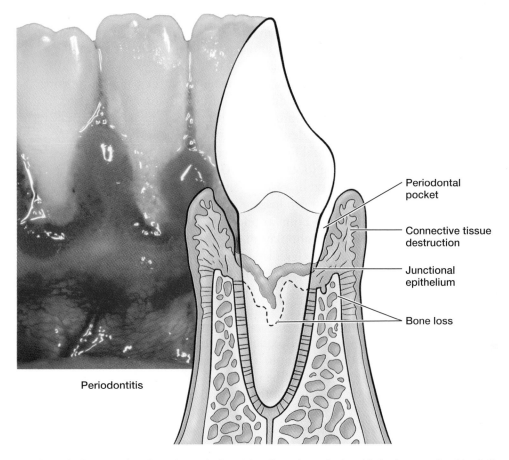

Figure 15.3. Clinical Changes in Chronic Periodontitis. Chronic periodontitis is characterized by inflammation within the supporting tissues of the teeth, progressive destruction of the periodontal ligament, and loss of supporting alveolar bone.

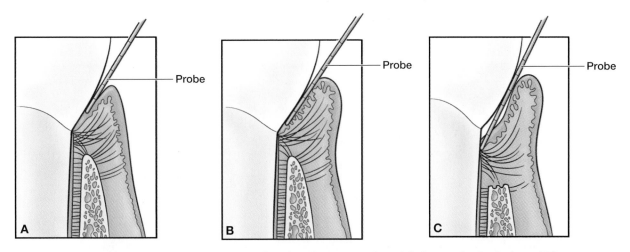

Figure 15.4. Diagrammatic Representation of Probe Tip Penetration Relative to the Periodontal Tissues. It has been established that the extent of probe penetration is influenced by the inflammatory status of the periodontal tissues [1–16]. **A:** In a normal sulcus, the probe penetrates about one-third of the length of the junctional epithelium. **B:** With moderate inflammation within the tissues, the probe tip penetrates approximately half the length of the junctional epithelium. **C:** Severe inflammation within the tissues, the probe tip penetrates through the length of the junctional epithelium, and only stops when it encounters the collagen fibers of the gingival connective tissue.

D. Loss of Attachment

1. The amount of tissue destruction seen in chronic periodontitis corresponds with the amount of plaque biofilm accumulation, local contributing risk factors, smoking, and systemic risk factors.

2. Clinical attachment loss is an estimate of the extent that the tooth supporting structures have been destroyed around a tooth. Loss of attachment occurs in periodontitis and is characterized by: (1) relocation of the junctional epithelium to the tooth root, (2) destruction of the fibers of the gingiva, (3) destruction of the periodontal ligament fibers, and (4) loss of alveolar bone support from around the tooth (FIG. 15-3). The changes that occur in the alveolar bone in periodontal disease are significant because loss of bone height eventually can result in tooth loss.

3. Clinical attachment loss of 1 to 2 mm at one or several sites can be found in nearly all members of the adult population.

4. Clinical attachment loss may be classified based on the estimated position of the tooth-supporting structures as measured with a periodontal probe (FIG. 15-4).
   a. Mild: clinical attachment loss = 1 to 2 mm
   b. Moderate: clinical attachment loss = 3 to 4 mm
   c. Severe: clinical attachment loss is equal to or greater than 5 mm

5. Clinical characteristics of attachment loss may include:
   a. Loss of alveolar bone support to the teeth
   b. Periodontal pockets or recession of the gingival margin
   c. Furcation involvement in multirooted teeth (FIG. 15-5)
   d. Tooth mobility and/or drifting

E. Localized or Generalized Inflammation

1. Localized inflammation may involve one site on a single tooth, several sites on a tooth, or several teeth. Generalized inflammation may involve the entire dentition.

2. A patient may simultaneously have areas of health and areas with chronic periodontitis with tissue destruction.

3. Chronic periodontitis is classified as localized when less than 30% of sites are affected and generalized when greater than 30% of sites are affected.

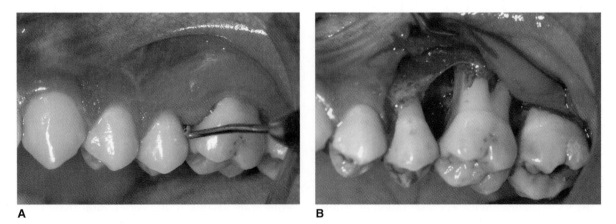

A   **B**

Figure 15.5. **Attachment Loss.** A: Assessment with a periodontal probe indicates severe loss of attachment on this molar tooth. B: The gingival tissue is lifted away from the molar during periodontal surgery to reveal the severe loss of alveolar bone and connective tissue attachment. (Courtesy of Dr Ralph Arnold, San Antonio, TX.)

F. **Contributing Factors.** Chronic periodontitis may be modified by and/or associated with local factors or systemic diseases such as diabetes mellitus. It can be modified by other factors, especially cigarette smoking.

G. **Symptoms**

1. Chronic periodontitis usually is painless. Therefore, an individual with chronic periodontits may be totally unaware of the disease, not seek treatment, and be unlikely to accept treatment recommendation.

2. Individuals may first become aware that something is wrong when they notice that their gums bleed when brushing; that spaces occur between the teeth; or that teeth have become loose.

3. Patients may complain of food impaction, sensitivity to hot or cold due to exposed roots, or dull pain radiating into the jaw.

H. **Chronic Periodontitis in Dental Implant Tissues.** Peri-implantitis is the term for chronic periodontitis in the tissues surrounding a dental implant.

3. **Onset and Progression Chronic Periodontitis**

A. **Gingivitis as a Risk Factor for Chronic Periodontitis**

1. Plaque-induced gingivitis precedes the onset of chronic periodontitis. Plaque-induced gingivitis may remain stable for many years and never progress to become periodontitis.

2. Bacterial plaque biofilms will induce gingivitis, but the host susceptibility and other contributing factors determine whether or not chronic periodontitis will develop.

3. Gingivitis manifests after only days or weeks of plaque biofilm accumulation. In most cases, chronic periodontitis requires longer periods (years) of plaque biofilm and calculus exposure to develop [17,18].

4. Findings from epidemiologic studies and clinical trials indicate that the presence of gingivitis may be regarded as a risk factor for chronic periodontitis [19,20].

B. **Age of Onset.** The onset of chronic periodontitis may be at any age. It is most commonly detected in adults older than age 35, but can occur in children and adolescents. The prevalence and severity of chronic periodontitis increases with age.

C. **Progression.** In most cases, chronic periodontitis progresses in a slow to moderate pace. Periods of rapid tissue destruction may, however, occur.

D. **Patient Education: The Warning Signs of Chronic Periodontitis**

1. The warning signs of periodontitis are red or swollen gingiva, bleeding during brushing, a bad taste in the mouth, persistent bad breath, sensitive teeth, loose teeth, and pus around teeth and gingiva.

2. Pain usually is not a symptom of periodontitis. This absence of pain may explain why periodontitis is often advanced before the patient seeks treatment and why a patient may avoid treatment even after receiving a diagnosis of periodontitis.

3. Tools such as oral health self-evaluations distributed at health fairs or other events can be helpful in increasing the public's awareness of the signs and symptoms of periodontal disease.

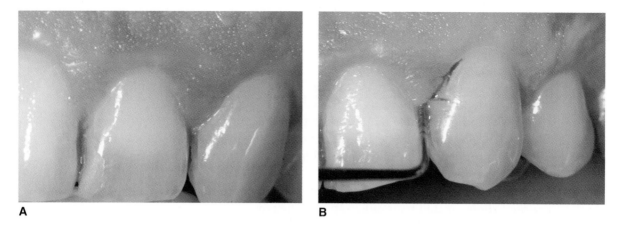

A   **B**

Figure 15.6. **Health or Disease?** A: The clinical appearance of the tissue in this photograph suggests health. B: When assessed with a probe, however, a deep 7 mm pocket reveals bone loss on the mesiofacial of the canine. This example underscores the importance of a thorough periodontal assessment. (Courtesy of Dr Don Rolfs, Wenachee, WA.)

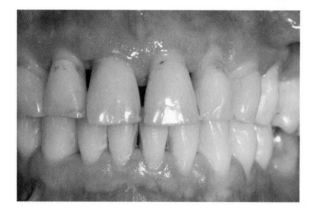

Figure 15.7. **Health or Disease?** This individual received periodontal treatment for chronic periodontitis several years ago. The assessment at today's appointment reveals meticulous patient self-care and no additional attachment loss since beginning periodontal maintenance several years ago. Therefore, this tissue is considered healthy. The attachment loss is simply an indicator of previous disease. (Courtesy of Dr Ralph Arnold, San Antonio, TX.)

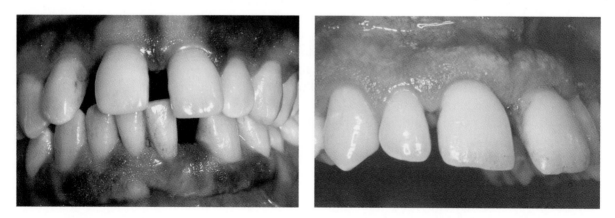

Figure 15.8. **Chronic Periodontitis.** Two examples of chronic periodontitis showing firm, nodular (fibrotic) tissue changes.

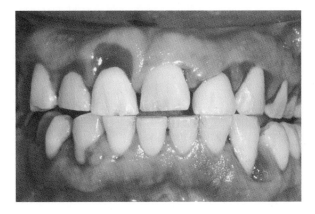

Figure 15.9. Chronic Periodontitis. Chronic periodontitis showing pronounced changes in the appearance of the gingiva.

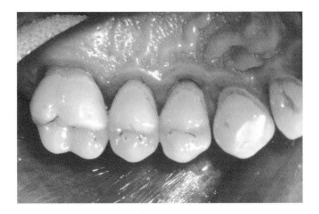

Figure 15.10. Chronic Periodontitis. Palatal gingiva in a patient with chronic periodontitis. Note the calculus deposits on the tooth surfaces and the rolled gingival margins. Clinical signs on the lingual aspect usually are not as evident as those seen on the facial aspect of the gingiva.

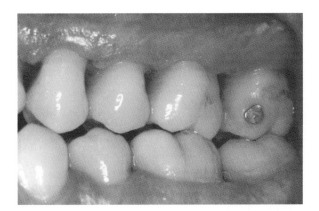

Figure 15.11. Chronic Periodontitis. Chronic periodontitis showing blunting of the interdental papillae and recession of the gingival margin.

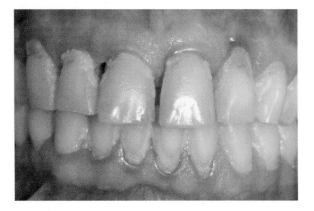

Figure 15.12. Chronic Periodontitis. Heavy accumulation of bacterial plaque biofilm in an individual with chronic periodontitis. (Courtesy of Dr Ralph Arnold, San Antonio, TX.)

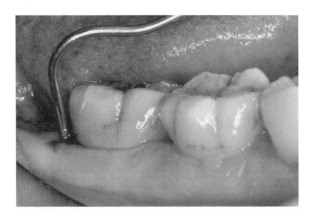

Figure 15.13. Chronic Periodontitis. Chronic periodontitis case with periodontal probe inserted in a pocket showing attachment loss.

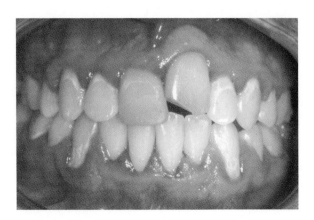

Figure 15.14. Chronic Periodontitis. Chronic periodontitis showing pronounced changes in the appearance of the gingiva. (Courtesy of Dr Ralph Arnold, San Antonio, TX.)

SEVERITY, EXTENT, AND PROGRESSION OF CHRONIC PERIODONTITIS

1. **Extent of Destruction in Chronic Periodontitis**
    A. **Overview.** Extent is the degree or amount of periodontal destruction and can be characterized based on the number of sites that have experienced tissue destruction.
        1. Localized inflammation may involve one site on a single tooth, several sites on a tooth, or several teeth. A patient may simultaneously have areas of health and areas with chronic periodontitis with tissue destruction.
        2. Generalized inflammation may involve the entire dentition.
    B. **Localized or Generalized Extent**
        1. Localized chronic periodontitis is chronic periodontitis in which 30% or less of the sites in the mouth have experienced attachment loss and bone loss.
        2. Generalized chronic periodontitis is chronic periodontitis in which more than 30% of the sites in the mouth have experienced attachment loss and bone loss.

2. **Disease Progression**
    A. **Overview.** Disease progression refers to the change or advancement of periodontal destruction. For example, how does the amount of attachment loss and bone destruction seen today compare with that seen several months ago? Is it the same, somewhat worse, or much worse?
    B. **Progression of Chronic Periodontitis.** In most cases, chronic periodontitis progresses at a slow to moderate pace. Periods of rapid tissue destruction may, however, occur.
        1. The current view is that the *progression of chronic periodontitis in most individuals and at most disease sites is a continuous process but that periods of exacerbation occasionally may occur.*
        2. Episodes of disease progression in chronic periodontitis occur randomly over time and at random sites in the mouth.
        3. Tissue destruction in chronic periodontitis does not affect all teeth evenly, but rather is a site-specific disease. That is, in the same dentition some teeth may have severe tissue destruction while other teeth are almost free of signs of attachment and bone loss.
        4. Chronic periodontitis does not progress at an equal rate in all affected sites throughout the mouth.
            a. Some disease sites may remain unchanged for long periods of time [21].
            b. Other disease sites may progress more rapidly. More rapidly progressing disease sites occur most frequently in interproximal areas and may be associated with areas of greater plaque biofilm accumulation and inaccessibility to plaque biofilm control measures (e.g., sites of malposed teeth, restorations with overhanging margins, areas of food impaction, deep periodontal pockets, furcation areas) [22].
        5. It is important to note that contributing factors (local and systemic) associated with the initiation of chronic periodontitis may also influence disease progression.
        6. The number of sites of attachment loss, bone loss, and/or deep pockets is a good predictor of future disease occurrence in an individual patient. The best predictor of disease progression is an individual's previous disease experience.

3. **Disease Severity**
    A. **Overview.** The severity, or seriousness, of the tissue destruction is determined by the rate of disease progression over time and the response of the tissues to treatment.

B. **Tissue Destruction.** Disease severity may be described as slight (mild), moderate, or severe. These terms may be used to describe the disease severity of the entire dentition, part of the mouth (sextant or quadrant), or the disease status of a single tooth.
  1. Slight (mild) periodontitis—no more than 1 to 2 mm of clinical attachment loss
  2. Moderate periodontitis—3 to 4 mm of clinical attachment loss has occurred.
  3. Severe periodontitis—5 mm or more of clinical attachment loss has occurred.

TREATMENT CONSIDERATIONS FOR INITIAL NONSURGICAL THERAPY

1. **Initial Therapy for Chronic Periodontitis**
   A. **Initial care includes:**
      1. Consultation with the patient's physician is indicated if systemic risk factors are present (such as: uncontrolled or poorly controlled diabetes, systemic diseases, or certain systemic medications).
      2. Individualized instruction, reinforcement, and evaluation of the patient's self-care skills.
      3. Smoking cessation counseling should be offered to patients who smoke.
      4. Periodontal instrumentation of tooth surfaces.
      5. Antimicrobial agents may be used as an adjunct to initial therapy.
      6. Removal or control of local factors contributing to inflammation.
   B. **Care Intervals.** A periodontal examination and re-evaluation of the initial therapy's outcomes should be performed after allowing an appropriate time interval for resolution of inflammation and tissue repair.
   C. **Treatment Goals.** The goals for treatment of patients with chronic periodontitis are to:
      1. Control bacterial plaque biofilm to a level that is compatible with periodontal health
      2. Alter or eliminate any local or systemic contributing risk factors for periodontitis
      3. Arrest the disease progression (*stop the attachment and bone loss from worsening*)
      4. Prevent the recurrence of periodontitis.
2. **Outcomes Assessment**
   A. **Desired Outcomes.** The desired outcomes of periodontal therapy for chronic periodontitis should result in:
      1. Significant reduction in gingival inflammation.
      2. Reduction of dental plaque biofilm to a level compatible with gingival health.
      3. Reduction of probing depths.
      4. *Prevention of further attachment loss.*
   B. **Determinates of Long-Term Outcome**
      1. The long-term outcome of periodontal therapy depends on patient compliance with self-care and periodontal maintenance (recall appointments) at appropriate intervals.
      2. Variables that influence the response to self-care and professional maintenance include an individual's host response to periodontal pathogens as well as local and systemic factors that influence both the quantity and quality of the bacterial challenge and the host response to periodontal pathogens.
      3. Not all patients or sites will respond equally to therapy. Disease sites that have not responded successfully to treatment are characterized by: (a) inflammation of the gingiva, (b) increasing clinical attachment loss, and (c) plaque biofilm levels that are not compatible with gingival health. In patients in whom the periodontal condition does not resolve, additional therapy may be required. In some cases, only specific sites in the dentition may require additional therapy.

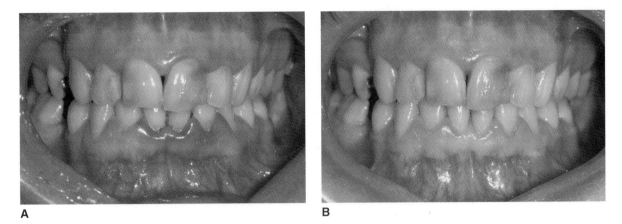

A   **B**

Figure 15.15. Chronic Periodontitis: Before and After Periodontal Therapy. A: Note the tissue changes before periodontal therapy. Clinical changes are particularly pronounced on the lower anterior sextant. **B:** The same individual after treatment. (Courtesy of Dr Ralph Arnold, San Antonio, TX.)

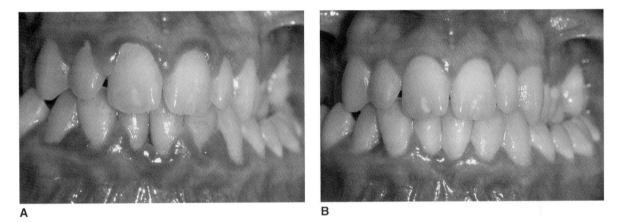

A   **B**

Figure 15.16. Chronic Periodontitis: Before and After Periodontal Therapy. A: Very pronounced tissue changes are evident prior to therapy. **B:** Much improved clinical picture at 3-month follow-up appointment. (Courtesy of Dr Ralph Arnold, San Antonio, TX.)

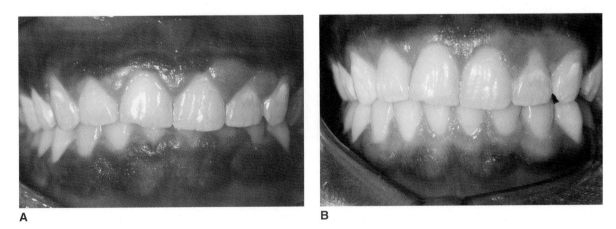

A   **B**

Figure 15.17. Chronic Periodontitis: Before and After Periodontal Therapy. A: Very swollen gingival tissues pre-treatment. **B:** The same individual after treatment. (Courtesy of Dr Ralph Arnold, San Antonio, TX.)

RECURRENT AND REFRACTORY FORMS OF CHRONIC PERIODONTITIS

1. Recurrent disease—new signs and symptoms of destructive periodontitis that reappear after periodontal therapy because the disease was not adequately treated and/or the patient did not practice adequate self-care.
2. Refractory disease—destructive periodontitis in a patient who, when monitored over time, exhibits additional attachment loss at one or more sites, despite appropriate, repeated professional periodontal therapy and a patient who practices satisfactory self-care and follows the recommended program of periodontal maintenance visits (Box 15-2).
   A. Under the 1989 classification system, "refractory periodontitis" was a separate disease category. It is now believed that refractory periodontitis is not a single disease entity, but rather that a small percentage of all forms of periodontitis may not respond to treatment.
   B. *In the new 1999 classification system, the designation "refractory" can be applied to all types of periodontal diseases that do not respond to treatment.* Cases of chronic periodontitis that do not respond to periodontal therapy are designated as refractory chronic periodontitis.

Box 15.2 Refractory Chronic Periodontitis

Additional attachment loss in a patient despite all of the following:

- Appropriate periodontal therapy
- Satisfactory self-care
- An appropriate program of periodontal maintenance visits

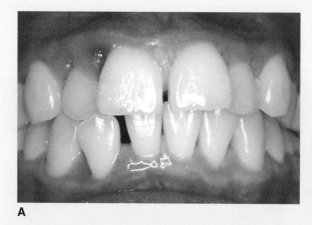
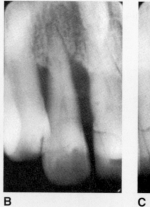
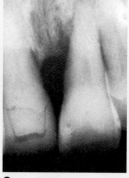

A   B   C

Figure 15.18. A–C: Refractory Chronic Periodontitis. Chronic periodontitis is considered refractory when the disease is not controlled by the conventional periodontal therapy normally recommended for patients with chronic periodontitis. In a refractory case, the patient experiences additional attachment loss despite appropriate periodontal therapy and satisfactory self-care. The dental radiographs of a patient with refractory periodontitis reveal *continuing evidence of bone loss over time despite appropriate therapy.*

Chapter Summary Statement

Chronic periodontitis is a bacterial infection resulting in inflammation within the supporting tissues of the teeth, progressive destruction of the periodontal ligament, and loss of supporting alveolar bone.

- Chronic periodontitis involves *irreversible* loss of attachment and bone and is the most frequently occurring form of periodontitis.
- Chronic periodontitis may involve one area of a tooth's attachment, several teeth, or the entire dentition. A patient can simultaneously have areas of health and areas with periodontitis.
- Chronic periodontitis usually is characterized by slow to moderate rates of disease progression and a favorable response to periodontal therapy.
- The desired outcome of periodontal therapy for chronic periodontitis is to stop the progression of the disease to prevent further attachment loss.

Section 3
Focus on Patients

Case 1

A new patient has a diagnosis of severe generalized chronic periodontitis. The patient tells you that it is hard for him to believe he has serious periodontal problems since he has never had any discomfort and has never even noticed any dental problems. How could you respond to this patient's comments?

Case 2

A patient who has recently moved to your city has an appointment with you regarding self-care instructions. The periodontal diagnosis is severe chronic periodontitis. In your discussion with the patient you learn that the patient is upset because she has been treated for periodontitis twice during the past decade in other dental offices. She is upset because now apparently she needs periodontal treatment again, and she states she is confused about how this might be possible. How could you respond to this patient's concerns?

References

1. Anderson GB, Caffesse RG, Nasjleti CE, Smith BA. Correlation of periodontal probe penetration and degree of inflammation. *Am J Dent.* 1991;4(4):177–183.
2. Armitage GC. Periodontal diseases: diagnosis. *Ann Periodontol.* 1996;1(1):37–215.
3. Carranza FA, Newman MG, Takei HH, Klokkevold PR. *Carranza's Clinical Periodontology.* 10th ed. St. Louis: Saunders Elsevier; 2006.
4. Caton J, Greenstein G, Polson AM. Depth of periodontal probe penetration related to clinical and histologic signs of gingival inflammation. *J Periodontol.* 1981;52(10):626–629.
5. Fowler C, Garrett S, Crigger M, Egelberg J. Histologic probe position in treated and untreated human periodontal tissues. *J Clin Periodontol.* 1982;9(5):373–385.
6. Hancock EB, Wirthlin MR. The location of the periodontal probe tip in health and disease. *J Periodontol.* 1981;52(3):124–129.
7. Hefti AF. Periodontal probing. *Crit Rev Oral Biol Med.* 1997;8(3):336–356.
8. Khan S, Cabanilla LL. Periodontal probing depth measurement: a review. *Compend Contin Educ Dent.* 2009;30(1):12–14, 6, 8–21; quiz 2, 36.
9. Lindhe J, Lang NP, Karring T, NetLibrary Inc. *Clinical Periodontology and Implant Dentistry.* Oxford; Ames, Iowa: Blackwell Munksgaard; 2008.
10. Listgarten MA. Periodontal probing: what does it mean? *J Clin Periodontol.* 1980;7(3):165–176.
11. Listgarten MA, Mao R, Robinson PJ. Periodontal probing and the relationship of the probe tip to periodontal tissues. *J Periodontol.* 1976;47(9):511–513.
12. Magnusson I, Listgarten MA. Histological evaluation of probing depth following periodontal treatment. *J Clin Periodontol.* 1980;7(1):26–31.
13. Moriarty JD, Hutchens LH, Jr., Scheitler LE. Histological evaluation of periodontal probe penetration in untreated facial molar furcations. *J Clin Periodontol.* 1989;16(1):21–26.
14. Robinson PJ, Vitek RM. The relationship between gingival inflammation and resistance to probe penetration. *J Periodontal Res.* 1979;14(3):239–243.
15. Spray JR, Garnick JJ, Doles LR, Klawitter JJ. Microscopic demonstration of the position of periodontal probes. *J Periodontol.* 1978;49(3):148–152.
16. Tessier JF, Ellen RP, Birek P, et al. Relationship between periodontal probing velocity and gingival inflammation in human subjects. *J Clin Periodontol.* 1993;20(1):41–48.
17. Lindhe J, Hamp SE, Loe H. Plaque induced periodontal disease in beagle dogs. A 4-year clinical, roentgenographical and histometrical study. *J Periodontal Res.* 1975;10(5):243–255.
18. Loe H, Anerud A, Boysen H, Smith M. The natural history of periodontal disease in man. The rate of periodontal destruction before 40 years of age. *J Periodontol.* 1978;49(12):607–620.
19. Schatzle M, Loe H, Lang NP, et al. The clinical course of chronic periodontitis. *J Clin Periodontol.* 2004;31(12):1122–1127.
20. Suda R, Cao C, Hasegawa K, et al. 2-year observation of attachment loss in a rural Chinese population. *J Periodontol.* 2000;71(7):1067–1072.
21. Lindhe J, Okamoto H, Yoneyama T, et al. Longitudinal changes in periodontal disease in untreated subjects. *J Clin Periodontol.* 1989;16(10):662–670.
22. Lindhe J, Okamoto H, Yoneyama T, et al. Periodontal loser sites in untreated adult subjects. *J Clin Periodontol.* 1989;16(10):671–678.

Suggested Reading

1999 International Workshop for a Classification of Periodontal Diseases and Conditions. Papers. Oak Brook, Illinois, October 30 to November 2, 1999. *Ann Periodontol.* 1999;4(1):1–112.

Aggressive Periodontitis

Learning Objectives

- Compare and contrast the clinical and radiographic features of chronic periodontitis and aggressive periodontitis.

- Discuss the differences between ideal and reasonable treatment goals for aggressive periodontitis.

- Given the clinical and radiographic features for a patient with a history of aggressive periodontitis, determine if the disease is localized or generalized aggressive periodontitis.

Key Terms

Aggressive periodontitis (AgP)
Episodic disease progression
Localized aggressive periodontitis (LAP)
Generalized aggressive periodontitis (GAP)

Section 1
Aggressive Periodontitis—Highly Destructive Form

Periodontitis is a bacterial infection that may have many different clinical presentations. This chapter discusses aggressive periodontitis. Aggressive periodontitis (AgP) is a bacterial infection characterized by a rapid destruction of the periodontal ligament, rapid loss of supporting bone, high risk for tooth loss, and a poor response to periodontal therapy. Fortunately, aggressive periodontitis is less common than chronic periodontitis.

GENERAL CHARACTERISTICS OF AGGRESSIVE PERIODONTITIS

1. **Alternative Terminology.** Until recently, aggressive periodontitis was defined as occurring in individuals under the age of 30 and was known as early-onset periodontitis (EOP). Features of AgP can present at any age and is not confined to individuals under the arbitrarily chosen age of 30.
2. **Characteristics**
   A. **Primary Features.** The primary features of aggressive periodontitis are [1]
      1. Rapid destruction of the attachment and rapid loss of supporting bone
      2. No obvious signs or symptoms of systemic disease
      3. Other family members (parents, siblings) with aggressive periodontitis
   B. **Secondary Features.** Secondary features that are generally but not always present are
      1. Relatively small amounts of bacterial plaque biofilm; the disease severity seems to be exaggerated given the light amount of plaque biofilm
      2. Elevated proportions of *Aggregatibacter actinomycetemcomitans* (*Aa*)
      3. Phagocyte abnormalities
      4. Elevated production of prostaglandin E2 (PGE2) and interleukin-1β (IL-1β) in response to bacterial endotoxins
      5. A lack of clinical signs of disease
         a. Affected tissue may have a normal clinical appearance
         b. Probing reveals deep periodontal pockets on affected teeth
      6. A poor response to periodontal therapy
      7. Episodic disease progression (FIG. 16-1)
         a. Chronic periodontitis is a very slowly progressing disease.
         b. In aggressive periodontitis, attachment loss is episodic, occurring in a succession of acute destructive phases with intermittent inactive phases.

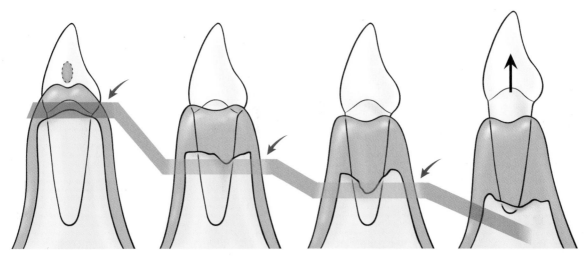

Figure 16.1. Episodic Disease Progression in Untreated Aggressive Periodontitis. Aggressive periodontitis progresses in a series of acute phases of tissue destruction followed by periods of disease inactivity.

LOCALIZED AND GENERALIZED AGGRESSIVE PERIODONTITIS

1. **Localized Aggressive Periodontitis (LAP)**
    A. **Features of Localized Aggressive Periodontitis** (Box 16-1)
        1. Onset of localized aggressive periodontitis around the time of puberty
        2. Localized attachment loss affecting the first molars and/or incisors and involving no more than two teeth other than first molars and incisors
        3. There is a lack of tissue inflammation and minimal amounts of plaque biofilms that seem inconsistent with the amount of periodontal destruction
        4. Frequently associated with *Aggregatibacter actinomycetemcomitans* (*Aa*)
        5. Vertical bone loss around the first molars and incisors, beginning around puberty is a classic radiographic sign of LAP.
    B. **Alternative Terminology.** Localized aggressive periodontitis was previously known as localized juvenile periodontitis (LJP).

Box 16.1 Localized Aggressive Periodontitis (LAP)

- Onset around the time of puberty
- Localized attachment loss involving the first molars and incisors
- Frequently associated with A*a*
- Previously called localized juvenile periodontitis

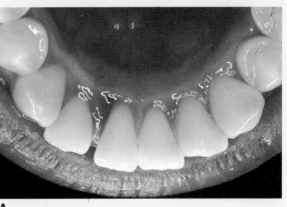

Figure 16.2A. Localized Aggressive Periodontitis. The photo shows a patient with LAP. Note that there are not any supragingival calculus deposits evident.

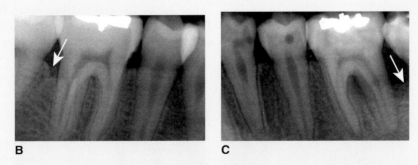

Figure 16.2B, C. Radiographic Characteristics of Localized Aggressive Periodontitis. Patients with LAP have bone loss on the *first molar and incisor teeth*. The radiographs shown here reveal a pattern of bone loss on the first molars that is similar on both sides of the mandibular arch.

2. **Generalized Aggressive Periodontitis (GAP)**
   A. **Features of Generalized Aggressive Periodontitis** (Box 16-2)
      1. Onset of generalized aggressive periodontitis occurs in persons younger than 30 years of age, but patients may be older. A survey of US adolescents age 14 to 17 reports that 0.13% had GAP [2].
      2. Generalized interproximal attachment loss affecting at least three permanent teeth other than the first molars and incisors. Destruction of attachment and alveolar bone is very episodic, occurring in a succession of acute phases rather than in a gradual progression.
      3. Small amounts of bacterial plaque biofilms that seem inconsistent with the amount of periodontal destruction.
      4. The appearance of the gingival tissues varies in GAP.
         a. The gingival tissues may be acutely inflamed, ulcerated, and fiery red. This tissue response is believed to occur during the destructive phase of disease progression.
         b. The gingival tissues may appear pink and free of inflammation. Deep pockets can be detected, however, with periodontal probing. This tissue response may coincide with periods of disease inactivity [3].
   B. **Alternative Terminology.** Generalized aggressive periodontitis (GAP) was previously known as generalized juvenile periodontitis (GJP) or generalized early-onset periodontitis (G-EOP).

Box 16.2 Generalized Aggressive Periodontitis (GAP)

- Disease onset usually occurs in persons under 30 years of age, but patients may be older
- Generalized interproximal attachment loss affecting at least three permanent teeth other than the first molars and incisors
- Associated with A*a*
- Previously known as generalized juvenile periodontitis

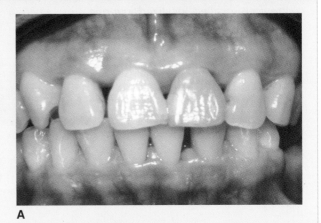

A

Figure 16.3A. **Generalized Aggressive Periodontitis.** The rate of attachment loss and bone loss is rapid in GAP compared to chronic periodontitis.

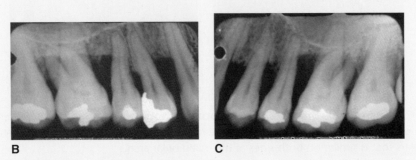

B   C

Figure 16.3B, C. **Radiographic Characteristics of Generalized Aggressive Periodontitis.** Radiographs of patients with GAP reveal severe alveolar bone loss *around most teeth*.

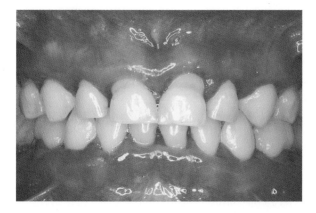

Figure 16.4. Child with Aggressive Periodontitis.
Aggressive periodontitis in a 5-year-old child with attachment loss on all teeth.

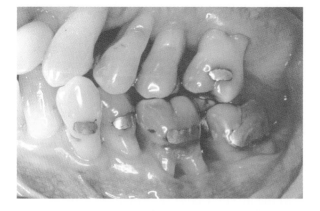

Figure 16.5. Aggressive Periodontitis. Aggressive periodontitis in a patient with good plaque biofilm control. In aggressive periodontitis, the disease severity typically seems exaggerated given the amount of bacterial plaque biofilm.

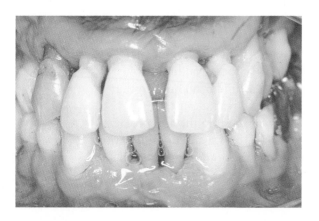

Figure 16.6. Aggressive Periodontitis. An example of AgP with continued disease progression despite good daily self-care by the patient. (Courtesy of Dr John S. Dozier.)

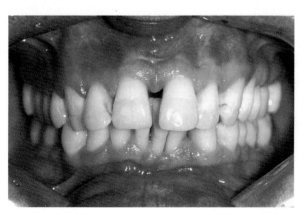

Figure 16.7. Aggressive Periodontitis. Aggressive periodontitis in a 30-year-old male with good daily self-care.

TREATMENT CONSIDERATIONS FOR AGGRESSIVE PERIODONTITIS

1. **Screening for Aggressive Periodontitis.** A small but significant proportion of children and young adults are thought to be affected by aggressive periodontitis. Early detection is important given the severity and progression of aggressive periodontitis.
    A. **Screening of Adolescents and Adults**
        1. Periodontal probing is the most accurate screening method for detecting attachment loss currently available. The measurement of attachment by probing is the screening method of choice for adolescents and adults.
        2. If aggressive periodontitis is suspected, the patient's medical history should be updated and reviewed to rule out possible systemic contributing factors. Periodontitis as a manifestation of systemic disease is the disease category used when the systemic condition is the major predisposing factor for periodontitis.
    B. **Screening of Primary and Mixed Dentitions**
        1. The measurement of attachment loss on primary teeth or partially erupted teeth may be difficult.
        2. Measurement of the distance between the CEJ and the alveolar bone crest on bitewing radiographs is a useful screening approach with children (FIG. 16-8). Bitewing radiographs routinely are taken on children for caries screening and these radiographs also should be screened for the presence of marginal alveolar bone loss.
        3. The "normal" distance between the CEJ and the alveolar bone crest has been evaluated by recent investigations [4,5].
            a. The median distances between the CEJ and the alveolar crest of primary molars in 7- to 9-year-old children is 0.8 to 1.4 mm.
            b. The CEJ of permanent molars is 0 to 0.5 mm coronal to the alveolar crest in 7- to 9-year-olds.
            c. Greater distances between the CEJ and alveolar crest are seen at sites with caries, restorations, or open contacts. These local conditions may contribute to localized bone loss in children in a similar manner to that seen in adults and are not indicative of aggressive periodontitis.
            d. A distance of 2 mm between the CEJ and alveolar crest, in the absence of local contributing factors, should cause the clinician to suspect periodontitis. If the measurement exceeds this value, periodontitis should be suspected and a comprehensive periodontal examination should be performed.

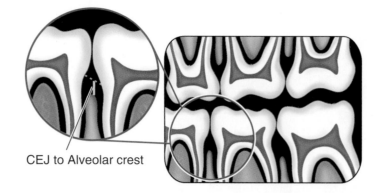

CEJ to Alveolar crest

Figure 16.8. Use of Bitewing Radiographs in Screening for LAP in Children. The distance from the CEJ and the alveolar bone crest is measured from a line connecting the CEJs of the two adjacent teeth. Measurements are taken for each mesial and distal surface. Normal CEJ-to-alveolar bone crest distances for 7- to 9-year olds are less than 2 mm.

2. **Initial Therapy for Aggressive Periodontitis.** Treatment methods for aggressive periodontitis are similar to those used for chronic periodontitis.
   A. Due to the potential genetic link in aggressive periodontitis, evaluation and counseling of other family members is indicated.
   B. Care plan should include
      1. Smoking cessation counseling should be offered to patients who smoke
      2. Individualized instruction, reinforcement, and evaluation of the patient's plaque biofilm control skills
      3. Periodontal instrumentation of tooth surfaces, combined with antimicrobial therapy
      4. Removal or control of local factors contributing to inflammation
      5. Surgical debridement of the soft tissue
   C. A periodontal examination and re-evaluation of the initial therapy's outcomes should be performed after allowing an appropriate time interval for resolution of inflammation and tissue repair.

3. **Treatment Goals.** Periodontitis is controlled if further attachment loss can be prevented—that is, no additional destruction of periodontal attachment and alveolar bone. *Control of attachment loss may not be possible in aggressive periodontitis. In such cases, a reasonable treatment goal is to slow the progression of the disease.*
   A. The desired outcome of periodontal therapy in patients with aggressive periodontitis is
      1. Significant reduction in gingival inflammation
      2. Reduction of dental plaque biofilm to a level compatible with periodontal health
      3. Prevention of further loss of attachment and supporting alveolar bone
   B. The best long-term outcome will be achieved when there is good patient compliance with self-care and periodontal maintenance (recall appointments) at appropriate intervals.
   C. Disease sites that *do **not** respond successfully to treatment* may occur and are characterized by
      1. Inflammation of the gingiva
      2. Increasing attachment loss
      3. Plaque biofilm levels that are not compatible with gingival health
      4. Increasing tooth mobility.

Chapter Summary Statement

Periodontitis is a bacterial infection of all parts of the periodontium that results in irreversible destruction of the periodontal ligament fibers and alveolar bone. Periodontitis is a bacterial infection that may have many different clinical presentations. The 1999 AAP Classification of Periodontal Diseases and Conditions reclassified the forms of periodontitis into chronic periodontitis, aggressive periodontitis, and less common types of periodontal diseases.

Aggressive periodontitis is a bacterial infection characterized by a rapid destruction of the periodontal ligament, rapid loss of supporting bone, high risk for tooth loss, and a poor response to periodontal therapy. Features of aggressive periodontitis can present at any age. The primary features of aggressive periodontitis are (1) rapid destruction of the attachment and rapid loss of supporting bone, (2) no obvious signs or symptoms of systemic disease, and (3) other family members (parents, siblings) with aggressive periodontitis.

Section 2
Focus on Patients

Case 1

While reading a journal article you find a reference to a periodontal disease called localized juvenile periodontitis (LJP). Since this is not a disease category in the currently accepted disease classification system, how does this terminology relate to modern periodontal diagnoses?

References

1. Lang NP, Bartold PM, Cullinam M, et al. International Classification Workshop. Consensus report: aggressive periodontitis. In: *Annals of periodontology*. vol. 4. Chicago: American Academy of Periodontology; 1999:53.
2. Loe H, Brown LJ. Early onset periodontitis in the United States of America. *J Periodontol.* 1991;62(10):608–616.
3. Page RC, Baab DA. A new look at the etiology and pathogenesis of early-onset periodontitis. Cementopathia revisited. *J Periodontol.* 1985;56(12):748–751.
4. Needleman HL, Ku TC, Nelson L, et al. Alveolar bone height of primary and first permanent molars in healthy seven- to nine-year-old children. *ASDC J Dent Child.* 1997;64(3):188–196.
5. Sjodin B, Matsson L. Marginal bone level in the normal primary dentition. *J Clin Periodontol.* 1992;19(9 Pt 1):672–678.

Other Periodontal Conditions

Learning Objectives

- Name and define the three major categories of periodontitis.

- Name and explain systemic or genetic factors that may contribute to the initiation and progression of periodontitis.

- Describe the impact of PMN (neutrophil) dysfunction on the periodontium.

- Define necrotizing periodontal diseases.

- Describe the tissue destruction that occurs in necrotizing periodontal diseases.

- Compare and contrast the clinical findings of necrotizing ulcerative gingivitis and necrotizing ulcerative periodontitis.

- Compare and contrast the tissue destruction in chronic periodontitis with that seen in necrotizing ulcerative periodontitis.

- Name several local factors that may contribute to the initiation and progression of periodontitis.

- Define secondary occlusal trauma and explain how it can lead to rapid bone loss.

Key Terms

Periodontitis as a manifestation of systemic disease
Neutropenia
Linear gingival erythema (LGE)
Necrotizing periodontal disease
Tissue necrosis

Necrotizing periodontal disease (NPD)
Necrotizing ulcerative gingivitis
Necrotizing ulcerative periodontitis
Pseudomembrane
Interproximal crater
Secondary occlusal trauma

LESS COMMON FORMS OF PERIODONTITIS

This group is composed of uncommon types of periodontitis including (1) periodontitis as a manifestation of systemic diseases, (2) necrotizing periodontal diseases (NPDs), (3) abscesses of the periodontium, (4) periodontitis associated with endodontic lesions, (5) developmental or acquired deformities and conditions, and (6) occlusal trauma. *Abscesses of the periodontium are discussed in the chapter on periodontal emergencies.*

Section 1
Periodontitis as a Manifestation of Systemic Diseases

A number of systemic diseases and conditions are a contributing factor in the development of periodontitis. Several hematologic (blood disorders) and genetic disorders are associated with the development of periodontitis (Box 17-1) [1,2]. *Refer to Chapter 10 for a detailed discussion of systemic disease as a contributing factor to periodontitis.* Periodontitis as a manifestation of systemic disease is the diagnosis used when the systemic condition is the major contributing factor for periodontitis and local factors such as heavy accumulations of dental plaque biofilm and calculus deposits are not evident.

Box 17-1. Periodontitis as a Manifestation of Systemic Diseases

A. Associated with hematological disorders
   1. Acquired neutropenia
   2. Leukemias
   3. Other

B. Associated with genetic disorders
   1. Familial and cyclic neutropenia
   2. Down syndrome
   3. Leukocyte adhesion deficiency syndrome
   4. Papillon-Lefèvre syndrome
   5. Chédiak-Higashi syndrome
   6. Histiocytosis syndromes
   7. Glycogen storage disease
   8. Infantile genetic agranulocytosis
   9. Cohen syndrome
   10. Ehlers-Danlos syndrome (Types IV and VIII)
   11. Hypophosphatasia
   12. Other

C. Not otherwise specified (NOS)

1. **Hematologic Disorders.** Hematologic disorders are abnormalities in the structure or function of the blood and blood-forming tissues such as red cells, white cells, platelets, or clotting factors. There are numerous rare hematologic disorders that may affect the periodontium (Box 17-2).
   A. **Acquired Neutropenia**
      1. Neutropenia is a blood disorder characterized by abnormally low level of neutrophils (PMNs) in the blood.
      2. Neutropenia has numerous causes. It may be genetic or may be seen with viral infections and after radiotherapy and chemotherapy. It affects as many as one in three patients receiving chemotherapy for cancer.
      3. Neutropenia lowers the immunologic barrier to bacterial and fungal infection.
      4. Neutrophil disorders that affect the production or function of polymorphonuclear leukocytes (PMNs) may result in severe periodontal destruction (Box 17-3).
   B. **Leukemia**
      1. Leukemia is cancer that begins in blood cells. In people with leukemia, the bone marrow produces a large number of abnormal white blood cells that do not function properly.
      2. At first, leukemia cells function almost normally. In time, they may crowd out normal white blood cells, red blood cells, and platelets.
      3. Periodontal manifestations of leukemia include gingival enlargement, bleeding, and infections (Box 17-4).
   C. **AIDS/HIV Infection**
      1. Linear gingival erythema (LGE) and necrotizing periodontal diseases (NPD) are the most common HIV-associated periodontal conditions reported in the literature [3].
         a. Linear gingival erythema (LGE) is a gingival manifestation of immunosuppression.
         b. The clinical appearance of LGE is characterized by a distinct linear erythematous (red) band that is limited to the free gingiva (Box. 17-5).
         c. LGE does not respond well to improved self-care or periodontal instrumentation.
      2. Periodontal attachment loss and alveolar bone destruction associated with HIV-infected individuals may be extremely rapid (Box 17-5) [4].

Box 17.2 Hemorrhagic Periodontitis Associated Blood Disorder

- Characterized by soft, swollen, gingival tissue. Bleeding occurs spontaneously or on the slightest provocation.

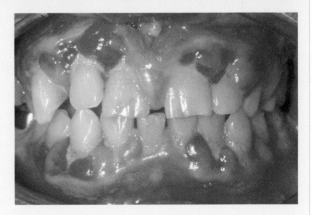

Figure 17.1. Periodontitis Associated with a Blood Disorder. This male patient has a rare blood disorder. His soft, swollen gingiva bleeds easily. (Courtesy of Dr Ralph Arnold, San Antonio, TX.)

Box 17.3 Periodontitis Associated with PMN Dysfunction

- Occurs in patients of any age
- Seen in young children beginning with the eruption of primary teeth
- Characterized by severe bone loss and tooth loss
- Associated with systemic conditions that interfere with the body's resistance to bacterial infection
- Previously known as generalized prepubertal periodontitis

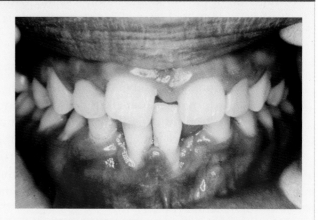

Figure 17.2. Periodontitis Associated with Immune Dysfunction. The dentition of a young patient with PMN dysfunction. Note the primary dentition is being lost and the permanent dentition is being exfoliated as soon as the permanent teeth erupt.

Box 17.4 Periodontitis Associated with Leukemia

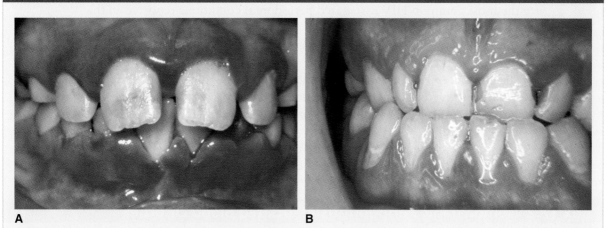

A   B

Figures 17.3. A,B: Periodontitis Associated with Leukemia. Two examples of periodontitis associated with leukemia. (Courtesy of Dr Ralph Arnold, San Antonio, TX.)

- Periodontal manifestations of leukemia include gingival enlargement, bleeding, and infections.

Box 17.5 Periodontitis Associated with HIV Infection

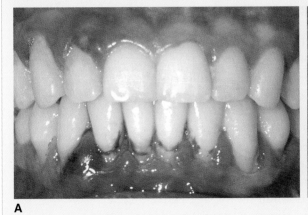

A

Figure 17.4A. Periodontitis Associated with HIV Infection. This HIV-positive individual exhibits a severe form of necrotizing ulcerative periodontitis with tissue necrosis of the gingival tissues combined with loss of attachment. Clinical signs are notable visible on the mandibular anterior sextant.

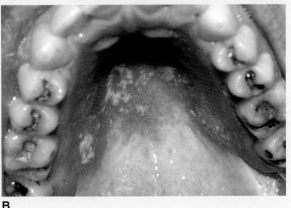

B

Figure 17.4B. Periodontitis Associated with HIV Infection. Palatal candidiasis on the palatal mucosa of an HIV-positive individual. (Courtesy of Dr Ralph Arnold, San Antonio, TX.)

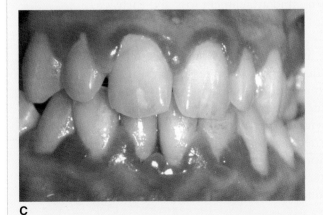

C

Figure 17.4C. Linear Gingival Erythema. Linear gingival erythema in an HIV-infected patient.

- The incidence and severity of chronic periodontitis are similar in HIV-positive and HIV-negative individuals [6–8].
- Immunocompromised individuals are slightly more susceptible to chronic periodontitis than those with a normal immune system [9].
- A necrotizing ulcerative, rapidly progressive form of periodontitis occurs more frequently among HIV-positive individuals.
- Oral manifestations of HIV infection include oral candidiasis, oral hairy Leukoplakia, oral hyperpigmentation, oral ulcers; red, purple, or blue edematous soft tissue lesions; and Kaposi sarcoma and other oral malignancies.

2. **Genetic Disorders.** A genetic disorder is a disease caused by the absence of a gene or by products of a defective gene. Genetic diseases are passed from one generation to the next but do not necessarily appear in each generation.

A. **Familial and Cyclic Neutropenia**
   1. Hereditary and congenital disorders that affect the bone marrow, resulting in abnormally low level of neutrophils (PMNs) in the blood.
   2. Individuals with cyclic neutropenia may experience severe periodontal destruction. Periodontal manifestations of this disease appear at a young age [5].

B. **Down Syndrome**
   1. A common birth defect caused by an error in cell division that results in the presence of an additional third chromosome 21 and presents mild to moderate mental retardation and associated medical problems.
   2. Individuals with Down syndrome often develop severe, aggressive periodontitis. Substantial plaque biofilm formation, deep periodontal pockets, and extensive gingival inflammation characterize periodontal disease in Down syndrome (Box 17-6).

C. **Leukocyte Adhesion Deficiency (LAD) Syndromes**
   1. An inherited disorder in which there is defective leukocyte chemotaxis. It is characterized by recurrent bacterial infections and impaired wound healing.
   2. Cases of periodontal disease attributed to LAD are rare. Periodontitis begins upon eruption of the primary teeth with rapid attachment loss and early tooth loss [10].

D. **Papillon-Lefèvre Syndrome**
   1. An inherited disorder characterized by hyperkeratosis of the palms of the hands and soles of the feet and severe destruction of the periodontium.
   2. Periodontitis causes bone loss and exfoliation of the teeth. Primary teeth are lost by 5 or 6 years of age. The permanent teeth erupt, but are lost due to bone destruction. By age 15 most individuals are edentulous.

E. **Chédiak-Higashi Syndrome.** A rare, inherited disease of the immune and nervous systems characterized by pale-colored hair, eyes, and skin. Impairment of neutrophil chemotaxis is a characteristic of this disease. Aggressive periodontitis has been described in individuals with this disease.

Box 17.6 Periodontitis Associated Down Syndrome

- Characterized by substantial plaque biofilm formation, deep periodontal pockets, and extensive gingival inflammation

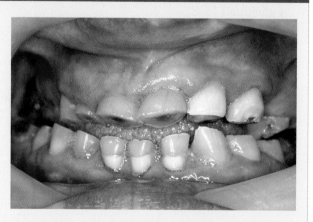

Figure 17.5. **Periodontitis Associated with Down Syndrome.** (Courtesy of Dr Richard Foster, Guilford Technical Community College, Jamestown, NC.)

F. **Glycogen Storage Disease**
1. One of the 14 recognized diseases that interfere with the storage of carbohydrates as glycogen in the body; characterized by neutropenia.
2. Periodontal manifestations of this disease appear at a young age with the potential for early tooth loss [11].

G. **Infantile Genetic Agranulocytosis (Kostmann syndrome)**
1. A rare inherited form of severe chronic neutropenia usually detected soon after birth.
2. Individuals with infantile genetic agranulocytosis experience severe periodontal disease [12].

H. **Cohen Syndrome**
1. An inherited disorder that affects many parts of the body and is characterized by neutropenia, developmental delay, mental retardation, small head size, and weak muscle tone.
2. Individuals with Cohen syndrome have increased susceptibility to early periodontal breakdown which is likely to be associated with neutropenia [13].

I. **Ehlers-Danlos Syndrome (Types IV and VIII)**
1. A heritable disorder of connective tissue with easy bruising, joint hypermobility (loose joints), skin laxity, and weakness of tissues.
2. Early-onset generalized periodontitis is one of the most significant oral manifestations of the syndrome. This can lead to the premature loss of deciduous and permanent teeth [14–16].

J. **Hypophosphatasia**
1. A genetic metabolic disorder of bone mineralization caused by a deficiency in alkaline phosphatase in serum and tissues; characterized by skeletal defects resembling those of rickets.
2. Periodontal manifestations include severe loss of alveolar bone and premature loss of primary and permanent teeth in the absence of an inflammatory response. Early exfoliation particularly affects the anterior teeth. Children with hypophosphatasia are at risk of developing oral complications during adolescent and adult life [17].

Section 2
Necrotizing Periodontal Diseases

Necrotizing periodontal diseases (NPD) include necrotizing ulcerative gingivitis (NUG) and necrotizing ulcerative periodontitis (NUP). To date, there is insufficient evidence to establish if necrotizing ulcerative gingivitis and necrotizing ulcerative periodontitis are two unique diseases or different stages of the same disease that progresses from NUG to NUP. Until a distinction between necrotizing ulcerative gingivitis and necrotizing ulcerative periodontitis can be clarified, NUG and NUP are classified together under the category of necrotizing periodontal disease. Both NUG and NUP appear to be related to diminished systemic resistance to bacterial infection.

1. Necrotizing periodontal disease (NPD) is an inflammatory destructive infection of periodontal tissues that involve tissue necrosis (localized tissue death). Both NUG and NUP are painful infections with ulceration, swelling, and sloughing off of dead epithelial tissue from the gingiva.
   A. Necrotizing ulcerative gingivitis (NUG)—tissue necrosis that is limited to the gingival tissues (Box 17-7).
   B. Necrotizing ulcerative periodontitis (NUP)—tissue necrosis of the gingival tissues combined with loss of attachment and alveolar bone loss (Box 17-8).
      1. NUP is a painful infection characterized by necrosis of gingival tissues, periodontal ligament, and alveolar bone.
      2. NUP is an extremely rapid and destructive form of periodontitis that can produce loss of periodontal attachment within days.
2. **Alternative Terminology.** These conditions previously have been known as trench mouth, Vincent infection, acute ulcerative necrotizing gingivitis (ANUG), and necrotizing ulcerative gingivostomatitis.
3. **Signs and Symptoms of Necrotizing Periodontal Disease**
   A. **Oral Signs and Symptoms.** The clinical appearance of necrotizing periodontal disease is noticeably different than that of any other periodontal disease [18–20].
      1. Necrotizing periodontal disease is a painful infection, primarily involving the interdental and marginal gingiva.
      2. Necrotizing periodontal disease is characterized by ulcerated and necrotic papillae and gingival margins, giving the appearance that the papillae and gingival margins have been "punched-out" or "cratered" (FIG. 17-8). The ulcerated margin is bounded by a red halo.

Box 17.7 Necrotizing Ulcerative Gingivitis (NUG)

- Sudden onset
- Pain
- Necrosis of interdental papillae (cratered, punched-out papillae)
- Yellowish white or grayish tissue slough
- Fiery red gingiva with spontaneous bleeding

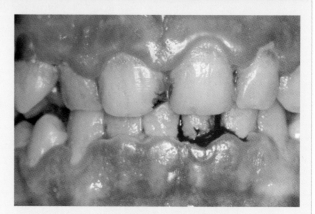

Figure 17.6. **Necrotizing Ulcerative Gingivitis.**

Box 17.8 Necrotizing Ulcerative Periodontitis (NUP)

- The same signs and symptoms of NUG
- Attachment loss

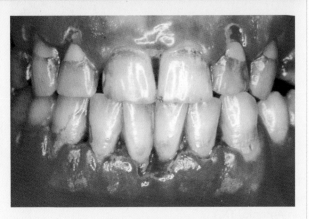

Figure 17.7. **Necrotizing Ulcerative Periodontitis.**

3. The necrotic areas of the gingiva are covered by a yellowish white or grayish tissue slough, which is termed a pseudomembrane.
   a. The pseudomembrane consists primarily of fibrin and necrotic tissue with leukocytes, erythrocytes, and masses of bacteria. (Fibrin is stringy protein formed during the process of blood clot formation.)
   b. The term, pseudomembrane, however, is misleading since the slough has no coherence and is not similar to a true membrane. It is easily wiped off with gauze, exposing an area of fiery red, shiny gingiva.
   c. The pseudomembrane may involve the gingiva of several teeth or it may cover the entire gingiva.
   d. The sloughing off of dead gingival epithelial tissue exposes the underlying connective tissue.
4. Fiery red gingiva with spontaneous gingival bleeding or bleeding to gentle touch.
5. *The necrotizing lesions develop rapidly and are painful.* Intense oral pain causes affected patients to seek dental treatment. This symptom is unusual since gingivitis and periodontitis normally are *not* painful.
6. The first lesions often are seen interproximally in the mandibular anterior sextant, but may occur in any interproximal papilla. Usually, the papillae swell rapidly and develop a rounded contour (FIG. 17-9).
7. A pronounced, fetid oral odor (bad breath) may be present, but can vary in intensity and in some cases is not very noticeable.
   a. The pain associated with necrotizing periodontal disease usually causes the individual to stop brushing.
   b. Materia alba, plaque biofilm, sloughed tissue, blood, and stagnant saliva to collect in the oral cavity causing the oral odor.
8. Necrotizing periodontal disease may be associated with excessive salivation.

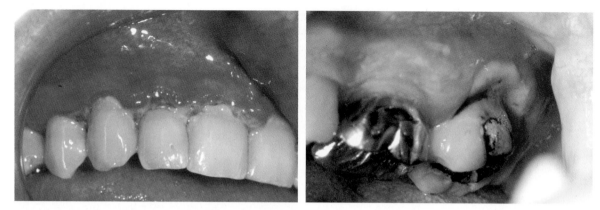

Figure 17.8. Necrotic Papillae and Gingival Margins. This patient with necrotizing periodontal disease exhibits the characteristic ulcerated, necrotic papillae, and gingival margins. (Courtesy of Dr Ralph Arnold, San Antonio, TX.)

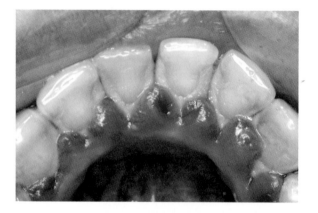

Figure 17.9. Swollen Papillae. Swollen papillae in the anterior regions of the mouth are characteristic of necrotizing periodontal disease. (Courtesy of Dr Richard Foster, Guilford Technical Community College, Jamestown, NC.)

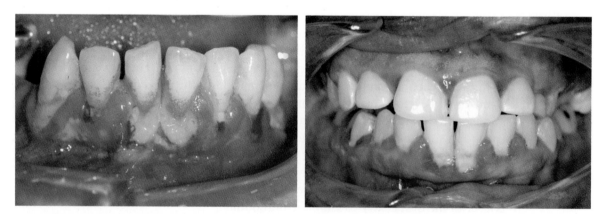

Figure 17.10. Necrotizing Ulcerative Periodontitis. Necrotizing ulcerative periodontitis is characterized by loss of attachment. (Figure 17-10A. Courtesy of Dr Ralph Arnold, San Antonio, TX; Figure 17-10B courtesy of Dr Richard Foster, Guilford Technical Community College, Jamestown, NC.)

9. As tissue necrosis progresses, interproximal craters are formed.
   a. Within a few days the involved papillae are often separated into one facial and one lingual portion with a necrotic depression between them.
   b. This central tissue destruction between the facial and lingual portions of a papilla results in an interdental crater.
   c. Once interproximal craters are formed, the disease process usually involves the periodontal ligament and alveolar bone, resulting in loss of attachment.
   d. Deep craters in the interdental alveolar bone characterize necrotizing ulcerative periodontitis.
   e. The deep periodontal pockets seen in other forms of periodontitis are not common in NUP because the tissue necrosis destroys the marginal epithelium and connective tissue, resulting in recession of gingival margin (Fig. 17-10). Progression of the interproximal disease process often results in destruction of most of the interdental bone.
10. As a result of pain it is often difficult for patients to eat.

B. **Systemic Signs and Symptoms**
   1. Swelling of the lymph nodes, especially the submandibular and cervical lymph nodes, may occur in NPD.
   2. Fever and malaise is not a consistent characteristic of NPD. Investigations indicate that fever is not common [21,22].

4. **Etiology of NPD**
   A. **Microorganisms.** Necrotizing periodontal diseases are associated with *Treponema* species, *Selenomonas* species, *Fusobacterium* species, and *Bacteroides melaninogenicus ss. intermedius* (*Provotella intermedia*).
   B. **Predisposing Factors for NPD**
      1. Systemic diseases which impair immunity, including HIV-infection, leukemia, measles, chicken pox, tuberculosis, herpetic gingivostomatitis, and malaria
      2. Poor self-care (plaque biofilm control)
      3. Emotional stress [23,24]
      4. Inadequate sleep, fatigue
      5. Alcohol use
      6. Caucasian background
      7. Cigarette smoking—most patients who experience NPD are smokers [22]
      8. Increased levels of personal stress
      9. Poor nutrition
         a. In North America, NUG is associated with poor eating habits of young adults, such as college students.
         b. In developing countries, NUG occurs in very young children and appears to be related to poor nutritional status, especially a low protein intake.
      10. Preexisting gingivitis or tissue trauma
      11. Young age—this disease can occur at any age, however, the reported mean age for NPD in industrialized countries is between 22 and 24 years [25].

5. **Treatment of Necrotizing Ulcerative Gingivitis.** The goal of acute phase treatment is to eliminate disease activity and relieve pain and discomfort.
   A. **Acute Care**
      1. Periodontal instrumentation, as thoroughly as can be tolerated by the patient. Ultrasonic instrumentation may be preferable. Use of minimal pressure against the tissues, an ultrasonic tip is used to remove soft and mineralized deposits.
      2. Patient self-care instruction: toothbrushing should be avoided in areas of open wounds to promote wound healing. Chemical plaque biofilm control can be used until healing is accomplished. Twice daily rinsing with 0.12% chlorhexidine solution is very effective.
      3. Adjunctive Oxygen Therapy with Hydrogen peroxide (3%):
         a. Used for mechanical cleaning of necrotic areas and as a mouth rinse (equal portions 3% hydrogen peroxide and warm water) [26–31]
         b. Adjunctive oxygen therapy results in early eradication of pathogenic anaerobic microorganisms and less damage to the periodontal tissues in cases of NPD [26].
      4. Pain control
      5. Supplemental antibiotic therapy as appropriate for the management of systemic manifestations (fever, swollen lymph nodes) or in patients with systemic disease.
         a. Metronidazole 250 mg (Flagyl) three times a day is the first choice for treatments of necrotizing ulcerative gingivitis [19,20]. Other antibiotics such as penicillin and tetracycline are also effective.
         b. In HIV-associated necrotizing ulcerative gingivitis, the adjunctive use of metronidazole is reported to be extremely effective in reducing acute pain and promoting rapid healing [32].
      6. Patients with necrotizing ulcerative gingivitis should be seen daily as long as acute symptoms persist. Appropriate treatment should alleviate symptoms within a few days. After symptoms subside, the patient should return in a week for complete periodontal clinical assessment and treatment planning.
   B. **Patient Education.** Patient counseling for patients with necrotizing ulcerative gingivitis should include instruction on proper nutrition, intake of fluids, and smoking cessation. A liquid dietary replacement, such as Ensure or Boost, can be recommended.

Section 3
Developmental or Acquired Deformities and Conditions

In general, this classification is comprised of local factors that contribute to the initiation and progression of periodontal disease. These factors fall into four subgroups (Box 17-9).

Box 17-9. Developmental or Acquired Deformities and Conditions

A. Localized tooth-related factors that modify or predispose to plaque-induced gingival diseases or periodontitis

   1. Tooth anatomic factors

   2. Dental restorations/appliances

   3. Root fractures

   4. Cervical root resorption and cemental tears

B. Mucogingival deformities and conditions around teeth

   1. Recession of the gingival margin

      a. Facial or lingual surfaces

      b. Interproximal (papillary)

   2. Lack of keratinized gingiva

   3. Decreased vestibular depth

   4. Aberrant frenum/muscle position

   5. Gingival excess

      a. Pseudopocket

      b. Inconsistent gingival margin

      c. Excessive gingival display

      d. Gingival enlargement

   6. Abnormal color

C. Mucogingival deformities and conditions on edentulous ridges

   1. Vertical and/or horizontal ridge deficiency

   2. Lack of gingiva/keratinized tissue

   3. Gingival/soft tissue enlargement

   4. Aberrant frenum/muscle position

   5. Decreased vestibular depth

   6. Abnormal color

D. Occlusal trauma

   1. Primary occlusal trauma

   2. Secondary occlusal trauma

TOOTH-RELATED FACTORS

Tooth anatomic factors that predispose to plaque-related gingival diseases or periodontitis include tooth anatomic factors, such as cervical enamel projections and enamel pearls, palatolingual grooves, or tooth malalignment (FIGS. 17-11 and 17-12). Faulty dental restorations can lead to plaque biofilm retention (FIGS. 17-13 and 17-14) and may impinge on the biologic width.

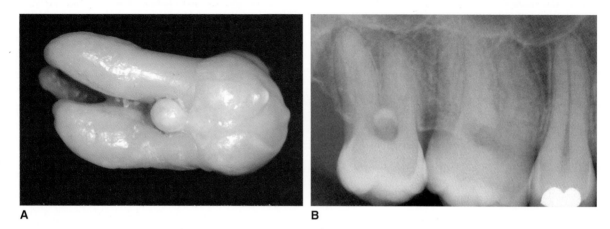

A   B

Figure 17.11. Enamel Pearl as Predisposing Factor. This maxillary second molar exhibits enamel pearl. Although not clear on the radiograph, this tooth experienced alveolar bone loss on the facial aspect. (Courtesy of Dr Ralph Arnold, San Antonio, TX.)

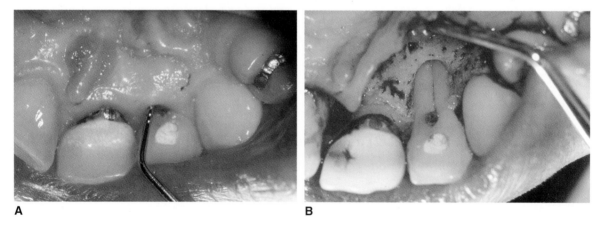

A   B

Figure 17.12. Palatolingual Groove. **A:** This patient has a deep periodontal pocket on the lingual of the maxillary lateral incisor. **B:** Periodontal surgery reveals a palatolingual groove as the predisposing factor for bone loss at this site. (Courtesy of Dr Ralph Arnold, San Antonio, TX.)

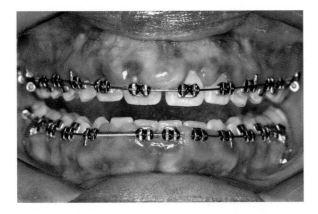

Figure 17.13. **Orthodontic Appliances as a Predisposing Factor**. Infrequent self-care and plaque biofilm accumulation results in periodontitis in this individual with orthodontic appliances. (Courtesy of Dr Richard Foster, Guilford Technical Community College, Jamestown, NC.)

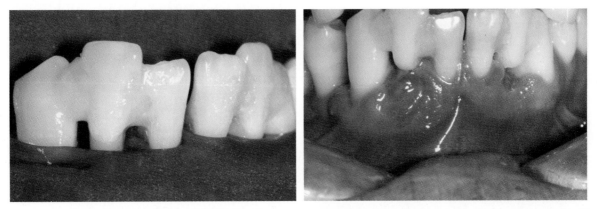

Figure 17.14. **Dentistry as Predisposing Factor**. The splinting of these mandibular anterior leads to plaque biofilm accumulation and was a predisposing factor for periodontitis. (Courtesy of Dr Ralph Arnold, San Antonio, TX.)

MUCOGINGIVAL DEFORMITIES AND CONDITIONS AROUND TEETH

A mucogingival deformity is a significant alteration of the morphology, size, and interrelationships between the gingiva and the alveolar mucosa that may involve the underlying bone. Recession of the gingival margin is the most common mucogingival deformity and it is characterized by the displacement of the gingival margin apically from the cementoenamel junction (FIGS. 17-15–17-18).

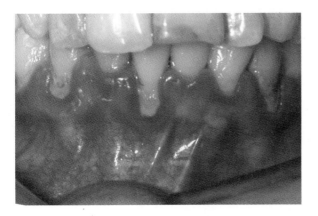

Figure 17.15. **Recession of the Gingival Margin**. Recession of the gingival margin on the mandibular central incisor extending to the mucogingival junction. (Courtesy of Dr Ralph Arnold, San Antonio, TX.)

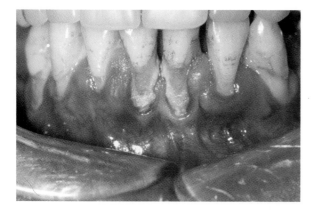

Figure 17.16. Recession of the Gingival Margin. Recession of the gingival margin on the mandibular central incisor extending to the mucogingival junction. (Courtesy of Dr Ralph Arnold, San Antonio, TX.)

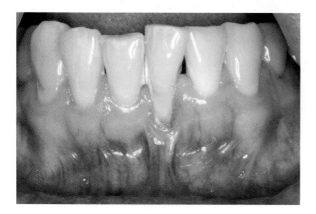

Figure 17.17. Frenum Attachments. Tension of a frenum may pull the gingiva away from the tooth and may be conducive to plaque biofilm accumulation and recession of the gingival margin. (Courtesy of Dr Richard Foster, Guilford Technical Community College, Jamestown, NC.)

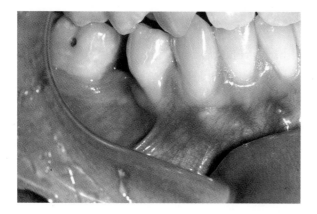

Figure 17.18. Frenum Attachments. Tension of a frenum may pull the gingiva away from the tooth and may be conducive to plaque biofilm accumulation and recession of the gingival margin. (Courtesy of Dr Ralph Arnold, San Antonio, TX.)

OCCLUSAL TRAUMA IN PATIENTS WITH PERIODONTITIS

1. Secondary occlusal trauma is injury as the result of occlusal forces applied to a tooth or teeth that have previously experienced attachment loss and/or bone loss.
2. *In this type of occlusal trauma, the periodontium was unhealthy before experiencing excessive occlusal forces* (Box 17-10).
3. Rapid bone loss and pocket formation may result when excessive occlusal forces are applied to a tooth that has previously experienced attachment loss and/or bone loss.

Box 17.10 Secondary Occlusal Trauma

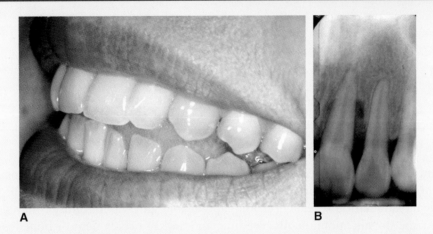

A   **B**

Figure 17.19A,B. Secondary Occlusal Trauma. A: The woman pictured above puts repeated heavy pressure against her central incisor tooth. **B:** A dental radiograph of her central incisor shows severe bone loss around the central incisor that is subjected to the heavy pressure.

Clinical indicators of occlusal trauma may include one or more of the following:
- Tooth mobility (progressive)
- Fremitis (vibration felt when palpating a tooth, as the patient taps the teeth together)
- Tooth migration
- Fractured tooth
- Thermal sensitivity on chewing or percussion

Radiographic indicators may include one or more of the following:
- Widened periodontal ligament space
- Bone loss
- Root resorption

Chapter Summary Statement

The 1999 AAP Classification of Periodontal Diseases and Conditions includes several less common types of periodontitis as well as other periodontal conditions. These are divided into the following subcategories:

- Periodontitis as manifestation of systemic disease
- Necrotizing periodontal diseases
- Abscesses of the periodontium
- Periodontitis associated with endodontic lesions
- Developmental or acquired deformities and conditions.

Section 4
Focus on Patients

Case 1

A new patient comes to the dental office on an emergency basis. The patient complains of severe pain in his gums and reports that he was unable to eat over the weekend due to the pain. A clinical examination reveals necrotic papillae and gingival margins, cratered papillae, a yellowish tissue slough, spontaneous bleeding, and no loss attachment or bone loss. Which type of periodontal disease does this patient exhibit? Outline the recommended acute treatment for this patient.

References

1. Kinane D. Blood and lymphoreticular disorders. *Periodontol 2000.* 1999;21:84–93.
2. Kinane DF. Periodontitis modified by systemic factors. *Ann Periodontol.* 1999;4(1):54–64.
3. Pistorius A, Willershausen B. Cases of HIV-associated characteristic periodontal diseases. *Eur J Med Res.* 1999;4(3):121–125.
4. Winkler JR, Grassi M, Murray PA. Clinical description and etiology of HIV-associated periodontal diseases. In Robertson PB, Greenspan JS, eds. *Perspectives on Oral Manifestations of AIDS: Diagnosis and Management of HIV-Associated Infections: Proceedings of a Symposium Held in January 18–20, 1988 in San Diego, California.* Littleton: PSG Pub. Co. 1988;216.
5. Rylander H, Ericsson I. Manifestations and treatment of periodontal disease in a patient suffering from cyclic neutropenia. *J Clin Periodontol.* 1981;8(2):77–87.
6. Mealey BL. Periodontal implications: medically compromised patients. *Ann Periodontol.* 1996;1(1):256–321.
7. Robinson PG, Adegboye A, Rowland RW, et al. Periodontal diseases and HIV infection. *Oral Dis.* 2002;8(Suppl 2):144–150.
8. Ryder MI. Periodontal management of HIV-infected patients. *Periodontol 2000.* 2000;23:85–93.
9. Robinson PG, Boulter A, Birnbaum W, et al. A controlled study of relative periodontal attachment loss in people with HIV infection. *J Clin Periodontol.* 2000;27(4):273–276.
10. Cox DP, Weathers DR. Leukocyte adhesion deficiency type 1: an important consideration in the clinical differential diagnosis of prepubertal periodontitis. A case report and review of the literature. *Oral Surg Oral Med Oral Pathol Oral Radiol Endod.* 2008;105(1):86–90.

11. Salapata Y, Laskaris G, Drogari E, et al. Oral manifestations in glycogen storage disease type 1b. *J Oral Pathol Med*. 1995;24(3):136–139.

12. Carlsson G, Andersson M, Putsep K, et al. Kostmann syndrome or infantile genetic agranulocytosis, part one: celebrating 50 years of clinical and basic research on severe congenital neutropenia. *Acta Paediatr*. 2006;95(12):1526–1532.

13. Alaluusua S, Kivitie-Kallio S, Wolf J, et al. Periodontal findings in Cohen syndrome with chronic neutropenia. *J Periodontol*. 1997;68(5):473–478.

14. Karrer S, Landthaler M, Schmalz G. Ehlers-Danlos type VIII. Review of the literature. *Clin Oral Investig*. 2000;4(2):66–69.

15. Letourneau Y, Perusse R, Buithieu H. Oral manifestations of Ehlers-Danlos syndrome. *J Can Dent Assoc*. 2001;67(6):330–334.

16. Moore MM, Votava JM, Orlow SJ, et al. Ehlers-Danlos syndrome type VIII: periodontitis, easy bruising, marfanoid habitus, and distinctive facies. *J Am Acad Dermatol*. 2006;55(2 Suppl): S41–S45.

17. Olsson A, Matsson L, Blomquist HK, et al. Hypophosphatasia affecting the permanent dentition. *J Oral Pathol Med*. 1996;25(6):343–347.

18. Scully C, Laskaris G, Pindborg J, et al. Oral manifestations of HIV infection and their management. I. More common lesions. *Oral Surg Oral Med Oral Pathol*. 1991;71(2):158–166.

19. Loesche WJ, Syed SA, Laughon BE, et al. The bacteriology of acute necrotizing ulcerative gingivitis. *J Periodontol*. 1982;53(4):223–230.

20. Proctor DB, Baker CG. Treatment of acute necrotizing ulcerative gingivitis with metronidazole. *J Can Dent Assoc (Tor)*. 1971;37(10):376–380.

21. Shields WD. Acute necrotizing ulcerative gingivitis. A study of some of the contributing factors and their validity in an Army population. *J Periodontol*. 1977;48(6):346–349.

22. Stevens AW Jr, Cogen RB, Cohen-Cole S, et al. Demographic and clinical data associated with acute necrotizing ulcerative gingivitis in a dental school population (ANUG-demographic and clinical data). *J Clin Periodontol*. 1984;11(8):487–493.

23. da Silva AM, Newman HN, Oakley DA. Psychosocial factors in inflammatory periodontal diseases. A review. *J Clin Periodontol*. 1995;22(7):516–526.

24. Hildebrand HC, Epstein J, Larjava H. The influence of psychological stress on periodontal disease. *J West Soc Periodontol Periodontal Abstr*. 2000;48(3):69–77.

25. Horning GM, Cohen ME. Necrotizing ulcerative gingivitis, periodontitis, and stomatitis: clinical staging and predisposing factors. *J Periodontol*. 1995;66(11):990–998.

26. Gaggl AJ, Rainer H, Grund E, Chiari FM. Local oxygen therapy for treating acute necrotizing periodontal disease in smokers. *J Periodontol*. 2006;77(1):31–38.

27. Lindhe J, Lang NP, Karring T. *Clinical Periodontology and Implant Dentistry*. Oxford; Ames, Iowa: Blackwell Munksgaard; 2008.

28. Marshall MV, Cancro LP, Fischman SL. Hydrogen peroxide: a review of its use in dentistry. *J Periodontol*. 1995;66(9):786–796.

29. Johnson BD, Engel D. Acute necrotizing ulcerative gingivitis. A review of diagnosis, etiology and treatment. *J Periodontol*. 1986;57(3):141–150.

30. MacPhee T, Cowley G. *Essentials of Periodontology and Periodontics*. 3rd ed. Oxford, St. Louis: Blackwell Scientific Publications; distributed in the United States by Blackwell Mosby Book Distributors; 1981.

31. Wennstrom J, Lindhe J. Effect of hydrogen peroxide on developing plaque and gingivitis in man. *J Clin Periodontol*. 1979;6(2):115–130.

32. Scully C, Laskaris G, Pindborg J, et al. Oral manifestations of HIV infection and their management. I. More common lesions. *Oral Surg Oral Med Oral Pathol*. 1991;71(2):158–166.

Suggested Reading

1999 International Workshop for a Classification of Periodontal Diseases and Conditions. Papers. Oak Brook, Illinois, October 30 to November 2, 1999. *Ann Periodontol*. 1999l;4(1):1–112.

Chapter 18

Periodontitis as a Risk Factor for Systemic Disease

Learning Objectives

- Educate patients at risk for cardiovascular diseases about the possible impact of periodontal infection on cardiovascular health and encourage oral disease prevention and treatment services.

- Educate pregnant women and those planning pregnancy regarding the possible impact of periodontal infection on pregnancy outcomes and encourage preventive oral care and treatment services.

- Educate patients with diabetes about the probable bidirectional association between periodontal disease and diabetes and encourage oral disease prevention and treatment services.

- Educate family members and caregivers about the association between periodontal disease and pneumonia in health-compromised seniors residing in hospitals and long-term care.

Key Terms

Atherosclerosis
Heat shock proteins (HSP)
C-reactive protein (CRP)
Low–birth-weight infant

Preeclampsia
Glycemic control
Hospital-acquired pneumonia

Section 1
Periodontitis and Systemic Disease

Research evidence emerging since the early 1990s suggests that there are two sides to the relationship between periodontitis and systemic health. First, as discussed in Chapter 10, the presence of systemic disease may increase the likelihood of disease initiation or the severity of periodontitis. On the other hand, the presence of a chronic oral infection (periodontitis) may have an adverse effect on an individual's systemic health.

This chapter discusses the possibility that periodontal disease may modify some aspect of certain systemic diseases to make those diseases more severe. Recent research studies show a connection between periodontal health and overall health, linking periodontitis to a variety of systemic problems. The influence of periodontal infections is documented in several systemic conditions including cardiovascular/cerebrovascular problems, diabetes mellitus, preterm labor, low–birth-weight delivery, and respiratory conditions (Box 18-1) [1–3].

Periodontal disease is a potentially modifiable risk factor. The possibility of an association between periodontal and systemic disease suggests that dental hygiene care and periodontal therapy may play roles in decreasing the incidence and severity of these systemic diseases. Interdisciplinary relationships between dental hygienists and other health professionals should be established to provide the highest standard of care for the patient.

Box 18-1. Systems Possibly Influenced by Periodontal Infection

Cardiovascular/cerebrovascular system
Coronary heart disease (CHD)
Atherosclerosis
Angina
Myocardial infarction (MI)
Cerebrovascular accident (stroke)

Endocrine system
Diabetes mellitus

Reproductive system
Preterm/low–birth-weight infants
Preeclampsia

Respiratory system
Hospital-acquired pneumonia

---

1. **Periodontitis as a Risk Factor for Cardiovascular Disease (CVD)**
   A. **Introduction to Periodontitis and CVD**
      1. Statistics: Cardiovascular Disease
         a. Cardiovascular disease made up 16.7 million, or 29.2% of total global deaths according to World Health Report 2003. By 2010, CVD will be the leading cause of death in developing countries [4].
         b. An estimated 80,700,000 American adults (1 in 3) have one or more types of CVD. Of these, 38,200,000 are estimated to be 60 years of age or older [5].
         c. Atherosclerosis, a major component of cardiovascular disease, is a process characterized by a thickening of artery walls. Complications that arise from atherosclerosis cause deaths from heart attack or stroke and have been reported to account for nearly three fourths of all deaths from CVD [5].

2. Plaque Biofilm as a Large Supply of Bacteria
   a. Subgingival plaque biofilm provides a large and persistent source of periodontal pathogens to the host.
   b. Waite and Bradley [6] estimated that a patient who has 28 teeth with pocket depths of 6 to 7 mm and bone loss has a large overall surface area of infection and inflammation that could be the size of the palm of an adult hand or larger.
   c. Bacteria and their by-products from the oral cavity are introduced into the blood stream (bacteremia) during toothbrushing, flossing, and subgingival irrigation. Periodontal infections result in bacteremias that could possibly have systemic effects on the vascular system.

B. **Summary of Research Studies**
   1. Findings from several research studies indicate consistent associations between periodontal disease and cardiovascular disease (Box 18-2).
   2. Evidence of the beneficial effects of periodontal therapy on CVD outcomes is limited. Several studies have demonstrated that periodontal patients with favorable clinical responses to nonsurgical periodontal therapy exhibited improvements in serum C-reactive protein (CRP) concentrations [7–9].
   3. It is important to note, however, insufficient evidence exists to show that treatment of periodontal disease can reduce the risk for cardiovascular disease. The impact of treatment for periodontitis on the cardiovascular disease is an area for ongoing research.

C. **Possible Biologic Explanations.** How is Periodontits Related to cardiovascular disease? Four biologic pathways have been proposed to explain the possible link between periodontits and cardiovascular disease. These biologic pathways include
   1. Pathway hypothesis 1: direct effect of periodontal pathogens on platelets
      a. In this proposed biologic pathway, periodontal pathogens induce clot formation by platelets, possibly leading to the blockage of a blood vessel by a blood clot (FIG. 18-1).
      b. Patients with periodontitis are at increased risk for thickening of the walls of the major coronary arteries [10]. In several studies of the fatty deposits on the inner walls of blood vessels obtained from humans, more than half of the lesions contained periodontal pathogens [11,12].
      c. *Porphyromonas gingivalis* and *Streptococcus sanguis* express virulence factors that induce clot and thrombus formation [11,12]. Thus, one possible pathway between periodontitis and CVD is that periodontal pathogens induce clot and thrombus formation.

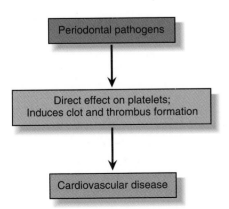

Figure 18.1. **Pathway Hypothesis 1: Direct Effect of Periodontal Pathogens on Platelets.** In this proposed biologic pathway, periodontal pathogens induce clot formation by platelets, possibly leading to the blockage of a blood vessel by a blood clot.

2. Pathway hypothesis 2: cross reactivity
    a. Introduction to heat shock proteins
        1) Heat shock proteins (HSPs), also called stress proteins, are a group of proteins that are present in all life forms. For the purpose of this discussion the reader should note that the cells of the human body produce heat shock proteins and that periodontal pathogens also produce heat shock proteins.
        2) Heat shock proteins are present in all life forms under normal conditions, but are expressed at high levels when a cell undergoes various types of environmental stresses like heat, cold, and oxygen deprivation.
        3) In the human body, extracellular stress proteins stimulate an immediate immune response designed to control an infection or disease.
    b. Periodontal infections and pathway hypothesis 2
        1) In this proposed pathway, periodontal pathogens induce a local immune response in the endothelial cells of the blood vessel walls.
        2) The endothelial cells react to the presence of periodontal pathogens by producing heat shock proteins.
    c. The Cross Reactivity Hypothesis proposes that the body's immune response to the heat stress proteins of the periodontal pathogens inadvertently cross-reacts with the heat shock proteins of host endothelial cells (Fig. 18-2).
        1) In this case, cross reactivity refers to the immune response mistakenly being directed at the heat shock proteins of host endothelial cells, rather than against the heat shock proteins of the periodontal pathogens.
        2) In this hypothesis, the misdirected immune response against the cells in blood vessels leads to vascular inflammation and atherosclerosis.

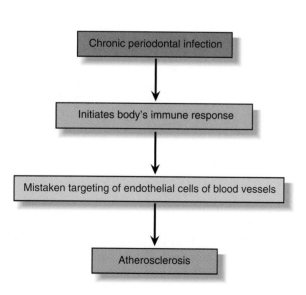

Figure 18.2. **Pathway Hypothesis 2: Cross Reactivity.** This proposed pathway suggests that the body's immune response to periodontal pathogens could mistakenly target cells in blood vessels leading to vascular inflammation and atherosclerosis.

3. Pathway hypothesis 3: periodontal pathogen invasion of vessels
   a. In this proposed biologic pathway, periodontal pathogens get into the bloodstream and invade the blood vessel walls leading to inflammation and atherosclerosis (FIG. 18-3).
   b. *Porphyromonas gingivalis* can invade the arteries. Several studies have identified periodontal pathogens in the fatty deposits on the walls of arteries.
   c. These studies show that periodontal pathogens can and do invade blood vessel walls. It is unclear, however, whether periodontal pathogens cause atherosclerosis or simply invade an already damaged artery.

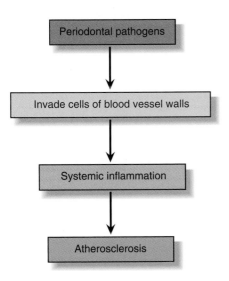

Figure 18.3. **Pathway Hypothesis 3: Periodontal Pathogen Invasion of Vessels.** In this proposed biologic pathway, periodontal pathogens get into the bloodstream and invade the blood vessel walls leading to inflammation and atherosclerosis.

4. Pathway hypothesis 4: triggering of proinflammatory cytokines
   a. Inflammation and The Chronic Diseases of Aging
      1) Recent research advances have led to the recognition that inflammatory mechanisms appear to be critical factors in the development and progression of most of the chronic diseases of aging.
      2) Inflammation plays a critical role in diseases that usually are not classified as inflammatory diseases, such as cardiovascular disease and Alzheimer disease.
      3) Overexpression of inflammation may be one of the key aspects of aging that influences and links different diseases in different individuals.
   b. Periodontal Infections and Pathway Hypothesis 4
      1) In this proposed pathway, periodontal infections may contribute to atherosclerosis by repeatedly challenging the blood vessel walls and arterial walls with proinflammatory cytokines (FIG. 18-4).
      2) Evidence from clinical and population studies suggest that inflammation is important in atherosclerosis and cardiovascular disease. As such, detection of systemic inflammatory markers plays an important role in risk assessment for cardiovascular disease.
      3) C-reactive protein (CRP) is a special type of plasma protein—produced by macrophages, endothelial cells, and smooth muscle—that

is present during episodes of acute inflammation or infection [13]. CRP is an important cardiovascular risk predictor [14–16]. Elevations in serum CRP are well-accepted risk factors for cardiovascular disease [17].

4) One hypothesis is that periodontitis is the source of the inflammation that triggers the production of CRP [18]. Serum CRP levels are elevated in individuals with periodontitis when compared to individuals without periodontitis [19–21].

D. **Implications for Dental Hygiene Practice.** Dental hygienists should educate patients at risk for cardiovascular diseases about the possible impact of periodontal infection on cardiovascular health and encourage oral disease prevention and treatment services. Treating periodontal inflammation may not only help manage periodontal diseases, but may also help with the management of other chronic inflammatory conditions, such as cardiovascular disease.

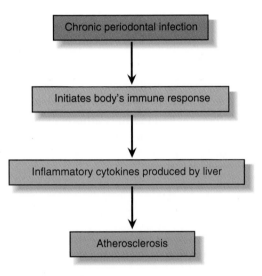

Figure 18.4. Pathway Hypothesis 4: Triggering of Proinflammatory Cytokines. In this proposed pathway, periodontal infections contribute to atherosclerosis by repeatedly challenging the blood vessel walls and arterial walls with proinflammatory cytokines.

Box 18-2. Summary of Studies Investigating an Association Between Periodontal Diseases and CVDs

Arbes et al. [22]	United States; 5,564 subjects (NHANES III); periodontal disease defined as attachment loss >3 mm on all teeth
	Reported a positive association between periodontal disease and coronary heart disease after adjusting for age, gender, race, and other risk factors
Abnet et al. [23]	29,584 rural Chinese subjects; periodontitis defined as tooth loss
	Reported tooth loss associated with increased odds for death from myocardial infarction and stroke
Beck et al. [24]	1,147 men
	Periodontal disease was associated with moderate risk for coronary heart disease and stroke after adjusting for age and cardiovascular disease risk factors
Beck et al. [10,25]; Elter, et al. [26]	United States; 6,017 subjects; severe periodontitis defined as clinical attachment loss ≥3 mm at 30% of more of the sites; presence of serum antibodies to periodontal pathogens was associated with carotid atherosclerosis
	Individuals with high attachment loss and tooth loss exhibited are more likely to experience cardiovascular disease when compared to individuals with low attachment loss and low tooth loss [26]; a significant association between severe periodontitis and thickened carotid arteries [10]; individuals with exposure to the periodontal pathogens *Campylobacter rectus* and *Peptostreptococcus micros* had almost twice the prevalence of carotid atherosclerosis as compared to those individuals with only a high *C. rectus* antibody [25].
DeStefano et al. [27]	9,760 subjects; subjects were classified as no periodontal disease, gingivitis, periodontitis, or edentulous
	Reported periodontitis associated with small increased risk for coronary heart disease among men
Desvarieux et al. [28]	United States; 1,056 subjects; tested subgingival plaque biofilm for the presence of 11 known periodontal pathogens using DNA techniques
	Cumulative periodontal bacterial burden was significantly related to risk of cardiovascular disease
Engebretson et al. [29]	203 subjects: periodontal disease defined as radiographic alveolar bone loss
	Severe periodontal bone loss was independently associated with carotid atherosclerosis

(continued)

Box 18-2. Continued

Hujoel et al. [30]	8,032 dentate adults; periodontal disease defined as periodontal pocketing and attachment loss
	Reported periodontitis was not associated with a significant increased risk for coronary heart disease
Hung et al. [31]	United States; 41,407 males followed for 12 years and 58,974 females followed for 6 years; self-reported periodontal disease and cardiovascular disease
	Individuals with a low number of teeth (10 or less) had a significantly higher risk of cardiovascular disease as compared to males with a high number of teeth (25 or more)
Janket et al. [32]	A meta-analysis of nine cohort studies
	Periodontal disease appears to be associated with a 19% increase in risk of future cardiovascular disease
Joshipura et al. [33]	United States; 468 males; evaluated the association between self-reported periodontal disease and serum biomarkers for cardiovascular disease (serum biomarkers are specific indicators found in a blood test that identifies a disease, in this case, cardiovascular disease)
	Self-reported periodontal disease was associated with significantly higher levels of CRP and LDL cholesterol. CRP is a protein that increases during systemic inflammation. These analyses suggest a significant association between self-reported periodontal disease and serum biomarkers for cardiovascular disease.
Khader et al. [34]	Meta-analysis of seven cohort studies and four studies of other designs.
	Subjects with periodontitis had an overall adjusted risk of coronary heart disease that was 1.15 times the risk for healthy subjects.
Mattila et al. [35]	Finland; case-control study of 100 subjects who had experienced a myocardial infarction (MI) and 102 control subjects with no history of MI
	The dental health of the subjects with a history of MI was significantly worse (periodontitis, periapical lesions, caries, pericoronitis) than that of control subjects. The association between poor dental health and history of MI was independent of other risk factors for heart attack such as age, social class, serum lipids, smoking, hypertension, and diabetes.
Mattila et al. [36]	100 cases; periodontal disease evaluated using the Dental Severity Index
	Significant association between dental infections and severe coronary atheromatosis (degeneration of the arteries) in men but not in women

(continued)

Box 18-2. Continued

Meurman et al. [37]	A meta-analysis of prospective and retrospective follow-up studies
	Reported a 20% increase in cardiovascular disease risk among patients with periodontal disease and an even higher risk ratio for stroke
Paraskevas et al. [38]	A meta-analysis of ten cross-sectional studies
	Reported strong evidence from cross-sectional studies that plasma C-reactive protein in periodontitis is elevated in periodontitis compared with healthy controls
Pussinen et al. [39,40,41]	Finland; 6,950 subjects [39]; 1,023 subjects [40]; 6,051 subjects followed for 10 years [41]; monitored serum antibodies to *P. gingivalis* and *A. actinomycetemcomitans*
	High-serum antibody levels to major periodontal pathogens were associated with risk of cardiovascular disease; periodontal pathogens or host response against them may contribute to the pathogenesis of CHD; exposure to periodontal pathogens or endotoxin induces systemic inflammation leading to increased risk for CVD
Wu et al. [20,21]	9,962 subjects (NHANES III and follow-up); subjects were classified as no periodontal disease, gingivitis, periodontitis, or edentulous
	Compared to periodontal health, the risk for stroke with periodontitis was 2.1 and significant

2. **Periodontitis as a Risk Factor for Adverse Pregnancy Outcomes**
    A. **Introduction to Periodontitis and Adverse Pregnancy Outcomes**
        1. Adverse pregnancy outcomes that have been linked to periodontal disease include miscarriage, preterm birth, low birth weight, preeclampsia.
            a. Preterm delivery of low–birth-weight infants is a leading cause of neonatal death and of long-term neurodevelopmental disturbances and health problems in children.
            b. Preeclampsia is a serious complication of pregnancy characterized by an abrupt rise in blood pressure, large amounts of the protein albumin into the urine and swelling of the hands, feet, and face. Preeclampsia occurs in the third trimester (the last third) of pregnancy.
        2. Adverse pregnancy outcomes have been linked to risk factors such as smoking, alcohol use, poor diet, genitourinary infections, and stress. Preterm low–birth-weight deliveries represent approximately 10% of annual births in industrialized nations. Of these births, 25% occur with no known risk factors. Recent findings suggest that periodontal diseases could represent a risk factor during pregnancy.
        3. The American Academy of Periodontology issued a statement in 2004, recommending, "Women who are pregnant or planning pregnancy undergo periodontal examinations. Appropriate preventive or therapeutic services, if indicated, should be provided. Preventive oral care services should be provided as early in pregnancy as possible. However, women should be encouraged to achieve a high level of oral hygiene prior to becoming pregnant and throughout their pregnancies" [42].
        4. Other groups who have approved the content of the American Academy of Periodontology statement regarding periodontal management of the pregnant patient include the American College of Obstetricians and Gynecologists, the US March of Dimes, and the US National Nursing Association [42].
    B. **Summary of Research Studies**
        1. Findings from several studies indicate an association between periodontal disease and adverse pregnancy outcomes (Box 18-3).
            a. Offenbacher et al. [43] found the women having low–birth-weight babies had greater clinical attachment loss than women having normal–birth-weight babies.
            b. Offenbacher et al. [43] found that periodontits contributed to more preterm low–birth-weight cases than did smoking or alcohol use during pregnancy.
        2. Further research is needed to establish pathogenic mechanisms of active periodontal disease and subgingival periodontal pathogens related to preeclampsia development.
        3. Additional research is needed to evaluate the efficacy and cost-effectiveness of different types of periodontal intervention on adverse pregnancy outcomes. Three intervention studies provide early evidence that periodontal treatment may reduce the likelihood of preterm low–birth-weight infants [44–46]. One study found that periodontal therapy does not significantly alter rates of preterm birth or low birth weight [47].
        4. At present, the US National Institute of Dental and Craniofacial Research (NIDCR) has made a significant investment in research on this topic with a $20 million dollar research project that includes two independent multicenter clinical trials, involving approximately 2,600 pregnant women.

C. Possible Biologic Explanations. How is Periodontits Related to Adverse Pregnancy Outcomes? Animal studies suggest that reservoirs of Gram-negative organisms, such as those found in periodontitis, may have a negative impact on pregnancy outcome (FIG. 18-5).

D. Implications for Dental Hygiene Practice. Dental hygienists should educate patients about the association between adverse pregnancy outcomes and periodontal infection and provide early oral hygiene services for pregnant women and those considering pregnancy. Understanding the mechanism of periodontal disease-associated adverse pregnancy outcomes could lead to interventions to improve fetal growth.

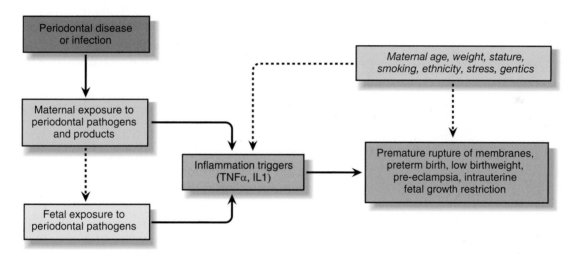

Figure 18.5. Proposed Biologic Pathway for Association Between Periodontal Disease and Adverse Pregnancy Outcomes. Reservoirs of Gram-negative organisms, such as those found in periodontitis, may have a negative impact on pregnancy outcome.

Box 18-3. Summary of Studies Investigating an Association Between Periodontal Diseases and Adverse Pregnancy Outcomes

Bassani et al. [48]	Brazil; 304 cases with periodontitis and 611 controls; periodontal disease defined as attachment loss >3 mm in at least three sites
	Concluded that periodontal disease alone was not a predictor of low birth weight in this case-control observational study
Boggess et al. [49]	United States; 1,017 subjects; periodontal disease defined as 15 or more sites with pocket depths 4 mm or greater
	Moderate or severe periodontal disease early in pregnancy is associated with delivery of a small-for-gestational-age infant
Boggess et al. [50]	United States; 763 subjects; periodontal disease defined as 15 or more sites with pocket depths 4 mm or greater
	After adjusting for other risk factors, active maternal periodontal disease during pregnancy is associated with an increased risk for the development of preeclampsia
Buduneli et al. [51]	Turkey; 53 cases and 128 controls; periodontal disease defined as presence of periodontal pocketing
	No statistically significant differences between the cases and the control subjects
Bosnjak et al. [52]	Croatia; 17 cases and 93 controls; periodontal disease defined as >60% of sites with clinical attachment loss of 4 mm or greater
	Periodontal disease represents an independent and clinically significant risk factor for preterm birth in the studied cohort
Conde-Agudelo et al. [53]	Systematic review of cohort, case-control, or cross-sectional studies with original data that evaluated the association between maternal periodontal disease and preeclampsia were included; six studies, representing a total of 3,420 women (493 preeclamptic and 2,927 non-preeclamptic control women) were pooled for meta-analysis
	Periodontal disease during pregnancy is associated with an increased risk of preeclampsia
Contreras et al. [54]	Columbia; 130 cases and 243 controls; periodontal disease defined as clinical attachment loss 4 mm or greater and bleeding on probing
	Chronic periodontal disease and the presence of *P. gingivalis*, *Tannerella forsythensis*, and *Eikenella corrodens* were significantly associated with preeclampsia in pregnant women.
Davenport et al. [55]	United Kingdom; 236 cases and 507 controls; periodontal disease defined as presence of periodontal pockets
	No association detected for periodontal disease and preterm birth

(continued)

Box 18-3. Continued

Goepfert et al. [56]	United States; 59 cases and 44 controls; periodontal disease defined as clinical attachment levels of 5 mm or greater
	Women with early spontaneous preterm birth were more likely to have severe periodontal disease than women with term birth
Holbrook et al. [57]	Iceland; 96 subjects; periodontal disease defined as pocket depth of >4 mm
	No association detected between periodontal disease and low birth weight
Jarjoura et al. [58]	United States; 83 cases and 120 controls; periodontal disease defined as five or more sites with clinical attachment levels of 3 mm or greater
	Periodontitis is independently associated with preterm birth and low birth weight
Jeffcoat et al. [59]	United States, 1,313 subjects; periodontal disease defined as 90 or more sites with clinical attachment levels of 3 m or greater
	Severe or generalized periodontal disease is associated with preterm delivery
Khader et al. [60]	Meta-analysis of periodontal disease in relation to the risk of preterm birth/low birth weight of two case-control studies and three prospective cohort studies
	Periodontal diseases in the pregnant mother significantly increase the risk of subsequent preterm birth or low birth weight
Lopez et al. [61]	Chile; 763 subjects; periodontal disease defined as 15 or more sites with pocket depths of 4 mm or greater
	Periodontal disease was associated with both preterm birth and low birth weight, independent of other risk factors
Meurman et al. [62]	Finland; 207 subjects; Community Periodontal Index for Treatment Needs
	No association detected between poor periodontal health and adverse pregnancy outcomes
Moore et al. [63]	United Kingdom; 3,738 subjects; periodontal disease defined as pocket depths >4 mm
	No association between either preterm birth or low birth weight and periodontal disease in this population
Moore et al. [64]	United Kingdom; 61 cases and 93 controls; periodontal disease defined as pocket depths >5 mm
	No association between the severity of periodontal disease and pregnancy outcome in this population

(*continued*)

Box 18-3. Continued

Moliterno et al. [95]	Brazil; 76 cases and 75 controls; periodontal disease defined as four or more sites with pocket depths >4 mm and clinical attachment levels of 3 mm or greater
	Periodontitis was considered a risk indicator for low birth weight in this sample
Moreu et al. [65]	Spain; 96 subjects; periodontal disease defined as pocket depths of 3 mm or greater
	Periodontal disease is a significant risk factor for low birth weight but not for preterm delivery
Offenbacher et al. [43]	United States; 93 cases and 31 controls; periodontal disease defined as 60% of sites with clinical attachment levels of 3 mm or greater
	Periodontal diseases represent a clinically significant risk factor for preterm low birth weight
Offenbacher et al. [66,67]	United States; 1,020 subjects; periodontal disease defined as four or more sites with pocket depths of 5 mm or greater and clinical attachment levels of 2 mm or greater
	Moderate-severe periodontal disease and progressive periodontal disease are significant risk factors for preterm delivery
Offenbacher et al. [68]	United States; controlled pilot study with 67 subjects
	Evidence supports the potential benefits of periodontal treatment on pregnancy outcomes. Treatment was safe, improved periodontal health, and prevented periodontal disease progression; preliminary data show a 3.8-fold reduction in the rate of preterm delivery
Pitiphat et al. [69]	United States; 1,635 middle-class women in the Project Viva cohort study of pregnant women
	Results suggest that periodontitis is an independent risk factor for adverse pregnancy outcome among middle-class women
Radnai et al. [70]	Hungary; 41 cases and 44 controls; periodontal disease defined as one or more sites with probing depth 4 mm or greater and bleeding on probing
	Early localized periodontitis of the patient during pregnancy can be regarded as an important risk factor for preterm low birth weight
Radnai et al. [71]	Hungary; 77 cases and 84 controls; periodontal disease defined as one or more sites with probing depth 4 mm or greater and bleeding on probing
	Significant association between periodontal disease and preterm low birth weight

3. **Periodontitis as a Risk Factor for Diabetes Complications**
  A. **Introduction to Periodontitis and Diabetes Complications.** Research suggests that there is a two-way relationship between diabetes and periodontal disease.
    1. First, it is clear that diabetes increases the risk for and severity of periodontal diseases [72,73]. The American Diabetes Association's Standard of Medical Care 2008 includes taking a history of past and current dental infections as part of the physician's examination [74,75].
    2. Second, periodontal disease may exacerbate diabetes mellitus by significantly worsening glycemic control over time [76].
  B. **Summary of Research Studies.** Periodontal disease may have an impact on glycemic control but the mechanism through which this occurs is not clear [72]. Further research is needed to clarify the relationship of periodontal diseases and diabetes.
  C. **Possible Biologic Explanations.** How is Periodontits Related to Diabetes Complications?
    1. Overview of glycemic control
      a. Glycemic control is a medical term referring to the typical levels of blood sugar (glucose) in a person with diabetes mellitus.
        1) Optimal management of diabetes involves patients measuring and recording their own blood glucose levels.
        2) Prolonged and elevated levels of glucose in the blood, which is left unchecked and untreated, will, over time, result in serious diabetic complications in those susceptible and sometimes even death.
      b. Blood sugar level is measured by means of a glucose meter, with the result either in mg/dL (milligrams per deciliter in the United States) or mmol/L (millimoles per liter in Canada and Europe) of blood.
        1) The average normal person should have a glucose level of around 4.5 to 7.0 mmol/L (80 to 125 mg/dL).
        2) In the diabetic patient a before-meal level of less than 6.1 mmol/L (<110 mg/dL) and a level 2 hours after the start of a meal of less than 7.8 mmol/L (<140 mg/dL) is acceptable.
      c. Poor glycemic control refers to persistently elevated blood glucose and glycosylated hemoglobin levels, which may range from 200 to 500 mg/dL (11 to 28 mmol/L) and 9% to 15% or higher over months and years before severe complications occur.
    2. Proposed biologic pathways
      a. Periodontal diseases may serve as initiators of insulin resistance, thereby aggravating glycemic control (Fig. 18-6).
      b. In recent years, interest has been growing in a possible inflammatory basis for diabetes and its complications (Box 18-4).
        1) Much of this research focuses on C-reactive protein (CRP) as a measure of circulating inflammatory biomarkers.
          a. Concentrations of CRP in individuals with long-term type 1 diabetes are significantly higher than those of healthy controls [77]. These findings suggest that the inflammatory process may play a role in the long-term progression of type 1 diabetes.
          b. Increases in inflammatory markers are detected in apparently healthy individuals who later go on to develop type 2 diabetes [78,79].

2) Further research is required to confirm the role of inflammation in diabetes and what role, if any, periodontitis—as source of inflammation that triggers the production of CRP—might play in the disease process.

D. Implications for Dental Hygiene Practice. Dental hygienists should educate patients with diabetes about the possible impact of periodontal infection on glycemic control and encourage oral disease prevention and treatment services.

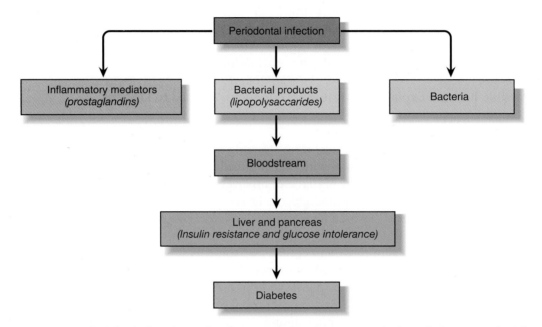

Figure 18.6. Proposed Biological Pathway for the Association Between Periodontal Disease and Diabetes. Periodontal diseases may serve as initiators of insulin resistance, thereby aggravating glycemic control.

Box 18-4. Summary of Studies Investigating an Association Between Periodontal Diseases and Diabetes

Collin et al. [80]	Finland; 25 patients with non–insulin-dependent diabetes (NIDDM)
	Advanced periodontitis seems to be associated with the impairment of the metabolic control in patients with NIDDM.
Janket et al. [32]	United States
	Meta-analysis of published studies and abstracts. Findings suggest that periodontal disease is a risk factor for cardiovascular and renal mortality in people with diabetes.
Mealey et al. [72]	United States
	Review of 200 articles. Inflammatory periodontal disease may increase insulin resistance, thereby aggravating glycemic control. Further research is needed to clarify the relationship between periodontitis and diabetes.
Saremi et al. [81]	United States; longitudinal study of 628 subjects
	Periodontal disease is a strong predictor of mortality form ischemic heart disease and diabetic nephropathy in Pima Indians with type 2 diabetes. The effect of periodontal disease is in addition to the effects of traditional risk factors for these diseases.
Scannapieco et al. [82]	United States
	Systematic literature review. Findings suggest that periodontal disease is a risk factor for cardiovascular and renal mortality in people with diabetes.
Taylor et al. [76]	United States
	Severe periodontitis at baseline was associated with increased risk of poor glycemic control at follow-up. These results support considering severe periodontitis as a risk factor for poor glycemic control and suggest that physicians treating patients with NIDDM should be alert to the signs of severe periodontitis in managing NIDDM.

4. Periodontitis as a Risk Factor for Respiratory Disease
   A. Periodontitis and Hospital-Acquired Pneumonia
      1. Pneumonia is a serious inflammation of one or both lungs. It is caused by the inhalation of microorganisms and can range in seriousness from mild to life threatening. There are two types of pneumonia: community-acquired and hospital-acquired.
      2. Community-acquired pneumonia is pneumonia that is contracted outside of the hospital setting.
         a. Most cases of community-acquired bacterial pneumonia are caused by aspiration of oropharyngeal organisms such as *Streptococcus pneumoniae*, *Haemophilus influenzae*, and *Mycoplasma pneumoniae* [83].
         b. Community-acquired bacterial pneumonia generally responds well to treatment. There is no evidence that periodontal disease or oral hygiene alters the risk for community-acquired pneumonia.
      3. Hospital-acquired pneumonia is an infection of the lungs contracted during a stay in a hospital or long-term care facility.
         a. Hospital-acquired pneumonia is not caused by the same organisms that cause community-acquired pneumonia.
            1) Hospital-acquired pneumonia usually results from organisms called *potential respiratory pathogens* (PRPs) that are generally found in the gastrointestinal tract, but may be passed into the oropharynx through gastroesophageal reflux.
            2) Gastroesophageal reflux disease (GERD) is the return of stomach contents back up into the esophagus. This reflux frequently causes heartburn because of irritation of the esophagus by stomach acid.
         b. Hospital-acquired pneumonia tends to be more serious, because a patient's defense mechanisms against infection are often impaired during a stay in a hospital or long-term care facility.
         c. Oral colonization with potential respiratory pathogens (PRPs) increases during hospitalization, and the longer a patient is hospitalized the greater their prevalence [84–86].
            1) Bacterial plaque biofilm can serve as reservoirs for PRPs, particularly during prolonged hospitalization [87].
            2) A patient with PRPs colonizing the mouth and oropharynx is at increased risk for pneumonia.
   B. Summary of Research Studies
      1. Evidence suggests that in certain at-risk individuals, periodontitis and poor oral hygiene may be associated with hospital-acquired pneumonia.
      2. Several studies provide early evidence that periodontal intervention may be beneficial in reducing the incidence of hospital-acquired pneumonia [88–90].
   C. Periodontitis and Chronic Obstructive Pulmonary Disease (COPD)
      1. COPD is a group of lung diseases, mainly emphysema and chronic bronchitis, characterized by an obstruction of airflow during exhalation.
      2. Several investigators have hypothesized that periodontal infections may increase the risk of COPD.
      3. Two recent systematic reviews of all of the current evidence, however, indicate that at present there is not sufficient evidence for an association between periodontal disease and COPD [91,92].

D. **Possible Biologic Explanations. How is Periodontits Related to Respiratory Disease?** Bacterial respiratory infections are thought to be acquired through aspiration (inhaling) of fine droplets from the oral cavity and throat into the lungs. These droplets contain germs that can breed and multiply within the lungs to cause damage.

E. **Implications for Dental Hygiene Practice.** Poor oral hygiene is common in hospitals or long-term care facilities, especially in patients who are quite ill [86,93]. Dental healthcare providers should advocate for programs that enhance the access of institutionalized elders to dental care services and to train medical healthcare providers on providing daily oral hygiene care.

   1. Studies show that improved oral hygiene measures can reduce the incidence of hospital-acquired pneumonia [94].

   2. Application of 0.2% chlorhexidine gel to the teeth, gingiva, and other oral mucosal surfaces has been shown to significantly decrease the risk for pneumonia, especially in patients who are on ventilators [88,89].

Chapter Summary Statement

Periodontitis is a chronic oral infection that may be a risk factor for systemic disease. It is possible that periodontitis may modify some aspect of certain systemic disease to make those diseases more severe. Periodontitis may be a modifiable risk factor in several systemic conditions including cardiovascular/cerebrovascular problems, diabetes mellitus, preterm labor, low–birth-weight delivery, and hospital-acquired pneumonia. Education to encourage better periodontal health, dental hygiene care, and periodontal therapy may play roles in decreasing the incidence and severity of these systemic diseases.

Section 2
Focus on Patients

Case 1

A new patient in your dental office is 3 months pregnant with her first child. She is 38 years old and has chronic periodontitis. What counsel would you provide this patient about the association between adverse pregnancy outcomes and periodontitis?

References

1. Chapple IL, Hamburger J. *Periodontal Medicine: A Window on the Body*. London; Chicago: Quintessence; 2006:258.
2. Mealey BL. Influence of periodontal infections on systemic health. *Periodontol 2000*. 1999;21:197–209.
3. Rose LF, NetLibrary Inc. *Periodontal Medicine*. Hamilton; London: B.C. Decker; 2000.
4. Walt G. WHO's world health report 2003. *Br Me J*. 2004;328(7430):6.
5. Rosamond W, Flegal K, Furie K, Go A, et al. Heart disease and stroke statistics—2008 update: a report from the American Heart Association Statistics Committee and Stroke Statistics Subcommittee. *Circulation*. 2008;117(4):e25–e146.
6. Waite DE, Bradley RE. Oral infections: report of two cases. *J Am Dent Assoc*. 1965;71:587–592.
7. D'Aiuto F, Ready D, Tonetti MS. Periodontal disease and C-reactive protein-associated cardiovascular risk. *J Periodontal Res*. 2004;39(4):236–241.
8. Elter JR, Hinderliter AL, Offenbacher S, Beck JD, et al. The effects of periodontal therapy on vascular endothelial function: a pilot trial. *Am Heart J*. 2006;151(1):47.
9. Seinost G, Wimmer G, Skerget M, Thaller E, et al. Periodontal treatment improves endothelial dysfunction in patients with severe periodontitis. *Am Heart J*. 2005;149(6):1050–1054.
10. Beck JD, Elter JR, Heiss G, Couper D, et al. Relationship of periodontal disease to carotid artery intima-media wall thickness: the atherosclerosis risk in communities (ARIC) study. *Arterioscler Thromb Vasc Biol*. 2001;21(11):1816–1822.
11. Chiu B. Multiple infections in carotid atherosclerotic plaques. *Am Heart J*. 1999;138 (5 Pt 2):S534–S536.
12. Haraszthy VI, Zambon JJ, Trevisan M, Zeid M, et al. Identification of periodontal pathogens in atheromatous plaques. *J Periodontol*. 2000;71(10):1554–1560.
13. Van Dyke TE, Kornman KS. Inflammation and factors that may regulate inflammatory response. *J Periodontol*. 2008;79(8 Suppl):1503–1507.
14. Haverkate F, Thompson SG, Pyke SD, Gallimore JR, et al. Production of C-reactive protein and risk of coronary events in stable and unstable angina. European Concerted Action on Thrombosis and Disabilities Angina Pectoris Study Group. *Lancet*. 1997;349(9050):462–466.
15. Liuzzo G, Biasucci LM, Gallimore JR, Grillo RL, et al. The prognostic value of C-reactive protein and serum amyloid a protein in severe unstable angina. *N Engl J Med*. 1994;331(7):417–424.
16. Ridker PM, Cushman M, Stampfer MJ, Tracy RP, et al. Inflammation, aspirin, and the risk of cardiovascular disease in apparently healthy men. *N Engl J Med*. 1997;336(14):973–979.
17. Ridker PM, Rifai N, Rose L, Buring JE, et al. Comparison of C-reactive protein and low-density lipoprotein cholesterol levels in the prediction of first cardiovascular events. *N Engl J Med*. 2002;347(20):1557–1565.
18. Ridker PM, Silvertown JD. Inflammation, C-reactive protein, and atherothrombosis. *J Periodontol*. 2008;79(8 Suppl):1544–1551.
19. Slade GD, Offenbacher S, Beck JD, Heiss G, et al. Acute-phase inflammatory response to periodontal disease in the US population. *J Dent Res*. 2000;79(1):49–57.
20. Wu T, Trevisan M, Genco RJ, Dorn JP, et al. Periodontal disease and risk of cerebrovascular disease: the first national health and nutrition examination survey and its follow-up study. *Arch Intern Med*. 2000;160(18):2749–2755.
21. Wu T, Trevisan M, Genco RJ, Falkner KL, et al. Examination of the relation between periodontal health status and cardiovascular risk factors: serum total and high density lipoprotein cholesterol, C-reactive protein, and plasma fibrinogen. *Am J Epidemiol*. 2000;151(3):273–282.
22. Arbes SJ Jr, Slade GD, Beck JD. Association between extent of periodontal attachment loss and self-reported history of heart attack: an analysis of NHANES III data. *J Dent Res*. 1999;78(12):1777–1782.
23. Abnet CC, Qiao YL, Dawsey SM, Dong ZW, et al. Tooth loss is associated with increased risk of total death and death from upper gastrointestinal cancer, heart disease, and stroke in a Chinese population-based cohort. *Int J Epidemiol*. 2005;34(2):467–474.
24. Beck J, Garcia R, Heiss G, Vokonas PS, et al. Periodontal disease and cardiovascular disease. *J Periodontol*. 1996;67(10 Suppl):1123–1137.
25. Beck JD, Eke P, Lin D, Madianos P, et al. Associations between IgG antibody to oral organisms and carotid intima-medial thickness in community-dwelling adults. *Atherosclerosis*. 2005;183(2):342–348.
26. Elter JR, Champagne CM, Offenbacher S, and Beck JD. Relationship of periodontal disease and tooth loss to prevalence of coronary heart disease. *J Periodontol*. 2004;75(6):782–790.

27. DeStefano F, Anda RF, Kahn HS, Williamson DF, et al. Dental disease and risk of coronary heart disease and mortality. *Br Med J.* 1993;306(6879):688–691.

28. Desvarieux M, Demmer RT, Rundek T, Boden-Albala B, et al. Periodontal microbiota and carotid intima-media thickness: the Oral Infections and Vascular Disease Epidemiology Study (INVEST). *Circulation.* 2005;111(5):576–582.

29. Engebretson SP, Lamster IB, Elkind MS, Rundek T, et al. Radiographic measures of chronic periodontitis and carotid artery plaque. *Stroke.* 2005;36(3):561–566.

30. Hujoel PP, Drangsholt M, Spiekerman C, and DeRouen TA. Periodontal disease and coronary heart disease risk. *JAMA.* 2000;284(11):1406–1410.

31. Hung HC, Joshipura KJ, Colditz G, Manson JE, et al. The association between tooth loss and coronary heart disease in men and women. *J Public Health Dent.* 2004;64(4):209–215.

32. Janket SJ, Baird AE, Chuang SK, and Jones JA. Meta-analysis of periodontal disease and risk of coronary heart disease and stroke. *Oral Surg Oral Med Oral Pathol Oral Radiol Endod.* 2003;95(5):559–569.

33. Joshipura KJ, Devine PC, Perez-Delboy A, Herrera-Abreu M, et al. Periodontal disease and biomarkers related to cardiovascular disease. *J Dent Res.* 2004;83(2):151–155.

34. Khader YS, Albashaireh ZS, Alomari MA. Periodontal diseases and the risk of coronary heart and cerebrovascular diseases: a meta-analysis. *J Periodontol.* 2004;75(8):1046–1053.

35. Mattila KJ, Nieminen MS, Valtonen VV, Rasi VP, et al. Association between dental health and acute myocardial infarction. *Br Med J.* 1989;298(6676):779–781.

36. Mattila KJ, Valle MS, Nieminen MS, Valtonen VV, et al. Dental infections and coronary atherosclerosis. *Atherosclerosis.* 1993;103(2):205–211.

37. Meurman JH, Sanz M, Janket SJ. Oral health, atherosclerosis, and cardiovascular disease. *Crit Rev Oral Biol Med.* 2004;15(6):403–413.

38. Paraskevas S, Huizinga JD, Loos BG. A systematic review and meta-analyses on C-reactive protein in relation to periodontitis. *J Clin Periodontol.* 2008;35(4):277–290.

39. Pussinen PJ, Alfthan G, Rissanen H, Reunanen A, et al. Antibodies to periodontal pathogens and stroke risk. *Stroke.* 2004;35(9):2020–2023.

40. Pussinen PJ, Nyyssonen K, Alfthan G, Salonen R, et al. Serum antibody levels *to Actinobacillus actinomycetemcomitans* predict the risk for coronary heart disease. *Arterioscler Thromb Vasc Biol.* 2005;25(4):833–838.

41. Pussinen PJ, Tuomisto K, Jousilahti P, Havulinna AS, et al. Endotoxemia, immune response to periodontal pathogens, and systemic inflammation associate with incident cardiovascular disease events. *Arterioscler Thromb Vasc Biol.* 2007;27(6):1433–1439.

42. American Academy of Periodontology statement regarding periodontal management of the pregnant patient. *J Periodontol.* 2004;75(3):495.

43. Offenbacher S, Katz V, Fertik G, Collins J, et al. Periodontal infection as a possible risk factor for preterm low birth weight. *J Periodontol.* 1996;67(10 Suppl):1103–1113.

44. Jeffcoat MK, Hauth JC, Geurs NC, Reddy MS, et al. Periodontal disease and preterm birth: results of a pilot intervention study. *J Periodontol.* 2003;74(8):1214–1218.

45. Lopez NJ, Da Silva I, Ipinza J, and Gutierrez J. Periodontal therapy reduces the rate of preterm low birth weight in women with pregnancy-associated gingivitis. *J Periodontol.* 2005;76 (11 Suppl):2144–2153.

46. Lopez NJ, Smith PC, Gutierrez J. Periodontal therapy may reduce the risk of preterm low birth weight in women with periodontal disease: a randomized controlled trial. *J Periodontol.* 2002;73(8):911–924.

47. Michalowicz BS, Hodges JS, DiAngelis AJ, Lupo VR, et al. Treatment of periodontal disease and the risk of preterm birth. *N Engl J Med.* 2006;355(18):1885–1894.

48. Bassani DG, Olinto MT, Kreiger N. Periodontal disease and perinatal outcomes: a case-control study. *J Clin Periodontol.* 2007;34(1):31–39.

49. Boggess KA, Beck JD, Murtha AP, Moss K, et al. Maternal periodontal disease in early pregnancy and risk for a small-for-gestational-age infant. *Am J Obstet Gynecol.* 2006;194(5): 1316–1322.

50. Boggess KA, Lieff S, Murtha AP, Moss K, et al. Maternal periodontal disease is associated with an increased risk for preeclampsia. *Obstet Gynecol.* 2003;101(2):227–231.

51. Buduneli N, Baylas H, Buduneli E, Turkoglu O, et al. Periodontal infections and pre-term low birth weight: a case-control study. *J Clin Periodontol.* 2005;32(2):174–181.

52. Bosnjak A, Relja T, Vucicevic-Boras V, Plasaj H, et al. Pre-term delivery and periodontal disease: a case-control study from Croatia. *J Clin Periodontol.* 2006;33(10):710–716.

53. Conde-Agudelo A, Villar J, Lindheimer M. Maternal infection and risk of preeclampsia: systematic review and metaanalysis. *Am J Obstet Gynecol.* 2008;198(1):7–22.

54. Contreras A, Herrera JA, Soto JE, Arce RM, et al. Periodontitis is associated with preeclampsia in pregnant women. *J Periodontol.* 2006;77(2):182–188.

55. Davenport ES, Williams CE, Sterne JA, Murad S, et al. Maternal periodontal disease and preterm low birthweight: case-control study. *J Dent Res.* 2002;81(5):313–318.

56. Goepfert AR, Jeffcoat MK, Andrews WW, Faye-Petersen O, et al. Periodontal disease and upper genital tract inflammation in early spontaneous preterm birth. *Obstet Gynecol.* 2004;104(4):777–783.

57. Holbrook WP, Oskarsdottir A, Fridjonsson T, Einarsson H, et al. No link between low-grade periodontal disease and preterm birth: a pilot study in a healthy Caucasian population. *Acta Odontol Scand.* 2004;62(3):177–179.

58. Jarjoura K, Devine PC, Perez-Delboy A, Herrera-Abreu M, et al. Markers of periodontal infection and preterm birth. *Am J Obstet Gynecol.* 2005;192(2):513–519.

59. Jeffcoat MK, Geurs NC, Reddy MS, Cliver SP, et al. Periodontal infection and preterm birth: results of a prospective study. *J Am Dent Assoc.* 2001;132(7):875–880.

60. Khader YS, Ta'ani Q. Periodontal diseases and the risk of preterm birth and low birth weight: a meta-analysis. *J Periodontol.* 2005;76(2):161–165.

61. Lopez NJ, Smith PC, Gutierrez J. Higher risk of preterm birth and low birth weight in women with periodontal disease. *J Dent Res.* 2002;81(1):58–63.

62. Meurman JH, Furuholm J, Kaaja R, Rintamaki H, et al. Oral health in women with pregnancy and delivery complications. *Clin Oral Investig.* 2006;10(2):96–101.

63. Moore S, Ide M, Coward PY, Randhawa M, et al. A prospective study to investigate the relationship between periodontal disease and adverse pregnancy outcome. *Br Dent J.* 2004;197(5):251–258; discussion 247.

64. Moore S, Randhawa M, Ide M. A case-control study to investigate an association between adverse pregnancy outcome and periodontal disease. *J Clin Periodontol.* 2005;32(1):1–5.

65. Moreu G, Tellez L, Gonzalez-Jaranay M. Relationship between maternal periodontal disease and low-birth-weight pre-term infants. *J Clin Periodontol.* 2005;32(6):622–627.

66. Offenbacher S, Boggess KA, Murtha AP, Jared HL, et al. Progressive periodontal disease and risk of very preterm delivery. *Obstet Gynecol.* 2006;107(1):29–36.

67. Offenbacher S, Lieff S, Boggess KA, Murtha AP, et al. Maternal periodontitis and prematurity. Part I: Obstetric outcome of prematurity and growth restriction. *Ann Periodontol.* 2001;6(1):164–174.

68. Offenbacher S, Lin D, Strauss R, McKaig R, et al. Effects of periodontal therapy during pregnancy on periodontal status, biologic parameters, and pregnancy outcomes: a pilot study. *J Periodontol.* 2006;77(12):2011–2024.

69. Pitiphat W, Joshipura KJ, Gillman MW, Williams PL, et al. Maternal periodontitis and adverse pregnancy outcomes. *Community Dent Oral Epidemiol.* 2008;36(1):3–11.

70. Radnai M, Gorzo I, Nagy E, Urban E, et al. A possible association between preterm birth and early periodontitis. A pilot study. *J Clin Periodontol.* 2004;31(9):736–741.

71. Radnai M, Gorzo I, Urban E, Eller J, et al. Possible association between mother's periodontal status and preterm delivery. *J Clin Periodontol.* 2006;33(11):791–796.

72. Mealey BL, Oates TW. Diabetes mellitus and periodontal diseases. *J Periodontol.* 2006;77(8):1289–1303.

73. Papapanou PN. Periodontal diseases: epidemiology. *Ann Periodontol.* 1996;1(1):1–36.

74. Report of the expert committee on the diagnosis and classification of diabetes mellitus. *Diabetes Care.* 2003;26 Suppl 1:S5–S20.

75. Standards of medical care in diabetes—2008. *Diabetes Care.* 2008;31 Suppl 1:S12–S54.

76. Taylor GW, Burt BA, Becker MP, Genco RJ, et al. Severe periodontitis and risk for poor glycemic control in patients with non-insulin-dependent diabetes mellitus. *J Periodontol.* 1996;67 (10 Suppl):1085–1093.

77. Treszl A, Szereday L, Doria A, King GL, et al. Elevated C-reactive protein levels do not correspond to autoimmunity in type 1 diabetes. *Diabetes Care,* 2004;27(11):2769–2770.

78. Pradhan AD, Manson JE, Rifai N, Buring JE, et al. C-reactive protein, interleukin 6, and risk of developing type 2 diabetes mellitus. *JAMA.* 2001;286(3):327–334.

79. Thorand B, Lowel H, Schneider A, Kolb H, et al. C-reactive protein as a predictor for incident diabetes mellitus among middle-aged men: results from the MONICA Augsburg cohort study, 1984–1998. *Arch Intern Med.* 2003;163(1):93–99.

80. Collin HL, Uusitupa M, Niskanen L, Kontturi-Narhi V, et al. Periodontal findings in elderly patients with non-insulin dependent diabetes mellitus. *J Periodontol*, 1998;69(9):962–966.

81. Saremi A, Nelson RG, Tulloch-Reid M, Hanson RL, et al. Periodontal disease and mortality in type 2 diabetes. *Diabetes Care*. 2005;28(1):27–32.

82. Scannapieco FA, Bush RB, Paju S. Associations between periodontal disease and risk for atherosclerosis, cardiovascular disease, and stroke. A systematic review. *Ann Periodontol*. 2003;8(1):38–53.

83. Ostergaard L, Andersen PL. Etiology of community-acquired pneumonia. Evaluation by transtracheal aspiration, blood culture, or serology. *Chest*. 1993;104(5):1400–1407.

84. Limeback H. Implications of oral infections on systemic diseases in the institutionalized elderly with a special focus on pneumonia. *Ann Periodontol*. 1998;3(1):262–275.

85. Russell SL, Boylan RJ, Kaslick RS, Scannapieco FA, et al. Respiratory pathogen colonization of the dental plaque of institutionalized elders. *Spec Care Dentist*. 1999;19(3):128–134.

86. Scannapieco FA, Mylotte JM. Relationships between periodontal disease and bacterial pneumonia. *J Periodontol*. 1996;67(10 Suppl):1114–1122.

87. El-Solh AA, Pietrantoni C, Bhat A, Okada M, et al. Colonization of dental plaques: a reservoir of respiratory pathogens for hospital-acquired pneumonia in institutionalized elders. *Chest*. 2004;126(5):1575–1582.

88. DeRiso AJ II, Ladowski JS, Dillon TA, Justice JW, et al. Chlorhexidine gluconate 0.12% oral rinse reduces the incidence of total nosocomial respiratory infection and nonprophylactic systemic antibiotic use in patients undergoing heart surgery. *Chest*. 1996;109(6):1556–1561.

89. Fourrier F, Cau-Pottier E, Boutigny H, Roussel-Delvallez M, et al. Effects of dental plaque antiseptic decontamination on bacterial colonization and nosocomial infections in critically ill patients. *Intensive Care Med*. 2000;26(9):1239–1247.

90. Yoneyama T, Yoshida M, Ohrui T, Mukaiyama H, et al. Oral care reduces pneumonia in older patients in nursing homes. *J Am Geriatr Soc*. 2002;50(3):430–433.

91. Scannapieco FA, Bush RB, Paju S. Associations between periodontal disease and risk for nosocomial bacterial pneumonia and chronic obstructive pulmonary disease. A systematic review. *Ann Periodontol*. 2003;8(1):54–69.

92. Azarpazhooh A, Leake JL. Systematic review of the association between respiratory diseases and oral health. *J Periodontol*. 2006;77(9):1465–1482.

93. Beck JD. Periodontal implications: older adults. *Ann Periodontol*. 1996;1(1):322–357.

94. Scannapieco FA, Stewart EM, Mylotte JM. Colonization of dental plaque by respiratory pathogens in medical intensive care patients. *Crit Care Med*. 1992;20(6):740–745.

95. Moliterno LF, Monteiro B, Figueredo CM, Fischer RG. Association between periodontitis and low birth weight: a case-control study. *J Clin Periodontol*. 2005;32(8):886–90.

Clinical Periodontal Assessment

Learning Objectives

- Explain which members of the dental team are responsible for the clinical periodontal assessment.
- Compare and contrast a periodontal screening examination and a comprehensive periodontal assessment.
- Describe how to perform one type of periodontal screening examination.
- Name the components of a comprehensive periodontal assessment.
- Describe how to evaluate each component of a comprehensive periodontal assessment.
- Explain how to calculate the width of attached gingiva.
- Explain how to calculate clinical attachment level given several different clinical scenarios.
- In a clinical scenario, calculate and document the clinical attachment levels for a patient with periodontitis.

Key Terms

Clinical periodontal assessment
Legal responsibility
Treatment outcomes
Baseline data
Periodontal screening examination
Periodontal Screening and Recording (PSR)
World Health Organization (WHO) probe
Color-coded reference mark
PSR code

Comprehensive periodontal assessment
Exudate
Recession of the gingival margin
Horizontal tooth mobility
Vertical tooth mobility
Fremitus
Gingival crevicular fluid
Attached gingiva
Clinical attachment level (CAL)

Section 1
Introduction to Periodontal Assessment

OVERVIEW OF THE ASSESSMENT PROCESS

1. The clinical periodontal assessment is a fact-gathering process designed to provide a comprehensive picture of the patient's periodontal health status.
   A. **Importance of the Periodontal Assessment**
      1. This assessment is one of the most important duties performed by a dental team.
         a. The dental team must complete and document a periodontal assessment for all patients when first encountered by the team and periodically thereafter.
         b. This assessment requires meticulous attention to detail since successful patient care is highly dependent on a thorough and accurate periodontal evaluation.
      2. The information gathered during the clinical periodontal assessment forms the basis of both a periodontal diagnosis and an individualized treatment plan for the patient.
   B. **Objectives.** The objectives of the clinical periodontal assessment include the following:
      1. Detect clinical signs of inflammation in the periodontium.
      2. Identify damage to the periodontium already caused by disease or trauma.
      3. Provide the dental team with data used to assign a periodontal diagnosis.
      4. Document features of the periodontium to serve as baseline data for the long-term patient monitoring.
   C. **Two Types of Periodontal Assessment.** Two commonly used types of periodontal assessment are the periodontal screening examination and the comprehensive periodontal assessment.
      1. **Periodontal Screening.** A periodontal screening examination is a rapid and efficient information-gathering process used to determine if a patient has periodontal health, gingivitis, or periodontitis.
      2. **Comprehensive Periodontal Assessment.** A comprehensive periodontal assessment is an intensive information-gathering process used to gather detailed data needed to make a periodontal diagnosis (e.g., chronic periodontitis or aggressive periodontitis) and to document the periodontal health status to allow for long term monitoring of the patient.
2. **Responsibilities and Legal Considerations**
   A. **Responsibilities of the Dentist and Dental Hygienist.** Although the dental team in each dental office will function differently, it is helpful to look at the typical responsibilities for the dentist and for the dental hygienist in the assessment, diagnosis, and treatment planning steps.
      1. Typically, the dentist and dental hygienist share the responsibility for periodontal screening and comprehensive periodontal assessment.
      2. The dentist has the responsibility of assignment of a periodontal diagnosis, and the dentist with input from the dental hygienist plans the nonsurgical periodontal therapy.
      3. It is important for members of the dental team to understand that the dentist has the legal responsibility for all of the diagnosis and treatment planning that occurs in the office.
      4. Because of the extensive special training received by the dental hygienist, many dentists place part of the periodontal data collection in the capable hands of the dental hygienist.
   B. **Legal Considerations: Standards of Care**
      1. *Dentists and dental hygienists have a legal responsibility to complete an accurate and thorough periodontal assessment on every patient.*

a. The failure to diagnose and properly treat periodontal disease may be one of the leading causes of dental malpractice.

b. Dentists and hygienists must perform a clinical periodontal assessment in a manner that is consistent with the current standards of care set forth by the dental profession.

2. Without a thorough clinical periodontal assessment, periodontal diseases are often not diagnosed or are misdiagnosed, leading to either undertreatment or overtreatment of the patient.

3. To be competent clinically, all dentists and dental hygienists must master the skills necessary to perform a thorough and accurate clinical periodontal assessment.

DOCUMENTATION

1. The clinical periodontal assessment is not complete until all of the information gathered during the assessment has been accurately recorded in the patient chart. Documentation is discussed in detail in Chapter 35.

2. Clinicians use the documented information to measure treatment outcomes and to monitor the patient's periodontal health status over time.

A. Findings documented during the clinical periodontal assessment often serve as baseline data against which to evaluate the success or failure of periodontal therapy. Baseline data refers to clinical information gathered prior to periodontal therapy that can be used for comparison to clinical information gathered at subsequent appointments.

B. Documented findings also provide the baseline data used in the long-term monitoring of the patient's periodontal health status. An example of when patient monitoring may occur is at periodontal maintenance visits following successful treatment. Periodontal maintenance is discussed in Chapter 32.

Section 2
The Periodontal Screening Examination

In some dental offices a periodontal screening examination is one of the first steps in evaluating the periodontal status of a patient. A periodontal screening examination is a periodontal assessment used to (i) determine the periodontal health status of the patient and (ii) identify patients needing a more comprehensive periodontal assessment. The Periodontal Screening and Recording (PSR) is an efficient, easy-to-use screening system for the detection of periodontal disease.

1. **Periodontal Screening and Recording (PSR)**
   A. **Characteristics of Periodontal Screening and Recording**
      1. The PSR can help to identify those patients who need a comprehensive periodontal assessment. The results of this screening examination are used to separate patients into broad categories: those that have periodontal health, gingivitis, or periodontitis.
      2. When the PSR screening examination indicates the presence of periodontal health or gingivitis, in many instances no further clinical periodontal assessment is needed beyond the PSR.
   B. **Techniques for Performing the PSR Screening Examination**
      1. Special Probe. A World Health Organization (WHO) probe is used for this examination. The WHO probe has a colored band (called the reference mark) located 3.5 to 5.5 mm from the probe tip. This color-coded reference mark is used when performing the PSR screening examination.
      2. One Code Per Sextant. Each sextant of the mouth is examined and assigned a PSR code. The unique aspects of the PSR screening system are the manner in which the probe is read and the minimal amount of information that is recorded.
         a. Instead of reading and recording six precise measurements per tooth, the clinician only needs to observe the position of the color-coded reference mark in relation to the gingival margin and a few other clinical features such as bleeding on probing, the presence of calculus, or the presence of an overhang on a restoration.
         b. Each of the sextants is examined as a separate unit during the PSR screening (i.e., only one PSR code number will be assigned to the entire sextant).
         c. *Only one PSR code is recorded for each sextant in the mouth.* Each sextant is assigned a single PSR code; the highest code obtained for the sextant is recorded. An "X" is recorded if a sextant is edentulous.
   C. **Probing Technique**
      1. The probe is walked circumferentially around each tooth in the sextant being examined.
      2. The color-coded reference mark is monitored continuously as the probe is walked around each tooth. At each site probed, the color-coded reference mark will be (a) completely visible, (b) partially visible, or (c) not visible at all.
2. **The PSR Codes**
   A. **Use of PSR Codes**
      1. A PSR code is assigned to each sextant according to the criteria shown in TABLE 19-1. *The code assigned to a sextant should represent the most advanced periodontal finding on any tooth in that sextant.*

2. The PSR codes are used to guide further clinical documentation.
   a. For some patients with low PSR codes in all sextants (codes 0, 1, or 2), the PSR screening is adequate documentation of the patient's periodontal health status (and a comprehensive periodontal assessment is not needed). Note, however, that occasionally the dentist may request a comprehensive periodontal assessment even when low PSR codes are found, since certain peridontal conditions must be monitored in more detail than that included in the PSR.
   b. For patients with higher PSR codes in one or more sextants (codes 3 or 4), a comprehensive periodontal examination should be preformed as outlined in Section 3 of this chapter.
B. **Cautions for Interpreting PSR Codes.** The PSR codes can occasionally mislead a clinician. As already pointed out, lower codes usually mean periodontal health or gingivitis, and higher codes usually mean periodontitis. *When interpreting the results of the PSR, the clinician must be alert for teeth with gingival enlargement or with recession of the gingival margin. In the presence of either of these conditions the PSR can give misleading results.*

TABLE 19-1. Criteria for Assigning PSR Codes	
CODE 0:	• Color-coded reference mark is *completely visible* in deepest sulcus or pocket of the sextant • No calculus or defective margins on restorations are present • Gingival tissues are healthy with no bleeding evident on gentle probing
CODE 1:	• Color-coded reference mark is *completely visible* in deepest sulcus or pocket of the sextant • No calculus or defective margins on restorations are present • Bleeding *is evident* on probing
CODE 2:	• Color-coded reference mark is *completely visible* in deepest sulcus or pocket of the sextant • Supragingival or subgingival calculus and/or defective margins are detected
CODE 3:	• Color-coded reference mark is *partially visible* in the deepest sulcus or pocket of the sextant • Code 3 indicates a probing depth between 3.5 and 5.5 mm
CODE 4:	• Color-coded referencae mark is *not visible* in the deepest sulcus of pocket of the sextant • Code 4 indicates a probling depth of >5.5 mm

CODE *:	• The * (star) symbol is added to the code of any sextant that exhibits any of the following:
	   1. Furcation involvement
	   2. Mobility
	   3. Mucogingival problems
	   4. Recession extending into the colored area of the probe
	 • The * (star) symbol is recorded next to the sextant code. For example, "4*"

Section 3
The Comprehensive Periodontal Assessment

A comprehensive periodontal assessment is an intensive clinical periodontal evaluation used to gather information about the periodontium. This section of the chapter outlines the clinical features that should be noted and documented during a comprehensive periodontal assessment. It is important to note that special precautions are necessary when examining dental implants. These examination techniques are not discussed in this chapter because they are presented in detail in Chapter 33.

The comprehensive periodontal assessment normally includes clinical features such as probing depth measurements, bleeding on probing, presence of exudate, level of the free gingival margin and the mucogingival junction, tooth mobility, furcation involvement, presence of calculus and bacterial plaque biofilm, gingival inflammation, radiographic evidence of alveolar bone loss, and presence of local contributing factors.

1. **Components of the Comprehensive Periodontal Assessment**
   A. **Probing Depth Measurements.** Probing depth measurements are made from the free gingival margin to the base of the pocket.
      1. Probing depths are recorded to the nearest full millimeter. Round up measurements to the next higher whole number (e.g., a reading of 3.5 mm is recorded as 4 mm, and a 5.5 mm reading is recorded as 6 mm).
      2. Probing depth measurements are recorded for six specific sites on each tooth: (i) distofacial, (ii) middle facial, (iii) mesiofacial, (iv) distolingual, (v) middle lingual, and (vi) mesiolingual.
   B. **Bleeding on Probing**
      1. Bleeding on gentle probing represents bleeding from the soft tissue wall of a periodontal pocket where the wall of the pocket is ulcerated (i.e., where portions of the epithelium have been destroyed; FIG. 19-1).
      2. Bleeding can occur immediately after the site is probed or can be slightly delayed in occurrence. An alert clinician will observe each site for a few seconds before moving on to the next site.
      3. Excessive probing force could cause bleeding. Probing pressure should be between 10 and 20 g of pressure. Sensitive scales, available from scientific supply companies, can be used to calibrate probing pressure.

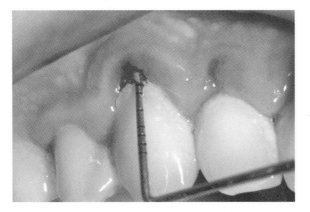

Figure 19.1. A Bleeding Site. Bleeding from the soft tissue wall is a sign of disease. This bleeding was evident upon gentle probing.

C. Presence of Exudate

1. Exudate, sometimes referred to as suppuration, is pus that can be expressed from a periodontal pocket. Pus is composed mainly of dead white blood cells and can occur in any infection, including periodontal disease.

2. Exudate can be recognized as a pale yellow material oozing from the orifice of a pocket. It is usually easiest to detect when the gingiva is manipulated in some manner. For example, light finger pressure on the gingiva can usually reveal exudate when present (FIG. 19-2). Figure 19-3 illustrates how to use a gloved finger to detect exudate by expressing it from a periodontal pocket.

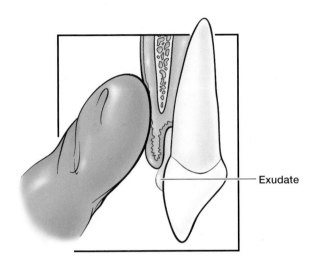

Exudate

Figure 19.2. Using Finger Pressure to Detect Exudate. Exudate can be detected in a periodontal pocket by placing an index finger on the soft tissue in the area of the pocket and exerting slight pressure. This slight pressure can force the exudate out of the pocket, making it readily visible to the clinician.

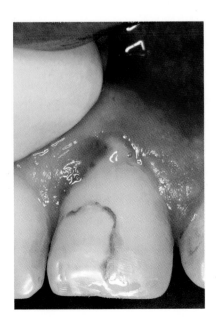

Figure 19.3. Exudate. Pressure with the clinician's finger on the gingiva reveals exudate from the gingival tissue adjacent to the lateral incisor. (Courtesy of Dr Don Rolfs, Periodontal Foundations, Wenatchee, WA.)

D. **Level of the Free Gingival Margin**
1. The level of the free gingival margin in relationship to the cementoenamel junction (CEJ) should be recorded on the dental chart. This level can simply be drawn on the facial and lingual surfaces of the dental chart.
2. Several possible relationships exist between the free gingival margin and the CEJ:
    a. **Free gingival margin can be slightly coronal to (above) the CEJ.** This is the natural level of the gingival margin and represents the expected position of the gingival margin in the absence of disease or trauma.
    b. **Free gingival margin can be significantly coronal to the CEJ.** The gingival margin can be coronal to the CEJ due to (1) swelling (edema), (2) overgrowth (as seen in patients taking certain medications), and/or (3) increase in fibrous connective tissue (as seen in long-standing inflammation of tissue).
    c. **Free gingival margin is apical to the CEJ.** This relationship, known as recession of the gingival margin, results in exposure of a portion of the root surface. Recession of the gingival margin is defined as the location of the gingival margin apical to the cementoenamel junction resulting in exposure of a portion of the root surface. [1]
3. Box 19-1 outlines the technique for determining the free gingival margin level.
4. When the gingival margin is apical to the CEJ (i.e., recession of the gingival margin is present), the severity of recession of the gingival margin is normally classified using the Miller classification system for recession of the gingival margin. This system is outlined in Figure 19-4A–D.

Box 19-1. Technique for Determining the Level of the Gingival Margin

When tissue swelling or recession is present, a periodontal probe is used to measure the distance the gingival margin is apical or coronal to the CEJ. Keep in mind that the natural or expected level of the gingival margin in the absence of disease or trauma is slightly coronal to the CEJ.

1. For recession of the gingival margin. If recession of the gingival margin is present, the distance between the CEJ and the gingival margin is measured using a calibrated periodontal probe. This distance is recorded as the gingival margin level.

2. For gingival enlargement. If gingival enlargement is present, the distance between the CEJ and the gingival margin is also measured using a calibrated periodontal probe. This distance is estimated using the following technique:

    a. Position the tip of the probe at a 45-degree angle to the tooth surface.

    b. Slowly move the probe beneath the gingival margin until the junction between the enamel and cementum is detected.

    c. Measure the distance between the gingival margin and the CEJ. This distance is recorded as the gingival margin level.

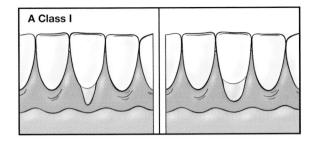

Figure 19.4A. Miller Class I Defect. In Miller Class I gingival defects the recession is isolated to the facial surface and the interdental papillae fill the interdental spaces. Class I recession does not extend to the mucogingival line. These Class I defects can be further subdivided into narrow or wide.

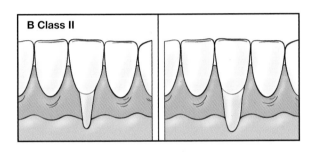

Figure 19.4B. Miller Class II Defect. In Miller Class II gingival defects the recession are isolated to the facial surface and the papillae remain intact. Class II recession does extend beyond the mucogingival line into the mucosa.

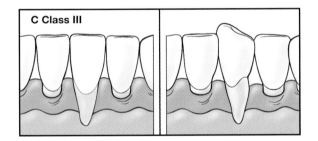

Figure 19.4C. Miller Class III Defect. In Miller Class III gingival defects the recession is quite broad with the interdental papillae missing due to damage from disease. Class III recession also extends beyond the mucogingival line into the mucosa.

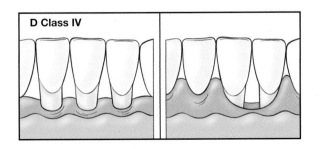

Figure 19.4D. Miller Class IV Defect. In Miller Class IV gingival defects the recession shows loss of hard (bone) and soft tissue around the entire tooth with open interdental areas.

E. **Level of Mucogingival Junction**
1. The level of the mucogingival junction represents the junction between the keratinized gingiva and the nonkeratinized mucosa. The level of the mucogingival junction is used in determining the width of the attached gingiva as will be described in fourth section.
2. The mucogingival junction is usually readily visible since the keratinized gingiva is normally pale pink and opaque while the surface of the mucosa is thin, translucent tissue (FIG. 19-5).
3. Occasionally, the mucogingival junction can be difficult to detect visually. In this case, the tissue can be manipulated by pulling on the patient's lip or pushing on the tissue with a blunt instrument to distinguish the moveable mucosa from the more firmly attached gingiva.

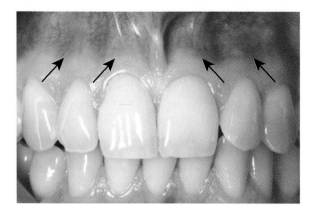

Figure 19.5. **Mucogingival Junction.** The mucogingival junction represents the junction between the keratinized gingiva with the nonkeratinized mucosa.

F. **Tooth Mobility and Fremitus**
1. Horizontal tooth mobility, movement of the tooth in a facial to lingual direction, is assessed by trapping the tooth between two dental instrument handles.
   a. Alternating moderate pressure is applied in the facial-lingual direction against the tooth first with one, then the other instrument handle.
   b. Mobility can be observed by using an adjacent tooth as a stationary point of reference during attempts to move the tooth being examined.
2. Vertical tooth mobility, the ability to depress the tooth in its socket, is assessed using the end of an instrument handle to exert pressure against the occlusal or incisal surface of the tooth (FIG. 19-6).
3. Even though the periodontal ligament allows some slight movement of the tooth in its socket, the amount of this natural tooth movement is so slight that it cannot be seen with the naked eye. Thus, when visually assessing mobility, the clinician should expect to find no visible movement in a periodontally healthy tooth.
4. There are many rating scales for recording clinically visible tooth mobility. One useful scale is indicated in TABLE 19-2.
5. In some dental offices, the dentist may also wish to assess fremitus.
   a. Fremitus is a palpable or visible movement of a tooth when in function.
   b. Fremitus can be assessed by gently placing a gloved index finger against the facial aspect of the tooth as the patient either taps the teeth together or simulates chewing movements.

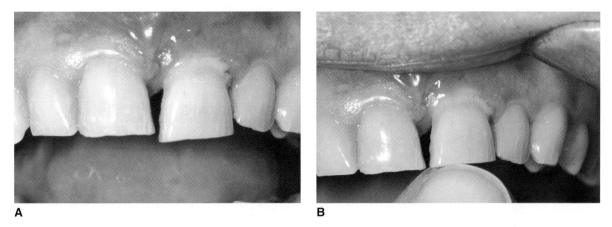

A   B

Figure 19.6. Vertical Tooth Mobility. A: The patient came to the dental office complaining of a loose tooth. Note the position of the maxillary left central incisor. **B:** The patient then demonstrated how he could push this tooth upward by applying pressure with his index finger against the incisal edge. This central incisor has vertical mobility. (Photographs courtesy of Dr Don Rolfs, Periodontal Foundations, Wenatchee, WA.)

TABLE 19-2.	Scale for Rating Visible Tooth Mobility
Classification	**Description**
Class I	Slight mobility, up to 1 mm of horizontal displacement in a facial-lingual direction
Class 2	Moderate mobility, >1 mm but <2 mm of horizontal displacement in a facial-lingual direction
Class 3	Severe mobility, >2 mm of displacement in a facial-lingual direction or vertical displacement (tooth depressible in the socket)

G. Furcation Involvement
   1. A furcation probe is used to assess furcation involvement on multi-rooted teeth. Most molar teeth are multi-rooted, but some maxillary premolar teeth also develop with two roots creating the potential for a furcation involvement on some premolars also.
   2. Furcation probes are curved, blunt-tipped instruments that allow easy access to the furcation areas.
   3. Furcation involvement occurs on a multi-rooted tooth when periodontal infection invades the area between and around the roots, resulting in a loss of attachment and loss of alveolar bone between the roots of the tooth.
      a. Mandibular molars are usually bifurcated (mesial and distal roots), with potential furcation involvement on both the facial and lingual aspects of the tooth (Fig. 19-7A).
      b. Maxillary molar teeth are usually trifurcated (mesiobuccal, distobuccal, and palatal roots) with potential furcation involvement on the facial, mesial, and distal aspects of the tooth (Fig. 19-7B).
      c. Maxillary first premolars can have bifurcated roots (buccal and palatal roots) with the potential for furcation involvement on the mesial and distal aspects of the tooth.

4. Furcation involvement frequently signals a need for periodontal surgery after completion of nonsurgical therapy, so detection and documentation of furcation involvement is a critical component of the comprehensive periodontal assessment.

5. Furcation involvement should be recorded using a scale that quantifies the severity (or extent) of the furcation invasion. TABLE 19-3 shows a commonly used scale for rating furcation invasions of multirooted teeth.

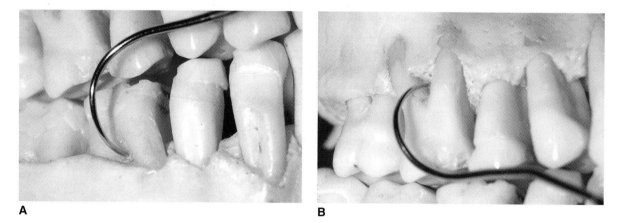

A   **B**

Figure 19.7. Use of Furcation Probes. A: Correct positioning of a furcation probe on a mandibular molar is demonstrated on a human skull. **B:** Correct positioning of a furcation probe on a maxillary molar is demonstrated on a human skull. (Courtesy of Dr Don Rolfs.)

TABLE 19-3.   Scale for Rating Furcation Involvement

Classification	Description
Class I	Curvature of the concavity can be felt with the probe tip; however the probe penetrates the furcation no more than 1 mm
Class II	The probe penetrates into the furcation >1 mm, but does not pass completely through the furcation
Class III	Probe will pass completely through the furcation
	In mandibular molars, the probe passes compleely through the furcation between the mesial and distal roots
	In maxillary molars, the probe passes between the mesiobuccal and distobuccal roots and will touch the palatal root
Class IV	Same as Class III furcation, except that the entrance to the furca is clinically visible because of the presence of recession of the gingival margin

H. **Presence of Calculus Deposits on the Teeth**
1. The presence of dental calculus on the teeth should be noted since these deposits must later be identified and removed as part of the nonsurgical therapy.
2. Calculus is a local contributing factor in both gingivitis and periodontitis; thus, the identification and removal of these deposits is a critical component of successful patient treatment.
3. Calculus deposits can be located through several techniques that include the following:
    a. Direct visual examination using a mouth mirror to locate supragingival deposits.
    b. Visual examination while using compressed air to dry the teeth to aid in locating supragingival deposits.
    c. Tactile examination using an explorer to locate subgingival calculus deposits.

I. **Presence of Plaque Biofilm on the Teeth**
1. The presence of bacterial plaque biofilm on the teeth should be noted during a comprehensive periodontal assessment since these deposits contain living periodontal pathogens that can lead to both gingivitis and periodontitis.
2. Plaque biofilm deposits can be identified using disclosing dyes or by moving the tip of an explorer or a periodontal probe along the tooth surface adjacent to the gingival margin.
3. There are many ways to record the presence of bacterial plaque biofilm, but most dental offices record the results of the plaque biofilm assessment in terms of the percentage of tooth surfaces with plaque biofilm evident at the gingival margin. A useful formula for recording plaque biofilm percentages is shown in Box 19-2.
    a. Note that in using the calculation shown in Box 19-2, a plaque biofilm score of 90% indicates that 90% of the total available tooth surfaces have plaque biofilm at the gingival margin.
    b. One goal of therapy would be for the patient to learn and perform plaque biofilm control measures that would bring the plaque biofilm score as close to 0% as possible (or at least to bring the percentage of tooth surfaces with plaque biofilm as low as possible).
4. As discussed previously in this book, bacterial plaque biofilm is the primary etiologic factor for both gingivitis and periodontitis. Identification of the presence and distribution of bacterial plaque biofilm on the teeth is a critical piece of information needed when planning appropriate therapy and patient education.

Box 19-2. Formula for Calculating Plaque Biofilm Percentages

$$\frac{\text{Number of tooth surfaces with plaque biofilm}}{\text{Total number of tooth surfaces}} \times 100 = \text{Percentage score}$$

J. **Gingival Inflammation**
1. A thorough periodontal assessment includes recording the overt signs of inflammation. The overt signs of inflammation of the gingiva include erythema (redness) and edema (swelling) of the gingival margins resulting in readily identifiable changes in gingival color and contour.
2. It is always important to be aware that inflammation can be present in the deeper structures of the periodontium without necessarily involving any obvious clinical signs of inflammation of the gingival margin.

    a. When assessing the presence of inflammation, it is important to remember that bleeding on probing also can be a sign of inflammation.

    b. Thus, when a clinician is identifying gingival inflammation for purposes of planning treatment, the visible signs such as color, contour, and consistency changes in the gingiva must be correlated with the other signs such as bleeding on probing or the presence of exudate.

K. Radiographic Evidence of Alveolar Bone Loss. Radiographic interpretation is discussed in Chapter 20, so it will not be discussed in this chapter.

    1. It is important for the clinician to remember, however, that radiographs play an important role in arriving at the periodontal diagnosis and in developing an appropriate plan for nonsurgical periodontal therapy.

    2. Radiographic evidence of alveolar bone loss is always an important part of a clinical periodontal assessment.

L. Presence of Local Contributing Factors

    1. A thorough periodontal assessment will always include identification of local contributing factors.

    2. These factors are discussed in Chapter 7. The plan for treatment for any periodontal patient will always include measures to eliminate or to minimize the impact of these local factors.

2. Supplemental Diagnostic Tests

A. Overview of Supplemental Diagnostic Tests

    1. Clinical periodontal assessment using the parameters discussed in Section 3 will result in an accurate periodontal diagnosis and can serve as a sound basis for designing an appropriate plan for therapy for the patient with gingival or periodontal disease. There are, however, a number of supplemental diagnostic tests that can be used for certain patients.

    2. Clinicians might consider using some of these supplemental tests for patients that have periodontitis that is failing to respond to conventional periodontal therapy or periodontitis that shows other unusual signs of disease progression.

    3. There are a number of supplemental tests that have been suggested for use, and much research is continuing related to these types of tests. Most of these tests fall into three general types:

        a. Tests related to bacteria

        b. Tests that analyze gingival crevicular fluid content

        c. Tests for genetic susceptibility to periodontal disease.

    4. It is critical for the clinician to realize that based upon current research, none of these supplemental diagnostic tests should be ordered routinely on all patients with periodontal disease.

B. Tests Related to Bacteria. TABLE 19-4 presents an overview of the tests related to bacteria. It is important to keep in mind that conventional periodontal therapy brings periodontal pathogens to low enough levels that disease progression can be halted without the need for identifying specific periodontal pathogens in most patients.

C. Tests that Analyze Gingival Crevicular Fluid Content

    1. Gingival Crevicular Fluid

        a. Gingival crevicular fluid is the fluid that flows into the sulcus from the adjacent gingival connective tissue; the flow is slight in health and increases in the presence of inflammatory disease.

        b. Gingival crevicular fluid originates in connective tissue and flows into periodontal pockets. It has long been believed that this gingival crevicular fluid can contain markers for periodontal disease progression, and quite a bit of research time has been devoted to the study of this fluid.

2. Examples of Gingival Crevicular Contents Being Studied

    a. Collagenase (an enzyme that breaks down collagen) is an example of one of the gingival crevicular fluid contents that has been studied, though no test for this is currently in use.

    b. Prostaglandin E2 is another such gingival crevicular fluid ingredient that has been studied. Prostaglandin E2 is associated with arachidonic acid that is involved with inflammatory reactions such as those seen in periodontal disease.

D. Tests for Genetic Susceptibility to Periodontal Disease

    1. Genetic Susceptibility

        a. It is obvious that a patient's genetic makeup affects susceptibility to many diseases including periodontal disease.

        b. This genetic makeup is inherited and cannot normally be altered.

    2. Tests for Interleukin-1

        a. One test for genetic susceptibility to periodontal disease has been studied extensively and has resulted in a test that has been marketed to clinicians (the PST Genetic Susceptibility Test from Interleukin Genetics Inc., Waltham, MA).

        b. This test identifies patients with genetic programming to produce high levels of interleukin-1 (an inflammatory mediator produced in response to the presence of periodontal pathogens).

            1) Higher levels of interleukin-1 in patients tend to predispose the patients to more inflammation in the periodontium.

            2) It has been reported that 30% of the people in the United States have the genetic makeup to produce high levels of interleukin-1 in response to periodontal pathogens.

E. The Future. It would be extremely helpful if clinicians had access to a diagnostic test that could indicate which patients are undergoing or are likely to undergo attachment loss. It is safe to assume that as more research is completed related to gingival crevicular fluid content, that some useful clinical tests will be developed in this area.

TABLE 19-4.	**Tests Related to Bacteria**	
Test Name	**Purpose of Test**	**Special Considerations**
Phase contrast microscopic study of plaque biofilm sample	Used for patient education and motivation	Test cannot identify specific bacterial species
Culture and sensitivity	Used to determine the sensitivity of bacteria to specific antibiotics	Sampling techniques for this test and the transport of bacterial samples to the laboratory are difficult
Deoxyribonucleic acid (DNA) probe analysis	Used to identify specific periodontal pathogens in a patient's mouth	Only a few bacterial species can be identified by this test

Section 4
Clinical Features that Require Calculations

Some judgments that are made as part of the clinical periodontal assessment will require some calculations. The most common are the width of the attached gingiva and attachment level.

1. **Determining the Width of Attached Gingiva**
   A. **Description.** The attached gingiva is the part of the gingiva that is firm, dense, and tightly connected to the cementum on the cervical-third of the root or to the periosteum (connective tissue cover) of the alveolar bone. The attached gingiva lies between the free gingiva and the alveolar mucosa, extending from the base of the sulcus (or pocket) to the mucogingival junction.
      1. The functions of the attached gingiva are to keep the free gingiva from being pulled away from the tooth and to protect the gingiva from trauma.
      2. The width of the attached gingiva is not measured on the palate since it is not possible to determine where the attached gingiva ends and the palatal mucosa begins.
      3. *The attached gingiva does not include any portion of the gingiva that is separated from the tooth by a crevice, sulcus, or periodontal pocket.*
   B. **Significance.** The width of the attached gingiva on a tooth surface is an important clinical feature for the dentist to keep in mind when planning many types of restorative procedures. If there is no attached gingiva on a tooth surface, the dentist is limited in the types of restorations that can be placed. Therefore, it is important to use the information collected during the comprehensive periodontal assessment to calculate this clinical feature.
   C. **Method of Calculation.** The method for calculation of the width of attached gingiva is shown in Box 19-3. Note that the information needed to calculate the width of the attached gingiva already would have been recorded during the periodontal assessment.

Box 19.3 Calculating the Width of Attached Gingiva

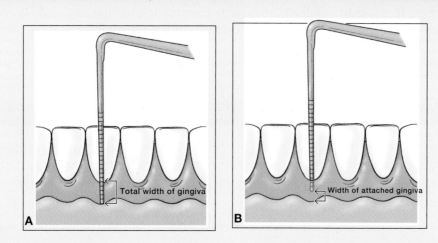

Formula: To calculate the width of attached gingiva at a specific site, measure the width of the gingiva and subtract the probing depth from the total that width using the steps below.
Step 1: Measure the total width of the gingiva from the gingival margin to the mucogingival junction.
Step 2: Measure the probing depth (from the gingival margin to the base of the pocket).
Step 3: Calculate the width of the attached gingiva by subtracting the probing depth from the total width of the gingiva.
(Used from Nield-Gehrig JS. *Fundamentals of Periodontal Instrumentation and Advanced Instrumentation.* 6th ed. Philadelphia: Lippincott Williams & Wilkins; 2008:454, with permission.)

2. **Calculating the Clinical Attachment Level (CAL)**
   A. **Definition.** The clinical attachment level (CAL) is an estimate of the true periodontal support around the tooth as measured with a periodontal probe. This measurement is only an estimation of the actual histologic level of attachment still present. It is a means of estimating the level of the junctional epithelium. Box 19-4 explains the rationale for using CAL as an accurate measurement of the periodontal support.
   B. **Significance of Clinical Attachment Levels**
      1. An attachment level measurement is a more accurate indicator of the periodontal support around a tooth than is a probing depth measurement.
         a. Probing depths are measured from the free gingival margin to the base of the sulcus or pocket. The position of the gingival margin may change with tissue swelling, overgrowth of tissue, or recession of tissue. Since the position of the gingival margin can change (move coronally or apically), probing depths do not provide an accurate means to monitor changes in periodontal support over time in a patient.
         b. CAL provides an accurate means to monitor changes in periodontal support over time. The CAL is calculated from measurements made from a fixed point on the tooth that does not change—the CEJ.
      2. The presence of loss of attachment is a critical factor in distinguishing between gingivitis and periodontitis.
         a. Inflammation with no attachment loss is characteristic of gingivitis.
         b. Inflammation with attachment loss is characteristic of periodontitis.
         c. When attachment loss is 5 mm or greater, most dental teams should refer the patient to a periodontist.

Box 19-4. Rationale for Using the CAL as an Accurate Measurement of the Periodontal Support

- Probing depths are not reliable indicators of the extent of bone support because these measurements are made from the gingival margin. The position of the gingival margin changes with tissue swelling, overgrowth of gingiva, and recession of the gingival margin.

- Clinical Attachment levels are calculated from measurements made from a fixed point that does not change (i.e., the CEJ). Since the bone level in health is approximately 2 mm apical to the CEJ, clinical attachment levels provide a reliable indication of the extent of bone support for the tooth.

   C. **Calculating the Clinical Attachment Level.** When the gingival margin is at its normal location, the probing depth and the Clinical Attachment Level readings are the same. When tissue swelling or recession is present, a periodontal probe is used to measure the distance the gingival margin is apical or coronal to the cementoenamel junction (Fig. 19-8A–C).
      1. **For recession of the gingival margin.** If recession of the gingival margin is present, the distance between the CEJ and the gingival margin is measured using a calibrated periodontal probe. This distance is recorded as the gingival margin level.
      2. **When the gingival margin is significantly coronal to the CEJ.** If the gingival margin significantly covers the cementoenamel junction, the distance between the margin and the CEJ is estimated using the following technique:
         a. Position the tip of the probe at a 45-degree angle to the tooth.

b. Slowly move the probe beneath the gingival margin until the junction between the enamel and cementum is detected.

c. Measure the distance between the gingival margin and the cementoenamel junction. This distance is recorded as the gingival margin level.

D. **Recording the Gingival Margin on a Periodontal Chart.** Customarily, the notations 0, –, or, + are used to indicate the position of the gingival margin on a periodontal chart (Box 19-5).

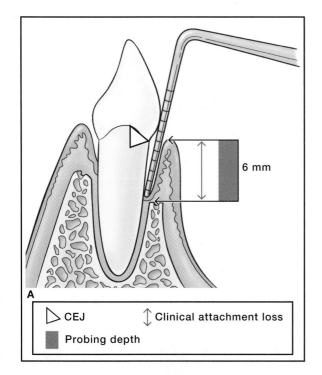

| △ CEJ | ↕ Clinical attachment loss |
| ■ Probing depth | |

Figure 19.8A. Calculating CAL when the Gingival Margin is Slightly Coronal to the CEJ. When the gingival margin is slightly coronal to the CEJ, no calculations are needed since the probing depth and the CAL are equal.

For example:
Probing depth measurement: 6 mm
Gingival margin level: 0 mm
Clinical attachment loss: 6 mm

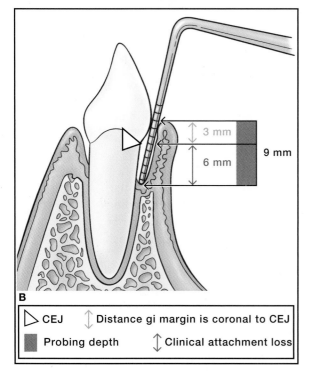

| △ CEJ | ↕ Distance gi margin is coronal to CEJ |
| ■ Probing depth | ↕ Clinical attachment loss |

Figure 19.8B. Calculating CAL when the Gingival Margin is Significantly Coronal to the CEJ. When the gingival margin is significantly coronal to the CEJ, the CAL is calculated by SUBTRACTING the gingival margin level from the probing depth.

For example:
Probing depth measurement: 9 mm
Gingival margin level: –3 mm
Clinical attachment loss: 6 mm

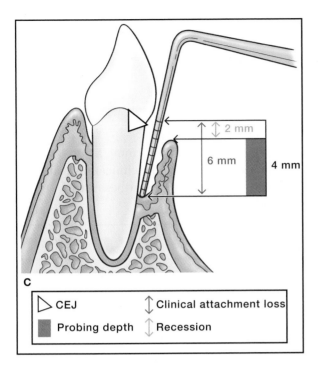

Figure 19.8C. **Calculating CAL in the Presence of Recession of the gingival margin.** When recession is present, the CAL is calculated by ADDING the probing depth to the gingival margin level.

For example:
Probing depth measurement: 4 mm
Gingival margin level: +2 mm
Clinical attachment loss: 6 mm

Box 19-5. Notations That Indicate the Position of the Free Gingival Margin

- A zero (0) indicates the free gingival margin is slightly coronal to the CEJ
- A negative number (–) indicates the free gingival margin significantly covers the CEJ
- A positive number (+) indicates the free gingival margin is apical to the CEJ (recession)

Chapter Summary Statement

The information gathered by the members of the dental team during the clinical periodontal assessment forms the basis for an individualized treatment plan for the patient. This chapter discusses two types of clinical periodontal assessment: a periodontal screening examination and the comprehensive periodontal assessment. The Periodontal Screening and Recording (PSR) is an efficient periodontal screening system for the detection of periodontal disease.

The comprehensive periodontal assessment is a complete clinical periodontal assessment used to gather information about the periodontium. The information collected in a comprehensive periodontal assessment includes probing depth measurements, bleeding on probing, presence of exudate, level of the free gingival margin and the mucogingival junction, tooth mobility, furcation involvement, presence of calculus and bacterial plaque biofilm, gingival inflammation, radiographic evidence of alveolar bone loss, and presence of local contributing factors. Supplemental diagnostic tests are indicated for certain patients. Some judgments made during a clinical periodontal assessment require calculation. These include the width of attached gingiva and clinical attachment levels. Detection of clinical attachment level is important in determining whether gingivitis or periodontitis is present at a site of inflammation.

Section 5
Focus on Patients

Case 1

While visiting a dental office, you observe a member of the dental team performing a periodontal assessment. You note that while searching for furcation invasion, the clinician is using a straight calibrated periodontal probe. What critical information might be lost because of instrument selection for this step in a periodontal assessment?

Case 2

During a comprehensive periodontal assessment you note severe inflammation of the gingiva over the facial surface of a lower right molar tooth. On the dental chart you are using there is no obvious mechanism to record this important piece of periodontal information. How should you proceed?

Case 3

During a periodontal assessment of a periodontitis patient, you are trying to determine the CAL on the facial surface of a canine tooth. On the facial surface of the canine tooth you have measured 3 mm of recession of the gingival margin and a probing depth of 6 mm. How much attachment has been lost on the facial surface of this canine tooth?

References

1. For the dental patient. Gingival recession: causes and treatment. *J Am Dent Assoc* 2007; 138(10):1404.

Suggested Readings

Armitage GC. Diagnosis of periodontal diseases. *J Periodontol.* 2003;74(8):1237–1247.

For the dental patient. Gingival recession: causes and treatment. *J Am Dent Assoc.* 2007;138(10):1404.

Jansson H, Norderyd O. Evaluation of a periodontal risk assessment model in subjects with severe periodontitis. A 5-year retrospective study. *Swed Dent J.* 2008;32(1):1–7.

Leisnert L, Hallstrom H, and Knutsson K. What findings do clinicians use to diagnose chronic periodontitis? *Swed Dent J.* 2008;32(3):115–123.

Sweeting LA, Davis K, and Cobb CM. Periodontal Treatment Protocol (PTP) for the general dental practice. *J Dent Hyg.* 2008;82 Suppl 3:16–26.

Van Aelst L, Cosyn J, and De Bruyn H. Guidelines for periodontal diagnosis in Belgium. *Rev Belge Med Dent.* 2008;63(2):59–63.

Ziada H, Irwin C, Mullally B, Allen E, et al. Periodontics: 1. Identification and diagnosis of periodontal diseases in general dental practice. *Dent Update.* 2008;34(4):208–210, 213–214, 217.

Chapter 20

Radiographic Analysis of the Periodontium

Learning Objectives

- Recognize the radiographic characteristics of normal and abnormal alveolar bone.
- Recognize and describe early radiographic evidence of periodontal disease.
- Distinguish between vertical and horizontal alveolar bone loss.
- Recognize potential etiologic agents for periodontal disease radiographically.
- Gain practical experience in radiographic assessment by applying information from this chapter in the clinical setting.

Key Terms

Radiolucent
Radiopaque
Cortical bone

Lamina dura
Crestal irregularities
Triangulation

Section 1
Radiographic Appearance of the Periodontium

Dental radiographs are an important adjunct to the clinical assessment of the periodontium. To recognize disease, the dental hygienist must be able to recognize the normal radiographic appearance of the periodontium. Periodontal anatomy visible on radiographs includes the alveolar bone, periodontal ligament space, and cementum. The gingiva is a noncalcified soft tissue that cannot be seen on a radiograph.

1. **Radiolucent and Radiopaque Structures and Materials**
    A. Radiolucent materials and structures are easily penetrated by x-rays.
        1. Most of the x-rays will be able to pass through these objects and structures to expose the radiograph. Radiolucent areas appear as dark gray to black on the radiograph.
        2. Examples of radiolucent structures are the tooth pulp, periodontal ligament space, a periapical abscess, marrow spaces in the bone, and bone loss defects.
    B. Radiopaque materials and structures absorb or resist the passage of x-rays.
        1. Radiopaque areas appear light gray to white on the radiograph. These structures absorb most of the x-rays so that very few x-rays reach the radiograph.
        2. Examples of radiopaque structures and materials are metallic silver (amalgam restorations) and newer composite restorations, enamel, dentin, pulp stones, and compact or cortical bone.
2. **Identification of the Periodontium on Radiographs.** The components of the periodontium that can be identified on radiographs include the alveolar bone, periodontal ligament space, and cementum (Fig. 20-1).
    A. **Cortical Bone**
        1. Cortical bone is the outer surface of the bone and is composed of layers of bone closely packed together.
            a. On the maxilla, the cortical bone is a thin shell.
            b. On the mandible, the cortical bone is a dense layer.
        2. Radiographic Appearance of Cortical Bone
            a. Inferior border of the mandible appears on the radiograph as a thick white border.
            b. Interdental alveolar crests between the teeth of both jaws appear on the radiograph as a thin white line on the outside of crestal bone.
            c. The lattice-like pattern of the cancellous bone that fills the interior portion of the alveolar process appears on the radiograph as a pattern of delicate white tracings within the bone.

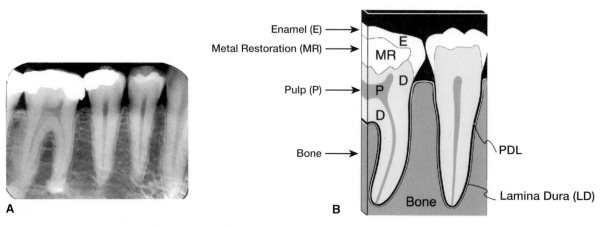

Figure 20.1. Radiographic Structures of the Periodontium.

B. **Alveolar Crest.** *The normal level of the alveolar bone is located approximately 2-mm apical to (below) the cementoenamel junction (CEJ).*
   1. If the coronal bone level is within 3 mm of the CEJ, the bone level is considered normal.
   2. It is unlikely that bone loss less than 3 mm can be detected on a radiograph.
C. **Crestal Contour of the Interdental Bone**
   1. The contour of the crest of the interproximal bone is a good indicator of periodontal health. *The contour of the interpoximal crest is parallel to an imaginary line drawn between the CEJs of adjacent teeth.*
   2. In posterior sextants, the contour of the interproximal crest is parallel to an imaginary line drawn between the CEJs of the adjacent teeth.
      a. Horizontal crest contour. The crest of the interproximal bone will have a horizontal contour when the CEJs of the adjacent teeth are at the same level (Fig. 20-2).
      b. Angular crest contour. The crest of the interproximal bone will have a vertical contour when one of the adjacent teeth is tilted or erupted to different height (Fig. 20-3).

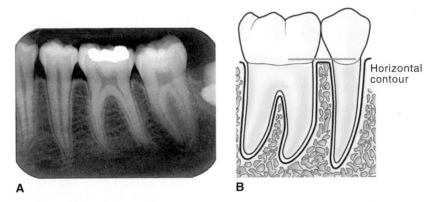

A   **B**

Figure 20.2. A: **Normal Alveolar Bone Height.** This radiograph shows a normal alveolar bone height that is 1.5 to 2 mm below and parallel to the cementoenamel junction. In this example, alveolar crest is a dense radiopaque line similar in density to the lamina dura surrounding the root of the tooth. B: **Horizontal Crest Contour.** The crest of the interproximal bone will have a horizontal contour when the CEJs of the adjacent teeth are at the same level.

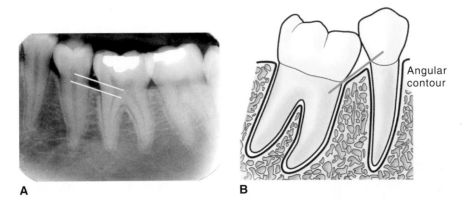

A   **B**

Figure 20.3. **Angular Crest Contour.** The crest of the interproximal bone will have a vertical contour when one of the adjacent teeth is tilted or erupted to different height.

D. **Alveolar Crestal Bone**
1. Alveolar bone is the part of the jawbone that supports the teeth.
2. The surfaces of the bony crests are smooth and covered with a thin layer of cortical (dense, hard) bone that may be seen as a thin, white line on a radiograph.
3. *The most important radiographic feature of the alveolar crest is that it forms a smooth intact surface between adjacent teeth with only the width of the periodontal ligament space separating it from the adjacent root surface.*
   a. The crest of the interdental septa between incisors is thin and pointed.
   b. The crest of the interdental septa between the posterior teeth is rounded or flat (Fig. 20-4).

E. **Lamina Dura**
1. The alveolar bone proper is the thin layer of dense bone that lines a normal tooth socket. In radiographs, the alveolar bone proper is identified as the lamina dura. On a radiograph, the lamina dura appears as a continuous white (radiopaque) line around the tooth root (Fig. 20-5).
2. On a radiograph, the lamina dura is continuous with the cortical bone layer of the crest of the interdental septa.

F. **Periodontal Ligament Space**
1. The space between the tooth root and the lamina dura of the socket is filled with the periodontal ligament tissue. The periodontal ligament tissue functions as the attachment of the tooth to the lamina dura of the socket.
2. Periodontal ligament tissue does not resist penetration of x-rays and, therefore, appears on the radiograph as a thin radiolucent black line surrounding the tooth root (Fig. 20-5).
3. In most cases, a widening of the periodontal ligament space (PDLS) on the radiograph indicates tooth mobility (Fig. 20-6).

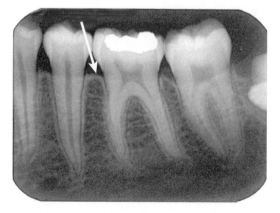

Figure 20.4. **Alveolar Crest**. The alveolar crest (indicated by an *arrow*) forms a smooth intact surface between adjacent teeth.

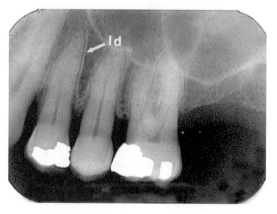

Figure 20.5. **Lamina Dura and Periodontal Ligament Space**. The lamina dura (ld) appears as a continuous white line around the tooth root.

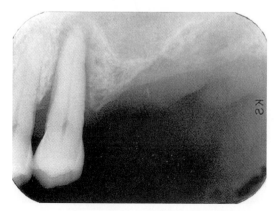

Figure 20.6. **Widening of the Periodontal Ligament Space**. This maxillary second premolar has a uniformly widened periodontal ligament space that is characteristic of tooth mobility.

Section 2
Use of Radiographs for Periodontal Evaluation

1. **Techniques for Good Radiographic Quality**
    A. **Long-Cone Paralleling Technique.** The long-cone paralleling technique provides a radiograph that is more anatomically accurate when compared with other intraoral techniques such as bisecting angle.
    B. **Long-Grayscale-Low Contrast Images.** Long-scale contrast radiographic images have many visible shades of gray that make it easier to see subtle changes such as bone loss in periodontal disease. These images can be obtained using high kVp exposures (70–100 kVp) or using digital imaging software adjustments to maximize the gray scale of normally exposed images.
2. **Limitations of Radiographs for Periodontal Evaluation.** There are limitations in the use of the radiograph in the diagnosis of periodontal disease.
    A. **A Two-Dimensional Image.** A radiograph provides a two-dimensional image of a complex three-dimensional structure. The fact that the radiograph is a two-dimensional image can be misleading to the viewer. For example, the buccal alveolar bone can hide bone loss on the lingual aspect of a tooth, and the palatal root makes it difficult to detect furcation involvement of a maxillary molar.
    B. **Information Limited to Noncalcified Structures.** In addition, radiographs do not provide any information about the noncalcified components of the periodontium.
    C. **Limited Information on Periodontium.** Radiographs *do not reveal* the following: the presence or absence of periodontal pockets, early bone loss, exact morphology of bone destruction, tooth mobility, early furcation involvement, condition of the alveolar bone on the buccal and lingual surfaces, or the level of the epithelial attachment.
        1. Periodontal Pockets
            a. *The only reliable method of locating a periodontal pocket and evaluating its extent is by careful periodontal probing.*
            b. The periodontal pocket is composed of soft tissue so it will not be visible on the radiograph.
        2. Early Bone Loss
            a. *The very earliest signs of periodontitis must be detected clinically, not radiographically.* By the time periodontal bone loss becomes detectable on the radiograph, it usually has progressed beyond the earliest stages of the disease.
                1) Interseptal bony defects smaller than 3 mm usually cannot be seen on radiographs.
                2) Bone height on the facial and lingual aspects is difficult to evaluate radiographically because the teeth are superimposed over the bone.
            b. *A radiograph cannot accurately display the shape of bone deformities because it is not three-dimensional.*
            c. A radiograph with poor technique and excessive vertical angulation can obscure bone loss (see Fig. 20-7).
                1) For this reason the bitewing radiograph should be the primary radiograph used to evaluate crestal bone height rather than the periapical radiograph.
                2) Proper long cone paralleling technique can prevent distortion of crestal bone height on periapical radiographs and improve their usefulness.

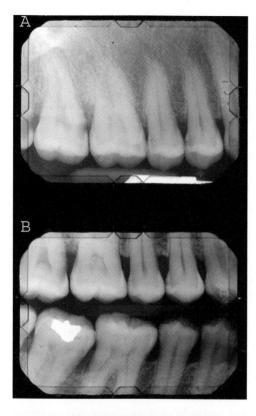

Figure 20.7A. Excessive Vertical Angulation. Note how the crestal bone height is exaggerated in the periapical radiograph shown here as opposed to the bitewing radiograph shown in Figure 20-7B.

Figure 20.7B. Bitewing Radiograph. The bitewing shown here reveals the true bone height of the teeth shown in Figure 20-7A.

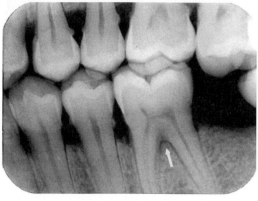

Figure 20.8. Furcation Involvement. The radiolucency on the mandibular first molar should be evaluated using a furcation probe.

3. Early Furcation Involvement
   a. Radiographs usually *show more interradicular bone*—bone between the roots of the teeth—than is actually present. The facial and lingual aspects of the alveolar bone will often be superimposed over the furcation and hide bone loss from view.
   b. *Variations in alignment of the x-ray beam may conceal the presence or extent of furcation involvement.*
   c. Furcation involvement (bone loss between the roots) is detected by clinical examination with a furcation probe. The furcation area of a tooth should be examined with a furcation probe even if the radiograph shows a very small radiolucency or an area of diminished radiodensity at the furcation (FIG. 20-8).
4. Extensive bone loss
   a. *Crestal bone loss of 5 mm or greater may cause the coronal bone to be poorly visualized or not seen at all on normal bitewing radiographs*
   b. Vertically oriented bitewings may be used in these situations
   c. An adaptor is available for most film holders to accomplish this
   d. The long axis of the film is rotated 90 degrees to be perpendicular to the occlusal plane instead of the short axis (FIG. 20-9).

e. Vertical bitewing radiographs show more of the coronal bone than regular bitewings especially when the teeth are widely separated by the film holder (FIG. 20-10).

5. Disease Activity

a. Just as clinical attachment levels only indicate past disease destruction, *radiographs do not show disease activity, but only the effects of the disease.*

b. Because of these limitations, the radiographic examination is never a satisfactory substitute for a clinical periodontal assessment.

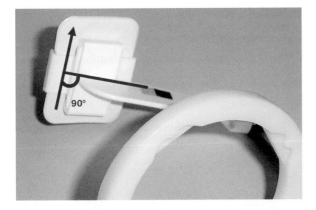

Figure 20.9. Film Placement for Vertical Bitewing. A #2 periapical film positioned for taking a vertical bitewing radiograph. Note how the film is rotated 90 degrees from the usual orientation.

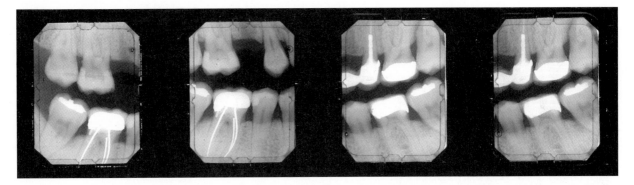

Figure 20.10. Four Film Vertical Bitewing Series. Note how much coronal bone is visible on these vertical bitewings despite the separation of the teeth by the positioning device.

3. **Benefits of Radiographs for Periodontal Evaluation.** Despite the radiograph's limitations, the periodontal examination is incomplete without accurate radiographs. Radiographs will demonstrate the following: most of the bony changes associated with periodontitis, the tooth root morphology, relationship of the maxillary sinus to the periodontal deformity, widening of periodontal ligament space, advanced furcation involvement, periodontal abscesses, and local factors such as overhanging restorations, marginal ridge height discrepancies, open contacts and calculus (TABLE 20–1).

A. **Assessment of Bony Changes.** Early radiographic signs of periodontitis are (1) fuzziness at the crest of the alveolar bone, (2) a widened periodontal ligament space, and (3) radiolucent areas in the interseptal bone (FIG. 20-11).

1. Crestal Irregularities. Crestal irregularities are the appearance of breaks or fuzziness instead of a nice clean line at the crest of the interdental alveolar bone.

TABLE 20-1. Benefits of Radiographs in the Detection of Periodontal Disease	
Condition	**Radiographic Sign(s)**
Early bony changes	Break or fuzziness at the crest of the interdental alveolar bone
	Widening of the periodontal ligament space at crestal margin
	Presence of finger-like radiolucent projections into the interdental alveolar bone
Horizontal bone loss	Can be measured from a plane that is parallel to a tooth-to-tooth line drawn from the CEJs of adjacent teeth
Vertical bone loss	Seen as more bone loss on the interproximal aspect of one tooth than on the adjacent tooth; bone level is at an angle to a line joining the CEJs
Bone defects	Are radiolucent due to bone loss and therefore visible on radiographs, although three-dimensional structure may be hard to determine
Furcation involvement	Loss of bone in furcation area may be detectable as triangular radiolucency especially on mandibular molars

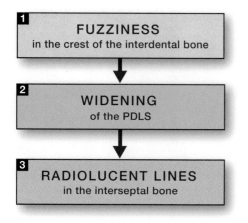

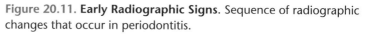

Figure 20.11. **Early Radiographic Signs.** Sequence of radiographic changes that occur in periodontitis.

2. **Triangulation (Funneling).** Triangulation is the widening of the periodontal ligament space caused by the resorption of bone along either the mesial or distal aspect of the interdental (interseptal) crestal bone (FIG. 20-12).

3. Interseptal Bone Changes
   a. Another radiographic sign of periodontitis is the existence of finger-like radiolucent projections extending from the crestal bone into the interdental alveolar bone (FIG. 20-13).
   b. These finger-like radiolucent lines represent a reduction of mineralized tissue (bone) adjacent to blood vessel channels within the alveolar bone.
   c. If chronic periodontitis goes untreated and much of the alveolar bone around the tooth is destroyed, the tooth will seem to "float in space"

on the radiograph. This represents the "terminal stage" of the disease process.

B. **Extent or Direction of Bone Loss.** The extent or direction of bone loss is determined using the cementoenamel junction (CEJ) of adjacent teeth as the points of reference.

  1. Horizontal Bone Loss
     Horizontal bone loss is bone destruction that is parallel to an imaginary line drawn between the CEJs of adjacent teeth (Fig. 20-14).
  2. Vertical Bone Loss
     Vertical (or angular) bone loss occurs when there is greater bone destruction on the interproximal aspect of one tooth than on the adjacent tooth (Fig. 20-15).

C. **Assessment of Bone Loss**

  1. The radiograph is an indirect method of detecting bone loss. *Periodontitis is a disease process with active and inactive periods, so the radiograph is only a snapshot of an instant in time in the disease process.*
  2. The radiograph reveals the bone *remaining* rather than the amount of bone actually lost. Bone loss occurs on all surfaces; however, the tooth root tends to mask (or hide) bone loss on the facial and lingual surfaces of the tooth.
  3. Mesial or distal bone loss is evaluated primarily by examining the interproximal septal bone on the radiograph. The amount of bone loss is *estimated* as the difference between the level of the remaining bone and the normal bone height.

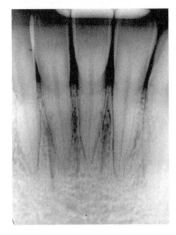

Figure 20.13. Finger-Like Radiolucent Projections. The nutrient canals within the bone are seen as finger-like projections extending between and beyond the roots of the mandibular incisors on this radiograph.

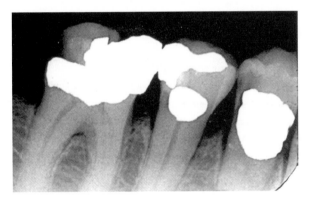

Figure 20.12. Triangulation. The crestal bone between these mandibular teeth demonstrates triangulation, a pointed, triangular appearance.

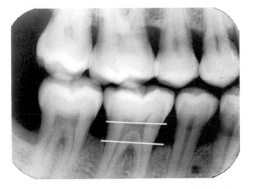

Figure 20.14. Horizontal Bone Loss. Horizontal bone loss is parallel to an imaginary line drawn between the CEJs of adjacent teeth.

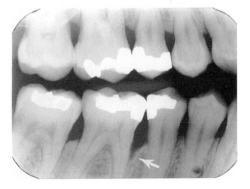

Figure 20.15. Vertical Bone Loss. The arrow points to vertical bone loss on the mesial surface of the mandibular first molar.

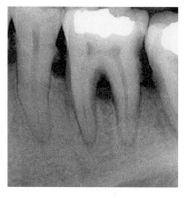

Figure 20.16. **Furcation Involvement**. The furcation involvement is easily visible on the mandibular first molar in this radiographic.

D. **Assessment of Furcation Involvement**
  1. Furcation involvement will not be seen on the radiograph until the bone resorption extends past the furcation area.
    a. Furcation involvement of mandibular molars is easier to detect on a radiograph than is furcation involvement of maxillary molars. This is because mandibular molars have only two roots, a mesial root and a distal root (FIG. 20-16).
    b. Furcation involvement on maxillary molars is more difficult to detect on a radiograph. Maxillary molars have three roots, a mesiobuccal, distobuccal, and palatal root. The palatal root is often superimposed over the furcation of the tooth on the radiograph and masks (hides) any radiolucency there.
  2. It is a general rule that furcation involvement is often *greater* than what the radiograph reveals.
  3. If using the radiograph to aid in the detection of furcation involvement, the following rules should be kept in mind:
    a. If there is a slight thickening of the periodontal ligament space in the furcation area, the area should be examined clinically with a furcation probe.
    b. If severe bone loss is evident on the mesial or distal surface of a multirooted tooth (especially maxillary molars), furcation involvement should be suspected.
E. **Recognition of Local Contributing Risk Factors.** Several local contributing risk factors that may be revealed by the radiograph are calculus deposits, faulty restorations, and food packing areas.
  1. Calculus Deposits
    a. *The only accurate way to detect calculus deposits is with an explorer,* however, large calculus deposits *may be visible* on a radiograph.
      1) The radiograph may show large, heavy interproximal calculus deposits.
      2) Calculus deposits may be visible on the facial and lingual surfaces of teeth when there is severe bone loss on these surfaces.
    b. The ability to visualize calculus radiographically depends on the degree of mineralization within the calculus and the angulation factors of the x-ray beam.
  2. Faulty Restorations. Inadequate dental restorations and prostheses are common causes of gingival inflammation, periodontitis, and alveolar bone resorption. In many cases, faulty restorations can be detected on a radiograph (FIG. 20-17).
  3. Trauma from Occlusion
    a. The radiograph is used only as a supplemental aid in recognizing trauma from occlusion.
    b. Radiographic signs of trauma from occlusion include the following:
      1) Increased width of the periodontal ligament spaces on the mesial and distal sides of the tooth due to resorption of the lamina dura.
      2) Vertical or angular bone destruction.

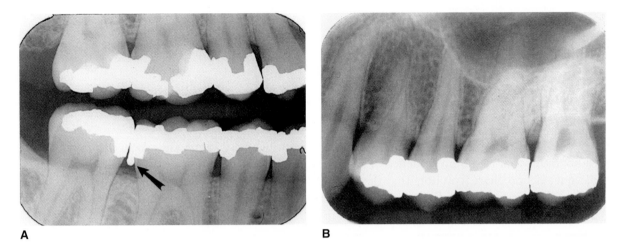

A   **B**

Figure 20.17. Faulty Restorations. A: The distal surface of the mandibular first molar, indicated by the arrow, has a faulty restoration that creates a food trap and harbors plaque biofilm. B: The distal proximal tooth surface of the maxillary first molar and the mesial tooth surface of the second molar have not been restored to their original shape and contour. These faulty contours create an open contact that can allow food impaction.

Chapter Summary Statement

When the limitations of radiographs are recognized, they can be an important diagnostic aid in the examination and diagnosis of patients with periodontitis. Radiographs are extremely useful tools in the detection of bony changes due to periodontitis such as crestal irregularities, triangulation, interseptal bone loss, assessment of bone defects, and furcation involvement.

Section 3
Focus on Patients

Case 1

Mr. Jones is a new patient in your dental office. He brings with him some recent full-mouth radiographs that reveal no evidence of alveolar bone loss. While studying a copy of the patient's dental chart, you note that there is a diagnosis of chronic periodontitis. How might you explain the apparent discrepancy between the lack of radiographic evidence of bone loss and the diagnosis of periodontitis?

Case 2

During a periodontal assessment for a new patient, you detect clinical attachment loss. When you suggest that the patient needs dental radiographs, the patient objects because she does not want to be exposed to "unnecessary x-rays." How should you respond?

Case 3

While reviewing a new set of dental radiographs for a patient, you note numerous sites of obvious bone loss. The bone loss appears to be vertical (or angular), where there is much more bone loss on one tooth surface compared with the immediately adjacent tooth surface. How might the dental team use this vertical pattern of bone loss when developing the periodontal diagnosis?

Chapter 21

Nutrition and Periodontal Disease

Learning Objectives

- Explain the possible relationship between vitamin D and calcium deficiency and periodontal disease.

- List some oral symptoms that can be seen in chronic or severe vitamin C deficiency.

- Define scurvy.

- Explain the term ascorbic acid-deficiency gingivitis.

- List several nutrient deficiencies that may increase the risk for periodontal disease.

- Name two dietary factors that may increase the risk for periodontal disease in addition to specific nutrient deficiencies.

- Name three general functions of nutrients in maintaining periodontal health.

- Explain how nutritional counseling might be accomplished with a patient.

Key Terms

Scurvy
Ascorbic acid-deficiency gingivitis
Kwashiorkor

Antioxidants
Omega-3 fatty acids

Section 1
The Influence of Diet and Nutrition on the Periodontium

Research evidence has not clarified the precise relationship between diet, nutrition, and periodontal disease at this point. Much of the scientific evidence relating nutrition and periodontal disease involves animal and laboratory studies with somewhat limited evidence from controlled human studies. In spite of this limitation, research does link some specific nutrient deficiencies and foods high in refined carbohydrates to increased inflammation—the very kind of inflammation that can trigger the host-mediated inflammatory response seen in periodontal disease [1]. As already discussed in several chapters of this book, periodontal disease is an inflammatory response to bacterial plaque biofilm. Though periodontal disease cannot be caused by nutritional deficiencies, some nutritional deficiencies do indeed appear to modify the severity and extent of the periodontal disease.

1. **Nutrient Deficiencies That May Increase Risk for Periodontal Disease.** There do appear to be specific dietary factors that may increase the risk for periodontal disease. When considering the relationship between nutritional deficiencies and periodontal disease, it is important to realize that certain deficiencies can be the result of disturbances in absorption, limitations in education, or geographic isolation as well as simply being the result of inadequate dietary intake.

   A. **Vitamin D and Calcium.** Diets deficient in vitamin D and calcium may play a role in increasing the risk for periodontal disease.

      1. Vitamin D (a group of steroid hormones) has an important influence in regulating plasma calcium levels.
      2. In addition to regulating body calcium levels, vitamin D also plays a role in host defense against infection by signaling macrophages to respond to and kill pathogens [2].
      3. In a large epidemiologic study the risk for attachment loss was increased in subjects with a low dietary calcium intake; the lower the intake the more attachment loss [3].
      4. In another interesting longitudinal study elderly adults with higher daily calcium intake had a smaller risk for tooth loss than adults consuming lower calcium levels [4].
      5. Vitamin D and calcium deficiencies have also been reported to result in bone loss and increased inflammation [5].
      6. Vitamin D is found in some foods but is mostly produced within the skin in response to sunlight; good sources of dietary vitamin D include egg yolk, liver and oily fish.
      7. In one study consumption of calcium-rich dairy products (especially yogurt and lactic acid drinks) correlated with periodontal health in nonsmokers [6].

   B. **Vitamin C (Ascorbic Acid)**
      1. Vitamin C deficiency has been studied extensively and has been associated with changes in the periodontium [7].
      2. Vitamin C is a water-soluble vitamin that cannot be stored by the body except in insignificant amounts.
      3. Since the human body lacks the ability to synthesize and make vitamin C, it depends on dietary sources to meet vitamin C needs.
      4. Vitamin C is found in fresh fruits and vegetables such as oranges, berries, tomatoes, leafy greens, and kiwifruit; consumption of fruits and vegetables or fortifying diets with vitamin C supplements are essential to avoid ascorbic acid deficiency.

5. Research conducted in the Netherlands on a group of Indonesian tea plantation workers found a small but statistically significant relationship between attachment loss and vitamin C deficiency [8].

6. An epidemiology study done in the United States involving over 12,000 adults showed a weak relationship between reduced vitamin C intake and the presence of periodontitis [9].

7. Prolonged and severe lack of vitamin C can result in scurvy.

    a. Scurvy is a systemic disorder caused by severe and prolonged deprivation of vitamin C, and scurvy can be accompanied by changes in the periodontium.

    b. Systemically scurvy results in poor wound healing, progressive anemia, muscle pain, internal bleeding, and a variety of other symptoms; scurvy in early childhood can cause musculoskeletal problems.

    c. In the periodontium scurvy can result in excessive swelling and bleeding of the gingiva, destruction of periodontal ligament, destruction of alveolar bone, tooth mobility, and tooth loss.

    d. Even though scurvy is uncommon in the United States and Canada, it still occurs in these countries and can affect adults and children who have chronic dietary vitamin C deficiency [10].

8. Ascorbic acid-deficiency gingivitis is an inflammatory response of the gingiva caused by dental plaque biofilm that is aggravated by chronically low vitamin C (ascorbic acid) levels.

    a. Ascorbic acid-deficiency gingivitis manifests clinically as bright red, swollen, ulcerated gingival tissue that bleeds with the slightest provocation [11,12].

    b. An example of infantile vitamin C deficiency is shown in Figures 21-1 and 21-2.

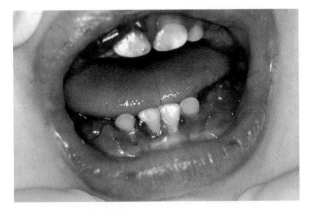

Figure 21.1. Ascorbic Acid-Deficiency Gingivitis. This 15-month-old boy had a history of unexplained gingival bleeding for several weeks and fever for 2 days. He had been fed only cow's milk and oatmeal since age 4 months. Laboratory blood tests revealed that his vitamin C levels were low. (Used with permission from Riepe FG, et al. Special feature: picture of the month. Infantile scurvy. *Arch Pediatr Adolesc Med.* 2001;155[5]:607–608; copyright 2001 American Medical Association. All rights reserved.)

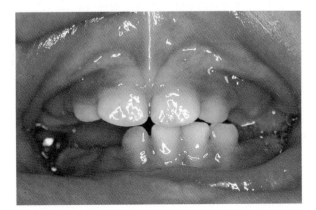

Figure 21.2. After Treatment with Vitamin C. The same boy shown in Figure 21-1 after 3 days treatment with vitamin C. (Courtesy of Dr Felix G. Riepe, MD, Christian Albrechts University, Kiel, Germany.)

C. **Refined Carbohydrates.** Diets rich in refined carbohydrates may play a role in increasing the risk for periodontal disease.

   1. Excess consumption of refined carbohydrates can affect the immune response and may lead to continued destruction of the periodontium in patients with existing periodontitis through mechanisms such as the action of enzymes (i.e., collagenase) and proinflammatory mediators (i.e., interleukin-1 and interleukin-6) [13]. These destructive mechanisms have been discussed in other chapters of this book.

   2. Diets high in refined carbohydrates and fats cause rapid release of glucose into the bloodstream (Table 21-1). High blood glucose levels increase triglyceride levels and stimulate the release of insulin, which decreases the ability of the body to break down fat stored in adipose depots. Diet-induced hyperlipidemia (excess lipids in the blood) can also increase inflammation [13].

D. **Proteins**

   1. Protein deficiency can have an effect on the host defenses that could modulate the progress of periodontitis.

   2. Cell-mediated immunity, the complement system, phagocyte activity, and production of cytokines are all impaired by protein deficiency [14].

   3. Severe protein deficiency is known as **kwashiorkor**; kwashiorkor can result in a shift in subgingival oral bacteria to include more periodontal pathogens [15].

   4. In animal studies severe protein deficiency has resulted in a greater incidence of periodontitis [16].

E. **Antioxidants**

   1. Though controversial, it has been suggested that diets deficient in antioxidants may play a role in increasing the risk for periodontal disease.

   2. **Antioxidants** are substances that occur naturally in the body and in certain foods; antioxidants can inhibit oxidation and thereby block damage to cells by free radicals.

      a. As part of their normal function, body cells make toxic molecules called free radicals. Oxygen damage (oxidation) to cells results when there are too many free radicals present in body tissues.

      b. Researchers surmise that cellular damage—as the result of free radicals— may be partly responsible for the effects of aging and certain diseases and that antioxidants may block this damage.

   3. Antioxidants include a number of enzymes and other substances such as vitamins A, C, E and the minerals zinc and selenium.

   4. Including antioxidants in the diet may modulate the inflammatory process [13].

TABLE 21-1. Refined Carbohydrates Versus Complex Carbohydrates

Refined Carbohydrates (Avoid)	Complex Carbohydrates (Choose)
White bread	Whole wheat break
Carbonated beverages, fruit juices	100% fruit juice
Table sugar, frosting, syrup, candy, cookies, cake	Cruciferous vegetables, celery, carrots, beans
Jelly and honey	Apples, blueberries, cherries, citrus fruit, plums
White rice	Brown rice
Boxed processed cereals	Oatmeal, barley

F. **Omega-3 Polyunsaturated Fatty Acids**
   1. It has also been suggested that diets deficient in omega-3 fatty acids may play a role in increasing the risk for periodontal disease.
   2. Omega-3 fatty acids are a type of polyunsaturated fat found in leafy green vegetables, vegetable oils, and cold-water fish; omega-3 fatty acids are capable of reducing serum cholesterol levels and having anticoagulant properties.
   3. Omega-3 fatty acids can reduce serum cholesterol and triglyceride levels and confer protective anti-inflammatory effects in the body [13].
   4. In one study rats fed diets rich in omega-3 polyunsaturated fats experienced less bone loss than those fed omega-6 polyunsaturated fats [13].

2. **Additional Dietary Factors and Periodontal Disease Risk**
   A. **Obesity and Periodontal Disease Risk**
      1. Obesity may be a predisposing factor to periodontal disease.
      2. Obese individuals who consume foods heavy in fat, sodium, and refined carbohydrates frequently avoid healthy, nutrient dense foods.
      3. Japanese researchers have discovered a possible association between obesity and periodontal disease. In one study overall abdominal obesity was associated with increased prevalence of periodontal disease [17].
      4. In a 2003 study, researchers found that obese adolescents with diets high in refined carbohydrates and deficient in vitamin C and calcium have an increased incidence of periodontal disease.
   B. **Physical characteristics of food**
      1. In animals fibrous foods have a tooth cleansing effect, and fibrous or hard foods can decrease plaque biofilm accumulation and decrease gingivitis, but in humans the physical characteristics of food appears unrelated to plaque biofilm accumulation and gingivitis [18].
      2. Study design between humans and animals is so different that this may account for this apparent contradiction; for example, it is impossible to place humans on hard diets for an extended time period.

3. **Nutrients That Can Promote Periodontal Health.** The human body requires daily nourishment to carry out body functions (Box 21-1). The more nutrient dense our diet, the greater the benefit to all body cells, and interactions between nutrition, infection, and the immune system may be of high importance in the oral cavity. It appears that to maintain periodontal health, we need specific nutrients to build new tissue, maintain an optimal immune system, and repair damaged tissue (TABLE 21-2).

BOX 21-1. How Does the Body Use Nutrients at a Cellular Level?

Every bite of food affects our body at the cellular level. For example, think of biting into a fresh sweet carrot. Everyone knows carrots are good for you and are rich in carotene, which is a precursor to vitamin A. The crunch, while chewing, is satisfying, stimulates saliva and can take the sensation of hunger away. But the real benefit of eating a carrot happens after digestion when micronutrients are delivered to all body cells. Vitamin A is used by the body's complex repair system to form new tissue where needed. If the sulcular epithelium is damaged by periodontal instrumentation, new epithelium must be formed. Ample amounts of vitamin A and other micronutrients must be present to repair the sulcular lining. Eating foods rich in vitamin A—like carrots—assure that the nutrient vitamin A is present when needed.

TABLE 21-2.	Function of Nutrients			
Nutrient	Tissue Synthesis	Healthy Immune System	Repair Damaged Tissue	Modulate Host Response
Vitamin A	x	x		
Vitamin B-complex	x	x		
Vitamin C		x	x	
Vitamin D	x			
Protein	x		x	
Calcium	x			
Iron	x		x	x
Zinc	x		x	x
Copper			x	
Selenium				x
Magnesium	x			

A. **Nutrients That Build a Healthy Periodontium**
   1. One example of a tissue within the periodontium that must be constantly renewed is sulcular epithelium, since sulcular epithelium has a very rapid turnover rate.
   2. Building and maintaining healthy sulcular epithelium is one of the body's first lines of defense against periodontal disease.
   3. To assist with continual generation of healthy sulcular epithelium the body needs protein, vitamins A, B-complex, D and minerals calcium and magnesium.
   4. In addition, strong alveolar bone is necessary for periodontal health, and vitamin D enhances the absorption of calcium and magnesium, giving strength to the alveolar process that supports the dentition.

B. **Nutrients That Build a Healthy Immune System**
   1. A healthy immune system, functioning at optimum performance, will help contain the bacterial assault that causes periodontal disease.
   2. Nutrients that help maintain a healthy immune system are vitamin A, vitamin B complex, and vitamin C.

C. **Nutrients That Help Tissue Repair**
   1. Periodontal infections might be compared to a "wound" that must be repaired and allowed to heal; inadequate nutrition may hinder this repair process.
   2. Vitamin C, iron, zinc, and copper all assist in collagen formation, a substance that helps with repair of all wounds including wounds in the periodontium.
   3. In addition, protein is the major nutrient that maintains and repairs diseased or injured tissue.

Section 2
Nutritional Counseling for a Healthy Periodontium

Making an appropriate connection between diet, nutrients, and periodontal disease can allow clinicians to make specific suggestions to improve a patient's diet. When indicated clinically, nutritional counseling, with an emphasis on periodontal health and root caries prevention, should be offered to periodontal patients. Teaching patients good dietary habits can be accomplished using standard diet forms, counseling techniques, and analysis procedures. The following information on nutritional counseling for a healthy periodontium is adapted from Sroda R. Diet, nutrition, and periodontal disease, Chapter 10. In *Nutrition for a Healthy Mouth*. 2 ed. Philadelphia: Lippincott Williams & Wilkins, 2009.

1. **Use of Diet Diaries**
   A. Diet diaries are varied. Choices are 24-hour recall—which is great for chair side counseling while waiting on a doctor-check—or 3-, 5-, or 7-day diet diaries for more in-depth counseling sessions.
   B. Involving the patient in the decision-making process as much as possible is the best counseling technique. Patient ownership of choices and decisions assures greater compliance and success.
   C. Following these five basic suggestions for good overall health will help all patients maintain good periodontal health.
      1. Follow the USDA My Pyramid for good overall health. (http://www.mypyramid.gov)
      2. Follow the USDA Guidelines for Healthy Americans, or guidelines appropriate for the patient's culture heritage. (http://www.health.gov/dietaryguidelines/)
      3. Take a daily multivitamin that contains no more than 100% of the US recommended daily allowance for both vitamins and minerals.
      4. Include at least one crunchy food at each meal.
      5. Include foods especially rich in antioxidants (vitamins A, C, E, selenium), vitamin D and calcium, omega-3 polyunsaturated fats.

2. **Steps That May Be Used for Nutritional Counseling**
   A. Review the medical and dental history, as well as intra/extra oral exam findings, for physical issues that relate to periodontal health (for e.g., anemia, use of multiple medications by a patient, hypertension, diabetes, new or recurrent caries, angular cheilitis, or denuded lingual papillae).
   B. Instruct the patient to keep a diet diary for several days. Educational institutions are usually willing to share diet intake forms and examples are available in nutrition textbooks.
   C. Analyze the patient-reported diet.
   D. Create a personalized nutritional profile for the patient at www.mypyramid.gov.
   E. Compare suggested servings for all food groups with recommendations based on the patient's lifestyle. Assure adequate dietary protein and dairy products.
   F. Evaluate frequency of eating crunchy foods.
   G. Evaluate inclusion of specific nutrients: antioxidants, vitamin D and calcium, omega-3 fats, etc.
   H. Make specific food suggestions according to TABLE 21-3 if a deficiency is noted.
   I. Explain the function of nutrients in the maintenance of periodontal health.

J. Evaluate frequency of consumption of refined carbohydrates and explain the difference between refined and complex carbohydrates. Explain the relationship between high consumption of refined carbohydrates and inflammatory periodontal disease.

K. Explain the benefit of eating foods rich in lactic acid and soy.

TABLE 21-3. Nutrient Food Sources	
Nutrient	**Food Source**
Antioxidants	
Vitamin A	Carrots, sweet potato, pumpkin, spinach, collards, kale, turnip greens
Vitamin C	Citrus fruits, kiwi, papaya, bell peppers, broccoli, strawberries, cauliflower, kale
Vitamin E	Fortified cereal, sunflower seeds, almonds, olives, papaya, swiss chard
Selenium	Snapper, halibut, cod, tuna, shrimp, lamb, barley
Zinc	Liver, beef, lamb, venison, pumpkin seeds, yogurt, green peas
Other vitamins	
B-Complex	Eggs, meat, legumes, milk
Vitamin D	Salmon, shrimp, cow's milk, cod
Major nutrients	
Protein	Meat, cow's milk, eggs, fish, legumes, peas, beans, grains
Omega-3	Tuna, salmon, mackerel, walnuts, flax seeds, canola oil
Minerals	
Calcium	Fortified cereal, soy, sardines, tofu, cow's milk, yogurt, sesame seeds, spinach, mozzarella cheese
Iron	Clams, oysters, organ meats, fortified cereal, white beans, soybeans, pumpkin
Copper	Liver, whole grains, nuts, legumes, vegetables, and fruits
Magnesium	Pumpkin, brazil nuts, fortified cereal, halibut, spinach, almonds
Soy isoflavones	Tofu, soymilk, tempeh, soy beans, soy sauce

Chapter Summary Statement

Though periodontal disease cannot be caused by nutritional deficiencies, some nutritional deficiencies do indeed appear to modify the severity and extent of the periodontal disease.

Research links specific nutrient deficiencies and foods high in refined carbohydrates to increased inflammation—the very kind that triggers the host-mediated inflammatory response seen in periodontal disease. It is wise to counsel patients with periodontal disease to be thoughtful food shoppers and to prepare meals and snacks that are rich in specific nutrients.

Section 3
Focus on Patients

Case 1: Mr. Phillip Burgess

Directions for Case 1: Review the assessment and 24-hour diet recall for fictitious patient Phillip Burgess located on pages 355 and 356. Answer the following questions regarding Mr. Burgess.

1. What are this patient's diet-related periodontal concerns?
2. Which food choices could be contributing to gingival inflammation?
3. What simple change could Mr. Burgess make that would decrease refined carbohydrates and add complex carbohydrates?
4. What food group is absent in the 24-hour diet recall?
5. Did Mr. Burgess' diet include any good sources of antioxidants?
6. As his dental hygienist, what nutritional advice would you give Mr. Burgess to help repair damage caused by the infection?

Assessment Information: Mr. Burgess

Phillip Burgess: 39-year-old single Caucasian male: cellular telephone sales representative

Periodontal Diagnosis: generalized mild chronic periodontitis

Purpose of Visit: "My gums are bleeding when I brush and sometimes when I eat hard foods."

Medical History:
- 5'10"; 190 lb
- Blood pressure: 125/86
- Has not seen physician for 3 years
- Currently not taking any medications; no known allergies

Dental History:
- No restorations; all third molars were extracted 20 years ago
- Carious lesions at gingival-third on facial of teeth No. 3 and 14, and 30 and 31
- Last dental visit about 6 years ago

Periodontal Chart:
- Generalized 4–6 mm pocket depths with no recession
- Generalized moderate to heavy bleeding
- Class I furcation involvement on facial of teeth #3, 14, 19, 30
- No mobility

Plaque Biofilm Record: O'Leary Plaque Biofilm Score is 100%

Oral Hygiene Assessment: Patient reports brushing once in the morning and rarely flosses.

Radiographs: Loss of interproximal lamina dura, slight horizontal bone loss in posteriors with generalized moderate calculus deposits (Case 1 continues on the next page)

Mr. Burgess' 24-Hour Diet Recall

Breakfast:

Two cups of coffee with nondairy creamer and two teaspoons of sugar

Scrambled eggs in flour tortilla

Four pieces of Canadian bacon

Lunch:

Wendy's double hamburger with cheese, lettuce, tomato, onion

Baked Potato with sour cream and butter

Regular Frosty

Large Coke

Snack:

One can regular Coke

One small bag chips

Dinner:

Large serving of Spaghetti with three medium-sized meatballs

Tossed salad with Italian dressing

Six black olives

Two pieces garlic toast

Water

Case 2

A 52-year-old male is new to your practice and presents with generalized 6- to 7-mm pockets in mandibular and maxillary posteriors. Tissues are marginally red with generalized slight to moderate bleeding upon probing. Oral examination reveals a bright red shiny tongue, extraction of all third molars and large carious lesions on third posterior teeth. He reports eating a soft diet due to broken carious teeth and is a practicing vegetarian. Last dental visit was over 10 years ago. Evaluation of oral hygiene practices reveals ineffective daily plaque biofilm removal with toothbrushing and no interproximal cleaning. What can be deducted about the relationship between his diet and oral condition, and what would you recommend during diet counseling?

References

1. Enwonwu CO. Cellular and molecular effects of malnutrition and their relevance to periodontal diseases. *J Clin Periodontol*. 1994;21(10):643–657.
2. Bikle DD. Vitamin D and the immune system: role in protection against bacterial infection. *Curr Opin Nephrol Hypertens*. 2008;17(4):348–352.
3. Nishida M, Grossi SG, Dunford RG, Ho AW, et al. Calcium and the risk for periodontal disease. *J Periodontol*. 2000;71(7):1057–1066.
4. Krall EA, Wehler C, Garcia RI, Harris SS, et al. Calcium and vitamin D supplements reduce tooth loss in the elderly. *Am J Med*. 2001;111(6):452–456.
5. Hildebolt CF. Effect of vitamin D and calcium on periodontitis. *J Periodontol*. 2005;76(9):1576–1587.
6. Shimazaki Y, Shirota T, Uchida K, Yonemoto K, et al. Intake of dairy products and periodontal disease: the Hisayama Study. *J Periodontol*. 2008;79(1):131–137.
7. Woolfe SN, Hume WR, Kenney EB. Ascorbic acid and periodontal disease: a review of the literature. *J West Soc Periodontol Periodontal Abstr*. 1980;28(2):44–56.
8. Amaliya TMF, Abbas F, Loos BG, Van der Weijden GA, et al. Java project on periodontal diseases: the relationship between vitamin C and the severity of periodontitis. *J Clin Periodontol*. 2007;34(4):299–304.
9. Nishida M, Grossi SG, Dunford RG, Ho AW, et al. Dietary vitamin C and the risk for periodontal disease. *J Periodontol*. 2000;71(8):1215–1223.
10. Leger D. Scurvy: reemergence of nutritional deficiencies. *Can Fam Physician*. 2008;54(10):1403–1406.
11. Moran JR, Greene HL. The B vitamins and vitamin C in human nutrition. II. 'Conditional' B vitamins and vitamin C. *Am J Dis Child*. 1979;133(3):308–314.
12. Riepe FG, Eichmann D, Oppermann HC, Schmitt HJ, et al. Special feature: picture of the month. Infantile scurvy. *Arch Pediatr Adolesc Med*. 2001;155(5):607–608.
13. Chapple IL. Potential mechanisms underpinning the nutritional modulation of periodontal inflammation. *J Am Dent Assoc*. 2009;140(2):178–184.
14. Woodward B. Protein, calories, and immune defenses. *Nutr Rev*. 1998;56(1 Pt 2):S84–S92.
15. Sawyer DR, Nwoku AL, Rotimi VO, and Hagen JC. Comparison of oral microflora between well-nourished and malnourished Nigerian children. *ASDC J Dent Child*. 1986;53(6):439–443.
16. Enwonwu CO, Phillips RS, Falkler WA Jr. Nutrition and oral infectious diseases: state of the science. *Compend Contin Educ Dent*. 2002;23(5):431–434, 436, 438 passim; quiz 448.
17. Al-Zahrani MS, Bissada NF, Borawskit EA. Obesity and periodontal disease in young, middle-aged, and older adults. *J Periodontol*. 2003;74(5):610–615.
18. Alfano MC. Controversies, perspectives, and clinical implications of nutrition in periodontal disease. *Dent Clin North Am*. 1976;20(3):519–548.

Best Practices for Periodontal Care

Learning Objectives

- Define the term best practice.
- Summarize how the explosion of knowledge is impacting practitioners and patients.
- Identify the three components of evidence-based decision making.
- Define a systematic review.
- Discuss the benefits and limitations of experience.
- Describe the role of the patient in the evidence-based model.
- List locations for accessing systematic reviews.
- Explain the difference between a peer-reviewed journal and trade magazine.
- State desired three outcomes from attending continuing education courses.
- Formulate a question using the PICO process.

Key Terms

Best practice
Evidence-based healthcare
Confirmation bias
Best evidence
Levels of evidence
Systematic review

PICO process
Databases
TRIP database
Cochrane collaboration
MEDLINE (PubMed)
Peer-reviewed journal

Section 1
What is Best Practice?

Providing the best possible care to patients is the foremost goal of all dental healthcare providers. Yet it is generally acknowledged that periodontal care may vary from office to office and even by regions of the country. *As new procedures and techniques become available, hygienists committed to excellence must regularly update and adapt their strategies for providing patient care.* The approach known as "best practice" is an important tool in helping hygienists provide high-quality care to their patients.

1. Overview of the Concept of Best Practice
   A. **Definition.** Best practice can be defined as clinical practices, treatments, and interventions that result in the best possible outcome for the patient [1].
   B. **Goals and Considerations.**
      1. The goal of best practice is consistent, superior patient outcomes.
         a. The outcomes should be measurable such as a reduction in probing depths.
         b. The outcome should be reproducible. For example, if a technique produces a certain result on one patient, it is reasonable to expect a similar outcome when the technique is used with other patients.
      2. How do we know what a best practice is? The process begins with understanding the common sources of information available to dental healthcare providers: (1) research data, (2) personal experience, and (3) expert opinion.
2. Circumstances That Prompted the Best Practice Approach to Patient Care
   A. **Direct Access to Rapidly Emerging Clinical Research Information**
      1. Explosion of Information
         a. Information about new techniques, tests, procedures, and products for periodontal care is emerging at an astonishing rate. Hundreds of articles are published in dental journals each year.
         b. In addition to the information in dental journals, relevant articles are published each year in medical and specialty journals. Examples of articles in other disciplines that are relevant to periodontal health are those on the topic of the oral/systemic link; important research on this topic is in journals such as the *New England Journal of Medicine* or *Diabetes Care*.
      2. Direct Access to Information
         a. In the past, dental healthcare providers relied on what they learned in school and the advice of recognized experts to determine how to provide care. Patients had little or no input into this process. Knowledge of new or cutting-edge research was limited to a few practitioners with access to an educational or healthcare institution.
         b. Today, with the Internet, clinicians have instant access to the results of federally funded clinical trials on treatment methods, equipment, and materials. PubMed, a gateway to more than 18 million research citations, can be accessed by anyone for free.
         c. *Practicing dental hygienists are expected to remain current with new techniques, devices, and materials that will result in improvements in periodontal care.* Dental hygienists in private practice cannot continue to use the same treatments and techniques learned in dental hygiene school year after year. The best practice 2 years ago may not represent the highest standard of care today.

B. **Active Patient Role in Decision Making**
   1. Today's patient expects to be a partner in the decision-making process about his or her own periodontal care. Patients arrive at the dental office with information downloaded from the Internet.
   2. Before the widespread use of information technology, patients depended on the expertise of a healthcare provider for advice and in most cases accepted that advice without question.

3. **Interpreting the Literature**
   A. **Not All Studies Are Significant to Clinical Care.** Even though hundreds of studies are published yearly, very few are significant enough on their own to merit a change in clinical care.
      1. The merit or weight of study is influenced by its design.
      2. No study is completely free of bias. Reputable journals require investigators to declare a conflict of interest and disclose corporate financial support for studies.
      3. Many studies either are not designed to provide an answer to the needs of the clinician or provide results that are too weak to merit implementation.
   B. **New Does Not Necessarily Mean Better**
      1. New treatments and products need to demonstrate consistent superiority to established methods.
      2. Some new products and therapies are also significantly more costly to implement, and these costs are ultimately passed down to patients.
   C. **Associations Are Not the Same as Cause and Effect.** Over the past several years, many studies have looked at the relationship between periodontal disease and a host of systemic conditions. While many studies do show that periodontal disease is more common in people with some conditions such as uncontrolled diabetes, at the time of this writing, a cause and effect between the two has not been established.

Section 2
The Role of Evidence-Based Care in Best Practice

1. **Introduction to Evidence-Based Care.** The American Dental Hygienists' Association (ADHA) advocates evidence-based, patient/client-centered *dental hygiene* practice.
   A. **Definition.** The ADHA defines evidence-based healthcare as the conscientious, explicit, and judicious use of current best evidence in making decisions about the care of individual patients. The practice of evidence-based dental hygiene requires the integration of individual clinical expertise and patient preferences with the best available external clinical evidence from systematic research [2].
   B. **Why is there a need for evidence-based care?**
      1. The goal of evidence-based healthcare is to assist healthcare professionals in applying the most current and best scientific evidence to patient care. In other words, to improve health outcomes by closing the gap between what is known—research—versus what is practiced (the care that patients receive in medical and dental offices) [3–6].
      2. Studies of appropriateness of dental and dental hygiene care confirm that there is a wide range of variability between what is known to be best practice and the care that patients actually receive [4,5]. Recent studies on dental hygienists' knowledge and practices relating to oral cancer detection and caries prevention showed variation in knowledge and practices [7–10].
      3. In addition, studies found that the longer healthcare providers were out of school, the less current their knowledge [11–13].
   C. **About Evidence-Based Care**
      1. Evidence-based care integrates the best research evidence with clinical expertise and patient values [13].
      2. Evidence-based healthcare includes three foundational elements: (1) incorporation of the best scientific evidence with (2) the healthcare provider's clinical expertise and (3) patient's preferences and values. Figure 22-1 illustrates these three foundational elements of evidence-based healthcare.
      3. There is a vast amount of dental literature published every year.
         a. In 1998, approximately 10,000 journal articles were published in English [14]. Considering this, it is not surprising that busy dental healthcare providers find it difficult to keep up with current research.
         b. Fortunately, there are numerous trustworthy resources and mechanisms for busy practitioners who want to implement high-quality science into patient care. Resources are discussed in Section 3 of this chapter.

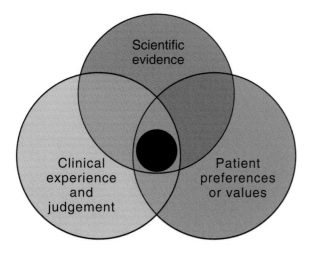

Figure 22.1. The Three Foundational Elements of Evidence-Based Healthcare. Evidence-based care has three equal components: scientific evidence, clinical experience, and patient preferences or values.

Box 22-1. Evidence-Based Practice: An Example

Evidence-based practice is built on information obtained from research.

For example, perhaps a dental hygienist was taught in school that ultrasonic instrumentation should be used sparingly and only for the removal of large supragingival calculus deposits. In addition, the hygienist learned in school that hand instruments produce the best results for periodontal information.

After reading current research on ultrasonic instrumentation, the hygienist learns that modern slim-tipped ultrasonic instruments can be used subgingivally and that a combination of ultrasonic and hand instrumentation leads to excellent results.

This evidence motivates the dental hygienist to attend a continuing education course on ultrasonic instrumentation and to incorporate ultrasonic instrumentation in treating periodontitis.

C. **Three Foundational Elements of Evidence-Based Care**
1. Evidence-based care recognizes that it is essential that all three foundational elements are present in order to obtain the best health outcomes [3,15].
    a. Over time, healthcare providers gain clinical expertise by engaging in clinical experiences (i.e., treating patients and observing the results).
    b. Patients' preferences may be the result of many factors including past dental experiences, perceived needs, health values, and economic considerations.
    c. The most challenging of the three elements for the healthcare professional is the systematic assessment of scientific evidence obtained from reliable sources (Box 22-1).
2. Clinical experience is both valuable and limiting. It signifies the ability of a clinician to grow in skill and knowledge through experience.
    a. Experience helps the practitioner make thoughtful clinical judgments about the applicability of research findings to individual patient situations. Yet all patients are different; they may present with complicated or complex medical and dental histories.
    b. Experience is valuable when it is used as a learning rather than reinforcement tool. Ideally, a clinician uses his or her clinical experiences in making better treatment decisions.
    c. Experience can be limiting. The limitation is that not all individuals are able to learn and grow from experience. To acquire "practical wisdom" the clinician needs to learn how to be reflective and analyze his or her own performance.
        1) There is a human tendency to look for or interpret information that confirms our beliefs. This tendency is called confirmation bias.
        2) Confirmation bias can lead practitioners to misinterpret information based on beliefs, positive or negative, about a treatment or device.
3. Patient preference is an important consideration in treatment selection. If due consideration is not given to the individual patient's preferences and concerns, the likelihood of the patient fully accepting the clinician's recommendation is diminished.

    a. It is the dental hygienist's responsibility to understand the evidence and its implications for periodontal treatment and communicate it effectively to a patient. Ultimately, it will be the patient who chooses which therapy he or she prefers.

    b. In helping a patient decide which treatment is right for him or her, there are several elements that should be discussed, including

        1) The evidence about a particular treatment option.

        2) The treatment of choice based on the evidence.

        3) All possible treatment alternatives.

        4) The risks of no treatment at all.

    c. In addition to the efficacy of a proposed treatment, a patient may place equal weight on other aspects of treatment such as

        1) Cost. Patients usually are concerned about what a treatment will cost. In addition, patients decide if the treatment has benefits that they perceive as being worth the cost.

        2) Pain. Assurances about pain control and management help lessen these concerns.

        3) Time lost from work. Different jobs and work environments have varying levels of flexibility in allowing employees time off for health-related matters.

        4) Impact on family. Caregivers of young children or elderly family members may feel that they do not have the time to devote to periodontal treatment. Individuals with chronic health problems may believe that periodontal care is no longer a priority.

        5) Insurance benefits. A practice reality is that patients will sometimes choose care based on what insurance will pay versus the full treatment recommendation.

2. Evaluation of Scientific Evidence. All scientific evidence is not created equal.

  A. Levels of Evidence. Best evidence is the highest level of evidence available for a specific clinical question.

    1. Levels of evidence is a ranking system used in evidence-based care to describe the strength of the results measured in a clinical trial or research study. In simple terms, one way of looking at levels of evidence is as follows (the higher the level, the better the quality; the lower, the greater the bias). Figure 22-2 illustrates the levels of evidence.

    2. Based on a hierarchy of levels of evidence, systematic reviews of randomized controlled trials constitute the highest level of current best evidence, and expert opinion is lower-level evidence.

    3. The highest level of evidence available represents the current best evidence for a specific clinical question.

  B. Systematic Reviews: The Highest Ranked Source of Evidence

    1. A systematic review is a concise summary of individual research studies on a treatment or device to determine the overall validity and clinical applicability of that treatment or device.

    a. The systematic review process strives to comprehensively identify and track down all the literature on a given topic. And then, to summarize, appraise, and communicate the results and implications in a concise form for healthcare professions who need this information to keep up-to-date.

    b. Internationally, the stimulus for systematic reviews has come from the Cochrane Collaboration, a worldwide group of subject and methodological specialists who aim to identify and synthesize the research in all aspects of healthcare.

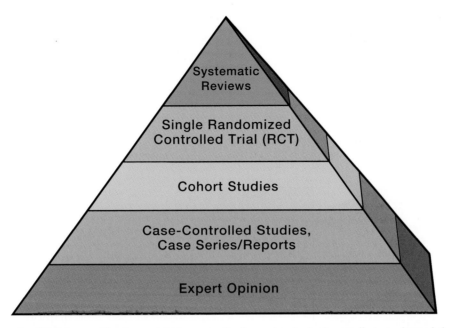

Figure 22.2. Levels of Evidence. The importance or merit of a research study usually is evaluated through its design. Systematic reviews and randomized controlled trails represent the best levels of evidence. Case reports and expert opinion are the lowest levels of evidence.

2. Systematic reviews are, by their very nature, efficient. As an information management tool they provide a way of coping with large volumes of data in a concise and manageable form.
   a. With more than 2 million articles published in medical and dental journals annually, it is impossible for any one healthcare provider to read and utilize all the new information.
   b. Systematic reviews provide a way to more efficiently keep up with current research and provide data for better decision making [16].
   c. Systematic reviews also facilitate the development of best practice guidelines by bringing together all that is known about a given topic in a non-biased manner.
3. Because of the emphasis on evidenced-based care, there are more systematic reviews conducted in dentistry than before.
4. The systematic review makes incorporating evidence-based care easier. In the past, practitioners were encouraged to do their own searching for research. Since most busy practitioners do not have the time or expertise to do this, the systematic review fills this gap.

Section 3
Finding Clinically Relevant Information

The Centre for Evidence-Based Medicine (CEBM) recommends a straightforward approach based on (1) formulating a question; (2) searching evaluated (secondary) resources—such as the TRIP database—and (3) then examining primary text documents—such as from PubMed [17,18]. Figure 22-3 illustrates this straightforward approach to finding clinically relevant information.

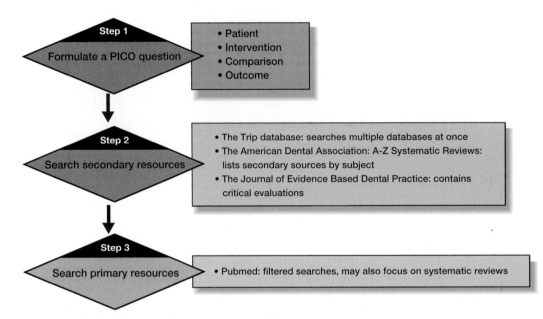

Figure 22.3. Best Strategy for Finding Evidence. The CEBM recommends a straightforward approach based on (1) formulating a question; (2) searching evaluated (secondary) resources, and (3) then examining primary text documents.

1. **Formulate a Question.** A clinical question may develop from questions that arise relative to patient care or from an area in which the hygienist wants up-dated knowledge. In order to find the best information to help patients, it is fundamental to learn how to ask the "right questions." This is more challenging than it seems. It involves converting problems into answerable questions.
   A. **Use Four Components to Structure The Question.** The structure for asking a clear and focused question entails four critical components, known as the PICO Process [19]. The PICO process involves the combination of four separate components to form an answerable question: "Patient, Intervention, Comparison, and Outcome."
      1. P (Patient or Problem). An example of the P component might be: "*A periodontal maintenance patient with bleeding and gingivitis.*"
      2. I (Intervention)
         a. An intervention is a specific diagnostic test, treatment, adjunctive therapy, medication, product, or clinical procedure.
         b. An example of an intervention being questioned is: "*brushing and daily home irrigation.*"
      3. C (Comparison)
         a. Identifies the specific alternative therapy or device that you wish to compare to the main intervention.

      b. An example of the "C" segment of the question is: *"compared to brushing and flossing."*

    4. O (Outcome)

      a. Identifies the measurable outcome you plan to accomplish, improve, or influence.

      b. An example of the "O" segment of the question is: *"reduce gingivitis and bleeding within four weeks."*

  B. Formulate the Question. Once each of the PICO components has been determined, the clinician combines them into an answerable question. Using the above examples, the question would read: *"For a periodontal maintenance patient with bleeding and gingivitis, will brushing and daily home irrigation OR brushing and flossing provide a better reduction in bleeding and gingivitis within four weeks?"*

2. Search Secondary Resources for Systematic Reviews

  A. Databases.

    1. The most efficient way to go about finding relevant research is to use an online index of published articles, such as PubMed, MEDLINE, or CINAHL (Cumulative Index of Nursing and Allied Health Literature).

    2. These indexes—known as databases—list all articles published in a given period of time by journals in a particular profession or group of professions.

  B. Systematic Reviews. Many dental healthcare providers do not have the time or expertise needed to do their own systematic reviews of a question. Fortunately, there are numerous trustworthy resources for busy practitioners who want to implement high-quality science into patient care. Box 22-2 lists some of the secondary resources for systematic reviews.

Box 22-2. Websites for Accessing Systematic Reviews

- TRIP Database: http://www.tripdatabase.com

- Cochrane Collaboration: http://www.cochrane.org

- Pubmed: http://www.pubmed.gov

- American Dental Association Center for Evidence-based Dentistry: http://ebd.ada.org/

  C. The TRIP Database

    1. The TRIP Database—one of the Internet's leading resources for Evidence-Based Medicine—allows users to rapidly identify the highest quality clinical evidence for clinical practice.

    2. The aims of the TRIP Database are to allow health professionals to easily find the highest-quality material available on the web—to help support evidence-based practice.

    3. The database is subdivided into specialist sites. The Oral Health Specialist site searches both the core TRIP content plus 14 of the leading dental journals.

    4. The Oral Health specialist site is accessed at http://www.tripdatabase.com/oral/specialismhomepage.html.

  D. The Cochrane Collaboration Database of Systematic Reviews

    1. The Cochrane Collaboration was established in 1993 by a British epidemiologist, who recognized that ready access to systematic reviews of available evidence would facilitate better-informed decisions by healthcare providers.

2. The Cochrane Database of Systematic Reviews includes systematic reviews of healthcare interventions that are produced and disseminated by The Cochrane Collaboration; a global not-for-profit organization.

   a. The Cochrane Library is published quarterly and is available on CD-ROM. Abstracts of reviews are free.

   b. Also, many health science libraries subscribe to the Cochrane databases so that faculty and students have free online access.

3. The Cochrane review group relevant to periodontics is the Oral Health Review Group. An example of a systematic review conducted by the Oral Health Group is on the topic of psychological interventions to improve adherence to oral hygiene instructions in adults with periodontal diseases.

4. A complete listing of topics and abstracts can be accessed at http://www.cochrane.org/reviews/index.htm.

E. **The MEDLINE Database: The National Library of Medicine**

1. MEDLINE (PubMed) that enable quick access to locate relevant clinical evidence in the published literature (FIG. 22-4) [20].

2. Anyone can access MEDLINE for free using PubMed—a gateway hosted by the National Library of Medicine.

   a. One feature is the PubMed Clinical Query, which provides specialized searches using evidenced-based filter.

   b. After plugging in traditional key words, practitioners have the options of selecting "Find Systematic Reviews." This streamlines searches by quickly and easily locating systematic review on a desired topic.

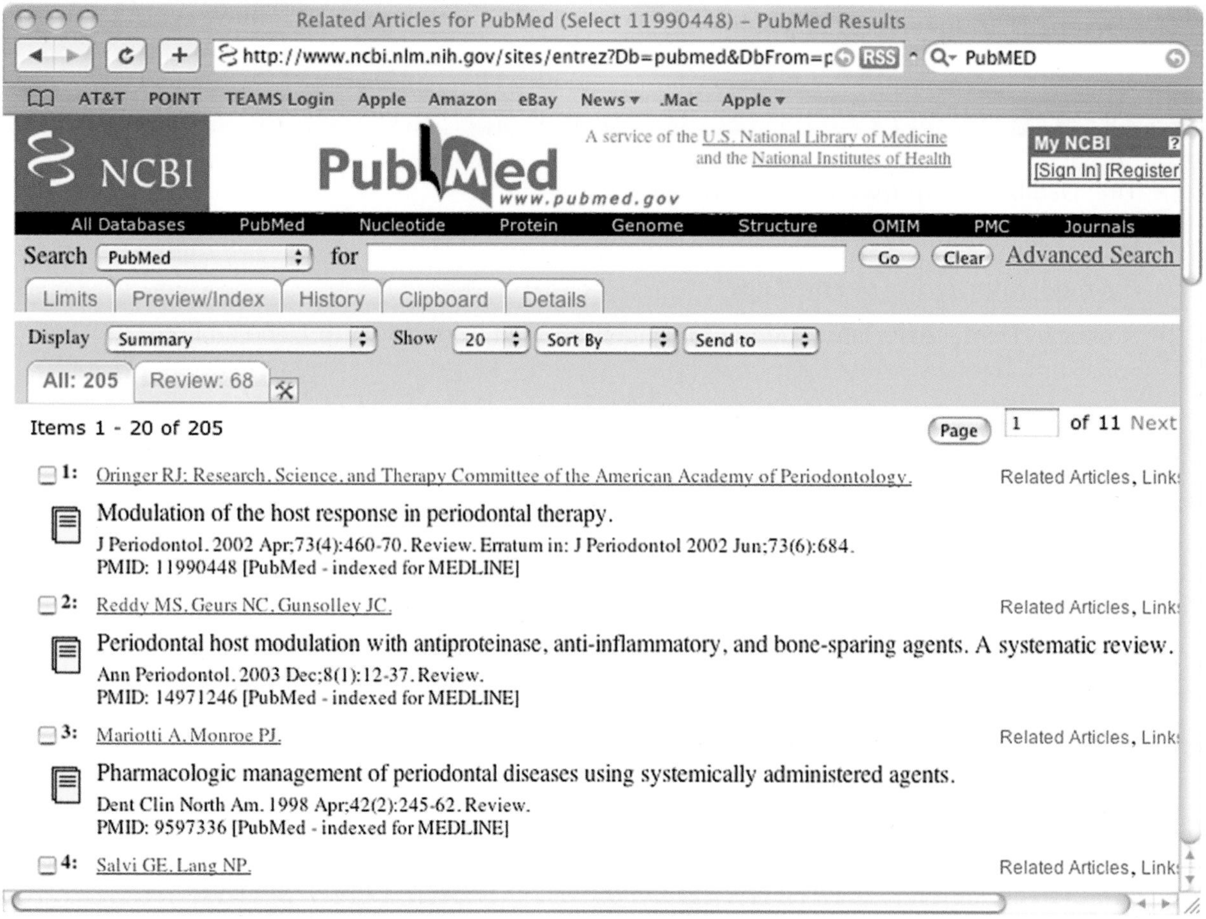

Figure 22.4. PubMed Website. PubMed search results for the topic "host modulation." (Courtesy of the US National Library of Medicine, Bethesda, MD.)

F. **Systematic Reviews by Professional Organizations.** Many professional organizations are developing systematic reviews. The American Dental Association recently developed a web-based Center for Evidenced-based Dentistry (http://ebd.ada.org)

G. **Systematic Reviews in Evidence-Based Journals**
1. Evidence-based journals publish summaries of valid research studies to simplify the evidence-based process for dental healthcare providers.
2. For example, The Journal of Evidence-Based Dental Practice scans the top dental journals and a panel reviews the selected articles for clinical relevance to practice.
3. Other examples of evidence-based journals include: Evidence-Based Dentistry, Evidence-Based Medicine, Evidence-Based Healthcare, and Evidence-Based Nursing.

3. **Examine Primary Text Documents.** The third step for finding evidence is to examine primary text documents. Abstracts and some full text journal articles are available on MEDLINE. Loansome Doc enables PubMed users to order documents found in MEDLINE. It is available to users in the US and internationally. A user can order articles from a list of citations retrieved from PubMed by sending requests to a library for the full-text documents. Users must register for this service; directions for using the Lonesome Doc service are found at http://www.nlm.nih.gov/pubs/factsheets/loansome_doc.html.

CLINICAL CASE EXAMPLE

A dental hygienist used the following steps to find evidence-based clinically relevant information.
1. Step 1: Formulate a PICO question.
   - Patient: adult female patient with chronic periodontitis; new patient in the dental office
   - Intervention: periodontal instrumentation
   - Comparison: full mouth disinfection versus quadrant instrumentation
   - Outcome: resolution of inflammation
   - Question: For a patient with chronic periodontitis, will full mouth disinfection OR quadrant instrumentation provide a better reduction in inflammation?
2. Step 2: Search online evidence-based sources in the following order:
   a. TRIP Database: Oral Health Section (Box 22-3)
   b. ADA Center for Evidence-Based Dentisty (Box 22-4)
   c. PubMed limited to systematic reviews (Box 22-4)
3. The results of the search suggest that both the traditional quadrant approach and the newer the full-mouth debridement could be equally effective.
4. In this instance, the dental hygienist presented both options to the patient, explaining that both treatment options are equally effective.
5. The patient chose full mouth debridement because it would be less disruptive for her to be away from work for 1 day rather than four shorter appointments over a period of several weeks.

Box 22-3. TRIP Database Results

Main Results

The search identified 216 abstracts. Review of these abstracts resulted in 12 publications for detailed review. Finally, seven randomized controlled trials (RCTs) which met the criteria for eligibility were independently selected by two review authors. None of the studies included reported on tooth loss. All treatment modalities led to significant improvements in clinical parameters after a follow-up of at least 3 months. For the secondary outcome, reduction in probing depth, the mean difference between full mouth disinfection and control was 0.53 mm (95% confidence interval [CI]: 0.28 to 0.77) in moderately deep pockets of single rooted teeth and for gain in probing attachment 0.33 mm (95% CI: 0.04 to 0.63) in moderately deep single and multirooted teeth. Comparing full mouth disinfection (FMD) and full mouth scaling (FMS) the mean difference in one study for gain in probing attachment amounted to 0.74 mm in favor of FMS (95% CI: 0.17 to 1.31) for deep pockets in multirooted teeth, while another study reported a mean difference for reduction in bleeding on probing of 18% in favor of FMD (95% CI: −34.30 to −1.70) for deep pockets of single rooted teeth. No significant differences were observed for any of the outcome measures, when comparing full mouth disinfection and control.

Authors' Conclusions

In patients with chronic periodontitis in moderately deep pockets slightly more favorable outcomes for pocket reduction and gain in probing attachment were found following full mouth disinfection compared to control. However, these additional improvements were only modest and there was only a very limited number of studies available for comparison, thus limiting general conclusions about the clinical benefit of full mouth disinfection.

Box 22-4. ADA Center for Evidence-Based Dentisty and PubMed Systematic Review Results

Results: The same results were found as on the TRIP Database.

Section 4
Lifelong Learning Skills for Best Practice

One of the most challenging but important aspects of getting to best practices involves self evaluation. Practitioners continually need to think about whether the care they are providing is still the best level care. There are several questions a dental hygienist should think about on a regular basis.

1. **How sure am I that what I do is right?**
   A. **Do I know where to access systematic reviews?**
   B. **Do I keep up with journal reading?**
      1. Peer-Reviewed Journals
         a. Peer-reviewed journals (also called refereed journals) use a panel of experts to review research articles for study design, statistics, and conclusions.
         b. Good sources for randomized clinical trials, and learning about new research findings. Sometimes will publish systematic reviews.
         c. Subscriptions may be expensive thus making access to the information difficult. In more recent years, some highly ranked peer-reviewed journals from professional associations have begun to allow free access to full studies 6 months after publication.
      2. Practice or Trade Magazines
         a. Can be commercial in nature
         b. May or may not be peer-reviewed; generally provide more of the "expert" opinion
         c. May or may not be supported with references
         d. Vary widely in quality
      3. Textbooks
         a. Provide a broad overview of a subject
         b. May not provide specifics on the research
         c. May be dated because of the amount of time involved in writing and publishing a textbook; always check the publication date
   C. **Do I attend continuing education courses?**
      1. Content: Is the subject matter something you like or something that you need? It is important to take the time to evaluate learning/practice needs. Conferring with co-workers or your employer can facilitate more objective choices.
      2. Speaker. Are they an expert, a facilitator, or both? A well-rounded speaker will provide information on the latest research findings along with providing some practical advice based on experience.
      3. Outcomes: A well-rounded continuing education course will do three things [21]:
         a. Reaffirm: The course information provides support for your current ways of providing treatment.
         b. Reenergize: The course supports changes in areas that you have previously identified, and provides the motivation and impetus to begin making those changes,
         c. Reexamine: The course addresses new research findings that merit further study and investigation as to the appropriateness of incorporation into practice.
   D. **Am I active in my professional association?**
      1. Networking with colleagues exposes dental hygienists to other practicing professionals who can provide guidance and mentoring to younger members.
      2. Membership in your professional organization can provide free access to peer-reviewed journals.

3. Active membership provides the opportunity to help shape evidence-based policies and guidelines for the organization.

E. **How well developed is my clinical judgment?** Am I able to combine evidence and clinical experience to make a good decision?

F. **Do I take into consideration what my patient wants?**
   1. Do I listen to my patients?
   2. Do I provide them with enough information and direction to make a good decision?
   3. Do I respect their autonomy and choices?

G. **Are there things that I should stop doing?**
   1. Am I holding on to what I do because "that's what I learned in school" even though it was several years ago?
   2. Is what I am doing making the best use of office and patient resources; both financial and human?

H. **Are there things I need to change?**
   1. Are there better, more efficient or cost effective tools available such as specific diagnostic tests, treatments, adjunctive therapies, medications, products, or procedures than what I am currently using?
   2. Do I have the appropriate amount of time scheduled or equipment provided for the highest level of patient care?

Chapter Summary Statement

Best practice is a process of care with the goal of achieving consistent, superior patient outcomes. Best practice is founded on evidence-based data. The highest ranked level of evidence today is the systematic review; an evaluation of a body of research on a treatment or device through rigorous scientific methods to determine the overall validity and clinical applicability of that treatment or device. In addition to scientific data, best practice incorporates sound clinical judgment and patient values into the process. Achieving best practice requires that dental hygienists question and think about what they are doing and be open to learning new techniques. By using this approach to periodontal care, hygienists can meet the challenges of continuing to provide quality care in a rapidly changing field of dental healthcare.

Section 5
Focus on Patients

Case 1

You have just started working in a new office and find that the other dental hygienist in the practice, Debbie, "doesn't believe" in using the ultrasonic equipment. Debbie states she has been practicing for 20 years, that is what she learned in school and she knows what she sees; good results with hand scaling. It is a little intimidating since you have less experience (only 5 years) but have routinely used ultrasonic instruments and mention to her "that is what you learned in school." For a while you pass it off as no big deal, a difference of opinions, but because Debbie didn't use the ultrasonic equipment, the equipment in the office is old and doesn't function at the level it should. You speak to your employer about getting a new machine, but he said, "Debbie doesn't use it, why do you?"

1. How would you answer your employer?
2. What types of evidence would you try to locate to justify your position?
3. Where would you search?
4. What types of key words would you use?
5. How would you manage your conflict with Debbie?

Case 2

Your patient, Ms. Karen Jones, is a healthy, nonsmoking 30-year-old. Her only medication is birth control pills of 5 years' duration, and a daily multi-vitamin. She has been coming in for regular maintenance every 6 months. She brushes two times per day and flosses when she remembers, perhaps once a week and she states she finds the procedure difficult. The exam shows some 4-mm probing depths and significant bleeding. As you have done several times in the past, you show the patient how to use the manual brush and floss and really "lay it on the line" about improving oral health and warn her she will need to come in more frequently if her habits do not improve. The patient states that "she tries" and is visibly upset when she leaves office. While you hate to see her upset, you hope she finally got the message.

About a month after her visit, you get a message that Karen Jones would like you call her. When you reach Karen, she tells you she has been "researching" her gum problem, and she has found out she has several alternatives to a manual toothbrush and floss. Karen reports she has looked on the Internet, and talked to a relative who is also a dental hygienist. She has learned about automatic toothbrushes, automatic flossing devices, and oral irrigators, and how they could help her. In fact, she has purchased one of everything, and feels her mouth is improving. Not only that, the power-flossing device makes the task so much easier. "Why didn't you tell me about this!" she demands. "I am unhappy, and going to have my records transferred elsewhere!"

1. What are some of the reasons the dental hygienist may have for not telling Karen about these products?
2. Ethically, is not telling a patient about all self-care products that have evidence to support their use the same as not telling a patient about all available professional treatment options? Why or why not?
3. What steps could the dental hygienist take to improve her knowledge on self-care products?

References

1. Lippincott Williams & Wilkins. *Best Practices: Evidence-Based Nursing Procedures.* 2nd ed. Philadelphia: Lippincott Williams & Wilkins; 2007.

2. ADHA Policy Manual, 2008. Available online at: http://www.adha.org/downloads/ADHA_Policies.pdf Accessed May 4, 2009.

3. Sackett DL, Rosenberg WM, Gray JA, Haynes RB, et al. Evidence based medicine: what it is and what it isn't. *Br Med J.* 1996;312(7023):71–72.

4. Bader JD, Shugars DA. Variation in dentists' clinical decisions. *J Public Health Dent.* 1995;55(3):181–188.

5. Bader JD, Shugars DA. Variation, treatment outcomes, and practice guidelines in dental practice. *J Dent Educ.* 1995;59(1):61–95.

6. Verdonschot EH, Angmar-Mansson B, ten Bosch JJ, Deery CH, et al. Developments in caries diagnosis and their relationship to treatment decisions and quality of care. ORCA Saturday Afternoon Symposium 1997. *Caries Res.* 1999;33(1):32–40.

7. Forrest JL, Drury TE, Horowitz AM. U.S. dental hygienists' knowledge and opinions related to providing oral cancer examinations. *J Cancer Educ.* 2001;16(3):150–156.

8. Forrest JL, Horowitz AM, Shmuely Y. Caries preventive knowledge and practices among dental hygienists. *J Dent Hyg.* 2000;74(3):183–195.

9. Forrest JL, Horowitz AM, Shmuely Y. Dental hygienists' knowledge, opinions, and practices related to oral and pharyngeal cancer risk assessment. *J Dent Hyg.* 2001;75(4):271–281.

10. Warren DP, Henson HA, Chan JT. A survey of in-office use of fluorides in the Houston area. *J Dent Hyg.* 1996;70(4):166–171.

11. Davidoff F, Case K, Fried PW. Evidence-based medicine: why all the fuss? *Ann Intern Med.* 1995;122(9):727.

12. Evans CE, Haynes RB, Birkett NJ, Gilbert JR, et al. Does a mailed continuing education program improve physician performance? Results of a randomized trial in antihypertensive care. *JAMA.* 1986;255(4):501–504.

13. Sackett DL. *Evidence-Based Medicine: How to Practice and Teach EBM.* New York; Edinburgh: Churchill Livingstone; 1997:250, xii.

14. Niederman R, Badovinac R. Tradition-based dental care and evidence-based dental care. *J Dent Res.* 1999;78(7):1288–1291.

15. Ismail AI, Bader JD. Evidence-based dentistry in clinical practice. *J Am Dent Assoc.* 2004;135(1):78–83.

16. Mulrow CD. Rationale for systematic reviews. *Br Med J.* 1994;309(6954):597–599.

17. Gillette J. Evidence-based dentistry for everyday practice. *J Evid Based Dent Pract.* 2008;8(3):144–148.

18. Gillette J. Answering clinical questions using the principles of evidence-based dentistry. *J Evid Based Dent Pract.* 2009;9(1):1–8.

19. Forrest JL, Miller SA. Evidence-based decision making in action: Part 1–Finding the best clinical evidence. *J Contemp Dent Pract.* 2002;3(3):10–26.

20. Rosenberg W, Donald A. Evidence based medicine: an approach to clinical problem-solving. *Br Med J.* 1995;310(6987):1122–1126.

21. Jahn CA. Product focus: continuing education. *Access.* 2008;22:30–32.

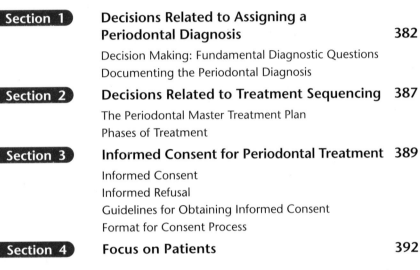

Chapter 23

Decision Making During Treatment Planning for Patients with Periodontal Disease

Learning Objectives

- List the three fundamental diagnostic questions used when assigning a periodontal diagnosis.
- Explain how to arrive at appropriate answers to each of the fundamental diagnostic questions.
- Explain the difference between the terms signs of a disease and symptoms of a disease.
- Explain the term silent disease.
- Describe what is meant by the term clinical attachment loss.
- Describe the elements of a well written diagnosis for periodontitis.
- List the phases of treatment.
- Explain the term informed consent.
- List guidelines for obtaining informed consent

Key Terms

Clinical decision-making
Signs of periodontal disease
Symptoms of periodontal disease
Silent disease
Overt signs
Hidden signs
Natural level of gingival attachment
Clinical attachment loss
Disease sites

Master treatment plan
Assessment and preliminary therapy phase
Nonsurgical periodontal therapy phase
Surgical therapy phase
Restorative phase
Periodontal maintenance phase
Informed consent
Informed refusal

Section 1
Decisions Related to Assigning a Periodontal Diagnosis

Clinical decision making and treatment planning is the process whereby the dentist and dental hygienist use the information gathered during the clinical periodontal assessment to identify treatment strategies that meet the individual needs of the patient.

DECISION MAKING: FUNDAMENTAL DIAGNOSTIC QUESTIONS

1. Overview of the Decision-Making Process for Periodontal Care
   A. Roles in the Decision-Making Process
      1. The Dental Team's Role
         a. It is the dentist's responsibility to arrive at a periodontal diagnosis; however, it is both the dentist's and the dental hygienist's responsibilities to plan the nonsurgical therapy.
         b. In an efficient dental practice, the entire team must be familiar with the diagnostic decision-making process and the fundamental principles for planning nonsurgical periodontal therapy.
      2. Patient's Role in Decision Making
         a. An equally important component of the treatment planning process is the patient's involvement in the decision-making process.
         b. Dental healthcare providers have an obligation to encourage patients to participate fully in all treatment decisions and goals.
   B. Decision Making Is an Ongoing Process
      1. Since most patients are monitored for many years or even decades by a dental team, clinical decision making and treatment planning can be an ongoing process over time.
      2. In addition, the periodontium consists of dynamic and continuously changing tissues, and an individual's periodontal care needs change over time.
      3. The dental team must be aware that a perfectly sensible periodontal diagnosis and plan for therapy at one point in time may require modification at a later date.
   C. Assigning a Periodontal Diagnosis. The first step in treatment planning is assigning a correct periodontal diagnosis.
      1. Determination of a periodontal diagnosis can be simplified by asking and answering three fundamental clinical questions in a systematic manner (FIG. 23-1).
      2. These three fundamental questions are used to guide the dental team through the diagnostic process.
      3. Many decisions, including assigning a periodontal diagnosis and planning nonsurgical therapy, revolve around the answers to these fundamental questions.
2. Assigning a Periodontal Diagnosis: Fundamental Diagnostic Questions
   A. The First Fundamental Diagnostic Question is: *"Does the clinical assessment indicate health or inflammatory disease in the periodontium?"*
      1. The answer to the first question should be based on the signs of inflammation that are noted and recorded during the clinical assessment, and by its very nature is not usually difficult for members of the dental team to answer.
         a. The dental team should be familiar with the difference between the signs of a disease and the symptoms of a disease. Signs of periodontal disease are the features of a disease that can be observed or are measurable by a clinician.
            1) Examples of periodontal disease signs might include gingival erythema (redness), gingival edema (swelling), bleeding on gentle probing, loss of attachment, tooth mobility, or loss of alveolar bone support.

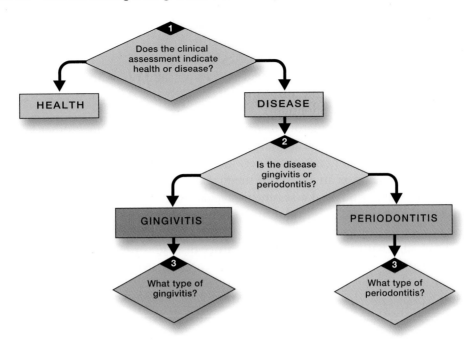

Figure 23.1. Decision **Tree.** A decision tree using three fundamental questions for determining an initial periodontal diagnosis.

2) Some of these signs are easy to detect by the clinician (i.e., gingival erythema (redness); some of these signs require careful assessment by the dental team (i.e., loss of attachment).

b. Symptoms of periodontal disease are features of a disease that are noticed by the patient.

1) Examples of symptoms of periodontitis might include difficulty chewing, itching gums, blood on the bed pillow, or a bad taste in the mouth.

2) In many patients periodontitis does not cause much in the way of obvious symptoms to the patients, and some clinicians refer to periodontitis as a silent disease because of this lack of or "silence" of obvious symptoms.

3) Calling periodontitis a silent disease underscores the frequent clinical observation that periodontitis can exist in patients who are totally unaware of its presence.

c. Members of the dental team should realize that signs of inflammation include both overt signs of inflammation (i.e., those signs that are readily visible) and hidden signs of inflammation (i.e., those signs that not readily visible) (TABLE 23-1).

1) Examples of overt signs of inflammation are changes in the color, contour, and consistency of the gingival tissue.

TABLE 23-1.   Signs of Inflammation in the Periodontium

Overt (Readily Visible) Signs	Hidden Signs
Color changes in the gingiva	Bone loss
Contour changes in the gingiva	Purulence (exudate)
Changes in consistency in the gingiva	Bleeding on probing

2) Examples of hidden signs of inflammation are alveolar bone loss, bleeding on probing, and purulence or exudate.

2. Health as an answer to the first diagnostic question
   a. If the clinical periodontal assessment reveals no signs of inflammation in the periodontium, then the answer to Question No. 1 is health (i.e., an inflammation-free periodontium).
   b. This means that inflammatory disease is not present and, though other problems in the periodontium may well be present, the patient certainly does not have either gingivitis or periodontitis.

3. Inflammatory disease as an answer to the first diagnostic question
   a. If the clinical periodontal assessment reveals either overt or hidden signs of inflammation in the periodontium, then the answer to Question #1 is, of course, inflammatory disease.
   b. This means that some type of inflammatory disease is present and that further diagnostic decisions related to this inflammatory disease will need to be made by the team.

4. Additional Diagnostic Measures
   a. Note that even in the absence of any inflammatory disease in the periodontium, some patients will require additional diagnostic measures.
   b. For example, a patient with no inflammation in the periodontium at all but with severe recession of the gingival margin accompanied by cervical abrasion of the teeth may need to be evaluated for possible use of traumatic toothbrushing techniques.

B. **The Second Fundamental Diagnostic Question is:** *"If the clinical assessment indicates inflammatory disease, is the disease gingivitis or is it periodontitis?"*
   1. Using Attachment Loss to Answer Question No. 2.
      a. The answer to this second fundamental question is based on clinical evidence of attachment loss as determined from the clinical findings recorded during the clinical assessment.
         1) The natural level of the gingival attachment to the tooth is at the cementoenamel junction (CEJ).
         2) Clinical attachment loss or attachment loss refers to migration of the junctional epithelium to a position apical to (below) the level of the CEJ (Fig. 23-2).
      b. Gingivitis. If the clinical assessment reveals no attachment loss in the presence of inflammation, then the answer to Question #2 is gingivitis.
      c. Periodontitis. If the clinical assessment revealed attachment loss in the presence of inflammation, then the answer to Question #2 is periodontitis.
   2. It is important for the dental team to use dental radiographs during the clinical assessment.
      a. In most patients with moderate to severe periodontitis, alveolar bone loss will be evident on the radiographs.
      b. However, even before radiographic changes occur, attachment loss will be detectable by the alert clinician.
      c. The members of the dental team must be able to detect periodontitis before there is obvious radiographic evidence of alveolar bone loss.

C. **The Third Fundamental Diagnostic Question is:** *"If the patient has gingivitis, what type of gingivitis?"* or *"If the patient has periodontitis, what type of periodontitis?"*
   1. The classification of various types of gingival disease and the various types of periodontitis was discussed in many other chapters in this textbook, and this discussion will not be repeated in this chapter.

2. The dentist will use these disease classifications to assign a specific periodontal diagnosis based on the clinical features outlined in those chapters.

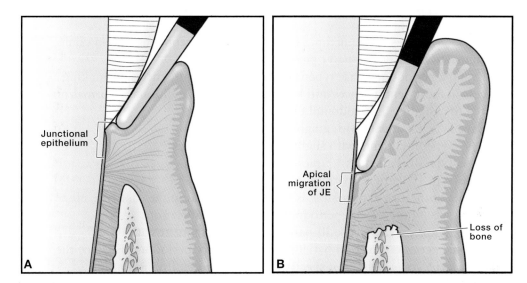

Figure 23.2. Level of Attachment. A: Natural Level of Attachment. The natural level of the junctional epithelium is at *the same level as* the cementoenamel junction CEJ. Note that the probe tip does not reach the CEJ if the attachment is at its natural level. **B:** Attachment Loss. In attachment loss, the junctional epithelium is *apical* to the level of the CEJ. Note that the probe tip extends beyond the CEJ if the attachment apparatus has migrated apically.

DOCUMENTING THE PERIODONTAL DIAGNOSIS

1. **Special Considerations Related to Documenting the Periodontal Diagnosis**
   A. **Guidelines for Documenting Periodontal Diagnoses.** Documenting the periodontal diagnosis is a critical skill for the dental team, and adhering to a standard format for such documentation is helpful. The following are some guidelines for documenting periodontal diagnoses.
   1. Diagnositc Term. As part of the diagnosis include the correct diagnostic term as outlined in the classification scheme, such as chronic periodontitis or aggressive periodontitis.
   2. Disease Severity. When assigning a diagnosis, then add descriptive modifiers such as slight (mild), moderate, or severe to describe the *severity* of the disease.
      a. TABLE 23-2 shows how the terms slight, moderate, and severe should be used as part of documentation of a periodontitis diagnosis.
      b. Note that the term *clinical attachment loss* (CAL) is used to underscore that these measurements are clinical measurements and may not coincide exactly with histologic measurements.
   3. Disease Extent. When assigning a diagnosis, also include descriptive modifiers such as localized or generalized to describe the *extent* of the disease.
      a. TABLE 23-2 also shows how the terms localized and generalized should be used as part of documentation of the extent of periodontal disease.
      b. Note that the term disease sites refers to the individual teeth or specific surfaces of a tooth that are experiencing periodontal destruction.
      c. Examples of appropriate periodontal diagnoses might be *generalized moderate chronic periodontitis* or *localized severe aggressive periodontitis.* TABLE 23-3 provides some examples of well written periodontal diagnoses.

B. Using the Case Type System for Periodontal Patients
1. Case Types
   a. Although the case type system is somewhat limited in value, it has been standard practice in the United States to assign a periodontal case type to all periodontal patients.
   b. These case types are sometimes used in insurance reporting and in communication with third-party payers.
2. Assigning a periodontal case type is included in the initial decision-making process in most dental offices and is included here as additional information related to assigning a periodontal diagnosis.
   a. Case Type I. Patients with gingivitis only
   b. Case Type II. Patients with slight (mild) periodontitis
   c. Case Type III. Patients with moderate periodontitis
   d. Case Type IV. Patients with severe periodontitis
3. The value of the case type system is very limited because the case type alone does not specify the precise periodontal disease classification.
   a. For example, a Case Type III patient could be a patient with either chronic periodontitis or a patient with aggressive periodontitis, since the Case Type system does not specify the precise type of periodontitis.
   b. Note that a designation of Case Type III only signifies that the disease is of moderate severity.
4. It is important for all members of the dental team to use the written periodontal diagnosis (e.g., generalized moderate chronic periodontitis) when describing the periodontal status of a patient and to use the case type only as a supplemental description.

TABLE 23-2. Use of Modifiers in Documenting Disease Severity and Extent

Descriptive Modifier	Definition
Disease severity	
Slight	1 to 2 mm clinical attachment loss
Moderate	3 to 4 mm clinical attachment loss
Severe	5 mm or more of clinical attachment loss
Disease extent	
Localized	30% or less of the sites in the mouth are involved
Generalized	More than 30% of the sites in the mouth are involved

TABLE 23-3. Examples of a Well Written Periodontal Diagnosis

Extent	Severity	Name of Disease
Localized	Slight	Chronic periodontitis
Localized	Moderate	Chronic periodontitis
Generalized	Moderate	Chronic periodontitis
Generalized	Severe	Chronic periodontitis
Localized	Moderate	Aggressive periodontitis

Section 2
Decisions Related to Treatment Sequencing

1. **The Periodontal Master Treatment Plan.** The master treatment plan is a sequential outline of the measures to be carried out by the dentist, the dental hygienist, or the patient to eliminate disease and restore a healthy periodontal environment. The master treatment plan is used to coordinate and sequence all treatment and educational measures to be employed. Although some of the treatment included in the master treatment plan does not involve the dental hygienist directly, it is important that the hygienist understand how all phases of treatment contribute to the goal of restoring a healthy periodontal environment. Refer to TABLE 23-4 for an overview of the classical (traditional) phases in the management of periodontal patients.

2. **Phases of Treatment.** The master treatment plan can be sequenced into phases. An overview of the phases of treatment is presented in Figure 23-3 as well as in the discussion below.

   A. **Assessment and Preliminary Therapy Phase**
      1. The assessment and preliminary therapy phase includes assessment data collection and needed care for immediate treatment needs such as emergency dental care. Details of the clinical periodontal assessment is discussed in Chapter 19.
      2. This stage of care also has been referred to as emergency therapy by some authors.

   B. **Nonsurgical Periodontal Therapy Phase**
      1. The nonsurgical periodontal therapy phase of treatment includes all the *nonsurgical* measures used to control gingivitis and periodontitis.
         a. This phase includes dental hygiene care and patient educational measures.
         b. It can also include measures to minimize the impact of local contributing factors.
      2. The nonsurgical periodontal therapy phase is also called *initial periodontal therapy*, *Phase I therapy*, *bacterial control*, and *anti-infective therapy*.

   C. **Surgical Therapy Phase**
      1. The surgical therapy phase of treatment includes any needed periodontal surgery and placement of dental implants.
      2. The surgical therapy phase of care is also known as *Phase II* therapy. Periodontal surgical procedures are discussed in other chapters of this book.
      3. Note that this phase of treatment is not needed for all patients.

   D. **Restorative Therapy Phase**
      1. The restorative therapy phase of treatment may include placement of dental restorations and replacement of missing teeth by fixed or removable prostheses.
      2. The restorative therapy phase of care is also called *Phase III* therapy.

   E. **Periodontal Maintenance Phase**
      1. The periodontal maintenance phase of treatment includes all measures used by the dental team and by the patient to keep periodontitis from recurring once the inflammatory disease is brought under control.
      2. The objective of the peridontal maintenance phase is to maintain the teeth functioning throughout life of the patient and may actually be needed for the rest of the patient's life.
      3. The periodontal maintenance phase of care is also known as *Phase IV* therapy. Periodontal maintenance is discussed in detail in Chapters 32 and 33.

3. **Documentation of Treatment.** Documentation of assessment data and all educational and treatment services performed should be entered in the patient record as they are performed. This documentation is referred to as the progress notes or chart notes. Documentation of periodontal care is presented in Chapter 35.

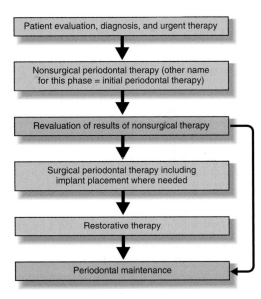

Figure 23.3. **Phases of Treatment.** This flow chart provides an overview of the sequence of the normal phases of treatment for a patient.

TABLE 23-4.	Classical Phases in the Management of Patients with Periodontitis
Phase	**Measures and Procedures**
Assessment phase and preliminary therapy	Health history
	Comprehensive oral examination
	Assessment data collection
	Radiographs as indicated
	Diagnosis of oral conditions
	Treatment of urgent conditions
	Planning of nonsurgical therapy
	Referral for care of medical conditions
	Extraction of hopeless teeth
Nonsurgical periodontal therapy (Phase I)	Self-care education
	Nutritional counseling
	Smoking cessation counseling
	Periodontal debridement (instrumentation)
	Antimicrobial therapy
	Correction of local risk factors
	Fluoride therapy
	Caries control and temporary restorations
	Occlusal therapy
	Minor orthodontic treatment
	Reevaluation of Phase I therapy
Surgical therapy (Phase II)	Periodontal surgery
	Endodontic surgery
	Dental implant placement
Restorative therapy (Phase III)	Dental restorations, fixed and removable prostheses
	Reevaluation of overall response to treatment
Periodontal maintenance (Phase IV)	Ongoing care at specified intervals

Section 3
Informed Consent for Periodontal Treatment

One critical decision in patient care is how to obtain informed consent for treatment. *The patient is a critical player in any plan involving periodontal therapy, and communications with the patient are vital as the treatment plan is developed.* A breakdown in communication often leads to lawsuits. According to experts on malpractice litigation, keeping the lines of communication open with the patient is a vital component in avoiding lawsuits. Studies demonstrate that patients who believe that they have been well informed regarding their condition and who have had their questions answered by members of the dental team, are more compliant with treatment recommendations, have a higher trust in their healthcare providers, and are more satisfied with their care. These factors lead to better treatment outcomes and reduced malpractice risk.

1. **Informed Consent.** Informed consent is a patient's voluntary agreement to proposed treatment after achieving an understanding of the relevant facts, benefits, and risks involved.

   A. **What Constitutes Informed Consent?**

      1. An individual's consent is informed only if the recommended treatment, alternate treatment options, and the benefits and risks of treatment have been thoroughly described to the person in language understood by the patient.

      2. Informed consent must be voluntary, and this informed consent originates from (i) a person's legal right to direct what happens to his or her body and (ii) the ethical duty of the dental healthcare provider to involve the individual in his or her own dental care.

      3. Informed consent is more than simply getting a patient to agree to a procedure or to sign a written consent form. It is *a process of communication between a patient and healthcare provider* that allows the patient to make a well-informed decision about his or her own dental care.

   B. **Goals of Informed Consent.** The most important goal of informed consent is to provide an individual an opportunity to be an informed participant in healthcare decisions, and it is generally accepted that complete informed consent includes a discussion of the following elements:

      1. The diagnosis and an explanation of the periodontal condition that warrants the proposed treatment.

      2. An explanation of the purpose of the proposed periodontal treatment.

      3. A description of the proposed treatment and the individual patient's role and responsibilities during and after periodontal treatment.

      4. A discussion of the known risks and benefits of the proposed periodontal treatment.

      5. An assessment of the likelihood that the proposed treatment will accomplish the desired objectives.

         a. When discussing treatment outcomes it is important not to appear to guarantee treatment outcomes to the patient.

         b. Remember that individual patients will respond differently to treatment.

      6. A presentation of alternative treatment options, if any, and the known risks and benefits of these options.

      7. The risks and benefits of not receiving the proposed periodontal treatment.

      8. A discussion of the prognosis (or outcomes expected) if no treatment is provided.

      9. A discussion of the actual costs associated with the proposed treatment.

10. Reinforcement of the individual's right to refuse consent to the proposed treatment.
    a. Patients often feel powerless when dealing with healthcare providers.
    b. To encourage the patient's voluntary consent, the dental healthcare provider should make it clear to the patient that she or he is participating in a decision, not merely signing a consent form.

2. **Informed Refusal.** Informed refusal is a person's right to refuse all or a portion of the proposed treatment after the recommended treatment, alternate treatment options, and the likely consequences of declining treatment have been explained in language understood by the patient. A patient always has a legal right to refuse proposed periodontal care.

3. **Guidelines for Obtaining Informed Consent.** The doctrine of informed consent reminds dental healthcare providers to respect patients by fully and accurately providing information relevant to their healthcare decisions. The following are some guidelines to use when obtaining informed consent from a patient.
   A. **Use Understandable Language.** Information should be provided in understandable language. It is the dental healthcare provider's responsibility to present all information necessary for informed consent to the individual in a way that is understood by the patient.
      1. Use simple, straightforward sentences.
      2. Use commonly recognizable terms. Avoid the use of jargon or technical terms, and explain terms that may not be easily understood.
      3. Use a translator if the patient does not speak English or speaks with little understanding.
   B. **Provide Opportunities for Patient Questions.** An opportunity should be provided for the patient to ask questions. Foster an open exchange of information and encourage the patient to ask questions. Using open-ended and nondirective questions such as those below can simplify this process.
      1. *"What more would you like to know?"*
      2. *"What are your concerns?"*
      3. *"What is your next question?"*
   C. **Assess Patient Understanding.** An assessment should be made of the patient's understanding of information provided.
      1. A simple strategy to assess understanding is to let patient know that *"MANY people have difficulty understanding the information that I give them or have questions that they need answered. So, please let's discuss anything you do not understand."*
      2. Another strategy is to make a comment such as: *"Most of my patients want to explain my treatment suggestions to another family member. What additional information can I give you to help you explain this treatment to your spouse?"*

4. **Format for Consent Process.** The format for the consent process may be either verbal or written. Some states have statutes or regulations requiring dentists to secure written informed consent from patients [1]. Dentists should ensure that they are familiar with and in compliance with the informed consent laws in their states.
   A. **Written Consent.** Many dental healthcare providers prefer to have the patient sign and date a written consent form for documentation of the consent process.
      1. In addition, the written consent document should be signed and dated by the dentist and a witness (generally, another staff member).
      2. Once signed, a written consent document becomes part of the individual's permanent dental record.

B. **Verbal Consent.** If a written consent document is not used, the patient's verbal consent should be documented in the patient chart. An example of documentation of verbal consent would be a written entry in the patient's chart that says, *"Discussed the diagnosis; purpose, description, benefits, and risks of the proposed treatment; alternative treatment options; the prognosis of no treatment; and costs. The patient asked questions and demonstrates that he understands all information presented during the discussion. Informed consent was obtained for the attached treatment plan."*

Chapter Summary Statement

When assigning a periodontal diagnosis, there are three fundamental diagnostic questions that should be asked and answered by the members of the dental team. These questions are:

(1) *"Does the clinical assessment indicate health or inflammatory disease in the periodontium?"*
(2) *"If the clinical assessment indicates inflammatory disease, is the disease gingivitis or is it periodontitis?"*
(3) *"If the patient has gingivitis, what type of gingivitis?"* or *"If the patient has periodontitis, what type of periodontitis?"*

It is important for the dental hygienist to understand how all phases of periodontal treatment contribute to the goal of restoring a healthy periodontal environment. The patient is a critical player in any plan involving periodontal therapy, and communications with the patient are vital as the treatment plan is developed. Informed consent is a patient's voluntary agreement to proposed treatment after achieving an understanding of the relevant facts, benefits, and risks involved.

Section 4
Focus on Patients

Case 1

Periodontal assessment of a new patient reveals generalized bleeding on probing but very little gingival erythema (redness) and very little gingival edema (swelling). How would you answer the first fundamental diagnostic question for this patient?

Case 2

Periodontal assessment of a new patient reveals definite signs of inflammation in the periodontium. Explain how to answer the second diagnostic question for this patient.

Case 3

Periodontal assessment of a new patient reveals localized signs of gingival inflammation but no attachment loss. The findings also include a site of recession of the gingival margin and toothbrush abrasion on the facial surface of a canine tooth. At this site of recession there is no sign of inflammation of the gingiva. How should this site of recession of the gingival margin due to traumatic brushing affect the basic diagnostic questions?

Reference

1. Sfikas PM. A duty to disclose. Issues to consider in securing informed consent. *J Am Dent Assoc.* 2003;134(10):1329–1333.

Suggested Reading

Glick M. Informed consent: a delicate balance. *J Am Dent Assoc.* 2006;137(8):1060, 1062, 1064.

Nonsurgical Periodontal Therapy

Learning Objectives

- Explain the term nonsurgical periodontal therapy.
- Name four goals for nonsurgical therapy.
- Write a typical plan for nonsurgical therapy for a patient with plaque-induced gingivitis.
- Write a typical plan for nonsurgical therapy for a patient with slight chronic periodontitis.
- Explain the terms periodontal debridement and deplaquing.
- Describe the type of healing to be expected following successful instrumentation of root surfaces.
- Explain the origin of the condition called dental hypersensitivity.
- Describe a strategy for managing dentinal hypersensitivity during nonsurgical therapy.
- Explain why reevaluation is a critical step during nonsurgical therapy.
- List steps in an appointment for reevaluation of the results of nonsurgical therapy.
- Describe three decisions made during the reevaluation appointment.
- Explain current American Academy of Periodontology recommendations for deciding which patients should be managed by a periodontist.

Key Terms

Nonsurgical periodontal therapy
Treatment plan
Periodontal maintenance
Periodontal debridement
Deplaquing
Long junctional epithelium
Dentinal hypersensitivity

Dentinal tubules
Odontoblastic process
Smear layer
Nonresponsive disease sites
Reevaluation
Comanagement

Section 1
Overview of Nonsurgical Periodontal Therapy

PRINCIPLES OF NONSURGICAL PERIODONTAL THERAPY

1. Nonsurgical periodontal therapy includes self-care measures, periodontal instrumentation, and use of chemical agents to prevent or control plaque-induced gingivitis or chronic periodontitis. It is convenient to view nonsurgical periodontal procedures as the initial steps in the periodontal treatment for a patient, but for many patients these initial steps are all that are needed to bring disease under control.

   A. *Nonsurgical periodontal therapy has the broad overall objective of eliminating inflammatory disease in the periodontium and returning the periodontium to a healthy state that can then be maintained by a combination of both professional care and patient self-care.*

      1. Many terms have been used to describe nonsurgical periodontal therapy, and this fact may create some confusion among novice clinicians. Other terms that have been used to describe this same treatment in the literature include initial periodontal therapy, initial therapy, hygienic phase, anti-infective phase, cause-related therapy, phase I treatment, and soft tissue management.

      2. Nonsurgical periodontal therapy, however, is the preferred terminology for this phase of periodontal care.

   B. **Philosophy for Developing a Plan for Nonsurgical Periodontal Therapy**

      1. The fundamental philosophy for developing a sensible plan for nonsurgical periodontal therapy should be to plan treatment that will provide for the control, elimination, or minimization of primary etiologic factors for periodontal disease, local risk factors for periodontal disease, and systemic risk factors for periodontal disease identified in a patient during the clinical assessment.

      2. Procedures included in a plan for nonsurgical periodontal therapy should be selected to meet the needs of each individual patient; therefore nonsurgical therapy plans can vary from patient to patient.

2. **General Indications for Nonsurgical Periodontal Therapy.** Nonsurgical periodontal therapy should be planned for all patients with plaque-induced gingivitis and for all patients with chronic periodontitis.

   A. **Plaque-Induced Gingivitis**

      1. Thorough nonsurgical therapy can normally bring plaque-induced gingivitis under control.

      2. Thorough nonsurgical therapy can also bring many cases of slight to moderate chronic periodontitis under control

      3. For many patients with more advanced periodontal disease, such as severe chronic periodontitis, control of the periodontitis will not only require thorough nonsurgical periodontal therapy, but it will also require more advanced periodontal procedures such as periodontal surgery.

   B. **Chronic Periodontitis and Other Forms of Periodontitis**

      1. Although periodontal surgery is frequently indicated for patients with more advanced periodontitis, it should be understood that *all patients with chronic periodontitis should undergo nonsurgical therapy prior to periodontal surgical intervention.*

      2. Nonsurgical periodontal therapy is frequently successful in minimizing the extent of any surgery subsequently needed and can improve the outcomes of that periodontal surgery.

3. Members of the dental team should be aware that nonsurgical periodontal therapy is not the treatment of choice for all patients with periodontitis.
   a. Nonsurgical periodontal therapy is not necessarily the best therapy for patients with other types of periodontitis, such as aggressive periodontitis.
   b. Patients with types of periodontitis other than chronic periodontitis should be referred to a periodontist for treatment; criteria for referral are discussed later in this chapter.

3. **Specific Goals of Nonsurgical Periodontal Therapy.** The goals of nonsurgical periodontal therapy are summarized in Box 24-1.
   A. **Goal 1: To minimize the bacterial challenge to the patient**
      1. Control of the bacterial challenge involves intensive training of the patient in appropriate techniques for self-care and professional removal of calculus deposits and bacterial products from tooth surfaces.
      2. Removal of calculus deposits and bacterial products contaminating the tooth surfaces is an important step in achieving control of the bacterial challenge. Calculus deposits are always covered with living bacterial biofilms that are associated with continuing inflammation if not removed.
   B. **Goal 2: To eliminate or control local contributing factors for periodontal disease**
      1. Local environmental risk factors can increase the risk of developing periodontitis in localized sites. For example, defective restorations can lead to plaque biofilm retention in the localized area of the defective restoration.
      2. Plaque biofilm retention in a site, over time, allows periodontal pathogens to live, multiply, and damage the periodontium.
      3. A thorough plan for nonsurgical periodontal therapy will always include minimizing the impact of local environmental risk factors.
   C. **Goal 3: To minimize the impact of systemic factors for periodontal disease**
      1. It is apparent that there are certain systemic diseases or conditions that can increase the risk of developing periodontitis or can increase the risk of developing severe periodontitis where periodontitis already exists. Two examples of systemic factors are uncontrolled diabetes mellitus and smoking.
      2. A thorough plan for nonsurgical therapy always includes measures to minimize the impact of systemic risk factors. For example, a periodontitis patient with a family history of diabetes mellitus should be evaluated to rule out undiagnosed diabetes as a contributing factor to the periodontitis. Another example would be a patient who smokes should receive smoking cessation counseling.
   D. **Goal 4: To stabilize the attachment level**
      1. The ultimate goal of nonsurgical periodontal therapy in chronic periodontitis patients is to stabilize the level of attachment.
      2. Stabilization of the attachment level involves control of all of the factors listed in the other goals of nonsurgical periodontal therapy.

Box 24-1. Goals of Nonsurgical Periodontal Therapy

Goal 1: To minimize the bacterial challenge to the patient

Goal 2: To eliminate or control local environmental risk factors for periodontal disease

Goal 3: To minimize the impact of systemic risk factors for periodontal disease

Goal 4: To stabilize the attachment level

4. **Procedures Included in Nonsurgical Periodontal Therapy**
   A. **Professional Care.** Box 24-2 shows a list of some of the nonsurgical therapy procedures that the dental team can utilize for patients.
      1. The list of procedures that may be included in this step is lengthy, but it should be evident that some of the procedures are included in the treatment of all patients and other procedures on the list are utilized only rarely.
      2. Since each patient presents unique treatment challenges, members of the dental team will need to customize the selection of the nonsurgical procedures included for each individual.
   B. **Patient Self-Care.** One important aspect of nonsurgical periodontal therapy, is that it includes self-care that is largely in the hands of a patient. This means that patients need to be taught self-care skills and also be motivated to use those skills. These important topics are discussed in Chapters 25, 26, and 27.

Box 24-2. Examples of Nonsurgical Therapy Procedures

1. Customized self-care instructions including
   a. Mechanical plaque biofilm control
   b. Chemical plaque biofilm control
2. Periodontal debridement (instrumentation) of tooth surfaces and pocket space
3. Correction of systemic risk factors
4. Correction of local contributing factors
5. Modulation of host defenses

TYPICAL TREATMENT PLANS FOR NONSURGICAL PERIODONTAL THERAPY

Although it is critical for a treatment plan for nonsurgical therapy to meet the needs of each individual patient, beginning clinicians often find it helpful to review examples of typical plans for nonsurgical therapy. Conceptually a treatment plan is simply a list of steps that addresses a patient's oral health needs. Thus a treatment plan for nonsurgical therapy is list of procedures or interventions that addresses a patient's oral health needs as identified during the periodontal assessment. A properly designed treatment plan for nonsurgical periodontal therapy would include procedures to be carried out by the dentist, by the dental hygienist, and by the patient.

1. **Examples of Typical Treatment Plans**
   A. **Plaque-Induced Gingivitis.** A typical plan for nonsurgical therapy for a patient with plaque-induced gingivitis might include the following:
      1. Customized self-care instructions including patient education and motivation.
      2. Periodontal debridement (typically a dental prophylaxis in American Dental Association [ADA] terminology).
      3. Elimination of plaque biofilm retentive factors such as overhanging restorations, caries, or ill-fitting dental prostheses.
      4. Correction of systemic risk factors.

5. Reevaluation of patient's periodontal status.
    a. Response to nonsurgical therapy is normally delayed, since it takes some time for the body defense mechanisms to respond to individual treatment steps and for the body to bring inflammation in the periodontium under control.
    b. Because of this delay time in healing, the dental team is always obligated to reevaluate the results of nonsurgical periodontal therapy after a period of healing to ensure that all appropriate measures have been included and to identify any other measures that might be needed.
    c. It is wise for the dental team to include this reevaluation step in the plan for nonsurgical therapy so that the patient has a clear understanding from the outset how future treatment decisions will be made.
B. **Slight to Moderate Periodontitis.** As already discussed, it is always important to customize the nonsurgical therapy for the needs of each patient, but again it may be helpful to look at a typical plan for a patient with slight to moderate periodontitis. This typical plan might include the following:
    1. Customized self-care instructions including patient education and motivation.
    2. Periodontal debridement (typically scaling and root planing in ADA terminology).
    3. Control of local risk factors to include steps such as removal of overhanging restorations, restoration of caries, or minimizing excessive occlusal forces.
    4. Correction of systemic risk factors to include steps such as smoking cessation counseling or referral for control of diabetes.
    5. Reevaluation of patient's periodontal status.
C. **Chronic Periodontitis.** Some patients with moderate chronic periodontitis and most patients with severe chronic periodontitis can include complicating factors such as deep probing depths, furcation involvements, or mucogingival problems that may require some more advanced procedures later in therapy. Periodontal surgery would not normally be part of a plan for nonsurgical periodontal therapy, but the dental team would be wise to document the possible need for this more advanced treatment and inform the patient when the need for such treatment appears likely. This can avoid confusion on the part of the patient later in the therapy.
    1. The members of the dental team should be aware of the possible need for periodontal surgical intervention in patients with more advanced periodontitis.
    2. As the severity of periodontitis increases, it becomes more likely that some periodontal surgery will be needed to bring the disease under control.
    3. The need for periodontal surgical therapy should be reevaluated after the completion of nonsurgical periodontal therapy. Surgical periodontal therapy is discussed in Chapter 30.

Section 2
Nonsurgical Instrumentation

PERIODONTAL INSTRUMENTATION

1. **Objective and Rationale for Periodontal Instrumentation**
   A. **Objective of Periodontal Instrumentation**
      1. The objective of the mechanical removal of calculus and bacterial plaque biofilm is the physical removal of microorganisms and their products to prevent and treat periodontal infections.
         a. *Because of the structure of biofilms, physical removal of bacterial plaque biofilm is the most effective mechanism of control.*
         b. Most subgingival plaque biofilm within pockets cannot be reached by brushes, floss, or mouth rinses.
            1) For this reason, frequent periodontal debridement of subgingival root surfaces to remove or disrupt bacterial plaque biofilm mechanically is an essential component of the treatment of periodontitis.
            2) In fact, periodontal debridement is likely to remain the most important component of nonsurgical periodontal therapy for the foreseeable future.
      2. Removal of deposits from tooth surfaces is a critical step in any plan for nonsurgical periodontal therapy.
         a. Calculus deposits harbor living bacterial biofilms; thus, if the calculus remains, so do the pathogenic bacteria, making it impossible to reestablish periodontal health.
         b. Calculus removal is always a fundamental part of nonsurgical periodontal instrumentation.
   B. **Rationale for Periodontal Instrumentation.** The scientific basis for performing periodontal instrumentation includes all points listed below.
      1. To arrest the progress of periodontal disease.
      2. To induce positive changes in the subgingival bacterial flora (count and content).
      3. To eliminate inflammation in the periodontium.
      4. To increase the effectiveness of patient self-care.
      5. To prevent recurrence of disease during periodontal maintenance (discussed in Chapters 31 and 32).
   C. **Instrument Selection for Periodontal Instrumentation**
      1. It is clear that periodontal instrumentation is a vital part of the therapy for all patients with plaque-induced gingivitis and for all patients with chronic periodontitis.
         a. The details of periodontal instrumentation techniques are not discussed in this chapter, since there are so many outstanding dental hygiene textbooks related to these important topics. The reader is referred to this wealth of information already available to dental hygienists.
         b. Research indicates that electronically powered devices are as effective as hand instrumentation and also have some advantages over hand instrumentation when used for periodontal debridement.
      2. Some advantages for the use of powered scalers over hand instruments during periodontal debridement are outlined below.
         a. Disruption and removal of plaque biofilm are important aspects of periodontal debridement, and powered scalers have been shown to be very effective in deplaquing of tooth surfaces.

   b. Many patients with moderate to severe periodontitis have furcation involvements as a result of the disease process, and slim diameter powered scaler tips have been demonstrated to be more effective in treating these furcation involvements than hand instruments.

   c. Using low to medium power settings with powered scalers seems to do less damage to root surfaces.

   d. Slim diameter tips on powered scalers can penetrate deeper into periodontal pockets than hand instruments.

   e. Water irrigation provided by powered scalers washes toxic products and free-floating bacteria from pockets and provides better vision during instrumentation by removing blood from the treatment site.

   f. The fluid stream flowing through a powered scaler tip produces two effects that are unique to these powered instruments, cavitation and acoustic turbulence. These actions are capable of disrupting bacterial cell walls and may even dislodge plaque biofilms slightly beyond the reach of the powered instrument tip.

   g. Several studies have shown that instrumentation time may be reduced when using powered instruments as compared with hand instruments.

2. **Periodontal Instrumentation Terminology.** There has been some evolution in the terminology associated with dental calculus removal and dental plaque biofilm removal over the past years. The careful reader will be wise to note that there are different sets of terminology that appear in the dental hygiene journals and textbooks compared to the terminology in dental journals and textbooks. The differences in this terminology revolve around the terms described below.

   A. **Traditional Instrumentation Terminology**

      1. Scaling is instrumentation of the crown and root surfaces of the teeth to remove plaque biofilm, calculus, and stains.

      2. Root planing is a treatment procedure designed to remove cementum or surface dentin that is rough, impregnated with calculus, or contaminated with toxins or microorganisms.

      3. Root planing is a fundamental treatment procedure for patients with chronic periodontitis.

         a. As traditionally defined, root planing involves the routine, intentional removal of cementum and the instrumenting of all root surfaces to a glassy smooth texture.

         b. Until relatively recently it was thought that bacterial products were firmly held in cemental surfaces exposed by attachment loss occurring as a result of periodontitis. It was believed that vigorous root planing with intentional removal of most cementum was always needed to ensure the removal of all calculus as well as all bacterial products from the root surfaces.

         c. It is now understood that vigorous root planing is not universally needed to reestablish periodontal health in all site of periodontitis. Rather than vigorous root planing and removal of most or all of the cementum, it is now known that the bacterial products can be removed from the root surfaces by using modern techniques with ultrasonic instruments combined with a minimal amount of actual root planing.

B. Emerging Terminology

1. Periodontal debridement is a newer term that has been used in the dental hygiene literature since 1993 to replace the term scaling and root planing. Periodontal debridement is defined as the removal or disruption of bacterial plaque biofilm, its byproducts, and plaque biofilm retentive calculus deposits from coronal tooth surfaces and tooth root surfaces to the extent needed to reestablish periodontal health and restore a balance between the bacterial flora and the host's immune responses.

   a. Periodontal debridement includes instrumentation of every square millimeter of root surface for removal of plaque biofilm and calculus, but does not include the deliberate, aggressive removal of cementum.

   b. Conservation of cementum is one goal of periodontal debridement.

      1) It is currently believed that conservation of cementum enhances periodontal healing in the form of either repair or regeneration. In periodontal health an important function of cementum is to attach the periodontal ligament fibers to the root surface. During the healing process after disease, cementum is thought to contribute to repair of the periodontium.

      2) In addition, research studies indicate that complete removal of cementum from the root surface, exposing the ends of dentinal tubules, may allow bacteria to travel from the pulp into the periodontal pocket in some instances. It is also possible that infusion of bacteria from the pulp may exacerbate alveolar bone loss.

   c. During periodontal debridement, the extent of instrumentation should be limited to that needed to obtain a favorable tissue response. Root surfaces should be instrumented only to a level that results in resolution of tissue inflammation in the peridontal tissues.

2. Deplaquing is the disruption or removal of subgingival microbial plaque biofilm and its byproducts from cemental surfaces and the pocket space.

C. Considerations Regarding Emerging Terminology. American Dental Association (ADA) insurance coding systems can frequently confuse clinicians. Insurance codes are entered on insurance forms, and all dental treatment procedures are associated with ADA procedure codes.

1. Although the term periodontal debridement as defined in the dental hygiene literature may describe modern periodontal therapy better than older terms, this term has not yet replaced the older terms as recognized by the ADA. Periodontal debridement is not a currently recognized ADA procedure name.

2. Study of the ADA codes will indeed reveal a procedure called "full mouth debridement to enable an examination and diagnosis." This procedure which does contain the word debridement should not be confused with the periodontal debridement discussed in this section.

3. Most dentists and periodontists have been reluctant to embrace the new terminology. Some authors and clinicians have redefined the term root planing so that its meaning is similar to that of periodontal debridement. This approach of redefining the term root planing can also be confusing because it is difficult to determine which definition any one person is using.

4. In the United States insurance codes for various nonsurgical periodontal procedures are published by the ADA in the book titled *Current Dental Terminology 2009/2010* [1]. These codes are very specific and should be reviewed carefully before specific dental treatment is coded. Insurance codes are discussed in detail in Chapter 34.

3. **End Point of Nonsurgical Instrumentation**
   A. **Tissue Health as an End Point**
      1. The end point for nonsurgical periodontal instrumentation is to return the periodontium to a state of soft tissue health.
      2. In this context soft tissue health means periodontal tissues free of inflammation.
   B. **Healing Following Nonsurgical Instrumentation**
      1. After thorough periodontal debridement, some healing of the periodontal tissues will normally occur.
         a. The primary type of healing after periodontal debridement is through the formation of a long junctional epithelium.
            1) As inflammation in the periodontium resolves, epithelial cells can readapt to the root surface as shown in Figure 24-1.
            2) This readaptation of the epithelial cells to the root surface is referred to as a long junctional epithelium.
         b. It is important to realize that following periodontal debridement, there is normally no formation of new alveolar bone, new cementum, or new periodontal ligament.
      2. Clinically, nonsurgical periodontal therapy, including instrumentation, can certainly result in reduced probing depths. Figure 24-2 shows examples of soft tissue responses to thorough periodontal debridement.
         a. The reduced probing depths result from the formation of a long junctional epithelium combined in many instances with resolution of gingival edema that is usually a part of the inflammatory process. Figure 24-3 shows how some of this reduction in probing depth can occur at the base of a periodontal pocket.
         b. Thus, one important clinical feature to monitor following periodontal debridement in addition to clinical attachment loss is the probing depths.

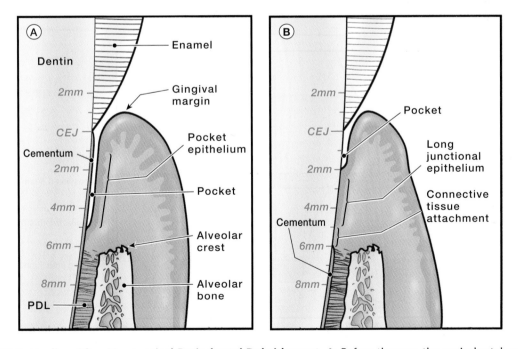

Figure 24.1. Healing After Nonsurgical Periodontal Debridement. A: Before therapy, the periodontal pocket has a probing depth of 6 mm. **B:** After periodontal therapy the tissue healing is through the formation of a long junctional epithelium. This results in a probing depth of 2 mm. Note that there is no formation of new bone, cementum, or periodontal ligament during the healing process that occurs after periodontal debridement.

    c. It should be noted at this point that there are other clinical signs that can correlate with inflammation that can be expected to change following periodontal debridement (i.e., bleeding on probing).

C. Assessing Tissue Healing. Tissue healing does not occur overnight, and in most cases it is not possible to assess the true tissue response for at least 1 month after the completion of instrumentation. Assessing tissue healing during and following nonsurgical therapy is discussed in Section 3 of this chapter.

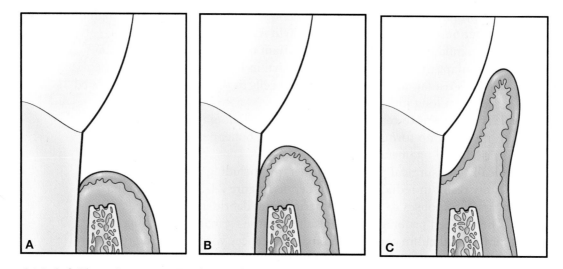

Figure 24.2. Soft Tissue Responses To Thorough Periodontal Debridement. This figure shows some of the possible tissue changes that can occur following thorough periodontal debridement. **A:** There can be complete resolution of the inflammation resulting in shrinkage of the tissue and a shallow probing depth. **B:** There can be readaptation of the tissues to the root surface forming a long junctional epithelium. **C:** There can be very little change in the level of the soft tissues resulting in a residual periodontal pocket.

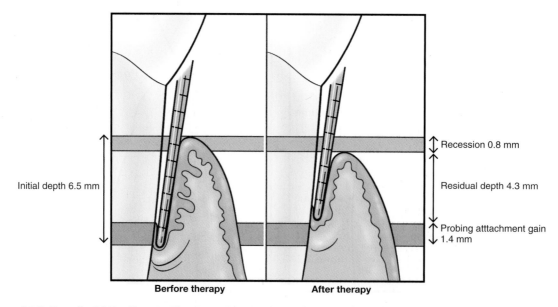

Figure 24.3. Details Of Healing At The Base Of A Pocket Following Periodontal Debridement. Since the tip of a periodontal probe can actually penetrate inflamed soft tissue in the base of periodontal pocket, the probing depth can decrease a small amount because the tissues at the base following debridement can be much more resistant to accidental penetration by the probe.

DENTINAL HYPERSENSITIVITY

Dentinal hypersensitivity as described in this section is not really a periodontal disease or a periodontal condition. However, dentinal hypersensitivity appears so frequently during successful nonsurgical periodontal therapy, that clinicians need to be aware of this condition, need to understand its origin, and need to be able to provide some of the therapies for the condition.

1. **Overview of Dental Hypersensitivity**
   A. **Description**
      1. Dentinal hypersensitivity is a short, sharp painful reaction that occurs when some areas of exposed dentin are subjected to mechanical (touch of toothbrush bristles), thermal (ice cream), or chemical (acidic grapefruit) stimuli. For example, an individual may experience pain when brushing a certain tooth or when eating sweet, sour, or acidic foods. In some patients with this condition breathing in cold air while walking outside on a cold day can produce a similar painful reaction.
      2. Dentinal hypersensitivity is associated with exposed dentin.
         a. Exposed dentin is dentin that is visible to the oral cavity due to the recession of the gingiva that normally covers the dentin or to an absence of the enamel due to damage to the tooth crown.
         b. Dentin may be exposed in a small area or exposed in an extensive area of a tooth.
         c. Since recession of the gingival margin is a very common condition, it is fortunate that not all exposed dentin is hypersensitive.
   B. **Precipitating Factors for the Sensitivity**
      1. As already stated, dentinal hypersensitivity is usually associated with recession of the gingival margin, though exposure of dentin can also occasionally result because of destruction of enamel.
      2. Resolution of inflammation in the periodontium following successful nonsurgical periodontal therapy in periodontitis patients frequently results in exposure of small areas of the tooth roots that can exhibit dentinal hypersensitivity.
      3. It is common for dentinal hypersensitivity to appear following periodontal surgical therapy, but sensitivity can also be associated with the nonsurgical periodontal therapy being discussed in this chapter.
      4. In the patient's eyes the increase in tooth sensitivity can appear to be a direct result of the nonsurgical treatment, but most often the sensitivity results from areas of clinical attachment loss which occurred prior to the actual treatment procedures.
   C. **Fundamental Origin of Hypersensitivity**
      1. Evidence suggests that the origin of dentinal hypersensitivity is explained by the hydrodynamic theory of dentin sensitivity. Important elements of this theory are outlined below.
         a. The dentinal tubules penetrate the dentin-like long, miniature tunnels extending throughout the thickness of the dentin. Figure 24-4 shows details of these dentinal tubules.
         b. As dentinal surfaces become exposed, the open dentinal tubules usually slowly close through a process of calcification that actually blocks the opening of each of the tubules.
         c. Sometimes the natural process of closure of dentinal tubules does not occur, leaving the tubule open or patent. These open or patent tubules contain fluids.

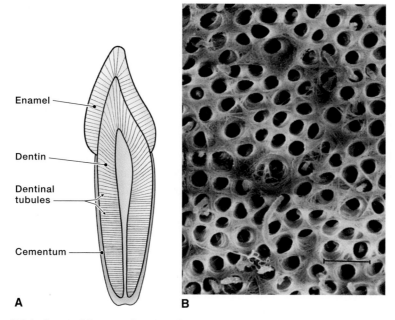

Figure 24.4. **Dentinal Tubules. A:** Diagram showing the numerous dentinal tubules that penetrate the dentin. **B:** A scanning electron micrograph of the cross section of dentinal tubules adjacent to the pulp chamber of a human tooth. The black line engraved in the lower right is 10 micrometers long. (Used with permission from Melfi RC. *Permar's Oral Embryology and Microscopic Anatomy.* 10th ed. Philadelphia: Lippincott Williams & Wilkins; 2000:120; Figure 5-8.)

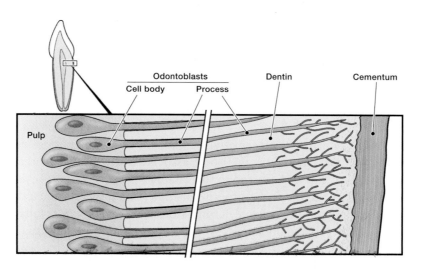

Figure 24.5. **Odontoblastic Process.** The odontoblastic cell process in the dentinal tubule often fills the part of the dentinal tubule closest to the pulp but can extend farther from the pulp toward the junction of the dentin with the enamel or cementum.

    d. The part of a dentinal tubule closest to the pulp contains an odontoblastic process which is a thin tail of cytoplasm from a cell in the tooth pulp called an odontoblast (FIG. 24-5).

    e. Disturbances to the surface of exposed dentin where the tubules remain open can result in movement of the fluids within the tubules themselves (FIG. 24-6). As already discussed, examples of disturbances to the surface of the tooth can be mechanical, thermal, or chemical stimuli. Cold temperature is one of the most common triggers for dentinal hypersensitivity.

    f. Fluid movement within open dentinal tubules can stimulate certain nerve endings that are associated with the odontoblastic processes resulting in a short, sharp pain in the tooth.

  2. Periodontal debridement and hypersensitivity can be closely related.

    a. For teeth with existing dentinal hypersensitivity instrumentation of root surfaces can result in eliciting the sharp pain. During instrumentation, local anesthesia can be used to control any discomfort that might arise during thorough instrumentation.

    b. It is fortunate that most commonly instrumentation of root surfaces does not result in dentinal hypersensitivity.

      1) Sensitivity may not occur in most instances because instrumentation of root surfaces can result in a smear layer of dentin covering the root surfaces.

      2) This so-called smear layer refers to crystalline debris from the tooth surface that covers or plugs the dentinal tubules and inhibits fluid flow, thus preventing the sensitivity.

  3. When dentinal tubules are exposed in the oral cavity such as through recession of the gingival margin, most tooth surfaces undergo a natural process of crystallization or occlusion (blocking) of the open dentinal tubules.

    a. Most dentinal hypersensitivity resulting from peridontal debridement is mild and resolves within a few weeks if the exposed root surfaces are kept plaque biofilm free.

    b. In its more severe forms, however, dentinal hypersensitivity can result in a patient's inability to perform complete self-care.

2. Strategies for Managing Dentinal Hypersensitivity

  A. Chemical Management

    1. Management of patients with dentinal hypersensitivity usually involves applying chemicals to the exposed root surface to occlude (or block) the dentinal tubules and applying chemicals to the root surface that can block the nerve receptors from activating a painful response.

    2. Chemicals can be used to occlude the dentinal tubules and to eliminate or minimize associated sensitivity. These chemicals have been reported to precipitate either minerals or proteins within open dentinal tubules resulting in sealing the openings of the tubules.

      a. There are toothpastes specifically formulated for desensitizing teeth. Toothpastes containing potassium nitrate, strontium chloride, sodium citrate, and fluorides as the active ingredients have been demonstrated to provide relief in some patients with dentinal hypersensitivity.

      b. There are also professionally applied in office products that contain chemicals that have been reported to decrease dentinal hypersensitivity. Examples of chemicals that have been reported to decrease hypersensitivity following in office applications are potassium oxalate, ferric oxalate, and fluorides solutions or fluoride varnishes.

    3. Chemicals can also be used to block the nerve receptors from activating a painful response.

      a. Potassium salts (such as potassium nitrate) found in some desensitizing toothpastes have been shown to be effective in decreasing sensitivity.

      b. Potassium can depolarize the nerve fiber and prevent pain signals from traveling to the brain.

4. Figure 24-7 illustrates the wide range of possibilities for dentinal tubules that become exposed in the oral cavity.

B. **Patient Education.** An appropriate strategy for managing patients undergoing nonsurgical periodontal therapy includes warning patients about the possibility of hypersensitivity even before beginning any treatment. Before initiating instrumentation, the dental hygienist can provide the patient with the following facts regarding dentinal hypersensitivity:

1. Sensitivity to cold can increase following periodontal debridement

2. If sensitivity resulting from periodontal debridement occurs, it usually gradually disappear over a few weeks.

3. Thorough daily plaque biofilm removal is one of the most important factors in the prevention and control of sensitivity. Without meticulous plaque biofilm control, treatments for dentinal hypersensitivity are usually not successful.

4. If dentinal hypersensitivity becomes a problem, recommendations for special toothpastes can be made that can enhance its resolution, but immediate results should not be expected.

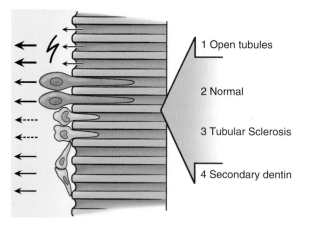

Figure 24.6. The Various Possibilities For Dentinal Tubules Both Before Therapy And Following Therapy. Dentinal tubules prior to therapy may be open, sclerosed, or insulated from the pulp itself by the formation of secondary dentin.

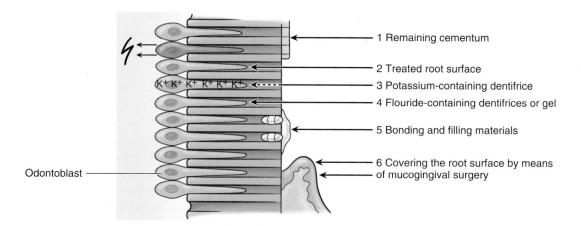

Figure 24.7. The Various Possibilities For Dentinal Tubules Following Therapy. Chemicals can be used to occlude the dentinal tubules and to eliminate or minimize associated dentinal sensitivity.

Section 3
Decisions Following Nonsurgical Therapy

THE RE-EVALUATION APPOINTMENT

Reevaluation refers to a formal step at the completion of nonsurgical therapy. During the reevaluation appointment, the members of the dental team perform another periodontal assessment to gather information about the patient's periodontal status. After comparison with the periodontal status at the time of the initial assessment, the team members make several critical clinical decisions regarding management of the patient's periodontal condition. The reevaluation is described in detail below.

1. **Reevaluation of Nonsurgical Periodontal Therapy**
   A. **Timing of a Reevaluation.**
      1. Periodontal tissue healing does not occur immediately, and in most cases it is not possible to reevaluate the true tissue response for at least 1 month after the completion of nonsurgical periodontal therapy.
      2. Members of the dental team should usually schedule an appointment for a reevaluation of a chronic periodontitis patient 4 to 6 weeks after completion of nonsurgical therapy.
   B. **Steps in a Reevaluation.** The steps in a typical reevaluation appointment include the following; these steps are also explained in Box 24-3.
      1. The first step in the reevaluation appointment is to do a medical status update for the patient. Of course this is the first step in any patient appointment.
      2. The second step is to perform a thorough periodontal assessment; the nature of a periodontal assessment has already been described in Chapter 19.
      3. The third step is to do a comparison of the results of the patient's initial assessment with the results of the patient's reevaluation assessment.
      4. The fourth step is to make appropriate decisions related to the next step in therapy. The next step may include any of the following.
         a. Additional nonsurgical therapy may be needed.
         b. The need for periodontal maintenance may be identified.
         c. The need for periodontal surgery may be evident.

Box 24-3. Steps in a Reevaluation Appointment

1. Update the medical status of the patient.
2. Perform a periodontal clinical assessment.
3. Compare the initial periodontal assessment with the reevaluation assessment.
4. Make decisions related to the next step in therapy.

   C. **Understanding Nonresponsive Disease Sites.** During the reevaluation, members of the dental team may identify nonresponsive disease sites.
      1. Nonresponsive disease sites are areas in the periodontium that show deeper probing depths, continuing loss of attachment, or continuing clinical signs of inflammation in spite of thorough nonsurgical therapy.

2. Nonresponsive sites should be carefully rechecked for thoroughness of self-care and rechecked with an explorer for the presence of residual calculus deposits.

3. If dental plaque biofilm is discovered at a nonresponsive site, the site should be thoroughly deplaqued with an ultrasonic instrument (unless ultrasonic instrumentation is contraindicated for this patient), and the patient should receive additional self-care motivation and training.

4. If calculus is found at a nonresponsite site, additional periodontal debridement should be performed.

5. When nonresponsive sites are encountered, the members of the dental team should also consider the possibility that other factors might be contributing to the disease process (such as undiagnosed diabetes or smoking).

D. **Documenting the Need for Additional Nonsurgical Therapy.** It is common for the reevaluation step to indicate the need for additional nonsurgical periodontal therapy by the dental team, and there are several reasons for this.

1. Self-care efforts by the patient, though improved, may be inadequate for control of inflammation in the periodontium.

2. Subgingival calculus deposits are difficult to remove especially in the presence of gingival edema which can make some deposits inaccessible because of deep probing depths.

3. An unsuspected systemic condition may be contributing to the disease process.

E. **Establishing a Program for Periodontal Maintenance**

1. Periodontal maintenance includes all measures used by the dental team and the patient to keep periodontitis under control; periodontal maintenance is discussed in Chapters 31 and 32.

2. The goal of periodontal maintenance is to prevent the recurrence of periodontal diseases.

3. All patients with periodontitis should be placed on an appropriate program of periodontal maintenance following nonsurgical periodontal therapy.

F. **Recognizing the Need for Periodontal Surgery**

1. The need for some types of periodontal surgery can be determined at the time of the initial periodontal assessment.

2. Periodontal surgery to control chronic periodontitis or to regenerate damaged periodontal tissues, however, is usually best identified at the time of the reevaluation; periodontal surgery and its indications are discussed in Chapter 30.

THE RELATIONSHIP BETWEEN NONSURGICAL THERAPY AND PERIODONTAL SURGERY

Periodontal surgery can play an important role in therapy for certain patients, and this topic will be discussed in other chapters of this textbook. However, at the time of reevaluation members of the dental team should be aware of the general relationship between nonsurgical periodontal therapy and periodontal surgery and should be able to discuss the possible need for periodontal surgery with patients.

1. **Indications for Surgical Therapy.** As a general rule, periodontal surgery will be needed by patients with more advanced periodontal conditions. Table 24-1 shows an overview of the relationship of nonsurgical periodontal therapy to surgical periodontal treatment for patients with various periodontal conditions.

> A. **Patients with Plaque-induced Gingivitis.** For most patients with plaque-induced gingivitis, the gingivitis can be controlled with nonsurgical therapy alone, and only rarely will periodontal surgery be a part of the treatment recommended.
>
> B. **Patients with Slight Periodontitis.** For most patients with slight (mild) chronic periodontitis, the periodontitis can be controlled with nonsurgical therapy alone.
>
> C. **Patients with Moderate Chronic Periodontitis.** For some patients with moderate periodontitis, the periodontitis can be controlled with nonsurgical therapy alone. For other patients with moderate chronic periodontitis, control of the periodontitis will require thorough nonsurgical periodontal therapy followed by periodontal surgery.
>
> D. **Patients with Severe Chronic Periodontitis.** For most patients with severe periodontitis, control of the periodontitis will require thorough nonsurgical periodontal therapy followed by periodontal surgery.

2. **Exceptions.** There will always be exceptions to the general rules described above.

> A. One example of an exception to the rule would be a patient with moderate plaque-induced gingivitis where the gingivitis has resulted in gingival enlargement. It is common for gingival enlargement to require periodontal surgery to reshape the enlargement to improve esthetics or to provide for improved access for effective self-care.
>
> B. Another example of an exception to the rule would be a patient with slight chronic periodontitis accompanied by severe recession of the gingival margin on a tooth. Though surgery is not normally needed in patients with slight chronic periodontitis, peridontal surgery may well be needed to correct the recession of the gingival margin.

TABLE 24-1. Indications for Nonsurgical and Surgical Therapy

Disease Status	Nonsurgical Therapy	Surgical Therapy
Plaque-associated gingivitis	Always indicated	Usually not indicated
Slight chronic periodontitis	Always indicated	Usually not indicated
Moderate chronic periodontitis	Always indicated	Sometimes indicated
Severe chronic periodontitis	Always indicated	Usually indicated

RECOGNIZING THE NEED FOR REFERRAL TO A PERIODONTIST

Although the general dental team can and should treat most patients with plaque-induced gingivitis and most patients with chronic periodontitis, the need for referral of some patients from a general dental office to a periodontist is always a possibility that should be considered. Making the important decision of where the patient should receive periodontal therapy is not always easy. Some recent recommendations from the American Academy of Periodontology (AAP) will be helpful for most dental teams. The members of the team should discuss this issue in detail to determine the comfort level for treating periodontitis patients within the general dental practice.

1. **American Academy of Periodontology Guidelines.** The American Academy of Periodontology recommendations for management of patients with periodontal diseases divides patients into three levels to aid a dental team in making the referral decisions [2].

    A. **Level 1: Patients Who *May Benefit* From Comanagement.** Level 1 includes patients who may benefit from comanagement by a referring dentist and the periodontist. Comanagement means management both in a general dental setting as well as in a periodontal specialist setting. Box 24-4 lists examples of patients that the AAP considers Level 1.

    B. **Level 2: Patients Who *Would Likely Benefit* from Comanagement.** Level 2 includes patients who would likely benefit from comanagement by a referring dentist and a peridontist. Box 24-5 lists examples of patients that the American Academy of Periodontology considers Level 2.

    C. **Level 3: Patients Who *Should Be* Treated by a Periodontist.** Level 3 includes patients who should be treated by a periodontist. Box 24-6 lists examples of patients that the American Academy of Periodontolgy considers Level 3.

2. **Individualizing AAP Recommendations.** It should be noted that each dental team should discuss the issue of comfort level for treating patients with periodontal conditions within the members of the team. Referral should be made for any patient with any periodontal condition which the referring dentist prefers not to treat.

Box 24-4. Examples of AAP Recommendations for Patients Who May Benefit From Comanagement by the Referring Dentist and the Periodontist (Level 1)

1. Patients with periodontal inflammation and any of the following conditions

    a. Diabetes

    b. Pregnancy

    c. Cardiovascular disease

    d. Chronic respiratory disease

2. Patients who are candidates for the following therapies who might be exposed to periodontal infection

    a. Cancer therapy

    b. Cadiovascular surgery

    c. Joint-replacement surgery

    d. Organ transplantation

Box 24-5. Examples of AAP Recommendations for Patients Who Would Likely Benefit from Comanagement by referring Dentist and the Periodontist (Level 2)

1. Patients who have onset of periodontitis prior to age 35
2. Patients with unresolved inflammation at the time of reevaluation
3. Patients with probing depths >5 mm at the time of reevaluation
4. Patients with vertical bone defects
5. Patients with radiographic evidence of progressive bone loss
6. Patients with progressive tooth mobility
7. Patients with progressive attachment loss
8. Patients with anatomic gingival deformities
9. Patients with exposed root surfaces
10. Patients with a deteriorating risk profile
11. Patients with medical or behavioral risk factors such as
    a. Smoking or tobacco use
    b. Diabetes
    c. Osteoporosis/osteopenia
    d. Drug related gingival conditions
    e. Compromised immune system
    f. A deteriorating risk profile

Box 24-6. Examples of AAP Recommendations for Patients Who Should be Treated by a Periodontist (Level 3)

1. Patients with severe chronic periodontitis
2. Patients with furcation involvement
3. Patients with vertical/angular bony defects
4. Patients with aggressive periodontitis
5. Patients with acute periodontal conditions
6. Patients with significant root surface exposure
7. Patients with progressive recession of the gingival margin
8. Patients with peri-implant disease

Chapter Summary Statement

Nonsurgical periodontal therapy refers to all the initial steps used by the dental team to bring gingivitis and periodontitis under control. The goals of nonsurgical periodontal therapy are to control the bacterial challenge to the patient, to minimize the impact of systemic risk factors, to eliminate or control local environmental risk factors, and to stabilize the attachment level. The precise steps included in nonsurgical periodontal therapy should depend on the precise needs of each individual patient.

A vital component of a plan for nonsurgical periodontal therapy is periodontal debridement. Biofilms are resistant to topical chemical plaque biofilm control; therefore, mechanical periodontal debridement of subgingival root surfaces is an essential component of successful nonsurgical periodontal therapy. Dentinal hypersensitivity may occur in some areas of exposed dentin. Thorough daily plaque biofilm removal is the most important factor in the prevention and control of hypersensitivity.

Reevaluation is an important step in nonsurgical periodontal therapy. During reevaluation the dental team determines the patient's need for additional nonsurgical therapy and/or periodontal surgery and establishes a program for periodontal maintenance.

The members of the dental team should be aware of the need for referral to a periodontist for some patients and should study the AAP recommendations for patient management.

Section 4
Focus on Patients

Case 1

A new patient for your dental team has obvious clinical signs of moderate chronic periodontitis with generalized dental plaque biofilm and dental calculus deposits. Though the patient denies having diabetes, the patient does report having several close family members with this disease. Make a list of steps your dental team might include in an appropriate plan for nonsurgical peridontal therapy for this new patient.

Case 2

At the time of reevaluation for a patient with a diagnosis of generalized moderate chronic periodontitis, your dental team identifies a few sites of residual subgingival calculus deposits and documents totally ineffective patient self-care. How should the members of your dental team manage the oral health needs of this patient?

Case 3

A new patient for your dental team is brought in for treatment in your general dental office by her parents. A screening examination reveals that this 16-year-old patient has advanced generalized attachment loss and severe alveolar bone loss. How should the members of your dental team manage the oral health needs of this young patient?

References

1. American Dental Association. *CDT-2009/2010: Current Dental Terminology*. Chicago: American Dental Association; 2008:287, vi.
2. Krebs KA, Clem DS III. Guidelines for the management of patients with periodontal diseases. *J Periodontol*. 2006;77(9):1607–1611.

Suggested Readings

Badersten A, Nilveus R, Egelberg J. Effect of nonsurgical periodontal therapy. I. Moderately advanced periodontitis. *J Clin Periodontol*. 1981;8:57–72.

Badersten A, Nilveus R, Egelberg J. Effect of nonsurgical periodontal therapy. III. Single versus repeated instrumentation. *J Clin Periodontol* 1984;11:114–124.

Bray KK. Innovations in periodontal debridement. *Dental Hyg Connect*. 1996;1:1–7.

Clifford LR, Needleman IG, Chan YK. Comparison of periodontal pocket penetration by conventional and microultrasonic inserts. *J Clin Periodontol*. 1999;26:124–130.

Cobb CM. Clinical significance of non-surgical periodontal therapy: an evidence-based perspective of scaling and root planing. *J Clin Periodontol*. 2002;29(Suppl 2):6–16.

Copulos TA, Low SB, Walker CB, et al. Comparative analysis between a modified ultrasonic tip and hand instruments on clinical parameters of periodontal disease. *J Periodontol*. 1993;64:694–700.

Cugini MA, Haffajee AD, Smith C, et al. The effect of scaling and root planing on the clinical and microbiological parameters of periodontal diseases: 12-month results. *J Clin Periodontol*. 2000;27:30–36.

Dragoo MR. A clinical evaluation of hand and ultrasonic instruments on subgingival debridement. 1. With unmodified and modified ultrasonic inserts. *Int J Periodontics Restorative Dent*. 1992;12:310–323.

Drisko CH. Nonsurgical periodontal therapy. *Periodontol 2000*. 2001;25:77–88.

Drisko CH: Root instrumentation. Power-driven versus manual scalers, which one? *Dent Clin North Am*. 1998;42:229–244.

Drisko CL, Cochran DL, Blieden T, et al. Position paper: sonic and ultrasonic scalers in periodontics. Research, Science and Therapy Committee of the American Academy of Periodontology. *J Periodontol*. 2000;71:1792–1801.

Drisko CH, Lewis LH. Ultrasonic instruments and antimicrobial agents in supportive periodontal treatment and retreatment of recurrent or refractory periodontitis. *Periodontol 2000*. 1996;12:90–115.

Greenstein G. Nonsurgical periodontal therapy in 2000: a literature review. *J Am Dent Assoc*. 2000;131:1580–1592.

Greenstein G. Periodontal response to mechanical nonsurgical therapy: a review. *J Periodontol*. 1992;63:118–130.

Haffajee AD, Cugini MA, Dibart S, et al. The effect of SRP on the clinical and microbiological parameters of periodontal diseases. *J Clin Periodontol*. 1997;24:324–334.

Hirsch RS, Clarke NG, Srikandi W. Pulpal pathosis and severe alveolar lesions: a clinical study. *Endod Dent Traumatol*. 1989;5:48–54.

Jansson LE, Ehnevid H. The influence of endodontic infection on periodontal status in mandibular molars. *J Periodontol*. 1998;69:1392–1396.

Kobayashi T, Hayashi A, Yoshikawa R, et al. The microbial flora from root canals and periodontal pockets of non-vital teeth associated with advanced periodontitis. *Int Endod J*. 1990;23:100–106.

Leon LE, Vogel RI. A comparison of the effectiveness of hand scaling and ultrasonic debridement in furcations as evaluated by differential dark-field microscopy. *J Periodontol*. 1987;58:86–94.

Lowenguth RA, Greenstein G. Clinical and microbiological response to nonsurgical mechanical periodontal therapy. *Periodontol 2000*. 1995;9:14–22.

Nield-Gehrig JS. *Fundamentals of Periodontal Instrumentation and Advanced Root Instrumentation*. 6 ed. Philadelphia: Lippincott Williams & Wilkins; 2000.

Nyman S, Sarhed G, Ericsson I, et al. Role of "diseased" root cementum in healing following treatment of periodontal disease. An experimental study in the dog. *J Periodont Res*. 1986;21:496–503.

Nyman S, Westfelt E, Sarhed G, Karring T. Role of "diseased" root cementum in healing following treatment of periodontal disease. A clinical study. *J Clin Periodontol*. 1988;15:464–468.

Oberholzer R, Rateitschak KH. Root cleaning or root smoothing. An in vivo study. *J Clin Periodontol*. 1996;23:326–330.

Rabbani GM, Ash MM Jr, Caffesse RG. The effectiveness of subgingival scaling and root planing in calculus removal. *J Periodontol*. 1981;52:119–123.

Stambaugh RV, Dragoo M, Smith DM, Carasali L. The limits of subgingival scaling, *Int J Periodontics Restorative Dent*. 1981;1:30–41.

Torfason T, Kiger R, Selvig KA, Egelberg J. Clinical improvement of gingival conditions following ultrasonic versus hand instrumentation of periodontal pockets. *J Clin Periodontol*. 1979;6:165–176.

Chapter 25

Using Motivational Interviewing to Enhance Patient Behavior Change

Learning Objectives

- Recognize the role of ambivalence in patient behavior change and explain the goal of motivational interviewing with respect to ambivalence.

- Describe the primary difference between how hygienists often approach patient education and the motivational interviewing approach.

- Be able to identify the three elements of the motivational interviewing philosophy and the four general principles.

- Give examples of specific motivational interviewing methods and how they are used to enhance patient motivation for change.

Key Terms

Motivational interviewing (MI)
Patient-centered
Guiding style
Ambivalence
Collaboration
Elicit
Autonomy
Empathy
Discrepancies

Rolling with resistance
Self-efficacy
Open-ended questions
Reflective listening
Affirm
Summarize
Change talk
Elicit, provide, elicit

Section 1
Introduction to Human Behavior Change

Patients with periodontal disease often are advised to change certain behaviors—use tuft-end toothbrushes or stop smoking—in order to promote periodontal health. The dynamics of behavior change are among the most rewarding and most challenging encounters for dental hygienists. Chronic periodontitis is largely preventable, but prevention often requires that the patient becomes actively involved in making and maintaining changes in his or her oral self-care habits.

Evidence suggests that patient adherence to recommendations is equally important as effective professional interventions (treatment) in controlling disease [1]. Behaviors such as effective, routine plaque biofilm removal, adherence to regular professional periodontal maintenance visits, and healthy lifestyle habits, therefore, are crucial issues for hygienists to address in their periodontal encounters. For this reason, effective management of the periodontal patient requires not only knowledge of the disease process and advanced instrumentation skills, but also an understanding of human behavior and motivation in order to effectively foster healthy oral self-care practices in patients.

It is very common for the dental hygienist to encounter periodontal patients who do not use effective oral self-care measures or adhere to recommendations for professional periodontal maintenance. In order to persuade patients to improve oral self-care or adhere to treatment recommendations, the dental hygienist often attempts to educate patients regarding the importance of these recommendations. Unfortunately the provision of education and expert advice is rarely sufficient to bring about the desired patient behavior change. All too often a dynamic develops in which the dental hygienist takes on the role of "the persuader" arguing for change, while the patient takes on the role of "the resistor," shooting down all suggestions, and providing a long list of reasons why he or she can't follow the recommendations. Patients may also resist passively by not engaging and simply ignoring the attempt to persuade them. In the end, patients may become more resistant while dental hygienists may become frustrated and even convinced that addressing behavior change is futile (FIG. 25-1).

Although it is tempting to simply blame the patient for being resistant, a wealth of research suggests the explanation for why patients struggle with health behavior change is far more complex. Patients' motivation is a function of numerous factors ranging from past life experiences (e.g., attitudes, beliefs, and habits developed over time); to current situational constraints (e.g., lack of time, financial resources, health literacy, and knowledge); to a lack of confidence and skills to make the necessary behavior change [2,3]. Furthermore, the interpersonal communication style of a healthcare provider can play an important role in fostering or undermining patient motivation [4,5].

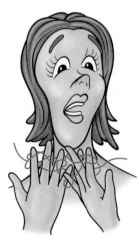

Figure 25.1. The Self-Care Struggle. Patients often struggle with professional recommendations for self-care—such as flossing—leading to frustration or even resistance to oral self-care routines.

Dental hygienists typically approach patient education in a persuasive, directive manner offering "knowledge" and prescriptive strategies to lead the patient in making required behavior change. The dental hygienist is the "expert" and the patient is the "recipient" of the expertise. When patients are not ready for behavior change, this directive, persuasive style can often lead patients to feel embarrassment, guilt, or even shame, if they are not willing or able to make the change being recommended. Not surprisingly the patient response is often defensive (FIG. 25-2) and he/she may tune out the hygienist's recommendations, or delay return for professional therapy [6–10]. Studies on adherence to health professionals' recommendations have shown that approximately 30% to 60% of health information provided in the clinician/patient encounter is forgotten within an hour, and that 50% of health recommendations provided by clinicians are not followed [11]. For patients lacking in readiness or motivation, alternatives to the expert-oriented, directive, educational approach are needed. One empirically supported alternative is Motivational Interviewing [6].

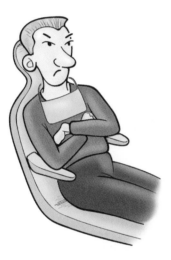

Figure 25.2. **Defensive Patient Response.** Health education advice alone usually creates defensiveness in the patient.

WHAT IS MOTIVATIONAL INTERVIEWING?

Motivational interviewing (MI) is defined as "a patient-centered method for enhancing a patient's motivation for behavior change by exploring the patient's mixed feelings about change" [8]. At its core, the Motivational Interviewing (MI) approach to counseling is "patient-centered" which means that the consideration of behavior change is viewed from the patient's perspective rather than the clinician's perspective. For example, the clinician may wish that a patient did not smoke, as smoking is an etiologic factor in periodontitis. The patient, on the other hand, might like to have healthier gums, but enjoys smoking too much to quit. The clinician's reasons why the patient should make a change—though they may be excellent—are considered far less important than the reasons the patient sees for and against change.

The clinician's goal is to develop a clear understanding of the patient's perspective on the possibility of change. Although the approach is client-centered, MI is not "non-directive" because the clinician DOES attempt to influence or encourage the patient toward healthy behavior change. One might think of this patient-centered approach as being somewhere along a continuum between "following," where the clinician mainly listens to the patient, and "directing," where the clinician tells or prescribes what the patient should do differently [12].

In MI, a guiding style is used to explore the ambivalence or pros and cons of change that the patient sees. Patients often feel ambivalent about behavior change—that is, they have mixed feelings and attitudes toward behavior change. Specific methods are used to foster the patient's intrinsic or "internal" motivation. Fostering the patient's internal motivation increases the likelihood that his or her ambivalence about changing will be resolved in the direction of change.

One of the underlying assumptions of MI is that ambivalence is typical in ANY change process (e.g., how do you feel about the need to eat at least five serving of fruit and vegetables every day, or exercise for 40 minutes 5 to 7 days a week?). It also assumed in MI that, when possible, patients tend to move naturally toward health. In other words the assumption is that most people WANT to be healthy, though they may not always feel motivated enough or capable enough of achieving it at any particular point in time. In MI the clinician attempts to tap in to and enhance any natural internal desire for healthy change in patients.

EMPIRICAL SUPPORT FOR MOTIVATIONAL INTERVIEWING

Meta-analyses indicate that MI interventions are as effective as other treatments and more effective than no-treatment or placebo controls for addictive behaviors (drugs, alcohol, and gambling), diet and exercise, treatment engagement, retention, and adherence [1,13–15]. Of particular relevance to oral self-care is evidence that MI is effective for changing overall dietary intake [16], fat intake [16,17], carbohydrate consumption [16], and consumption of fruits and vegetables [18,19]. Also, there is encouraging support for the efficacy of MI in smoking cessation, although the evidence is less strong than in other areas. MI has been found to increase readiness to quit [20], increase quit attempts [21,22], reduce smoking level [21], and in some studies to enhance cessation [23–26].

Few studies have addressed oral self-care. One study, however, compared MI to traditional health education among mothers of young children at high risk for dental caries. This study found a greater improvement in oral health among those receiving MI counseling [27,28]. Almomani et al. [29] examined the efficacy of MI for improving oral self-care in a sample of individuals with severe mental illness. Results revealed that at a single MI session prior to an oral health education session significantly enhanced motivation for regular brushing, increased oral health knowledge, and reduced plaque biofilm scores compared to oral health education alone.

Similar effects were achieved in two experimental single case studies of chronic periodontal patients. At baseline, these two patients had bleeding on probing values of 68% and 83%, respectively. Over multiple baselines these values stayed relatively stable; however when MI and oral care practice were instituted after the 4-week baseline period, both patients had statistically significant reductions in plaque biofilm and gingival index scores, with changes being maintained over a 24-month period [30].

One concern of many health practitioners is whether MI can be effective in a healthcare setting where clinicians are not trained counselors and time is short. Meta-analysis indicates that noncounselors can be effective when using MI with a significant effect in 80% of studies where MI was delivered by physicians [15]. With respect to time, as little as 15 minutes has been shown to be effective in the majority of studies [15].

Section 2
Components of Motivational Interviewing

The philosophy or "spirit" of MI is captured in three key elements. First, the approach is collaboration between the patient and clinician. In the MI approach, the clinician actively attempts to diminish his or her expert role. It is necessary to collaborate because the patient, not the clinician, is viewed as the expert on his or her life and the challenges of the behavior change in question. Second, the goal is to elicit (encourage the patient to disclose) the patient's perspective and internal motivation rather than attempting to persuade or instill motivation "from the outside." Third, MI emphasizes respect for the patient's autonomy, placing responsibility for change with the client.

Although it is sometimes easy for a healthcare provider to feel responsible for a patient's decisions, it is ultimately not the clinician's choice or life. Patients are far more likely to choose and succeed with behavior change when they have voiced their own reasons for change and made their own decision to commit. In MI, the focus of the clinician is not on the desired healthcare outcome but on facilitating a meaningful conversation that provides the greatest opportunity for a patient to consider change. The final decision for change rests with the patient. The clinician may communicate respect for the patient's autonomy directly such as *"So how would you like to proceed?"* or indirectly such as at the beginning of the visit by asking permission to talk about oral self-care (FIG. 25-3).

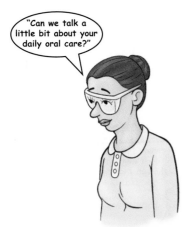

"Can we talk a little bit about your daily oral care?"

Figure 25.3. Asking Permission. Motivational Interviewing should start with asking the patient's permission.

FOUR GENERAL PRINCIPLES OF MOTIVATIONAL INTERVIEWING

Moving beyond the general philosophy or spirit, there are four general principles of Motivational Interviewing: express empathy, develop discrepancy, roll with resistance, and support self-efficacy.

1. **Express Empathy**

   Empathy is the ability to identify with and understand another person's feelings or difficulties. In MI, the clinician's expression of empathy and acceptance is critically important. In contrast to traditional patient education, this requires the clinician to explore the patient's perspective and to communicate an understanding of this view. The clinician needs to be nonjudgmental and communicate warmth and acceptance of the patient regardless of his or her choices. Open-ended questions and reflective listening—two excellent ways to express empathy—are discussed later in this chapter.

2. Develop Discrepancy

Inconsistencies between a patient's (1) current periodontal health status and self-care behaviors and (2) his or her values and goals may provide motivation for change. For example, most patients want to be healthy even though they may have chronic periodontitis and poor oral self-care. Similarly, they may want to avoid painful or unpleasant visits for dental care yet have poor oral self-care habits. These discrepancies between what would be ideal (e.g., be healthy or have no pain) and the status quo (poor self-care that results in periodontitis or pain and unpleasant visits for dental care) represent the discrepancy that can be developed or highlighted through open-ended questions and reflective listening (FIG. 25-4). For example the hygienist might highlight the discrepancy with this reflection: *"It sounds like you find it hard to stick with the thorough brushing and flossing each day, but you would really like to have healthy gums."*

3. Roll with Resistance

Another key component is to avoid confrontation and arguing by "rolling with resistance." When the patient expresses resistance to change, this is an ideal opportunity to listen well and explore the patient's perspective rather than attempting to persuade or provide counter arguments. Rolling with resistance can be accomplished in various ways but most simply by using reflective listening (FIG. 25-5). Typically patients who have been validated after expressing their reasons for not changing are then much more ready to talk about reasons why they might want to change.

4. Support Self Efficacy

Self-efficacy is a person's belief in his or her ability to perform specific tasks (e.g., public speaking, studying, etc.) to attain a goal. Many individuals avoid change because they don't believe they can succeed. Supporting self-efficacy involves seeking ways to enhance the patient's belief that he/she is capable of change. A wealth of research indicates that self-efficacy is essential for health behavior change to occur [2]. The MI clinician communicates belief in the patient's ability to change should he or she decide to do so and provides support and encouragement for this to occur.

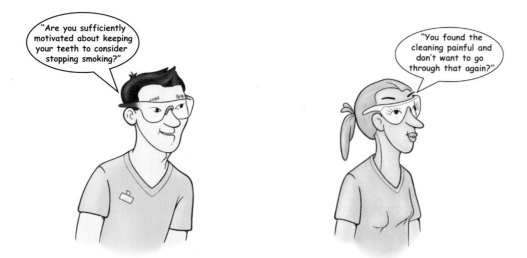

Figure 25.4. Develop Discrepancy. Open-ended questions and reflective listening can highlight discrepancies between what would be ideal (e.g., improved periodontal health) and the status quo (continuing to smoke).

Figure 25.5. Rolling with Resistance. When the patient is resistant to change, the clinician should listen well and explore the patient's point of view rather than attempting to persuade the patient that change is needed.

SPECIFIC MOTIVATIONAL INTERVIEWING METHODS

In order to implement these principles of MI, specific methods can be used which are described below.

Open-Ended Questions

Open-ended questions (questions that are framed to avoid a simple yes/no response) are preferred in MI. For example, "*How do you feel about using dental floss?*" "*How does brushing and flossing fit into your routine*" rather than "*Do you use dental floss?*" or "*Do you brush twice a day?*" The open-ended style of questioning encourages patients to elaborate and provides much more information to the clinician regarding the patient's perspective (FIG. 25-6).

Reflective Listening

Reflective listening is the process in which the healthcare provider listens to the patient's remarks and then paraphrases what the clinician heard the patient say. This allows the clinician to check with the patient that he or she is "getting the patient's message right," ensuring that the clinician is developing a good picture of the patient's perspective (FIG. 25-7). Reflective listening has the effect of validating the patient, expressing understanding (or empathy), and typically encourages the patient to elaborate so that the clinician can learn more.

Through the process of open-ended questioning and reflective listening, the clinician can begin to shift from a clinician-centered approach to oral health education to a patient-centered view of oral health education. Research has shown that the average healthcare provider interrupts patient disclosures after 18 seconds [11]. When this occurs, it sends a clear message that the patient's input is not respected nor seen as relevant. Affirming the patient's efforts and interest or willingness to seek care increases the patient's sense of trust. Once trust is established the patient can honestly express him/herself and begin to openly resolve ambivalence (mixed feelings) about change.

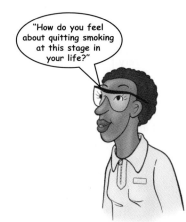

Figure 25.6. Use of Open-Ended Questions. Open-ended questions—that cannot be answered with a simple "yes" or "no" response—encourage the patient to provide additional information.

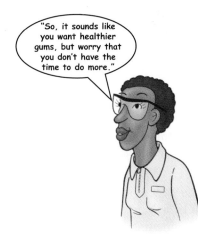

Figure 25.7. Reflecting Listening. By paraphrasing the patient's remarks, the clinician can double check if she understands the meaning of the patient's comments correctly.

Affirm

In MI, the patient's strengths and efforts should be affirmed (acknowledged) to communicate support to the patient for discussing something difficult (i.e., a change about which they may feel embarrassed, guilty, and ambivalent). Expressing appreciation for the patient taking the time to be there, or being willing to discuss their smoking, or taking some small steps toward change can enhance the therapeutic relationship and encourage the patient to engage further in the counseling process.

Summarize

Brief summaries are used in MI to link and reinforce what has been discussed and provide an opportunity for the clinician to demonstrate empathy (e.g., *"So I think I now have a fairly good picture of how you view your smoking…"*). Summaries can be used to move the conversation in a new direction (e.g., the summary can lead to a statement like "So given what we've talked about so far, what are your thoughts about the next step…" or tie different elements of the conversation together (e.g., after summarizing the patient's perspective on the difficulties of brushing regularly, the clinician might link to an earlier part of the conversation on the patient's dislike of the pain that he is experiencing: *"So it sounds like it's a real challenge to get a good brushing routine but at the same time you are really unhappy with the pain you are experiencing…"*).

Eliciting Change Talk

An integral component of MI is encouraging the expression of statements in the direction of change, referred to as change talk (i.e., the opposite of resistance). Research indicates that change talk is predictive of actual behavior change [31]. As indicated above, the assumption is that most individuals have mixed feelings about change. That patients have mixed feelings (pro and con) about change implies that they do have some reasons or desire for change. The task of the clinician is to evoke, facilitate, and strengthen this desire for change. Change talk can be elicited with simple open-ended questions such as *"What advantages do you see of cutting back on sugary foods?"*

Another approach is to use the "motivation" or "importance ruler" in which the clinician asks *"On a scale of 1 to 10 with 10 being most important, how important is to you to improve your oral self-care habits?"* (Fig. 25-8).

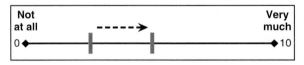

Figure 25.8. A Motivation Ruler. A motivation ruler is a method for learning a patient's level of readiness for behavior change.

Once the patient identifies the self-rated importance of change, the clinician elicits change talk by asking, *"What made you pick 3 rather than zero."* Rather than asking why the patient is NOT at 10, this open-ended question encourages the patient to express any importance that he or she DOES place on improving oral self-care behaviors. After eliciting and reflecting change talk, barriers to change can also be explored by asking, *"What would it take for you to increase the importance 2 or 3 additional levels?"* This approach can also be used to explore confidence (or self-efficacy) in engaging in a new behavior, which is also often a key contributor to an individual's motivation to change.

In general, once the clinician has elicited change talk the goal is to encourage even more change talk (Fig. 25-9). Reflective listening is very effective means of achieving this goal and the skilled MI clinician can use reflective statements to roll with resistance and highlight change (e.g., a reflection that ends with the change talk such as *"On the one hand you really love sugary foods, but on the other hand you really want to set a good example to your children"* encourages elaboration by the patient of the desire to set a good example rather than the love of sugary foods because the change talk is reflected at the end of the reflective statement.

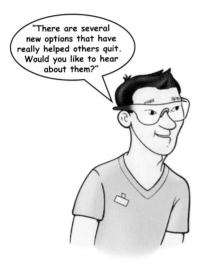

Figure 25.9. **Change Talk**. In this example the clinician engages in change talk while supporting the patient's right to make his or her own decision.

Providing Information and Advice

Although the provision of information and advice should be done with caution—to avoid taking the expert role and to avoid the pitfall of pressing for change—there are nevertheless occasions when providing information is appropriate. For example, providing information may be necessary when the patient asks for information, or when motivation might be enhanced by new information that might help in overcoming obstacles to change. To avoid "taking on the expert role," the clinician can ask permission first: *"Would you be interested in hearing some more information about the benefits of quitting smoking for your oral health?"* The clinician avoids the "expert role" by referring to other sources for the information such as *"Many patients tell me..."* or *"Research seems to indicate..."* rather then saying *"I have found..."* or *"I would recommend...."*

A three-step process known as "Elicit, Provide, Elicit" is also a useful method for delivering information and advice in an MI consistent manner. The first step (Elicit) involves enquiring what the patient already knows. For example, *"What have you heard about the benefits of flossing on a daily basis?"* The second step (Provide) involves the providing relevant information and advice: *"Yes you are right, those are some good reasons to floss daily. There are also some other reasons dental hygienists encourage flossing for cases like yours, such as..."* The final step (Elicit) involves checking back with the patient to see what they have taken from the information or advice provided. For example, *"So I'm wondering you think about that research and how it applies to you?"*

Section 3
Implications for Dental Hygiene Practice

Moving from the clinician-centered perspective of oral health education to the patient-centered view of behavior change can enhance the patient's internal motivation for healthy behavior change. If the hygienist judges, lectures, and directs, the patient ceases to engage in dialog and be part of the solution. Ironically, this can result in yet more directive advice given by the clinician. Using MI, the hygienist can engage in a more productive interaction in which he or she no longer feels responsible (and frustrated!) about the patient's decisions. Instead, the hygienist focuses on encouraging the patient to examine his or her attitudes about periodontal disease or the periodontal maintenance schedule.

EXAMPLE 1

Mrs. J. is a 50-year-old attorney who has been referred to your periodontal dental office for evaluation and treatment. Mrs. J. has type 2 diabetes, a glycosylated hemoglobin value of 8, and moderately severe chronic periodontitis. Mrs. J. has been sporadic in visiting her regular dentist and the letter from the referring dentist states that after a 1-year absence Mrs J. presented recently with increased bleeding on probing and evidence of increasing attachment loss. The general dentist is concerned that without periodontal therapy, Mrs. J. will likely lose several teeth.

Hygienist: I see that your general dentist has referred you here for periodontal treatment. Can you tell me a little about your past dental care and why you are here today?"

Mrs. J.: Yes, Dr. Smith thinks that if I don't get specialty treatment I'm going to lose some of my back teeth. I take care of my teeth and I think he's over reacting to my gums bleeding a bit more than usual.

Hygienist: I am very happy you followed up with Dr. Smith and came in to see us. [Affirmation] So if it's okay with you, I'd like to spend a little time talking about the health of your gums. [Getting permission]

Mrs. J.: That's fine with me.

Hygienist: Good. So, if you would, can you tell me what is a typical day like for you and how taking care of your teeth fits into your normal day? [Open-ended question]

Mrs. J.: Sure. Most days I need to be at my office by 8:30, so I generally get up around 7, shower, have some coffee and toast, check emails, brush my teeth, and drive my 20-minute commute to the office. Once I'm at my office, my schedule is really full. I'm currently working on three really difficult cases that take up most of my time. I'm pretty stressed out! I don't eat a regular lunch but will usually snack on a granola bar to hold me over to dinner. I'm usually home around 6:30, have dinner, and then catch up on reading documents for the next day. Sometimes I brush my teeth before bed, but mostly I'm just too exhausted to care at night. I do try, but don't always succeed. The dental hygienist at Dr. Smith's is always on my case about not brushing enough, not flossing enough, and not coming in every 3 months.

Hygienist: It sounds like you have a really busy schedule that makes it difficult for you to keep up with recommendations given by Dr. Smith's hygienist. If I understand you, though, you do make a concerted effort to brush at least every morning. [Reflective listening]

Mrs. J.: Yes, I am very good about brushing in the morning.

Hygienist: That's great. It's important to have a routine that works well for you. [Affirmation] You mentioned that the hygienist at Dr. Smith's office is concerned about your not flossing enough or coming in every 3 months. Tell me about that. [Open-ended questioning]

Mrs. J.: Shelley, that's her name, says that if I don't floss every day and come in to have my teeth scraped every 3 months that I'll end up losing my teeth. She lectures me every time I go in, and I really dread going to see her. I don't think she understands how busy my schedule is. The only reason I agreed to come here was that Dr. Smith thought you might be able to do something to get rid of my pockets.

Hygienist: So, it sounds like you are interested in improving your gum health but don't like being lectured when you go to the dentist. [Reflective listening]

Mrs. J.: That's right. I also read in a magazine that diabetes might make my gum disease worse, so I figured it's worth finding out. Is that true? Can my diabetes make my gums worse? Can you get rid of my pockets so this gum disease will stop?

Hygienist: There is quite a bit of new information about diabetes and periodontal disease, and there are some things that we can do at our office to reduce pockets. Research has shown that controlling gum disease, especially in diabetics, requires professional care but also requires patients to be actively involved in helping control the disease on a day to day basis. We have had many patients who have had very good success using this approach. Would you like to know more about it? [Providing information that was requested/Supporting autonomy]

Mrs. J.: I would like to know more, but I'm skeptical that it's going to be more of the same that I hear from Shelley—"brush—floss—come to see me—brush—floss—come to see me."

Hygienist: Right… you want help but worry that it will still involve more effort on your part than you really have time for. [Reflect]

Mrs. J.: Exactly!

Hygienist: Well, I want to emphasize that how we move forward is up to you. The time and effort you put in brushing and flossing is something you will need to determine based on what's most important to you. [Support autonomy] If it's ok with you [Support autonomy/Ask permission], I'd like to try to go slowly, try to work with your busy schedule, and help you keep your teeth. After I conduct my exam, I'd also like to give you some information on diabetes and gum disease that you can read before your next visit and then we can talk more about how that might be contributing to your gum disease. Are you interested in that? [Support autonomy/Ask permission]

Mrs. J.: That sounds good—the magazine article didn't give much detail, but it did say that diabetes can make gum disease worse. I'll make it a point of adding it to my evening reading tonight.

Hygienist: Excellent! I think you might find the information helpful as we work toward getting your gum disease under control.

EXAMPLE 2

Mr. A. is a 58-year-old banker who has come to the dental office wanting an implant for a first molar that was lost to periodontal disease last year. At the time, he was not interested in discussing a replacement but has made an appointment today, as he wants to get an implant for replacement. Although he contends that he brushes and flosses regularly, his oral self-care has only been fair for many years, he has a 30-year tobacco habit, and is currently smoking about 1½ pack of cigarettes a day.

Hygienist: Good morning Mr. A. What brings you in today? [Open ended questioning]

Mr. A.: Well, you know, I have this missing tooth here and when I chew it really bothers me. You know, food gets stuck up in there and on top of that it just doesn't look good when I smile. A buddy at work told me about implants and I'm seriously interested in getting one.

Hygienist: So where that tooth is missing is causing you some problems and you aren't happy with the appearance of that gap. [Reflective listening]

Mr. A.: Yeah, every time I eat I get food caught. It doesn't hurt but it's gotten really irritating. I know we talked about it when you took the tooth out, but I don't want a partial. I really want the implant. You mentioned then that my smoking might be a problem with getting an implant.

Hygienist: Your friend told you about dental implants and you think it's the right choice for replacing that tooth. [Reflective listening]

Mr. A.: That's right. I know when I was here before you said that my smoking might be a problem with getting an implant.

Hygienist: Yes, smoking is a major barrier for using implants because it makes it much harder for healing to occur and then maintain the health of tissues around the implant. But it sounds like you are really interested in getting an implant [Providing information in response to an implied question/Reflective listening].

Mr. A.: I am!

Hygienist: Well, can we spend a few minutes talking about your smoking, and what your thoughts and feelings about smoking are? [Asking permission]

Mr. A.: Sure, I'm a smoker and not ashamed of it.

Hygienist: Okay, let me put it another way. Are you sufficiently motivated about the implant to consider stopping smoking? [Developing discrepancy]

Mr. A.: No. I've tried to do that before and it wasn't any fun. I'm not sure I could quit if I wanted to.

Hygienist: Okay. It sounds like you have tried before and you have the sense that even if you wanted to quit, you don't think you could. It's something that is very hard for you. [Reflective listening]

Mr. A.: I went though that agony before and it didn't work. I can't see any reason to put myself through that again.

Hygienist: Trying to quit would be too painful and it's not important enough to you to stop right now. [Rolling with resistance]

Mr. A.: Yes, I enjoy it and haven't had any ill effects from smoking. I'm pretty happy to continue as I am.

Hygienist: Well, other than the possible disadvantage that smoking has to getting this implant, are there any other disadvantages that you see to smoking? [Eliciting change talk]

Mr. A.: Taxes keep going up, and it's an expensive habit, but I'm willing to pay the price. It's one of my luxuries in life.

Hygienist: Anything else? [Eliciting change talk]

Mr. A.: Only one thing—my kids really want me to quit. They are afraid I'm going to end up with something bad, but I haven't had any ill effects from smoking.

Hygienist: So, it sounds like the cost of smoking bothers you, but not too much, but you really haven't had any health problems. Your family worries though. [Reflective listening to elicit more change talk]

Mr. A.: Yes, that's right.

Hygienist: I have the sense that you're not ready to quit right now, but I'd like to learn more regarding your thoughts about smoking if that's ok with you. Where would you put yourself on a scale of 0 to 10 where 0 is "no motivation at all to quit" and 10 is "very motivated"? I know you aren't a 10, but where would you be. [Eliciting change talk using the motivation ruler]

Mr. A.: Hmmmm. I'd probably put myself at a 2 or 3, somewhere in there.

Hygienist: So you have some small amount of motivation to quit—what gives you that level of motivation? [Elicit change talk using the motivation ruler]

Mr. A.: Well I know that smoking isn't good for me, I'm not dumb. And like I said before, my family really wants me to quit. It would be a nice gesture to do that for my family. They really do have my best interests in mind.

Hygienist: You mentioned that you know smoking isn't good for you and your family worries about health effect. Can you tell me what ill health effects worry you? [Elicit change talk]

Mr. A.: Sure—cancer and lung disease.

Hygienist: So, there are some disadvantages besides the implant that you've thought about but you still aren't sufficiently motivated to quit. Earlier, though, you mentioned that you weren't sure that you would be able to quit even if you wanted to. [Reflective listening to explore influence of confidence on motivation] How motivated would you be if you were more confident that you could quit?

Mr. A.: I guess if I knew I could succeed with quitting I'd be more motivated.

Hygienist: If we could help you with improving your confidence in quitting, would you find that helpful? [Elicit change talk/assess interest before providing information or advice to support autonomy]

Mr. A.: Yes, it might.

Hygienist: There are several options that we could work on to improve your confidence to quit smoking. We could focus on doing that while also discussing the feasibility of the implant. Do you think you might be interested in pursuing this? [Elicit commitment/change talk while supporting autonomy]

Mr. A.: Sure. I guess I don't have anything to lose.

EXAMPLE 3

Ms. S. is a 35-year-old administrative assistant at the local community college. She has come to the dental office as a new patient and desires tooth whitening for her "yellowed teeth." During the routine dental evaluation no caries are found; however, there is generalized moderate gingival inflammation with slight bone loss in the interproximal posterior regions. The patient reports that she had a partial "deep cleaning" 2 years ago at her previous dentist but had really sensitive teeth and didn't return for completing treatment.

Hygienist: Hello Ms. S. What brings you to our office? [Open-ended questioning]

Ms. S.: My friend recently came to see you to have his teeth whitened and they look terrific. I haven't been happy with the color of my teeth for a long time, so I thought you could make my smile whiter too.

Hygienist: Okay. Can we first spend a few minutes talking about your mouth and oral health? [Getting permission]

Ms. S.: Sure, that's fine.

Hygienist: Good. Can you tell me a little about problems you have had and how taking care of your teeth fits into your regular days events? [Open-ended questioning]

Ms. S.: I have really healthy teeth and have never had any cavities. I'm really not happy with the yellow color of my teeth and want to do something about that.

Hygienist: Anything else?

Ms. S.: Well, the last dentist I went to said I had some gum disease. My gums have always bled when I brush, but they made a big deal out of it. I had to see the hygienist for a deep cleaning, but my teeth got so sensitive afterward, I didn't go back.

Hygienist: Tell me a little more about your gum treatment. [Open-ended questioning]

Ms. S.: The dentist and hygienist told me I had to have that deep cleaning or I could lose my teeth. Everyone in my family has gum disease and they still have most of their teeth. I must have inherited it. I'm really only interested in tooth whitening. I don't want any more deep cleanings.

Hygienist: It sounds like the deep cleaning you had was unpleasant and you don't see that gum disease is very important. [Reflective listening]

Ms. S.: I didn't say it wasn't important—I just want my teeth to look better. My teeth were so sensitive after having half of my mouth deep cleaned, I could barely drink anything with ice in it. If that is what it takes to have healthy gums, I'm happy just as I am.

Hygienist: The effects of the deep cleaning treatment were so bad that you don't want to go through it again even if it means not having healthy gums. [Rolling with resistance using reflective listening]

Ms. S.: It's not that it isn't important. I don't want to lose my teeth, but I also don't want all of that sensitivity. I was thinking that getting my teeth whitened will make me look better and wouldn't hurt as much.

Hygienist: Avoiding pain is really important to you. [Rolling with resistance by expressing empathy through reflective listening]

Ms. S.: Yeah, I guess I sound pretty wimpy. My teeth are important but if I have to be in pain for a long time afterward it's not worth it to me.

Hygienist: You want healthy teeth and if you could get your teeth whitened and gum disease treated without a lot of pain afterward, it might be worth doing. [Reflective listening]

Ms. S.: If I knew that I could get my gums healthy and not have to go through what I did before, I might be willing to discuss gum treatments. Is that possible?

Hygienist: There are several things that have worked for others to reduce the temperature sensitivity after deep cleaning. Are you interested in learning a little bit more? [Ask permission]

Ms. S.: I might be.

Hygienist: All right, let me give you some information and we can talk about strategies for controlling the sensitivity after treatment. [Provide] We can also talk about a plan for whitening your teeth once we get the gum disease under control. How would that meet your need for appearance and health? [Support autonomy]

Chapter Summary Statement

A key challenge for dental hygiene practitioners is working with patients to foster behavior change to improve oral self-care. MI provides an empirically supported approach to the challenges of counseling patients for health behavior change. It rests on a foundation of empathy and uses specific methods such as open-ended questions and reflective listening to encourage patients to consider their own reasons for change. Use of this patient-centered approach to behavior change can enhance the quality of encounters between hygienists and their patients by diminishing patient resistance, fostering greater patient motivation for change, and strengthening the patient-provider relationship.

Section 4
Focus on Patients

Case 1

Refer to the case of Mrs. J. the 50-year-old attorney to answer the following questions:
1. Why does the hygienist begin with the question "Can you tell me a little about… why you are here today?"
2. Describe Mrs. J's ambivalence regarding behavior change (i.e., what cons AND pros for change does SHE see?).
3. What examples of "change talk" can you identify in the dialogue.

Case 2

Refer to the case of Mr. A. the 58-year-old banker to answer the following questions:
1. When the conversation first turns to smoking the hygienist asks Mr. A. "Are you sufficiently motivated about the implant to consider stopping smoking?" This is labeled as an example of "developing discrepancy." What discrepancy does this refer to and how is this meant to foster motivation for change?
2. What is Mr. A's ambivalence regarding behavior change (i.e., what cons AND pros for change does HE see?)
3. Mr. A. provided lots of change talk in the dialogue but what turns out to be the key barrier for change that if the hygienist: can help address will significantly increase his motivation?

Case 3

Using the information in the case of Ms. S., the 35-year-old administrative assistant, try the following:
1. With a classmate take turns assuming the role of Ms. S. and the hygienist. Practice asking an open-ended question to begin the visit followed by a reflection of Ms. S's response.
2. Ms. S. could benefit from information on how to get her gums healthy while reducing sensitivity. With a classmate practice using the three step "Elicit, Provide, Elicit" process to give her some relevant information.

References

1. Hettema J, Steele J, Miller WR. Motivational interviewing. *Ann Rev Clin Psychol*. 2005;1: 91–111.
2. Bandura A. *Self-efficacy: The Exercise of Control*. New York: WH Freeman; 1997.
3. Fishbein M, Triandis HC, Kanfer FH, et al. *Factors influencing behavior and behavior change*, in *Handbook of Health Psychology*. In Baum A, Revenson TA, Dinger JE, eds. Mahwah: Lawrence Erlbaum; 2001:3–17.
4. Ryan RM, Deci EL. Self-determination theory and the facilitation of intrinsic motivation, social development, and well-being. *Am Psychol*. 2000;55(1):68–78.
5. Williams GC, McGregor HA, Zeldman A, et al. Testing a self-determination theory process model for promoting glycemic control through diabetes self-management. Health psychology: official journal of the Division of Health Psychology. *Am Psychol Assoc*. 2004;23(1):58–66.
6. Miller WR, Rollnick S. *Motivational Interviewing: Preparing People for Change*. 2nd ed. New York: Guillford Press; 2002.
7. Resnicow K, DiIorio C, Soet JE, et al. Motivational interviewing in health promotion: it sounds like something is changing. *Health Psychol*. 2002;21(5):444–451.
8. Rollnick S, Miller WR. What is motivational interviewing?. *Behav Cognitive Psychother*. 1995;23:325–334.
9. Shinitzky HE, Kub J. The art of motivating behavior change: the use of motivational interviewing to promote health. *Public Health Nurs*. 2001;18(3):178–185.
10. Freeman R. The psychology of dental patient care. 10. Strategies for motivating the non-compliant patient. *Br Dent J*. 1999;187(6):307–312.
11. Prounis C. *Doctor-patient communication*. **Pharmaceutical** executive. Advanstar Communications, Inc; 2005.
12. Rollnick S, Miller WR, Butler CC. *Motivational Interviewing in Health Care*. New York: The Guilford Press; 2008.
13. Burke BL, Arkowitz H, Menchola M. The efficacy of motivational interviewing: a meta-analysis of controlled clinical trials. *J Consult Clin Psychol*. 2003;71(5):843–861.
14. Burke BL, Dunn CW, Atkins DC, and Phelps JS. The emerging evidence base for motivational interviewing: A meta-analytic and qualitative inquiry. *J Cognitive Psychother*. 2004;18(4):309–322.
15. Rubak S, Sandbæk A, Lauritzen T, et al. Motivational interviewing: a systematic review and meta-analysis. *Br J Gen Pract*. 2005;55(513):305–312.
16. Mhurchu CN, Margetts BM, Speller V. Randomized clinical trial comparing the effectiveness of two dietary interventions for patients with hyperlipidaemia. *Clin Sci (Lond)*. 1998;95(4):479–487.
17. Bowen D, Ehret C, Pedersen M, et al. Results of an adjunct dietary intervention program in the Women's Health Initiative. *J Am Diet Assoc*. 2002;102(11):1631–1637.
18. Resnicow K, Jackson A, Wang T, et al. A motivational interviewing intervention to increase fruit and vegetable intake through Black churches: results of the Eat for Life trial. *Am J Public Health*. 2001;91(10):1686–1693.
19. Richards A, Kattelmann KK, Ren C. Motivating 18- to 24-year-olds to increase their fruit and vegetable consumption. *J Am Diet Assoc*. 2006;106(9):1405–1411.
20. Butler CC, Rollnick S, Cohen D, et al. Motivational consulting versus brief advice for smokers in general practice: a randomized trial. *Br J Gen Pract*. 1999;49:611–616.
21. Borrelli B, Novak S, Hecht J, et al. Home health care nurses as a new channel for smoking cessation treatment: outcomes from project CARES (Community-nurse Assisted Research and Education on Smoking). *Prev Med*. 2005;41(5–6):815–821.
22. Wakefield M, Olver I, Whitford H, et al. Motivational interviewing as a smoking cessation intervention for patients with cancer: randomized controlled trial. *Nurs Res*. 2004;53(6):396–405.
23. Curry SJ. Youth tobacco cessation: filling the gap between what we do and what we know. *Am J Health Behav*. 2003;27(Suppl 2):S99–S102.
24. Pbert L, Osganian SK, Gorak D, et al. A school nurse-delivered adolescent smoking cessation intervention: a randomized controlled trial. *Prev Med*. 2006;43(4):312–320.
25. Soria R, et al. A randomised controlled trial of motivational interviewing for smoking cessation. *Br J Gen Pract*. 2006;56(531):768–774.
26. Valanis B, Lichtenstein E, Mullooly JP, et al. Maternal smoking cessation and relapse prevention during health care visits. *Am J Prev Med*. 2001;20(1):1–8.
27. Weinstein P, Harrison R, Benton T. Motivating parents to prevent caries in their young children: one-year findings. *J Am Dent Assoc*. 2004;135(6):731–738.

28. Weinstein P, Harrison R, Benton T. Motivating mothers to prevent caries: confirming the beneficial effect of counseling. *J Am Dent Assoc*. 2006;137(6):789–793.

29. Almomani F, Williams K, Catley D, and Brown C. Effects of an oral health promotion program in people with mental illness. *J Dent Res*. 2009;88:648–52.

30. Jonsson B, Ohrn K, Oscarson N, and Lindberg P. An individually tailored treatment programme for improved oral hygiene: introduction of a new course of action in health education for patients with periodontitis. *Int J Dent Hyg*. 2009;7(3):166–175.

31. Amrhein PC, Miller WR, Yahne CE, et al. Client commitment language during motivational interviewing predicts drug use outcomes. *J Consult Clin Psychol*. 2003;71(5):862–878.

Chapter 26

Patient's Role in Nonsurgical Periodontal Therapy

Learning Objectives

- Discuss the concept of self-care and the roles of the patient and provider.
- State the benefits of power toothbrushes.
- In the clinical setting, recommend and teach power brushing to an appropriate patient.
- Give examples of oral conditions that might prompt a dental hygienist to recommend a power toothbrush.
- State the rationale for tongue cleaning.
- In the clinical setting, recommend and teach tongue cleaning to an appropriate patient.
- Explain why interdental care is of special importance for a patient with periodontitis.
- Define the term gingival embrasure space and explain its importance in selecting effective interdental aids.
- Define the term root concavity and explain its importance in selecting effective interdental aids.
- In a classroom or laboratory setting, explain the criteria for selection and correctly demonstrate the use of the following to an instructor: power toothbrush and all the interdental aids presented in this chapter.
- In a clinical setting, recommend, explain, and demonstrate appropriate interdental aids to a patient with type III embrasure spaces. Assist the patient in selecting an appropriate interdental aid that the patient is willing to use on a daily basis.

Key Terms

Nonsurgical periodontal therapy (NSPT)
Co-therapist
Volatile sulfur compounds (VSC)
Gingival embrasure space

Type I embrasure space
Type II embrasure space
Type III embrasure space
Root concavity

Section 1
Patient Self-Care

1. **The Patient's Role in Nonsurgical Therapy.** Nonsurgical periodontal therapy (NSPT) includes all nonsurgical treatment and educational measures used to help control gingivitis and periodontitis, such as patient self-care, periodontal instrumentation, and chemical plaque biofilm control.

    A. **Patient as Co-therapist.** Because the primary etiologic factor for periodontitis is bacterial plaque biofilm, much of nonsurgical periodontal therapy must be directed toward its daily control by the patient.

        1. Successful nonsurgical periodontal therapy always involves the patient in an intensive program of self-care techniques.

        2. The patient's efforts at self-care are so critical to the control of periodontitis that some dental teams refer to the patient as having the role of co-therapist in the process of nonsurgical periodontal therapy.

            a. This concept of the patient as co-therapist is used to underscore the vital role the patient plays in establishing control of periodontitis.

            b. The patient should be actively involved in making decisions about his or her own healthcare and be willing to make a long-term commitment to meticulous self-care and regular professional care.

    B. **Goals of Mechanical Plaque Biofilm Control.** The goal of mechanical plaque biofilm control is the physical removal or disruption of bacteria and their products. Mechanical plaque biofilm control includes self-care by the patient on a daily basis and subgingival periodontal instrumentation by the dental hygienist at regular intervals.

2. **Self-Care**

    A. **What Is Self-Care?** There is no single accepted definition of self-care. According to one medical dictionary, it is the personal care performed by the patient usually in collaboration with and after instruction by a healthcare professional [1]. This may include activities related to both disease prevention and health maintenance.

        1. Self-care involves instruction on the use and frequency of a product. For example, the addition of a product such as interdental aid to the daily routine.

        2. Self-care includes collaboration between the dental hygienist and patient.

            a. The dental hygienist needs to provide input and support while at the same time encouraging patient participation in the final decision on self-care devices.

            b. The optimal device must take patient preference into consideration. Recommending a device that the practitioner likes but that the patient dislikes will not contribute to patient motivation and compliance.

            c. Collaboration hinges on good communication so the dental hygienist needs to provide education and instruction using words that the patient understands.

    B. **Goals of Self-Care.** The goal of self-care is improved oral health via optimal biofilm removal and the elimination of bleeding and inflammation.

        1. Toothbrushing is the most frequently used and often the only used device by most patients for daily self-care.

        2. Tongue cleaning on a daily basis helps control halitosis and may contribute to a healthy periodontal environment.

        3. Interdental aids are necessary for most patients and critical for periodontal maintenance patients as this area is generally not accessible to toothbrushing.

Section 2
Toothbrushing and Tongue Cleaning

1. Toothbrushing
   A. **Manual Toothbrushing**
      1. Ensuring that the periodontitis patient uses a sulcular brushing technique with a soft bristle brush is central to most self-care programs.
      2. Manual toothbrushing techniques are not covered in detail here because these topics are covered fully in other courses in the dental hygiene curriculum.
   B. **Power Toothbrushing.** Power brushes have been in existence for many years. In the past, powered brushes were recommended for those individuals with special needs or a disability. Today, there is a power brush available to fit multiple needs in a wide range of prices.
      1. Rationale for Recommending a Power Toothbrush
         a. While any individual could benefit from a power toothbrush, patients with poor biofilm control, orthodontic appliances, implants, aesthetic restorations, gingival overgrowth, crowns and bridges, or physical disabilities are ideal candidates to use power toothbrush.
         b. Some power brushes feature timers. This feature is particularly beneficial for helping patients increase brushing time. Longer brushing times have been shown to enhance biofilm removal [2].
      2. Considerations for Recommending a Power Toothbrush
         a. Brush head size should be appropriate to the size of the patient's mouth. Patient preference should guide brush head configuration. Configurations are varied depending on manufacturer. Popular shapes are round or elliptical [2].
         b. Handle designs vary in size and ergonomics. Selection should be appropriate to the age and dexterity of the user [2].
         c. Power sources may come from rechargeable or replaceable (i.e., AA alkaline) batteries.
      3. Benefits
         a. Certain power toothbrushes have been shown to remove biofilm and reduce gingivitis better than a manual toothbrush. They may also provide better stain reduction and enhance patient compliance with a self-care regimen [2,3].
         b. One systematic review of power brushes found a rotation oscillation toothbrush was consistently superior to a manual toothbrush [4].
      4. Technique
         a. *Whether manual or power, thorough brushing is dependent on correct technique.*
            1. As with a manual toothbrush, the patient needs to properly angle the power toothbrush in the mouth. Once in place, however, the brush head motion on a power toothbrush will do all the work.
            2. Since a power brush generates more strokes per minute than a manual brush, the individual may remove more biofilm in the same amount of brushing time [2].
         b. Power brushes have a different sound and sensation than a manual brush.
            1. It may take some time for a patient to get adjusted to a new product.
            2. Additionally, some power brushes may increase the foaming action of toothpaste. Patients should be instructed to use a small amount of toothpaste and to place the brush head in the mouth before turning on the unit.

c. The dental hygienist should read the manufacturer's users guide prior to recommending and/or demonstrating a power brush to a patient. *Patients should also be counseled to follow the manufacturer's instructions for the best outcome.*

2. **Tongue Cleaning.** Many patients have coated tongues that make it difficult to maintain fresh breath and cause a lessened sense of taste. Daily tongue cleaning controls halitosis and may help to maintain a healthy periodontal environment.

   A. **Rationale for Tongue Cleaning**
      1. The tongue coating is made up of bacteria and other putrefied debris that produces hydrogen sulfide and methyl mercaptan.
      2. Periodontal patients have been shown to have significantly higher prevalence of tongue coating [5].
      3. Tongue coating also can contribute to a lessened sense of taste. Tongue cleaning should be recommended to geriatric patients who have a low desire to eat due to depressed taste sensation.
      4. Most patients are concerned about controlling halitosis and therefore are receptive to the introduction of tongue cleaning to their self-care routine. The practice of tongue cleaning may not only make a patient feel more confident, but may actually help in maintaining a healthy periodontal environment.

   B. **Role of Volatile Sulfur Compounds in Halitosis.**
      1. Volatile sulfur compounds (VSC) are a family of gases that are responsible for halitosis.
      2. Two members of the VSC family of gases, hydrogen sulfide and methyl mercaptan, are principally responsible for mouth odor. Methyl mercaptan is produced primarily by periodontal pathogens. Some studies have suggested that at low concentrations these gases may be toxic to tissues; however the research in this area is limited [6].
      3. Tongue cleaning is recommended because the bulk of bacteria and debris—especially the periodontal pathogens that produce methyl mercaptan—accumulate mostly within the filiform papillae and on the back of the tongue.
      4. Methyl mercaptan gases have been shown to increase the permeability of intact mucosa and stimulate the production of cytokines associated with periodontal disease.

   C. **Manual Tongue Cleaners.** Manual tongue cleaners come in a variety of styles. The two most common types are (1) specialized toothbrushes with a thin brush head and (2) tongue scrapers (FIG. 26-1).

   D. **Technique**
      1. The tongue brush or scraper is positioned as far back on the tongue as possible.
      2. Once the brush or scraper is in position, it is pulled forward gently over the tongue. This procedure is repeated two or three times or until the tongue is clean.
      3. When first learning tongue cleaning, many patients gag and find the process unpleasant.
         a. In the beginning, encourage the patient to place the cleaner wherever it is most comfortable on the tongue.
         b. Initially, it is helpful to encourage the patient by reminding him or her of the benefits of tongue cleaning, such as improved breath, improved taste sensation, and of course, better oral health.
         c. With regular use, most patients become accustomed to the sensation of the tongue brush or scraper and are able to clean further back on the tongue. Over time, most patients become skilled at tongue cleaning.

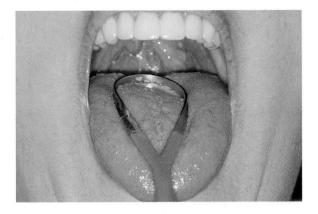

Figure 26.1. Manual Tongue Scraper. Daily tongue cleaning controls halitosis and may help to maintain a healthy periodontal environment.

TABLE 26-1. Aids for Interdental Plaque Biofilm Removal

Interdental Aid	Description/Example	Indications for Use
Dental Floss	Unwaxed or waxed thread made of silk and nylon or plastic monofilament fibers	A patient with type I embrasure spaces and excellent compliance to self-care regime
Floss holders	Hand held device to hold the floss or single use device containing a segment of dental floss (Reach Access Flosser, Glide Floss Picks)	A patient with type I embrasure spaces who is motivated but has dexterity issues
Tufted dental floss	Thickened yarn-like dental floss (J & J Superfloss)	Type II embrasure spaces, fixed bridges, distal surface of last tooth in the arch, proximal surfaces of widely spaced teeth
Interdental brush	Tiny nylon brushes on a handle (Butler Gum Proxibrush) Some brands come in varying sizes (TePe Interdental Brushes)	Type II or Type III embrasure spaces. Distal surface of last tooth in the arch, exposed furcation areas that permit easy insertion of the brush Embrasure spaces with exposed proximal root concavities
End-tuft brush	Small bristle tuft on a toothbrush like handle (Butler End-Tuft Brush)	Type III embrasure spaces, distal surface of the last tooth in arch, lingual surfaces of mandibular teeth, crowded or malaligned teeth, exposed furcation areas
Pipe cleaner	Standard pipe cleaner cut into 3-in lengths	Type III embrasure spaces, exposed furcation areas that permit insertion
Toothpick in holder	A round toothpick in a plastic handle (Marquis Perio-Aid)	Type II or III embrasure spaces, plaque biofilm removal at gingival margin, furcation areas or root concavities
Triangular wooden wedge	A triangular shaped toothpick generally made of Basswood (J & J Stim-U-Dent)	Type II or III embrasure spaces
Powered flossers or interdental cleaners	A powered flossing device (Waterpik power flosser)	Type I embrasure spaces Orthodontic appliances Lingual bar retainers Tight contacts

Section 3
Interdental Care

1. **Introduction to Interdental Care**
   A. **Importance of Interdental Care**
      1. For the periodontal patient, interdental care takes on special importance since periodontitis usually begins as inflammation in the interdental area first.
      2. While floss tends to be the primary recommendation of most dental hygienists, patient compliance is low. It has also been shown that a significant number of those that do floss are not able to perform the function effectively [7].
         a. Evidence indicates that a variety of alternative interdental aids are as effective as dental floss in removing biofilm and reducing bleeding and gingivitis [8].
         b. When given a choice, patients often prefer other types of interdental cleaners to dental floss [8].
         c. Flossing may not be as effective for periodontal patients; recession, attachment loss, and size of the gingival embrasure space are limiting factors [8].
         d. A dental water jet has also been shown to be an effective alternative to dental floss; appropriate for patients with many types of oral anatomy and conditions [8]. The topic of irrigation is discussed in detail in Chapter 27.
         e. Some mouthrinses have been shown to be an effective alternative to dental floss. Mouthrinses are discussed in detail in Chapter 28.
   B. **Indications for Use.** Indications for the use of interdental aids are summarized in TABLE 26-1.
      1. The type of interdental aid recommended to a patient should take into consideration patient dexterity and preference along with interdental anatomy
      2. When guiding patients to the appropriate alternative to dental floss, it is important to first identify the issues related to difficulty with flossing.
         a. Different patient challenges will require different products. For example, a patient who struggles with getting floss through the contact point will continue to have frustrations with a floss holder.
         b. In comparison, a patient who is unable to manipulate floss around the teeth but has no issues getting the floss through the contact area is a good candidate for a floss holder.
      3. It is advisable to keep a supply of the various interdental cleaners in the dental office for recommending and dispensing to patients. Local drug stores or pharmacies offer many choices that can be confusing to patients. Some interdental cleaners often are *not available* at these retail locations.
2. **Anatomical Challenges in Interdental Care for the Periodontitis Patient**
   A. **Gingival Embrasure Space.** The gingival embrasure space is the small triangular open space (apical to the contact area) between the curved proximal surfaces of two teeth.
      1. In health, the interdental papilla fills the gingival embrasure space. Dental floss is effective in areas of normal gingival contour.
      2. *The tissue destruction characterized by periodontitis usually results in an interdental papilla that is reduced in height or missing, resulting in an open embrasure space. Dental floss is not effective in areas with open embrasure spaces.*
      3. Analysis of the gingival embrasure spaces is critical in determining which interdental aid is likely to be most effective in plaque biofilm control.

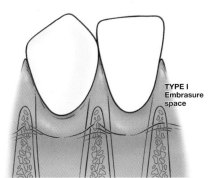

Figure 26.2. **Type I Embrasure**—space filled by the interdental papilla. Dental floss is effective.

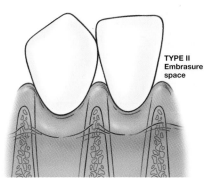

Figure 26.3. **Type II Embrasure**—height of interdental papilla is reduced. Interdental brushes, wooden interdental cleaners, and toothpicks are effective.

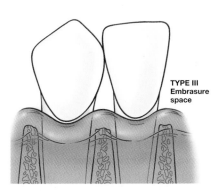

Figure 26.4. **Type III Embrasure**—the interdental papilla is missing. Interdental brushes and end-tuft brushes are effective.

    a. Type I embrasure—space filled by the interdental papilla. Dental floss is effective (FIG. 26-2).

    b. Type II embrasure—height of interdental papilla is reduced. Interdental brushes, wooden interdental cleaners, and toothpicks are effective (FIG. 26-3).

    c. Type III embrasure—interdental papilla is missing so that there is an open triangular space visible between the two teeth. Interdental brushes and end-tuft brushes are effective (FIG. 26-4).

B. Root Concavities. A root concavity is a trench-like depression in the root surface. Root concavities commonly occur on the proximal surfaces of anterior and posterior teeth and the facial and lingual surfaces of molar teeth.

    1. In health, root concavities are covered with alveolar bone and help to secure the tooth in the bone.

    2. Periodontitis results in the apical migration of the junctional epithelium, loss of connective tissue, and destruction of alveolar bone. This tissue destruction results in the exposure of root concavities to the oral environment (either in the presence of tissue recession or, frequently, within a periodontal pocket).

3. In Figure 26-5A–E, the root of a mandibular canine is covered with a colored powder that represents bacterial plaque biofilm on the root surface. This series of figures compares the effectiveness of dental floss and an interdental brush in removing bacterial plaque biofilm from the root concavity.
   a. Dental floss is not successful in removing plaque biofilm from the root concavity.
   b. The interdental brush is effective in removing bacterial plaque biofilm from the root concavity.

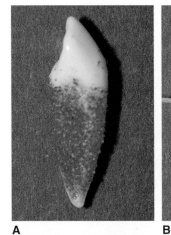
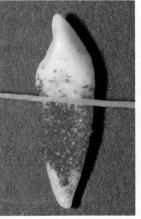
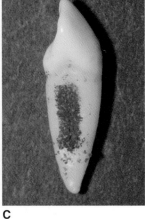

A   B   C

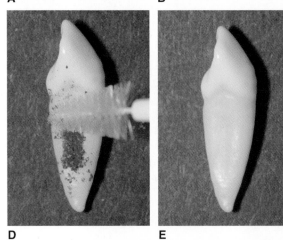

D   E

Figure 26.5. Plaque Biofilm Removal from Root Concavity. A: The proximal surface of this mandibular canine is covered with colored powder. **B, C:** Dental floss is used to clean the proximal surface; the floss is unable to remove the powder from the root concavity. **D, E:** An interdental brush effectively removes the colored powder from the root concavity.

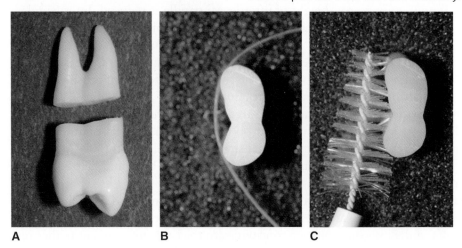

A   B   C

Figure 26.6. Application of Interdental Aids to Root Concavity. A: A maxillary premolar (side view) is cut to expose a cross section of the root. **B:** The root of the same maxillary premolar viewed in cross section; dental floss is unable to clean the root concavity. **C:** The bristles of the interdental brush extend into the root cavity for successful plaque biofilm removal.

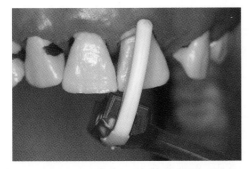

Figure 26.7. Technique for Use of Floss Holder. Flossing via a floss holder is as effective as handheld flossing provided the patient uses proper technique. The dental floss should be wrapped around the proximal tooth surface in a similar manner to the technique employed with handheld floss.

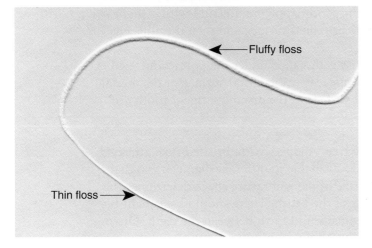

Fluffy floss

Thin floss

Figure 26.8. Tufted Dental Floss. This aid is a specialized type of floss consisting of a fluffy segment of yarn-like floss attached to a segment of thin floss.

4. Figure 26-6A–C compares the effectiveness of dental floss and an interdental brush in cleaning the root concavity of a maxillary premolar. Note that only the interdental brush is effective in reaching the concave surface of the root concavity.

3. Selecting Interdental Aids

A. Dental Floss

1. Description. Dental floss is unwaxed or waxed thread made of silk, nylon, or plastic monofilament fibers used to remove dental plaque biofilm from the proximal surfaces of teeth.

   a. When added to toothbrushing, dental floss has been shown to significantly increase the reduction in bleeding compared to toothbrushing alone [9].

   b. It may be easier for some individuals to use floss via a floss holder. Flossing via floss holder has been shown to be as effective as handheld floss and a mechanism for increasing the development of a flossing habit [10]. There are many variations of floss holder. Some require manually wrapping the floss onto the holder. Others may be single use devices with the floss already in place (FIG. 26-7).

2. Indications

   a. Type I embrasures. Dental floss is effective in removing plaque biofilm from tooth crowns and the convex root surfaces in the region of the cementoenamel junction (CEJ). Dental floss is not effective in removing plaque biofilm from root concavities and grooves.

   b. Recommended for patients with excellent compliance with self-care. Patient compliance with dental flossing is low with many patients being unable or unwilling to perform daily flossing [7].

   c. Power flossing devices may improve patient compliance with daily flossing.

B. **Tufted Dental Floss**
   1. Description. A specialized type of dental floss that has a segment of ordinary floss attached to a thicker, fluffy, yarn-like segment of floss (FIG. 26-8).
   2. Indications
      a. For type II embrasures.
      b. To clean under the pontic of a fixed bridge.
      c. To clean the distal surface of the last tooth in the arch.
      d. To remove plaque biofilm from the proximal surfaces of widely spaced teeth.
   3. Technique
      a. For interdental proximal surfaces, the fluffy part of the floss is used interdentally in a C-shape against the tooth, applying pressure with a slight sawing motion against first one proximal surface and then the adjacent proximal tooth surface.
      b. For fixed bridges, the tufted floss is threaded under the pontic and used to clean the undersurface of pontic. Next, the distal surface of the mesial abutment tooth and the mesial surface of the distal abutment tooth are cleaned using the tufted floss.

C. **Interdental Brush**
   1. Description. Tiny conical or "pine tree"-shaped nylon bristle brush attached to a handle (FIG. 26-9). Brushes are available in different diameters so that the best size can be selected. The size of the embrasure space determines the correct diameter of the bristle part of the brush. There should be a slight bit of resistance as the brush is moved back and forth between the teeth. Often it is necessary to use different size brushes within one mouth.
   2. Indications
      a. Interdental brushes have been shown to remove plaque biofilm as effectively as dental floss [11,12].
      b. Excellent for plaque biofilm removal in type II and III embrasure spaces (FIG. 26-10). Interdental brushes should not be used where the interdental papilla fills the interdental space.
      c. *The bristles of an interdental brush are very effective at cleaning root concavities.*
   3. Technique. The brush is inserted into the open interdental space and slid in and out of the embrasure space for several strokes. *Always use the interdental brush without toothpaste.* Figure 26-11 shows techniques for use of interdental brushes.

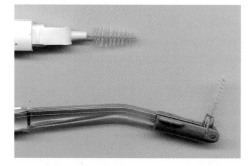

Figure 26.9. Interdental Brushes. Interdental brushes are one of the most useful aids for cleaning root concavities.

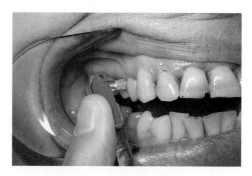

Figure 26.10. Use of Interdental Brush. (Courtesy of Dr Deborah Milliken, South Florida Community College.)

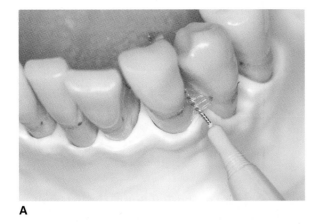

A

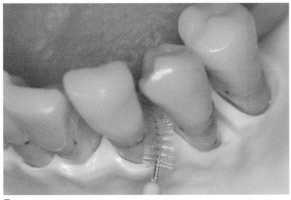

B

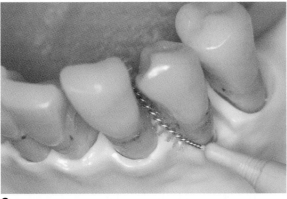

C

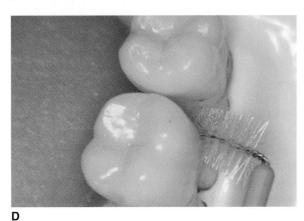

D

Figure 26.11. Procedure for Use of an Interdental Brush. A: The brush handle is held between the thumb and index finger and the brush gently pushed between the teeth. The brush should be maintained at a 90-degree angle to the long axis of the tooth. **B:** The bristles can be adapted to tooth surfaces with slight pressure and varying the angle of insertion. For optimal plaque biofilm removal, the brush is slid in and out of the space using the entire length of the bristle part of the brush. **C:** By changing the angle of insertion, the bristles can be adapted to the mesial surface of the first premolar. Slight pressure with the brush against the gingiva allows the bristles to clean slightly beneath the gingival margin. **D:** For posterior areas, advise the patient to close his or her mouth slightly to relax the cheek. The brush may be bent to facilitate insertion between posterior teeth.

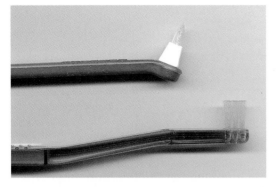

Figure 26.12. **End-Tuft Brushes**. End-tuft brushes are used to clean areas that are difficult to access with a standard brush.

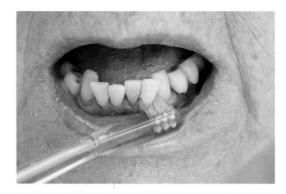

Figure 26.13. **Use of End-Tuff Brush**. End-tuff brush used around crowded anterior teeth. (Courtesy of Dr Deborah Milliken, South Florida Community College.)

D. **End-Tuft Brush**
   1. Description
      a. An end-tuff brush is similar to a standard toothbrush except that the brush head has only a small tuft of bristles (Fig. 26-12).
      b. A standard toothbrush easily can be modified to create a customized end-tuft brush by removing some of the bristles.
   2. Indications
      a. Effectively reaches sites around teeth that are difficult for patients to clean, such as the distal surface of the last tooth in the arch, lingual surfaces of mandibular teeth, and crowded or malaligned teeth (Fig. 26-13).
      b. Works well to remove plaque biofilm from type III embrasure spaces.
      c. Useful in removing plaque biofilm from an exposed furcation area since the small size of the bristle tufts allows them to partially enter the furcation site.
   3. Technique
      a. The end of the tuft is directed into the embrasure space or furcation area. Gentle circular strokes are used to clean the area.
      b. For difficult-to-reach mandibular lingual tooth surfaces, the brush is used like a standard brush with a sulcular brushing technique.
E. **Wooden Toothpick in a Holder**
   1. Description. This device consists of a round toothpick in a plastic handle.
   2. Indications
      a. The toothpick in a holder has been shown to reduce biofilm and bleeding as effectively as dental floss [13].
      b. Can be used gently along or slightly below the gingival margin for plaque biofilm removal.
      c. Effective in type II embrasures if the toothpick is easily inserted between the teeth; however, this aid is not effective in cleaning root concavities unless the teeth are widely spaced.
      d. Can be directed into furcation areas.
   3. Technique for Use of a Wooden Toothpick in a Holder
      a. A toothpick is secured in the holder and the long end is broken off flush with the holder so that it will not scratch the inside of the cheek (Fig. 26-14).
      b. The end of toothpick is moistened with saliva.

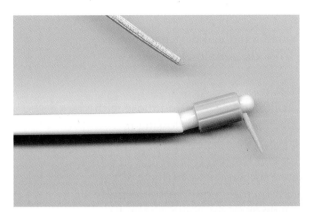

Figure 26.14. **Toothpick Holder**. To prepare this aid for use, secure a toothpick in the holder and break off the long end so that it is flush with the plastic holder.

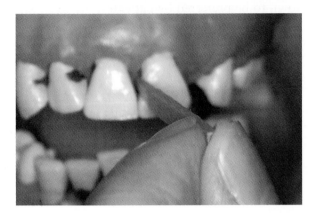

Figure 26.15. **Use of Wooden Wedge**. The wedge is held between the thumb and index finger with the flat side toward the gingiva. In the upper arch the flat surface faces up, and in the lower arch the flat surface faces down.

    c. The tip is applied at right angles to the gingival margin or directed just beneath the gingival margin at a less than 45-degree angle. The tip should not be directed against the epithelial attachment. The tip is used to trace the gingival margin around each tooth.

    d. Next, the tip is angled into embrasure spaces or exposed furcation areas and moved gently back and forth to sweep the area free of accumulated plaque biofilm.

F. Wooden Wedge

   1. Description. This aid is a triangular wooden stick usually made of soft wood. These wedges are triangular, wedge-shaped sticks and should not be confused with round or rectangular toothpicks.

   2. Indications

     a. Wooden wedges are used for interdental plaque biofilm removal in type III embrasures.

     b. To use a wedge there must be sufficient interdental space available to allow easy placement of the wooden wedge. Long term use of wooden wedges in type I embrasures may cause a permanent loss of the papillae.

   3. Technique for Use of Wooden Wedge

     a. The wooden wedge should be moistened thoroughly in the mouth to soften the wood prior to use.

     b. The wedge is inserted between the teeth with the *flat side next to the gingiva* (FIG. 26-15).

     c. The wedge is used with gentle in and out motion to clean between the teeth. The wedge should not be forced into tightly spaced teeth.

     d. During use, the wedge should be discarded as soon as the first signs of splaying are evident.

G. Powered Flossing Devices
1. Description. A powered flossing device is a small handheld device with a nylon filament for removing plaque biofilm from the proximal surfaces of the teeth (FIG. 26-16).
2. Benefits of Powered Flossing Devices
   a. In recent research studies, linear tip power flossing devices and those with floss holders have been shown to be as effective as manual flossing in reducing biofilm, bleeding, and gingivitis [14,15].
   b. Indications for Recommending Power Flossing Devices
      1) In general, a powered device is indicated for patients who have difficulties such as holding the floss correctly, maneuvering floss effectively around teeth, or manipulating the floss through the contact area. Use of power flossing devices has been shown to be preferred by patients over manual flossing [12].
      2) Patients who are reluctant to place their fingers in their mouth or who are gadget-oriented may find these products user-friendly.
      3) Indications for both types of flossing tips are similar to those for manual dental floss. Additionally, this is a user-friendly product for patients with orthodontic appliances, crown and bridge, or implants.
3. Directions. Technique is dependent on the type or brand of product. Dental hygienists should read the manufacturer's users guide before recommending and/or demonstrating a powered flossing device to a patient. Patients should be counseled to follow the manufacturer's instructions for the best outcome.

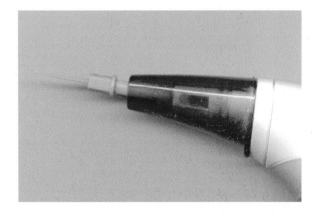

Figure 26.16. **Power Dental Flossing Device.** An example of a powered dental flossing device.

Chapter Summary Statement

The patient plays a vital role in the successful control of periodontal disease. The patient's efforts at self-care are critical to the control of periodontitis. Since the importance of mechanical plaque biofilm control is quite high for the patient with periodontitis, the dental hygienist should be knowledgeable about biofilm control measures and be prepared to recommend appropriate aids based on the individual needs of each patient.

Interdental plaque biofilm control has special importance for the periodontal patient since periodontitis usually damages the interdental tissues first. Interdental aids that are especially useful for patients with Type II or III embrasure spaces include interdental brushes and end-tuft brushes. Daily tongue cleaning results in reduced amounts of tongue coating and improvements in breath freshness.

Section 4
Focus on Patients

Case 1

A patient with slight (or mild) chronic periodontitis has generalized recession of the interdental gingival papillae. What options would you have for training this patient in interdental plaque biofilm control?

Case 2

You are discussing self-care for plaque biofilm removal with a patient with chronic periodontitis. You point out to the patient how the plaque biofilm control on the facial and lingual surfaces of his teeth is greatly improved and praise him for this success. The patient comments that he likes using his powered toothbrush and has been brushing longer. Unfortunately, you note that there is heavy plaque biofilm on the proximal surfaces of most teeth. The patient tells you that there is "No way that I am going to use that string. It is just too hard to use." The patient has Type II embrasure spaces throughout his mouth. What suggestions might you make for interdental plaque biofilm control?

Case 3

A patient with chronic periodontitis has generalized bone loss and recession of the gingival margin so that the cervical-thirds of the roots are exposed to the oral cavity. What interdental aids would you recommend to clean interproximally (between the roots).

References

1. Mosby Inc. Mosby's medical dictionary. 9th ed. St. Louis: Mosby/Elsevier; 2009.

2. Clayton NC. Current concepts in toothbrushing and interdental cleaning. *Periodontol 2000.* 2008;48:10–22.

3. Jahn CA. Evidence for self-care products: Power brushing and interdental aids. *J Pract Hyg.* 2004;13:24–29.

4. Robinson PG, Deacon SA, Deery C, et al. *Manual Versus Powered Toothbrushing for Oral Health (Cochrane Review).* Chichester: John Wiley & Sons, Ltd; 2005. The Cochrane Library, Issue 2.

5. Yaegaki K, Sanada K. Volatile sulfur compounds in mouth air from clinically healthy subjects and patients with periodontal disease. *J Periodontal Res.* 1992;27:223–238.

6. Ratcliff PA, Johnson PW. The relationship between oral malodor, gingivitis, and periodontitis: a review. *J Periodontol.* 1999;70(5):485–489.

7. Lang WP, Ronis DL, Farghaly MM. Preventive behaviors as correlates of periodontal health status. *J Public Health Dent.* 1995;55(1):10–17.

8. Asadoorian J. Canadian Dental Hygienists' Association Position Statement: Flossing. *CJDH.* 2006;40:1–10.

9. Graves RC, Disney JA, Stamm JW. Comparative effectiveness of flossing and brushing in reducing interproximal bleeding. *J Periodontol.* 1989;60:243–247.

10. Kleber CJ, Putt MS. Formation of flossing habit using a floss-holding device. *J Dent Hyg.* 1990;64:140–143.

11. Kiger RD, Nylund K, Feller RP. A comparison of proximal plaque removal using floss and interdental brushes. *J Clin Periodontol.* 1991;18:681–684.

12. Christou V, Timmerman MF, Van der Velden U, Van der Wiejden FA. Comparison of different approaches of interdental oral hygiene: interdental brushes versus dental floss. *J Periodontol.* 1998;69:759–764.

13. Lewis MW, Holder-Ballard C, Selders RJ, et al. Comparison of the use of a toothpick holder to dental floss in improvement of gingival health in humans. *J Peiodontol.* 2004;75:551–556.

14. Anderson NA, Barnes CM, Russell CM. A clinical comparison of the efficacy of an electromechanical flossing device or manual flossing in affecting interproximal gingival bleeding and plaque accumulation. *J Clin Dent.* 1995;6:105–107.

15. Shibly O, Ciancio S, Shostad S, et al. Clinical evaluation of an automated flossing device versus manual flossing. *J Clin Dent.* 2001;12:63–66.

Chapter 27

Supragingival and Subgingival Irrigation

Learning Objectives

- Discuss the oral health benefits from using a dental water jet.

- Identify the types of patients who would benefit from using a dental water jet.

- Compare the use of the dental water jet to traditional dental floss.

- Distinguish the depth of the delivery between the dental water jet, a toothbrush, dental floss, and other interdental aids.

- Name the types of agents that can be used in a dental water jet.

- Instruct patients in the use of the dental water jet including how to use the standard irrigation tip, subgingival tip, and orthodontic tip.

- Summarize research findings that relate to using professional irrigation to deliver chemicals to periodontal pockets.

Key Terms

Dental water jet
Hydrokinetic activity
Impact zone
Flushing zone

Standard irrigation tips
Subgingival irrigation tips
Orthodontic irrigation tips
Professional subgingival irrigation

Section 1
Patient-Applied Home Irrigation

This chapter addresses the role of supragingival and subgingival irrigation in the treatment of periodontal diseases. The primary objective of *supra*gingival irrigation is to diminish gingival inflammation by disrupting bacterial biofilms coronal to the gingival margin. The goal of *sub*gingival irrigation is to reduce the number of bacteria in the periodontal pocket space.

1. **What Is a Dental Water Jet?** The dental water jet is a generic term for a device that delivers a pulsed irrigation of water or other solution around and between teeth (supragingivally) and into the gingival sulcus or periodontal pocket (subgingivally). This process is commonly referred to as home or oral irrigation. A dental water jet may also be referred to as a dental water irrigator, home irrigator, or water flosser.

   A. **Mechanism of Action of a Dental Water Jet**
      1. A dental water jet creates a pulsating fluid stream to flush an area with water or an antimicrobial agent. Figure 27-1 shows examples of devices used for home oral irrigation.
         a. The pulsating fluid delivered by a dental water jet incorporates a compression and decompression phase that efficiently displaces biofilm, bacteria, and debris [1,2].
         b. The pulsating fluid creates two zones of fluid movement termed hydrokinetic activity (Fig. 27-2).
            1) The area of the mouth of initial fluid contact is called the impact zone.
            2) The depth of fluid penetration within a subgingival sulcus or pocket is called the flushing zone [3].
      2. Hydrokinetic fluid movement results in subgingival and interdental fluid penetration.

   B. **Fluid Penetration**
      1. A dental water jet produces subgingival fluid penetration regardless of the type of tip or attachment used [4,5].
      2. A dental water jet has the greatest potential for reaching deeper into a sulcus or pocket over other types of devices including toothbrushes and interdental aids (Table 27-1) [4,5].

2. **Benefits of Home Oral Irrigation.** Studies demonstrate that the dental water jet is clinically proven to remove biofilm and reduce bleeding, gingivitis, periodontal pathogens, and inflammatory mediators [6–20].

   A. **Removal of Biofilm**
      1. Studies as early as the 1970s demonstrate biofilm removal by the dental water jet [16]. Examination under a scanning electron microscope confirms that a three second application of water pulsation at a medium pressure using either the standard irrigation tip or orthodontic tip removes 99% of plaque biofilm from extracted teeth (Figs. 27-3 and 27-4) [15].
      2. A dental water jet used in combination with manual toothbrushing removes biofilm as well as traditional brushing and flossing [7].

   B. **Reduction in Bleeding.** Studies consistently show that the dental water jet is a valuable tool for helping patients reduce bleeding [6–10,13,14,18,19].
      1. A dental water jet used in combination with manual toothbrushing is more effective in the reduction of bleeding than manual toothbrushing and flossing [7].
      2. Daily irrigation with water significantly reduced bleeding in 14 days [10].
      3. Daily irrigation with water was significantly better than rinsing with 0.12% chlorhexidine at reducing marginal bleeding and bleeding on probing [14].

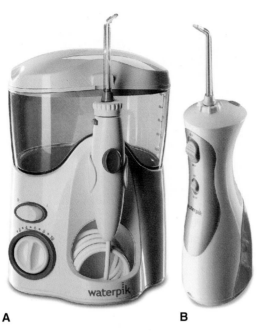

A   **B**

Figure 27.1. **Dental Water Jets**. A: A countertop dental water jet that plugs into an electrical outlet. B: A portable dental water jet that works off of a rechargeable battery. (Courtesy of Water Pik, Inc., Fort Collins, CO.)

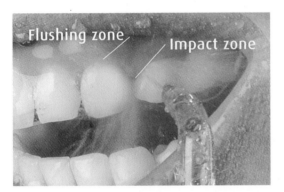

Figure 27.2. **The Impact and Flushing Zones**. A dental water jet creates a pulsating water stream to flush an area with fluid. The area of the mouth where the fluid initially contacts is called the impact zone. The depth of fluid penetration within the subgingival sulcus or pocket is called the flushing zone. (Courtesy of Water Pik, Inc., Fort Collins, CO.)

TABLE 27-1.	Depth of Delivery of Various Self-Care Products	
Oral Hygiene Aid	**Penetration**	**Comments**
Toothbrush	1 to 2 mm	No manual or power toothbrush has clinically proven subgingival access
Rinsing	2 mm	Can reach less accessible areas, but penetrates subgingival areas minimally [4]
Toothpick/wooden wedge	Depends on embrasure size	Effectiveness depends on sufficient interdental space
Interdental brush	Depends on embrasure size	Most effective with an open interdental space
Dental Floss	3 mm	Cannot reach into deeper pockets
Waterpik dental water jet	6 mm and beyond	Clinically proven to remove supragingival and subgingival plaque biofilm and bacteria [4,5]

Courtesy of Water Pik, Inc., Fort Collins, CO.

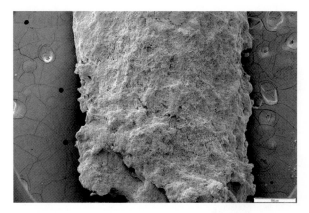

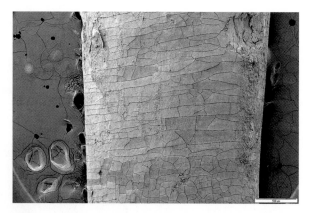

Figure 27.3. Tooth Surface Prior to Treatment. Untreated tooth surface (in vivo) covered with plaque biofilm as seen under a scanning electron microscope. (Courtesy of Water Pik, Inc., Fort Collins, CO.)

Figure 27.4. Same Tooth Surface After Treatment. Tooth treated with a 3-second pulsating spray at medium pressure removed significant amounts of (in vivo) plaque biofilm. (Courtesy of Water Pik, Inc., Fort Collins, CO.)

C. **Reduction in Gingival Inflammation.** The dental water jet has been shown to reduce the clinical signs of gingivitis [6–8,10,12–14,17,18,20].
   1. A dental water jet used in combination with manual toothbrushing is more effective in the reduction of gingivitis than manual toothbrushing and flossing [7].
   2. Daily irrigation with water significantly reduces the clinical signs of gingivitis [8].
D. **Reduction of Periodontal Pathogens.** Studies show that the dental water jet can reduce subgingival bacteria [3,8,11,21].
   1. The dental water jet has demonstrated the ability to reduce periodontal pathogens at up to a 6-mm level within a periodontal pocket [3,11].
   2. Daily irrigation with either water or 0.04% chlorhexidine significantly reduces subgingival bacteria compared to toothbrushing and 0.12% chlorhexidine rinsing [8].
E. **Reduction in Inflammatory Mediators and Destructive Host Response**
   1. Recent studies show that home oral irrigation is effective in significantly reducing inflammatory cytokines Il-1β and PGE$_2$ implicated in attachment loss and alveolar bone loss [8,10,22,23].
   2. Irrigation may produce these effects by flushing out loosely adherent plaque biofilm and toxins or inflammatory substances, although the exact mechanism of action of irrigation is still speculative [8,18].
3. **Indications for Recommending Home Oral Irrigation**
A. **Individuals on Periodontal Maintenance.** Studies have shown that daily use of the dental water jet may be beneficial for patients with gingivitis or for those in periodontal maintenance [6–10,13,14,18,20].
   1. Daily irrigation over a 6-month period reduces bleeding on probing by 50% [13].
   2. Patients with 5 mm pockets and bleeding who added daily irrigation to traditional home care achieved significant reductions in gingival inflammation and bleeding on probing when compared to patients using only traditional self-care methods [18].
B. **Individuals Noncompliant with Dental Floss.** While previously considered an adjunctive to brushing *and* flossing, new information indicates that home oral irrigation can be considered an effective *alternative* to daily flossing.

1. The addition of a dental water jet once daily with plain water to either a manual or power brushing routine was an effective alternative to dental floss for the reduction of bleeding, gingivitis, and biofilm [7].

2. The addition of a dental water jet to manual toothbrushing reduced 3.76 times more biofilm than flossing using a floss threader and 5.83 times more biofilm than manual toothbrushing alone.

3. The dental water jet also provided a significantly better reduction in bleeding; 84.5% from baseline. This was 26% better than the results achieved with dental floss [19].

C. **Individuals with Special Needs.** Home irrigation has been shown to be safe and effective for patients with special needs.

1. **Dental Implants.** For improving the health of peri-implant tissues, daily irrigation using the soft rubber tip and 0.06% chlorhexidine was more effective in reducing bleeding than rinsing with 0.12% chlorhexidine [12]. Although often recommended, to date no research studies have been conducted on the use of the standard irrigation tip on dental implants.

2. **Individuals with Diabetes.** For individuals living with diabetes, twice daily water irrigation using the soft rubber tip provided a 44% better reduction in bleeding over routine oral hygiene [6].

3. **Individuals with Orthodontic Appliances.** For those with orthodontic appliances, the dental water jet with the orthodontic tip provided 3.76 times better biofilm removal than flossing using a floss threader [19].

4. **Prosthetic Bridgework and Crowns.** For individuals with bridgework and/or crowns, daily irrigation produced significant reductions in inflammation [24].

4. **Patient Instruction**

A. **Considerations for Irrigator Use: Product Safety**

1. Dental water jets have been extensively studied on thousands of people with more than 50 studies since the 1960s. Examination with a scanning electron microscope of chronic periodontal pockets immediately following irrigation found no evidence of trauma or injury to the tissue [3].

2. The incidence of bacteremia from a dental water jet is similar to other healthcare devices [25].

a. The American College of Cardiology/American Heart Association 2008 Guideline Update on Valvular Heart Disease: Focused Update on Infective Endocarditis states: "Maintenance of optimal oral health and hygiene may reduce the incidence of bacteremia from daily activities and is more important than prophylactic antibiotics for a dental procedure to reduce the risk of infective endocarditis" [26].

b. Before recommending a dental water jet or any device to a patient who is at high risk for infective endocarditis, it is imperative that dental healthcare providers consider both the patient's overall medical and oral health status. Consultation with a physician is advisable in order to assess the patient's overall risk for infective endocarditis.

B. **Irrigant Solutions.** Most solutions can be used in a dental water jet. The most effective agent is one that is acceptable to the patient.

1. **Water**

a. Simple tap water has been demonstrated as highly effective in numerous clinical trials [3,6,7,10,13,15–17,19]. Therefore, the addition of any antimicrobial agent for home oral irrigation should be considered carefully.

TABLE 27-2. Common Dilutions for Chlorhexidine Rinse	
0.02% dilution	Five parts water to one part chlorhexidine rinse
0.04% dilution	Three parts water to one part chlorhexidine rinse
0.06% dilution	One part water to one part chlorhexidine rinse

  b. Water has several advantages; it is readily available, cost-effective and has no side effects.
  2. Antimicrobial Solutions
    a. Chlorhexidine (CHX)
      1) For home irrigation, chlorhexidine can be diluted with water (TABLE 27-2). Use of diluted solutions of chlorhexidine has been studied in concentrations from 0.02% to 0.06% [8,12,14,20].
      2) Because of better interproximal and subgingival penetration with irrigation compared to rinsing, a diluted solution of chlorhexidine is acceptable for daily irrigation. In some cases, dilution can minimize staining.
      3) CHX is available by prescription only. In the US, the maximum strength is 0.12%. In Europe, it is available at 0.2%.
    b. Essential Oils
      1) For home irrigation, the effectiveness of an essential oil mouth rinse has been demonstrated only when used at full-strength [9].
      2) Essential oil mouthrinses are available over the counter in both brand name and generic forms.
  3. Other Irrigation Solutions
    a. It is best to check with the manufacturer of an irrigation device for information on recommended solutions and dilutions. Some manufacturers do not recommend certain agents or mouthwashes as these solutions may damage the device.
    b. Some manufacturers sell premixed solutions for use in their equipment.
  C. **Criteria for Equipment Selection.** Selection of an irrigation device may be confusing because there are many types on the market. The commercial and scientific claims of some devices have yet to be evaluated.
  1. Only pulsating dental water jets have clinical research supporting safety and efficacy.
  2. As each device operates differently in respect to pressure and pulsation, outcomes from studies on one brand of product cannot be transferred to another product brand. Therefore, before recommending any device, it is important to evaluate the research unique to that brand of product.
5. **Technique for Use of Irrigation Tips**
  A. **General Instructions**
  1. It is important for both dental healthcare providers and patients to read all instructions thoroughly before using a dental water jet.
  2. The fluid reservoir can be filled with water, a solution of water and mouthwash, or a solution of an antimicrobial and water. The irrigating solution should be at room temperature for maximum patient comfort.

3. The unit should be flushed after using any solution other than water. After using a diluted solution, such as diluted chlorhexidine, the unit is cleaned by filling the reservoir with warm water and running the unit while holding the handle in the sink until the reservoir is empty.

4. Most patients seem to comply with recommendations to use a dental water jet and find a standard irrigation tip easy to use for supragingival irrigation [13,17]. For subgingival irrigation, it is important to provide patients with clear instructions on its use including the specific areas where the tip should be used.

B. **Irrigation Tips.** Irrigation is accomplished using a standard irrigation tip, a subgingival soft rubber tip, or a soft tapered brush orthodontic tip.

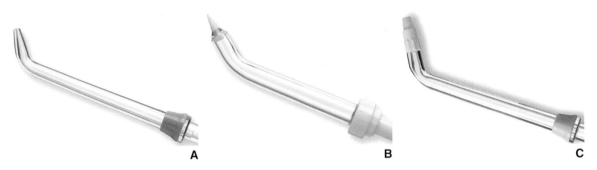

Figure 27.5. **Irrigation Tips.** Three examples of irrigation tip designs. A: Standard irrigation tip. B: Subgingival tip. C: Orthodontic tip.

1. Standard irrigation tips are usually made of a plastic material (FIG. 27-5A).
   a. The standard tip is used by placing the tip at a 90-degree angle at the neck of the tooth near the gingival margin.
   b. Dental water jet devices with standard irrigation tips may deliver solution that penetrates a depth of 50% or more of the pocket [5].
   c. This type of tip is recommended for generalized, full-mouth irrigation.
2. Subgingival irrigation tips usually have a soft rubber-tipped end (FIG. 27-5B).
   a. The soft rubber tip is gently placed beneath the gingival margin.
   b. Subgingival placement of the tip allows the water or antimicrobial agent to penetrate deeper into a pocket.
      1) In periodontal pockets 6 mm or less in depth, the subgingival tip may deliver water that penetrates up to 90% of the pocket depth.
      2) In deeper pockets—7 mm or more—depth of penetration is somewhat less at 64% of the depth of the pocket [4].
   c. Subgingival irrigation tips are recommended for use in areas such as deep pockets, furcation areas, dental implants, or areas that are difficult to access with a standard tip.
3. Orthodontic irrigation tips have a soft tapered brush end that enhances biofilm removal and provides for simultaneous irrigation (FIG. 27-5C).
   a. These tips are used in a similar manner to a standard irrigation tip by placing the tip at a 90-degree angle at the neck of the tooth near the gingival margin.
   b. The bristles should come in light contact with the tooth, implant, or orthodontic appliances to facilitate biofilm removal.
      1) The orthodontic tip when used in conjunction with toothbrushing was 3.76 times as effective as dental floss at removing plaque biofilm.
      2) When compared to toothbrushing only, the toothbrushing and orthodontic tip combination was 5.83 times as effective [19].

    c. Orthodontic tips can be used for full mouth irrigation and are recommended for people with orthodontic appliances, implants, or who need additional help with biofilm removal.

C. Procedure for Use of a Standard Tip

1. Initially the pressure setting should be adjusted to its lowest setting.
2. Over time as the condition of the gingival tissue improves, pressure should be increased to at least the medium setting as this setting is where clinical efficacy has been demonstrated [1,2].
3. The water spray is used to "trace" along the gingival margin with the tip positioned at a 90-degree angle almost touching the gingiva (FIG. 27-6).
4. The tip should be held briefly at each interproximal area.

D. Procedure for Use of a Subgingival Irrigation Tip

1. The dental hygienist should instruct the patient on the areas of his or her mouth where use of a subgingival irrigation tip would be beneficial, such as pockets, dental implants, or furcation areas. The patient should be instructed on use of the tip in each area or these areas.
2. The pressure setting is adjusted to its lowest setting. *The subgingival tip is designed for use only at the lowest pressure setting.*
3. The manufacturer's recommendations should be followed for use of the tip. Some tips are placed at the gingival margin, others can be placed 2 mm below the gingival margin.
4. The tip should be placed at the site prior to starting the irrigation unit. The subgingival tip is directed at a 45-degree angle and placed at the gingival margin or slightly beneath the gingival margin as recommended by the manufacturer (FIG. 27-7).
5. Once the tip is in place, the irrigation unit is turned on and the fluid is allowed to flow briefly in the area.
6. After a site has been irrigated, the unit is paused and the subgingival tip is repositioned in the next area of the mouth.

E. Procedure for the Use of an Orthodontic Tip

1. Initially, the pressure setting should be adjusted to its lowest setting.
2. Over time as the condition of the gingival tissue improves, pressure should be increased to at least the medium setting as this setting is where clinical efficacy has been demonstrated [1,2].
3. The water spray is used to "trace" along the gingival margin with the tip positioned at a 90-degree angle touching the gingiva (FIG. 27-8).
4. The tip should be held briefly in each interproximal area.
5. This tip can also be placed around orthodontic brackets or wires to enhance cleaning.

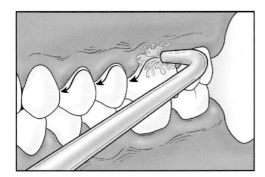

Figure 27.6. Placement of the Standard Irrigation Tip. The water spray is used to "trace" along the gingival margin with the tip positioned at a 90-degree angle almost touching the gingiva.

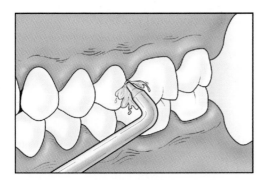

Figure 27.7. Placement of the Subgingival Irrigation Tip. The tip should be placed at the site prior to starting the irrigation unit. The subgingival tip is directed at a 45-degree angle and placed at the gingival margin or slightly beneath the gingival margin as recommended by the manufacturer.

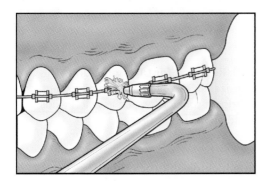

Figure 27.8. Placement of the Orthodontic Tip. The special orthodontic tip is used with the tip positioned at a 90-degree angle.

Section 2
Professional Subgingival Irrigation

1. **Introduction to Professional Irrigation**
   A. **Description of Subgingival Irrigation.** Professional subgingival irrigation is the in-office flushing of pockets performed by the dental hygienist or dentist using one of three systems:
      1. A blunt-tipped irrigating cannula that is attached to a handheld syringe (FIG. 27-9)
      2. Ultrasonic unit equipped with a reservoir (FIG. 27-10)
      3. A specialized air-driven handpiece that connects to the dental unit airline
   B. **Goal of Subgingival Irrigation.** The purpose of supragingival irrigation is the disruption and dilution of the bacteria and their products from within periodontal pockets.

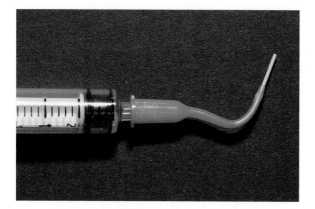

Figure 27.9. **Handheld Syringe.** Close up view of the tip of a handheld syringe used for subgingival irrigation. The tip is positioned subgingivally for delivery of an antimicrobial solution.

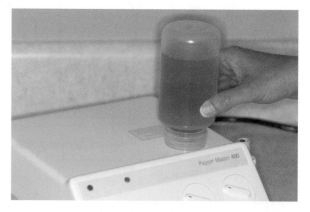

Figure 27.10. **Reservoir for Ultrasonic Unit.** This ultrasonic device has an optional reservoir system for dispensing irrigant solutions—such as chlorhexidine gluconate—to an ultrasonic tip.

   C. **Irrigant Solutions.** Solutions used for subgingival irrigation include chlorhexidine gluconate, povidone-iodine and water, stannous fluoride, tetracycline, or Listerine. Chlorhexidine gluconate and essential oil mouthrinses can be used full-strength. Povidone-iodine can be diluted as one part povidone-iodine to nine parts water. Stannous fluoride is diluted as one part stannous fluoride to one part water.
2. **Effectiveness of Professional Subgingival Irrigation**
   A. **Single Professional Application**
      1. The status of professional subgingival irrigation in the treatment of periodontitis remains controversial [27,28].
      2. In-office subgingival irrigation with an antimicrobial agent has been shown to have only limited or no beneficial effects over nonsurgical periodontal instrumentation alone.
         a. Several research studies indicate that irrigation did not enhance the therapeutic effect over that attained by nonsurgical periodontal instrumentation alone [29–34].
         b. Other studies found a minimal improvement. However, after 6 months there was no significant difference between irrigation versus nonsurgical periodontal instrumentation regarding probing depths or inflammatory status [35–39].

3. There is no long-lasting substantivity of the antimicrobial agent in the periodontal pocket due to the continuous flow of gingival crevicular fluid from the pocket, and the presence of serum and proteins in the pocket. A substantive antimicrobial agent, such as chlorhexidine gluconate, would have to be retained in the pocket and be released slowly over a period of time to interfere with the repopulation of bacteria within the pocket.

B. **Conclusions Regarding Professional Irrigation.** A position paper [40] on the role of supragingival and subgingival irrigation in the treatment of periodontal diseases concludes:

1. "...there currently is insufficient evidence to indicate that subgingival irrigation routinely should be used as a supplemental in-office procedure."

2. "However, preliminary data using high concentrations [35,38] and prolonged or multiple applications [29,32,33,38,41,42] of antimicrobials have shown some promise in improving periodontal status. Consequently, additional studies are needed to ascertain the full potential of subgingival irrigation as an adjunct to periodontal therapy" [40].

C. Subgingival irrigation performed before periodontal instrumentation may reduce the incidence of bacteremia and reduce the number of microorganisms in aerosols.

Chapter Summary Statement

When used daily for at-home self-care, supragingival and subgingival irrigation via a dental water jet can be beneficial for periodontal patients. A well-established body of evidence indicates that pulsating devices have the ability to remove biofilm and reduce bleeding, gingivitis, periodontal pathogens, and inflammatory mediators. Irrigation via a dental water jet also benefits patients with special oral health needs and considerations including those in periodontal maintenance or with implants, crowns, bridges, orthodontic appliances, and diabetes.

The status of professional subgingival irrigation in the treatment of periodontitis remains controversial. In-office subgingival irrigation with an antimicrobial agent has been shown to have only limited or no beneficial effects over nonsurgical periodontal instrumentation alone.

Section 3
Focus on Patients

Case 1

You have just recommended a dental water jet to your patient, and he has accepted, but he has no idea how to use the product. The patient is in periodontal maintenance, has two 5 mm pockets (No. 3M and No. 18D), one 6 mm pocket (No. 14M), and a furcation area on No. 30. He also has an implant replacing No. 19. What type of instructions would you provide for the patient?

Case 2

A new patient comes to your practice from another state. She has had periodontal therapy in the past. The patient uses a power toothbrush and flosses irregularly. Supragingival plaque biofilm control looks good but several areas of the mouth bleed upon probing. The medical history indicates that the patient has had type 2 diabetes for 7 years. How would you make a recommendation for the dental water jet to this patient?

References

1. Bhaskar SN, Cutright DE, Gross A, et al. Water jet devices in dental practice. *J Periodontol.* 1971;42(10):658–664.
2. Selting WJ, Bhaskar SN, Mueller RP. Water jet direction and periodontal pocket debridement. *J Periodontol.* 1972;43(9):569–572.
3. Cobb CM, Rodgers RL, Killoy WJ. Ultrastructural examination of human periodontal pockets following the use of an oral irrigation device in vivo. *J Periodontol.* 1988;59(3):155–163.
4. Braun RE, Ciancio SG. Subgingival delivery by an oral irrigation device. *J Periodontol.* 1992;63(5):469–472.
5. Eakle WS, Ford C, Boyd RL. Depth of penetration in periodontal pockets with oral irrigation. *J Clin Periodontol.* 1986;13(1):39–44.
6. Al-Mubarak S, Ciancio S, Aljada A, et al. Comparative evaluation of adjunctive oral irrigation in diabetics. *J Clin Periodontol.* 2002;29(4):295–300.
7. Barnes CM, Russell CM, Reinhardt RA, et al. Comparison of irrigation to floss as an adjunct to tooth brushing: effect on bleeding, gingivitis, and supragingival plaque. *J Clin Dent.* 2005;16(3):71–77.
8. Chaves ES, Kornman KS, Manwell MA, et al. Mechanism of irrigation effects on gingivitis. *J Periodontol.* 1994;65(11):1016–1021.
9. Ciancio SG, Mather ML, Zambon JJ, and Reynolds HS. Effect of a chemotherapeutic agent delivered by an oral irrigation device on plaque, gingivitis, and subgingival microflora. *J Periodontol.* 1989;60(6):310–315.
10. Cutler CW, Stanford TW, Abraham C, et al. Clinical benefits of oral irrigation for periodontitis are related to reduction of pro-inflammatory cytokine levels and plaque. *J Clin Periodontol.* 2000;27(2):134–143.
11. Drisko CL, White CL Killoy WJ, and Mayberry WE. Comparison of dark-field microscopy and a flagella stain for monitoring the effect of a Water Pik on bacterial motility. *J Periodontol.* 1987;58(6):381–386.
12. Felo A, Shibly O, Ciancio SG, et al. Effects of subgingival chlorhexidine irrigation on peri-implant maintenance. *Am J Dent.* 1997;10(2):107–110.

13. Flemmig TF, Epp B, Funkenhauser Z, et al. Adjunctive supragingival irrigation with acetylsalicylic acid in periodontal supportive therapy. *J Clin Periodontol.* 1995;22(6):427–433.

14. Flemmig TF, Newman MG, Doherty FM, et al. Supragingival irrigation with 0.06% chlorhexidine in naturally occurring gingivitis. I. 6 month clinical observations. *J Periodontol.* 1990;61(2):112–117.

15. Gorur A, Lyle DM, Schaudinn C, and Costerton JW. Biofilm removal with a dental water jet. *Compend Contin Educ Dent.* 2009;30 Spec No 1:1–6.

16. Hoover DR, Robinson HB. The comparative effectiveness of a pulsating oral irrigator as an adjunct in maintaining oral health. *J Periodontol.* 1971;42(1):37–39.

17. Lainson PA, Bergquist JJ, Fraleigh CM. A longitudinal study of pulsating water pressure cleansing devices. *J Periodontol.* 1972;43(7):444–446.

18. Newman MG, Cattabriga M, Etienne D, et al. Effectiveness of adjunctive irrigation in early periodontitis: multi-center evaluation. *J Periodontol.* 1994;65(3):224–229.

19. Sharma NC, Lyle DM, Qaqish JG, et al. Effect of a dental water jet with orthodontic tip on plaque and bleeding in adolescent patients with fixed orthodontic appliances. *Am J Orthod Dentofacial Orthop.* 2008;133(4):565–571; quiz 628 e1–e2.

20. Walsh TF, Glenwright HD, Hull PS. Clinical effects of pulsed oral irrigation with 0.2% chlorhexidine digluconate in patients with adult periodontitis. *J Clin Periodontol.* 1992;19(4):245–248.

21. Newman MG, Flemmig TF, Nachnani S, et al. Irrigation with 0.06% chlorhexidine in naturally occurring gingivitis. II. 6 months microbiological observations. *J Periodontol.* 1990;61(7):427–433.

22. Offenbacher S, Heasman PA, Collins JG. Modulation of host PGE2 secretion as a determinant of periodontal disease expression. *J Periodontol.* 1993;64(5 Suppl):432–444.

23. Tsai CC, Ho YP, Chen CC. Levels of interleukin-1 beta and interleukin-8 in gingival crevicular fluids in adult periodontitis. *J Periodontol.* 1995;66(10):852–859.

24. Krajewski J, Giblin J, Gargiulo A. Evaluation of a water pressure cleaning device as an adjunct to periodontal treatment. *J Am Soc Periodont.* 1964;2:76–78.

25. Wilson W, Taugert KA, Gewitz M, et al. Prevention of infective endocarditis: guidelines from the American Heart Association. *Circulation.* 2007;116:1736–1754.

26. Nishimura RA, Carabello BA, Faxon DP, et al. ACC/AHA 2008 guideline update on valvular heart disease: focused update on infective endocarditis: a report of the American College of Cardiology/American Heart Association Task Force on Practice Guidelines: endorsed by the Society of Cardiovascular Anesthesiologists, Society for Cardiovascular Angiography and Interventions, and Society of Thoracic Surgeons. *Circulation.* 2008;118(8):887–896.

27. Hallmon WW, Rees TD. Local anti-infective therapy: mechanical and physical approaches. A systematic review. *Ann Periodontol.* 2003;8(1):99–114.

28. Shiloah J, Hovious LA. The role of subgingival irrigations in the treatment of periodontitis. *J Periodontol.* 1993;64(9):835–843.

29. Braatz L, et al. Antimicrobial irrigation of deep pockets to supplement non-surgical periodontal therapy. II. Daily irrigation. *J Clin Periodontol.* 1985;12(8):630–638.

30. Herzog A, Hodges KO. Subgingival irrigation with Chloramine-T. *J Dent Hyg.* 1988;62(10):515–521.

31. Krust KS, Drisko CL, Gross K, et al. The effects of subgingival irrigation with chlorhexidine and stannous fluoride. A preliminary investigation. *J Dent Hyg.* 1991;65(6):289–295.

32. Listgarten MA, Grossberg D, Schwimer C, et al. Effect of subgingival irrigation with tetrapotassium peroxydiphosphate on scaled and untreated periodontal pockets. *J Periodontol.* 1989;60(1):4–11.

33. MacAlpine R, Magnusson I, Kiger R, et al. Antimicrobial irrigation of deep pockets to supplement oral hygiene instruction and root debridement. I. Bi-weekly irrigation. *J Clin Periodontol.* 1985;12(7):568–577.

34. Shiloah J, Patters MR. DNA probe analyses of the survival of selected periodontal pathogens following scaling, root planing, and intra-pocket irrigation. *J Periodontol.* 1994;65(6):568–575.

35. Christersson LA, Norderyd OM, Puchalsky CS. Topical application of tetracycline-HCl in human periodontitis. *J Clin Periodontol.* 1993;20(2):88–95.

36. Khoo JG, Newman HN. Subgingival plaque control by a simplified oral hygiene regime plus local chlorhexidine or metronidazole. *J Periodontal Res.* 1983;18(6):607–619.

37. Rosling BG, Slots J, Webber RL, etc. Microbiological and clinical effects of topical subgingival antimicrobial treatment on human periodontal disease. *J Clin Periodontol.* 1983;10(5):487–514.

38. Southard SR, Drisko CL, Killoy WJ, et al. The effect of 2% chlorhexidine digluconate irrigation on clinical parameters and the level of *Bacteroides gingivalis* in periodontal pockets. *J Periodontol*. 1989;60(6):302–309.
39. Wolff LF, Bakdash MB, Pilhlstrom BL, et al. The effect of professional and home subgingival irrigation with antimicrobial agents on gingivitis and early periodontitis. *J Dent Hyg*. 1989;63(5):222–225, 241.
40. Greenstein G. Position paper: The role of supra- and subgingival irrigation in the treatment of periodontal diseases. *J Periodontol*. 2005;76(11):2015–2027.
41. Macaulay WJ, Newman HN. The effect on the composition of subgingival plaque of a simplified oral hygiene system including pulsating jet subgingival irrigation. *J Periodontal Res*. 1986;21(4):375–385.
42. Wennstrom JL, Dahlen G, Grondahl K, and Heijl L. Periodic subgingival antimicrobial irrigation of periodontal pockets. II. Microbiological and radiographical observations. *J Clin Periodontol*. 1987;14(10):573–580.

Chapter 28

Chemical Agents in Plaque Biofilm Control

Learning Objectives

- Describe the difference between systemic delivery and topical delivery of chemical agents.
- Explain the term systemic antibiotic.
- Explain why systemic antibiotics are not used routinely in the treatment of patients with plaque-associated gingivitis and patients with chronic periodontitis.
- Describe three examples of mouth rinse ingredients that can help reduce the severity of gingivitis.
- Define the term controlled-release delivery device.
- List three antimicrobial agents that can be delivered with controlled-release delivery devices.
- Explain why toothpastes are nearly ideal delivery mechanisms for chemical agents.
- List two toothpaste ingredients that can reduce the severity of gingivitis.

Key Terms

Systemic delivery
Topical delivery
Microbial reservoir
Antibiotics
Systemic antibiotics
Antibiotic resistance
Conventional mechanical periodontal therapy
Controlled-release delivery device

Therapeutic mouth rinses
Efficacy
Stability
Substantivity
Safety
Active ingredient
Inactive ingredient
Essential oils

Section 1
Introduction to Chemical Agents in Plaque Biofilm Control

As discussed in other chapters of this textbook, it is clear that periodontal diseases are caused by bacterial infections, and that bacteria that can be found in dental plaque biofilm are the primary causative agents in these diseases. Many bacterial infections that have affected mankind have been brought under control using various chemical agents to attack germs that cause those diseases. It is quite natural for researchers and clinicians alike to search for chemical agents or medications to help in the difficult task of controlling periodontal diseases. This chapter discusses some of the more important chemical agents that can be used in dental plaque biofilm control.

1. **Delivery of Chemical Agents in Periodontal Patients.** Chemical agents useful in plaque biofilm control can be delivered by using either systemic delivery or topical delivery.
   A. **Systemic Delivery**
      1. In dentistry systemic delivery usually refers to administering chemical agents in the form of a tablet or capsule. When a tablet is taken by the patient, the chemical agent contained is released as the tablet dissolves, and the agent subsequently enters the blood stream—thus the chemical agent is circulated "systemically" throughout the body.
      2. As the chemical agent circulates throughout the body, it is also incorporated into the tissues of the periodontium including the gingival crevicular fluids where it can come into contact with bacteria causing periodontal diseases.
      3. An example of systemic delivery of a chemical agent would be for a patient to take a tablet or capsule of the antibiotic penicillin. The penicillin passes through the wall of the gastrointestinal track and enters body tissues. In medical care systemic delivery of chemical agents can also be administered by injection into a muscle or into a blood vessel, though this mode of systemic delivery has little to do with the control of dental plaque biofilm.
   B. **Topical Delivery**
      1. In dentistry topical delivery usually refers to placing a chemical agent into the mouth or even into a periodontal pocket where the chemical agent then comes into contact with plaque biofilm forming either on the teeth or in the periodontal pocket.
      2. Examples of topical delivery in dentistry would be using a mouth rinse or toothpaste that contains a chemical agent that can kill bacteria growing in dental plaque biofilm. In this instance the chemical agent would come into contact with the teeth, oral mucous membranes, and the surface of dental plaque biofilm.
      3. It should be noted that when chemical agents come into contact with oral mucous membranes, some of the agent enters the blood stream by passing through the mucous membranes, but the bulk of the agent contacts the bacteria topically.
      4. Chemical agents can also be delivered topically by using controlled-release devices that are placed into a periodontal pocket. See TABLE 28-1 for an overview of topical and systemic delivery mechanisms for chemical agents used in dental plaque biofilm control.
2. **Considerations for Use of Chemical Agents in Periodontal Patients**
   A. **Resistance of the Dental Plaque Biofilm to the Delivery of Chemical Agents**
      1. Research shows that dental plaque biofilm is covered by a slime layer that acts as a barrier to prevent chemical agents from contacting the bacteria on the plaque biofilm

TABLE 28-1. Systemic and Topical Delivery Mechanism for Chemical Agents Used in Dental Plaque Biofilm Control

Delivery Type	Specific Mechanisms	Possible Patient Benefits
Topical	Therapeutic mouth rinses	Reduce the severity of gingival inflammation
Topical	Therapeutic dentifrices	Reduction in dentinal hypersensitivity Reduction in gingival inflammation Reduction of supragingival calculus Reduction in surface stains on teeth
Topical	Subgingival irrigation	Disruption and dilution of bacteria and their products within dental plaque biofilm
Topical	Controlled-release delivery devices	Subject subgingival bacteria to therapeutic levels of a drug for a period of a week or longer
Systemic	Tablets, capsules	Help control aggressive periodontitis Fight acute oral infections

2. The barrier nature of the slime layer limits the extent to which chemical agents delivered to the oral cavity can be expected to control plaque biofilm and therefore to affect an oral disease such as gingivitis.

3. Because of the protective nature of the surface slime layer, mechanical plaque control is essential to allow the chemical agents to reach the bacterial themselves.

B. **Microbial Reservoirs for Periodontal Pathogens.** In the oral cavity there are a variety of microbial reservoirs that can lead to rapid repopulation of bacterial pathogens in a treated periodontal patient.

1. A microbial reservoir is a niche or secure place in the oral cavity that can allow periodontal pathogens to live undisturbed during routine therapy and subsequently repopulate periodontal pockets quickly.

2. An example of a microbial reservoir would be a residual calculus deposit following periodontal debridement. Living bacteria found within the calculus deposit can reproduce in periodontal pockets and continue to promote disease even after what appears to be thorough nonsurgical therapy.

3. Box 28-1 provides an overview of some of the many microbial reservoirs for periodontal pathogens in the oral cavity.

C. **Chemical Agents Effective Against Periodontitis.** At this point, there is no chemical biofilm control agent that can halt periodontitis, but there are a number of different chemical agents that can be used as part of comprehensive treatment for patients with periodontal diseases. An overview of some of the types of chemical agents that have been suggested for use in plaque biofilm control in periodontal patients is presented in TABLE 28-2.

Box 28-1. Microbial Reservoirs for Periodontal Pathogens

- Bacterial plaque biofilm in protected sites such as furcation areas
- Bacteria in residual calculus deposits that are not removed during nonsurgical therapy
- Bacteria living within the connective tissue adjacent to a periodontal pocket
- Bacteria that have penetrated dentinal tubules
- Bacteria protected by irregularities in tooth surfaces after mechanical treatment
- Bacteria protected by bulky restoration margins

TABLE 28-2. Overview of Some of the Chemical Agents Used in Dental Plaque Biofilm Control

Type of Agent	Example of Agent	Common Forms of Administration
Antibiotics	Tetracyclines	Tablet/capsule Local delivery mechanism
Bisbiquanide antiseptics	Chlorhexidine	Mouth rinse Local delivery mechanism
Fluorides	Stannous fluoride	Mouth rinse Toothpaste
Metal salts	Tin/zinc	Mouth rinse Toothpaste
Oxygenating agents	Hydrogen peroxide	Mouth rinse
Phenolic compounds	Essential oils	Mouth rinse
Quaternary ammonium	Cetylpyridinium chloride	Mouth rinse

Section 2
Use of Systemic Antibiotics to Control Dental Plaque Biofilm

1. **Overview of Systemic Antibiotics**
    A. **Definitions**
        1. Antibiotics are medications used to help fight infections either because they kill bacteria or because they can inhibit the growth of bacteria.
        2. Systemic antibiotics refer to those antibiotics that can be taken orally or that can be injected and are in widespread use in fighting bacterial infections throughout the world. In North America, healthcare providers such as physicians and dentists have access to a broad range of antibiotic drugs for use in patients with infections. These drugs have been used for many years to help the body fight certain bacterial infections and have undoubtedly been responsible for saving countless lives.
    B. **Systemic Antibiotics Studied for Use in Periodontal Diseases.** Systemic antibiotics have also been studied for their use in controlling periodontal diseases. Box 28-2 lists some examples of systemic antibiotics that have been studied by researchers for use in periodontal patients.
    C. **Plaque-Induced Gingivitis and Chronic Periodontitis**
        1. *For most patients with the more common forms of periodontal diseases (i.e., either plaque-induced gingivitis or chronic periodontitis) current recommendations are for clinicians to avoid the routine use of systemic antibiotic drugs to control these diseases.* There are two major reasons for recommendations to avoid their routine use in these patients.
            a. One reason dentists do not use systemic antibiotics routinely to control the more common forms of periodontal diseases is antibiotic resistance. Antibiotic resistance refers to the ability of a bacterium to withstand the effects of an antibiotic by developing mechanisms to protect the bacterium from the killing or inhibiting effects of the antibiotic. When antibiotic resistant strains of bacteria develop, they are generally not affected by the antibiotic, survive, and continue to cause more damage.
                1) According to the National Science Foundation and the Centers for Disease Control, antibiotic resistance is a serious public health problem throughout the world, and the problem is increasing in scope.
                2) An example of how antibiotic resistance can be a public health problem is the high incidence of penicillin resistant microorganisms that have already limited the usefulness of this important drug. As more and more bacteria develop resistance to the antibiotic penicillin, the usefulness of this antibiotic as a life saving drug will continue to decrease.

Box 28-2. Examples of Systemic Antibiotics That Have Been Studied for Use in Periodontal Care

- Penicillin and amoxicillin
- Tetracyclines
- Erythromycin
- Metronidazole
- Clindamycin

    b. Another reason dentists do not use systemic antibiotics routinely to control periodontal diseases is that studies indicate that in most patients these diseases respond to conventional mechanical periodontal therapy just as well as they respond to the systemic administration of antibiotics. Conventional mechanical periodontal therapy is a term that refers to self-care, periodontal instrumentation, and control of local contributing factors.

2. When antibiotics are being considered for use in periodontal patients, careful patient selection is necessary.

    a. When tempted to use systemic antibiotics to control either plaque-induced gingivitis or chronic periodontitis, dental healthcare providers must weigh potential benefits and disadvantages. At this point, most clinicians have decided that the potential harm outweighs the benefits.

    b. In patients with chronic periodontitis the efficacy of using antibiotic therapy is not completely clear, and antibiotic therapy in these patients should usually be limited to those patients that have continued periodontal breakdown after thorough conventional mechanical periodontal therapy.

    c. It should be noted that even though systemic antibiotics are rarely indicated for routine treatment of patients with plaque-induced gingivitis or chronic periodontitis, they are frequently indicated in the treatment of patients with the rarer forms of periodontitis such as aggressive periodontitis.

3. Patient Education. Even though systemic antibiotic drugs are not normally used for patients with plaque-induced gingivitis or chronic periodontitis, systemic antibiotics are discussed here because periodontal patients can ask why antibiotics are not being recommended for them.

    a. This question may arise when the patient learns that periodontitis is a bacterial infection. This is a natural question for a patient to ask given the widespread use of antibiotics in fighting infections of all sorts.

    b. When confronted with a question from a patient about why antibiotics are not being recommended, the dental hygienist can explain the following facts:

        1) Most cases of gingivitis and periodontitis can be readily controlled with treatments that do not require the use of potentially life saving systemic antibiotics.

        2) In the oral cavity bacteria grow so quickly and so readily that to control a chronic or long term disease such as periodontitis with a systemic antibiotic would require that the drug be taken for many years.

        3) Overuse of systemic antibiotics often results in the development of antibiotic-resistant strains of bacteria, simply compounding a complex dental problem. This is a major public health concern, since many antibiotics can be rendered useless for life saving measures through the development of antibiotic resistance.

D. Aggressive Periodontitis

1. *It is important to realize that the use of antibiotics in conjunction with mechanical therapy is usually indicated in patients with aggressive forms of periodontitis.*

2. When antibiotics are being considered for use, microbiologic analysis is a wise clinical step.

    a. Microbiologic analysis involves sampling the bacteria associated with the disease process and testing cultures of the bacteria for specific antibiotic susceptibility.

    b. Utilizing microbiologic analysis can avoid prescribing inappropriate antibiotics that can lead to a poor clinical response. Figure 28-1 illustrates the relationship between periodontal diagnoses and the use of systemic antibiotics.

2. **Use of Tetracyclines in Periodontal Patients.** One of the antibiotic groups, the group of drugs called tetracyclines, has received special attention by researchers because it has some specific properties that make it attractive to consider for use in selected periodontal patients. Box 28-3 outlines these special properties exhibited by tetracyclines.

   A. **Tetracyclines tend to be concentrated in the gingival crevicular fluids.**

      1. When tetracycline drugs are administered orally, the drugs permeate body tissues and reach a certain concentration in the blood serum.

      2. However, the level of tetracycline drugs is more concentrated within the gingival crevicular fluids that are found flowing into periodontal pockets than the level found in the blood serum. This results in a higher concentration of the drug in exactly the site it might be needed in a periodontal patient.

   B. **The tetracyclines are effective against most strains of *Aggregatibacter actinomycetemcomitans*.** *Aggregatibacter actinomycetemcomitans* is one of the periodontal pathogens thought to be a primary player in many patients with periodontitis.

   C. **The tetracyclines have other effects in addition to their antimicrobial properties.**

      1. Tetracyclines inhibit the action of collagenase—one of the enzymes responsible in part for breakdown of the periodontium in periodontitis patients.

      2. Any drug that can inhibit the action of collagenase can be expected to slow the progress of breakdown of the periodontium that is seen in periodontitis.

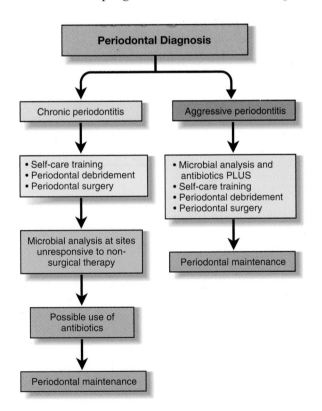

Figure 28.1. The Relationship between Periodontal Diagnoses and the Use of Systemic Antibiotics.

Box 28-3. Special Properties of the Tetracycline Antibiotics

- Tetracyclines are concentrated in the gingival crevicular fluid
- Tetracyclines are effective against many strains of *Aggregatibacter actinomycetemcomitans*
- Tetracyclines inhibit the action of collagenase

Section 3
Use of Topically Delivered Chemical Agents

1. **Controlled-Release of Antimicrobial Chemicals**
   A. **Overview of Controlled-Release Mechanisms**
      1. A controlled-release delivery device usually consists of an antibacterial chemical that is imbedded in a carrier material. It is designed to be placed directly into the periodontal pocket where the carried material attaches to the tooth surface and dissolves slowly, producing a steady release of the antimicrobial agent over a period of several days within the periodontal pocket.
      2. The earliest version of these products involved coating carrier fibers with chemical agents that would be released following placement of the fibers within periodontal pockets. Use of this early example of these products involved a return patient office visit for removal of the fibers.
      3. The latest versions of these products involve imbedding antimicrobial agents into carrier materials which dissolve slowly over approximately 1 week. The carrier material can be placed into a periodontal pocket, and as it dissolves it releases the antimicrobial agent slowly.
      4. Antimicrobial agents currently used in controlled-release delivery devices include chlorhexidine and some of the antibiotic drugs such as the tetracyclines. In the future, other drugs may be used for this purpose.
   B. **Rationale for Use.** The goal of the use of these controlled-release delivery devices is to subject subgingival bacteria to therapeutic levels of an antibacterial drug for a sustained period. Most of these controlled-release devices continue to deliver chemicals into the pockets for approximately 1 week.
   C. **Benefits of Controlled-Release Delivery Devices**
      1. Use of controlled-release delivery devices has been shown to result in a small increase in attachment level in a periodontal pocket.
      2. Unfortunately, very few controlled studies are available to guide dental healthcare providers in the appropriate use of these new devices.
         a. Controlled-release devices may be indicated for use in localized periodontal pockets that are nonresponsive after thorough nonsurgical and surgical periodontal therapy.
         b. When these products were used along with periodontal instrumentation, they can result in both an improvement in probing depth reduction and a clinical attachment gain. The clinical significance of the small amount of improvement is unclear at this point.
         c. Currently most clinicians use these devices in combination with periodontal debridement rather than as a substitute for periodontal debridement.
   D. **Controlled-Release Mechanisms.** Several controlled-release delivery products have been introduced in the United States over the last few years, and it is likely that more will be available within the next few years. The chemical agents that have been incorporated into these devices and marketed over the past few years are outlined below.
      1. Tetracycline Hydrochloride
         a. One of the first of these products released for use involved tetracycline hydrochloride containing fibers that were to be inserted into the periodontal pocket to deliver a high concentration of tetracycline to the site for several days.
            1) Marketed under the brand name Actisite, *this product is no longer available in the United States.*

      2) *This mechanism represents the first successful product of this type, and is discussed here for historical purposes.*

   b. Technique for Fiber Placement and Stabilization

      1) A gingival retraction cord-packing instrument was used to insert the tetracycline containing fibers into a pocket, but the insertion was time consuming.

      2) The fiber was placed under the gingival margin around an entire tooth, and the pocket was filled by layering the fiber back and forth upon itself (Fig. 28-2).

      3) Finally, adhesive was applied along the gingival margin to keep the fiber in the pocket.

      4) A return patient visit to the dental office was needed for fiber removal.

   c. Adverse reactions that were reported for this product included discomfort on fiber placement, oral candidiasis, allergic response, gingival inflammation, and pain.

2. Minocycline Hydrochloride Microspheres

   a. Another example of a controlled-release mechanism delivers the antibiotic minocycline hydrochloride in a powdered microsphere form. Minocycline hydrochloride is a broad-spectrum, semisynthetic tetracycline derivative that is bacteriostatic.

   b. Application

      1) A cannula tip is used to expel the microspheres into the pocket (Fig. 28-3) where, because of the sticky nature of the carrier material, it binds to the tooth surface.

      2) Over 5 to 7 days, the powdered microspheres dissolve releasing the embedded minocycline, so there is nothing to remove from the pocket.

   c. Adverse Reactions. Possible adverse reactions include oral candidiasis or an allergic response. In addition, the use of antibiotic preparations may result in the development of resistant bacteria.

   d. Contraindications for Use. This product is a tetracycline derivative, and should not be used in patients who are hypersensitive to any tetracycline or in women who are pregnant or nursing.

3. Doxycycline Hyclate Gel

   a. This product is a gel system that delivers the antibiotic doxycycline (also a tetracycline derivative) to the periodontal pocket (Fig. 28-3).

   b. Application

      1) The gel is expressed into the pocket with a cannula, and after placement the gel solidifies into a waxlike substance.

      2) The cannula tip is placed near the pocket base and gel is expressed using a steady pressure until the gel reaches the top of the gingival margin.

      3) A problem with this delivery system is that the gel tends to cling to the cannula when it is withdrawn from the pocket. This problem can be reduced by using a moistened dental hand instrument to hold the gel in place while slowly withdrawing the cannula tip from the pocket.

      4) The gel is biodegradable (it dissolves) so there is nothing to remove from the pocket.

   c. Adverse Reactions

      1) Possible adverse reactions include oral candidiasis or an allergic response.

      2) The use of antibiotic preparations may result in the development of resistant bacteria.

    d. Contraindications for Use. This product is a tetracycline derivative, and should not be used in patients who are hypersensitive to any tetracycline or in women who are pregnant or nursing.

4. Chlorhexidine Gluconate Chip

    a. Another example of a controlled-release device is a tiny gelatin chip containing the antiseptic chlorhexidine that is inserted into a periodontal pocket that is 5 mm or greater in depth (FIG. 28-4).

    b. Application

       1) The gelatin chip is inserted into the periodontal pocket.

       2) The gelatin chip can be difficult to insert into some pockets due to the size and shape of the chip.

       3) The gelatin chip is bioabsorbed so there is no need to have it removed after placement.

    c. Since chlorhexidine is not an antibiotic, there is no risk of antibiotic resistance with use of the chlorhexidine gluconate gelatin chip.

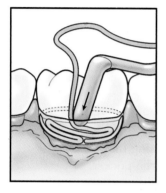

Figure 28.2. Fibers Inserted into the Pocket. One of the first local delivery mechanisms used involved a tetracycline-containing fiber. The tetracycline-containing fiber was inserted into the periodontal pocket, and the entire pocket was filled by layering the fiber back and forth upon itself. The fiber released the tetracycline slowly over several days, and required removal after 5 to 7 days. *This product is no longer available in the United States.*

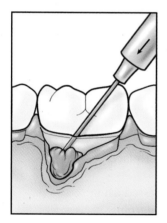

Figure 28.3. Products Expelled into the Pocket. Some local delivery mechanisms involve placing the carrier material into a periodontal pocket with a cannula tip. Minocycline hydrochloride containing microspheres and doxcycline gel are examples of such products. These carrier materials adhere to the tooth surfaces and dissolve slowly—releasing the antimicrobial agents trapped in the carrier material.

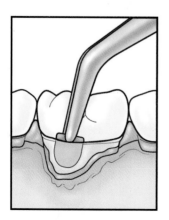

Figure 28.4. Gelatin Chip Inserted into Pocket. The gelatin chip is inserted into periodontal pockets 5 mm or greater in depth. The gelatin chip adheres to the tooth surface and dissolves slowly—releasing the chlorhexidine antimicrobial agent trapped in the gelatin.

2. **Mouth Rinses as Aids in Plaque Biofilm Control**
   A. **Introduction to Mouth Rinses**
      1. Many mouth rinses available today are therapeutic mouth rinses. Therapeutic mouth rinses are mouth rinses that have some actual benefit (provide some therapeutic action) to the patient in addition to the simple goal of making the breath smell a bit better.
         a. In the context of this chapter therapeutic mouth rinses would be rinses that decrease dental plaque biofilm enough to also decrease the severity of gingivitis (FIG. 28-5).
         b. Over the last few decades, researchers have been searching for chemicals that can be added to mouth rinses that might actually help reduce dental plaque biofilm build up on the tooth surface and thereby help control gingivitis or even periodontitis.
      2. It should be noted that in addition to therapeutic mouth rinses that can aid in the control of gingivitis, there are other therapeutic mouth rinses available that can benefit the patient in a variety of ways such as decreasing the risk of developing dental caries.

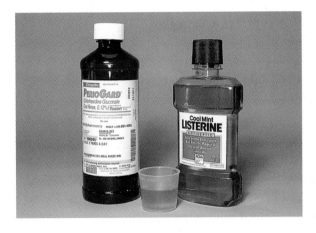

Figure 28.5. **Therapeutic Mouth Rinses**. Two examples of therapeutic mouth rinses used to aid in dental plaque biofilm control. The mouth rinses pictured on the left contains chlorhexidine gluconate as its active ingredient and requires a prescription for purchase. The mouth rinse pictured on the right contains essential oils as the active ingredient and is available over the counter.

   B. **Characteristics That an Ideal Mouth Rinse Should Possess.** Investigations into chemical plaque biofilm control have not yet produced a mouth rinse that can be used as a total substitute for mechanical plaque biofilm control. However, these investigations have indeed produced mouth rinses that can be useful components of a comprehensive program of patient self-care. An ideal mouth rinse would possess four characteristics that are described below. Box 28-4 provides an overview of the characteristics of the ideal mouth rinse.
      1. Efficacy. The active ingredient in the rinse should be effective in inhibiting or killing periodontal pathogens.
      2. Stability. The ingredients in the mouth rinse should be stable at room temperature and have a reasonable shelf life.
      3. Substantivity (sub-stan-tiv-ity). The active ingredient in the rinse should display the property of substantivity. This means that the active ingredient would be retained in the oral cavity for a while following rinsing and would be released slowly over time (usually several hours), resulting in a continuing antimicrobial effect against periodontal pathogens.

   a. Substantivity is an important characteristic, since dental plaque biofilm grows and matures continuously.

   b. An active ingredient that displays the property of substantivity would continue to kill periodontal pathogens over an extended number of hours following rinsing.

   4. Safety. The ingredients in the mouth rinse should not produce any harmful effects to the tissues in the oral cavity or systemically to the patient.

Box 28-4. Characteristics of an Ideal Mouth Rinse

- Efficacy

- Stability

- Substantivity

- Safety

C. Ingredients of Mouth Rinses

   1. Products such as mouth rinses contain both active ingredients and inactive ingredients.

   a. An active ingredient is a component that produces some benefit for the patient (such as a reduction in the severity of gingival inflammation associated with gingivitis).

   b. All mouth rinses also contain inactive ingredients.

   1) Inactive ingredients are included in mouth rinse formulations simply to add other properties such as to enhance the color, to improve the taste, to increase the shelf life, or to keep components in a liquid state.

   2) Though these ingredients are called "inactive," there can be associated side effects with some of these ingredients in certain patients. It is important that clinicians maintain familiarity with the inactive ingredients of rinses as well as the active ingredients.

   2. Many chemicals that might be placed in mouth rinses have been investigated for their effect against both plaque biofilm and gingivitis.

   a. Chemicals that reduce plaque biofilm formation to only a minor degree usually have little or no clinically significant effect against gingivitis, and therefore may not be very useful in controlling a disease such as gingivitis. Many mouth rinses marketed today fall into this category.

   3. Among the many ingredients tested for efficacy against gingivitis, three mouth rinse ingredients that have some effect against gingivitis have been studied extensively. These ingredients are listed below.

   a. Chlorhexidine gluconate

   b. Essential oils

   c. Cetylpyridinium chloride

D. Mouth Rinses Containing Chlorhexidine Gluconate

   1. One group of mouth rinses currently available contains chlorhexidine gluconate as the active ingredient. These rinses are only available through prescriptions in the United States, but they can be purchased over the counter in some other countries.

   a. Mouth rinses containing chlorhexidine gluconate as the active ingredient have been demonstrated to reduce the severity of gingivitis in numerous clinical studies.

b. In the United States the concentration of chlorhexidine gluconate used in prescription mouth rinses is 0.12%, but it should be noted that a higher concentration is used in mouth rinses in some other countries.

2. Investigations have demonstrated that the overall severity of *gingivitis* can be reduced by approximately 50% when patients use chlorhexidine gluconate containing rinses as recommended.

   a. At this point, chlorhexidine is the most effective antimicrobial agent for long-term reduction of plaque biofilm and gingivitis. For this reason, it is often regarded as the standard against which all other topical chemical plaque biofilm control agents are judged.

   b. The effectiveness of chlorhexidine gluconate mouth rinses is due to the following characteristics.

      1) Chlorhexidine is bactericidal agent that is effective against both Gram-positive and Gram-negative bacteria.

      2) Chlorhexidine binds with oral tissues in the mouth and is slowly released over time (several hours) in a concentration that will continue killing bacteria. Thus these rinses display the property of substantivity.

      3) Chlorhexidine has a very low level of toxicity and shows no permanent retention in the body.

3. The primary mechanism of action for chlorhexidine gluconate is disruption of the integrity of the cell walls of bacteria.

4. Chlorhexidine containing mouth rinses are useful adjuncts to plaque biofilm control in many patients. Current recommendations for use of this mouth rinse (0.12% chlorhexidine gluconate) are to rinse with one-half ounce for 30 seconds twice daily.

5. In addition to routine use of these rinses as part of a patient's self-care program, there are several groups of patients that should be considered for use of chlorhexidine gluconate mouth rinse. Some of these are outlined below.

   a. Special Needs Patients. The use of a chlorhexidine mouth rinse is suggested for specific groups of patients who have special needs. Two examples of such patients are those with immunodeficiencies that might be more susceptible to infections in general and patients who are unable to perform plaque biofilm control because of some impairment.

   b. Postsurgical Care Patients. Following periodontal surgery, it is frequently difficult for patients to perform adequate mechanical plaque biofilm control during the healing period without damaging the surgical site. In these patients chlorhexidine mouth rinses can be used for postsurgical rinsing as a temporary adjunct to mechanical plaque biofilm control. Use of a chlorhexidine mouth rinse following periodontal surgery for 4 to 6 weeks can be effective in many patients in facilitating postsurgical healing.

   c. Patients with Candida Infections. It should be noted that a variety of medications are used to control Candida infections, but chlorhexidine mouth rinses can be used as a disinfectant for dental appliances such as complete dentures or partial dentures in patients with these infections.

   d. Patients with Dental Caries. Chlorhexidine is also effective against the bacteria responsible for dental caries. Rinsing with chlorhexidine mouth rinses has been used to reduce the counts of caries causing bacteria in certain patients.

   e. Patients with Oral Piercings. Chlorhexidine mouth rinses have also been recommended for use by patients for aftercare of oral piercings.

E. **Mouth Rinses Containing Essential Oils**
   1. Chemicals referred to as essential oils have been used as active ingredients in some mouth rinses for many years. Chemical agents included in the group of chemicals called essential oils include thymol, menthol, eucalyptol, and methyl salicylate.
   2. Mouth rinses containing essential oils are available over the counter (i.e., available without a prescription). Listerine mouth rinse is one example of a rinse containing essential oils, but there are other products on the market with similar ingredients.
   3. There are numerous investigations related to the efficacy of essential oils in controlling gingivitis published in the literature.
      a. This group of chemicals can indeed help control plaque biofilm, and they have received the Seal of Acceptance from the American Dental Association for their effect against *gingivitis*.
      b. Investigations have demonstrated that when used in mouth rinses, the essential oils can reduce the severity of gingivitis by approximately 35% if used as recommended.
      c. The mechanism of action of essential oils appears to be disruption of the integrity of the cell wall and inhibition of certain bacterial enzymes.
      d. Mouth rinses containing essential oils are less effective than chlorhexidine gluconate mouth rinses. However, these mouth rinses are much less expensive than chlorhexidine gluconate mouth rinses and can be purchased without a prescription.
   4. Essential oil mouthrinses have also been evaluated related to their effectiveness as a preprocedural rinse for dental office procedures producing aerosols. The bacteria in aerosols produced by ultrasonic scalers can be reduced by more than 90% by using these rinses prior to the office procedure.

F. **Mouth Rinses Containing Quaternary Ammonium Compounds**
   1. Some mouth rinses currently marketed contain the quaternary ammonium compound cetylpyridinium chloride as the active ingredient.
   2. This surface active agent also kills bacteria by disrupting bacterial cell walls.
   3. This chemical agent binds to oral tissues, but is released so rapidly that it has very limited substantivity, limiting its effectiveness in controlling dental plaque biofilm.
   4. Investigations have shown that cetylpyridinium chloride can reduce the severity of gingivitis but the level of reduction is less than either chlorhexidine gluconate or the essential oils.

G. **The Use of Povidone Iodine as a Mouthrinse**
   1. Povidone iodine is a water soluble antimicrobial agent that has been used in medicinal practice as a presurgical scrub for skin disinfection.
   2. Povidone iodine has been studied as a mouth rinse and found to be comparable in results to some other chemical agents. It has been used in conjunction with basic nonsurgical therapy, and when combined with hydrogen peroxide as a mouthrinse, it can reduce papillary bleeding scores.
   3. Concerns related to the safety of the daily use of this chemical agent have been raised, however.
   4. This chemical agent should not be used in patients with sensitivity to iodine, patients with allergy to shellfish, women who are lactating or pregnant, and patients with thyroid dysfunction.

H. **Problems with Mouth Rinse Ingredients**
1. No chemicals are completely safe for all patients, and most mouth rinses have produced unwanted side effects in some patients. Reported side effects for some of the active ingredients discussed above are outlined in Boxes 28-5 and 28-6.
2. As already discussed, in addition to the active ingredients mouth rinses contain inactive ingredients such as flavoring agents and preservatives that can create problems for some patients. Two of these ingredients are listed below.
    a. Alcohol. Some mouth rinses have rather high levels of alcohol content, and these should be avoided in patients addicted to alcohol.
    b. Salt. Some mouth rinses have rather high levels of sodium, making them questionable for use in certain patients with hypertension (high blood pressure).

Box 28-5. Possible Side Effects of Essential Oils

- Burning sensation in the mouth
- Bitter taste
- Drying out of mucous membranes

Box 28-6. Possible Side Effects for Chlorhexidine Gluconate

- Allergic reaction
- Extrinsic staining of teeth
- Discoloration of tongue
- Alterations of taste
- Increase in calculus formation

---

3. **Toothpastes as Delivery Mechanisms for Plaque Biofilm Control Agents.** Dentifrices such as toothpastes and gels would appear to be nearly ideal delivery mechanisms for chemical agents that might benefit patients, since most patients use these products daily. Originally dentifrices were simply aids to brushing deposits off tooth surfaces, but today there are a variety of chemical agents that can be added to toothpastes as active ingredients that may actually benefit some patients in other ways.
    A. **Categories of Toothpastes.** The American Dental Association loosely classifies toothpastes as falling into one of the following categories:
        1. Antitartar activity
        2. Caries prevention
        3. Cosmetic effects
        4. Gingivitis reduction
        5. Plaque reduction
        6. Reduction of tooth sensitivity

B. **Active Chemical Ingredients.** This American Dental Association classification of toothpastes underscores the broad range of benefits that can be derived from active ingredient chemical agents added to some toothpastes.

1. Some of these chemical agents are added to toothpastes impart special benefits to periodontal patients. See Table 28-3 for some examples of the chemical agents that can be used as active ingredients in toothpastes for their periodontal benefits.

2. Stannous fluoride has been used successfully as an anticaries agent for many years. Studies indicate that stannous fluoride also affects dental plaque biofilm and can also reduce the severity of gingivitis when used as an active ingredient in toothpastes.

3. Triclosan is a topical antimicrobial agent used in many products and is now available as the active ingredient in a toothpaste.

   a. Triclosan can be combined with copolymers to enhance its substantivity (binding and subsequent slow release).

   b. Studies indicate that when combined with copolymers, triclosan (when delivered in toothpaste form) can decrease the severity of gingivitis approximately 20%.

   c. Triclosan can also be combined with zinc citrate to reduce dental calculus formation.

C. **The Future.** Toothpastes appear to be ideal delivery mechanisms for chemical agents that might be expected to control certain periodontal conditions, such as gingival inflammation. It is reasonable to expect that additional research in this area will result in additional toothpaste formulations that target periodontal conditions such as gingivitis.

TABLE 28-3. Examples of Tooth Active Ingredients Used for Periodontal Benefits

Ingredients	Actions
Pyrophosphates	Reduces *supra*gingival calculus
Stannous fluoride	Reduces gingival inflammation
Triclosan	Reduces *supra*gingival calculus Reduces gingival inflammation
Zinc citrate	Reduces *supra*gingival calculus

Chapter Summary Statement

Chemical agents that can be used to control dental plaque biofilm can be delivered both systemically and topically. Since dental plaque biofilm is covered by a protective slime layer, chemical agents will not necessarily contact all of the targeted bacteria, and their use must be accompanied by mechanical plaque biofilm control that can disrupt the structure of the plaque biofilm. Systemic antibiotics are not normally used to control dental plaque biofilm in patients with the most common periodontal conditions (plaque-associated gingivitis and chronic periodontitis) because of the high risk of developing antibiotic-resistant strains. Mouth rinses can be useful adjuncts in the treatment of patients with periodontal diseases. Thus far the most effective ingredients to control plaque biofilm that can be incorporated into mouth rinses include chlorhexidine and the essential oils. Controlled release delivery devices are also available to help control bacterial plaque biofilm in periodontal patients. Toothpastes are widely used by patients and appear to be an ideal mechanism for delivery of chemical agents to aid in plaque biofilm control.

Section 4
Focus on Patients

Case 1

A patient shows you a bottle of mouth rinse and asks you if it would be all right to use this mouth rinse instead of brushing and flossing so frequently. You study the label on the bottle of mouth rinse and find that the active ingredients are the essential oils. How should you respond to this patient about substituting this rinse for other self-care efforts such as brushing and an interdental brush?

Case 2

A patient being treated by the members of your dental team has generalized chronic periodontitis. Following your thorough explanation of the nature of chronic periodontitis and your emphasis that this disease is indeed a bacterial infection, the patient asks this question, "If periodontitis is an infection, can you ask the dentist to give me a prescription for an antibiotic?" How should you respond to this patient's question?

Case 3

A new patient being seen by your dental team has recently moved into your city. She has previously been treated for chronic periodontitis and has been on periodontal maintenance for several years. She is now having trouble with mechanical plaque biofilm control because of increasing dexterity problems. What chemical agents can you recommend that might help reduce the patient's gingival inflammation?

Suggested Readings

American Academy of Periodontology. Chemical agents for control of plaque and gingivitis. Committee on Research, Science and Therapy. Position Paper. Chicago: The Academy; 1994.

American Academy of Periodontology. The role of controlled drug delivery for periodontitis. *J Periodontol.* 2000;71:125–140.

Andrews LW. Commentary: the perils of povidone-iodine use. *Ostomy Wound Manage.* 1994;40: 68–73.

Anwar H, Strap J, Costerton J. Establishment of aging biofilms: Possible mechanism of bacterial resistance to anti-microbial therapy. *Antimicrob Agents Chemother.* 1992;36:1347–1351.

Banting D, Bosma M, Bollmer B. Clinical effectiveness of a 0.12% chlorhexidine mouthrinse over two years. *J Dent Res.* 1989;68:1716.

Beiswanger BB, Doyle PM, Jackson RD, et al. The clinical effect of dentifrices containing stabilized stannous fluoride on plaque formation and gingivitis—a six-month study with ad libitum brushing. *J Clin Dent.* 1995;6:46–53.

Christersson LA, Norderyd OM, Puchalsky CS. Topical application of tetracycline-HCL in human periodontitis. *J Clin Periodontol.* 1993;20:88–95.

Ciancio SG. Agents for the management of plaque and gingivitis. *J Dent Res.* 1992;71:1450–1454.

Ciancio S. Expanded and future uses of mouthrinses. *J Am Dent Assoc.* 1994;125(Suppl 2):29S–32S.

Cubells AB, Dalmau LB, Petrone ME, et al. The effect of a triclosan/copolymer/fluoride dentifrice on plaque formation and gingivitis: a six-month study. *J Clin Dent.* 1991;2:63–69.

DeSalva SJ, Kong BM, Lin YJ. Triclosan: a safety profile. *Am J Dent.* 1989;2:185–196.

Drisko C, Cobb C, Killoy R, et al. Evaluation of periodontal treatments using controlled-release tetracycline fibers. Clinical response. *J Periodontol.* 1995;66:692–699.

Drisko CH. Review/ Non-surgical periodontal therapy: pharmacotherapeutics. In: *Annals of Periodontal Therapy 1996 World Workshop in Periodontics.* Chicago: American Academy of Periodontology; 1996:493–506.

Drisko CH. Nonsurgical periodontal therapy. *Periodontol 2000.* 2001;25:77–88.

Fleischer W, Reimer K. Povidone iodine antisepsis. State of the art. *Dermatology.* 1997;195 (Suppl 2):3–9.

Garrett S, Johnson L, Drisko CH, et al. Two multi-center clinical studies evaluating locally delivered doxycycline hyclate, placebo control, oral hygiene, and scaling and root planing in the treatment of periodontitis. *J Periodontol.* 1999;70:490–503.

Gilbert P, Das J, Foley I. Biofilm susceptibility to antimicrobials. *Adv Dent Res.* 1997;11:160–167.

Gjermo P. Chlorhexidine and related compounds. *J Dent Res.* 1989;68:1602.

Goodson JM, Cugini MA, Kent RL, et al. Multi-center evaluation of tetracycline fiber therapy. I. Experimental design, methods, and baseline data. *J Periodont Res.* 1991;26:361.

Goodson JM, Cugini MA, Kent RL, et al. Multi-center evaluation of tetracycline fiber therapy: II. Clinical response. *J Periodont Res.* 1991;36:371.

Goodson JM. Pharmacokinetic principles controlling efficacy of oral therapy. *J Dent Res.* 1989;68: 1625–1632.

Gordon JM, Lamster IB, Seiger MC. Efficacy of Listerine antiseptic in inhibiting the development of plaque and gingivitis. *J Clin Periodontol.* 1985;12:697.

Greenstein G. Povidone-iodone's effects and role in the management of periodontal diseases: a review. *J Periodontol.* 1999;70:1397–1405.

Grossman E, Reiter G, Sturzenberger OP, et al. Six-month study on the effects of a chlorhexidine mouthrinse on gingivitis in adults. *J Periodont Res.* 1986;21:33.

Henke CJ, Villa KF, Aichelmann-Reidy ME, et al. An economic evaluation of a chlorhexidine chip for treating chronic periodontitis: The CHIP (chlorhexidine in periodontitis) study. *J Am Dent Assoc.* 2001;132:1557–1569.

Hanes PJ, Purvis JP. Local anti-infective therapy: pharmacologic agents. A systematic review. *Ann Periodontol.* 2003;8:79–98.

Jeffcoat M, Bray KS, Ciancio SG, et al. Adjunctive use of a sub-gingival controlled release chlorhexidine chip reduces probing depth and improved attachment level compared with scaling and root planing alone. *J Periodontol.* 1998;69:989–997.

Kinane DF, Radvar M. A six-month comparison of three periodontal local antimicrobial therapies in persistent periodontal pockets. *J Periodontol.* 1999;70:1–7.

Killoy WJ. The clinical significance of local chemotherapies. *J Clin Periodontol.* 2002;29:22–29.

Killoy WJ, Polson AM. Controlled local delivery of antimicrobials in the treatment of periodontitis. *Dent Clin North Am.* 1998;42:263.

Lamster IB, Alfano MC, Seiger MC, et al. The effect of Listerine antiseptic on reduction of existing plaque and gingivitis. *Clin Prev Dent.* 1983;5:12.

Lang NP, Brecx MC. Chlorhexidine digluconate—an agent for chemical plaque control and prevention of gingival inflammation. *J Periodont Res.* 1986;21(Suppl):74–89.

Lobene RR, Lovene S, Soparker PM. The effect of cetylpyridinium chloride mouthrinse on plaque and gingivitis. *J Dent Res.* 1977;56:595.

Newman JC, Kornman KS, Doherty FM. A 6-month multicenter evaluation of adjunctive tetracycline fiber therapy used in conjunction with scaling and root planing in maintenance patients: clinical results. *J Periodontol.* 1994;65:685.

Paquette DW, Ryan ME, Wilder RS. Locally delivered antimicrobials: clinical evidence and relevance. *J Dent Hyg.* 2008;82 Suppl 3:10–15.

Perlich MA, Bacca LA, Bollmer BW, et al. The clinical effect of a stabilized stannous fluoride dentifrice on plaque formation, gingivitis, and gingival bleeding: a six month study. *J Clin Dent.* 1995;6:54–58.

Quirynen M, Teughels W, De Soete M, et al. Topical antiseptics and antibiotics in the initial therapy of chronic adult periodontitis: microbiological aspects. *Periodontol 2000.* 2002;28:72–90.

Radvar M, Pourtaghi N, Kinane DF. Comparison of 3 periodontal local antibiotic therapies in persistent periodontal pockets. *J Periodontol.* 1996;67:860–865.

Scheie AAA. Modes of action of currently known chemical antiplaque agents other than chlorhexidine. *J Dent Res.* 1989;68:1609.

Slots J. Selection of antimicrobial agents in periodontal therapy. *J Periodont Res.* 2002;37:389–398.

Slots J, Ting M. Systemic antibiotics in the treatment of periodontal disease. *Periodontol 2000.* 2002;28:106–176.

Socransky SS, Haffajee AD. Dental biofilms: difficult therapeutic targets. *Periodontol 2000.* 2002;28:12–55.

Soskolne WA, Heasman PA, Stabholz A, et al. Sustained local delivery of chlorhexidine in the treatment of periodontitis: a multicenter study. *J Periodontol.* 1997;68:32–38.

Sweeting LA, Davis K, Cobb CM. Periodontal Treatment Protocol (PTP) for the general dental practice. *J Dent Hyg.* 2008;82 Suppl 3:16–26.

Systemic antibiotics in periodontics. *J Periodontol.* 1996;67:831–838.

Thomas J, Walker C, Bradshaw M. Long-term use of subantimicrobial dose doxycycline does not lead to changes in antimicrobial susceptibility. *J Periodontol.* 2000;71:1472–1483.

van der Ouderaa FJG. Anti-plaque agents. Rationale and prospects for prevention of gingivitis and periodontal disease. *J Clin Periodontol.* 1991;18:447–454.

van Steenberghe D, Bercy P, Kohl J, et al. Subgingival minocycline hydrochloride ointment in moderate to severe chronic adult periodontitis: a randomized, double-blind, vehicle-controlled, multicenter study. *J Periodontol.* 1993;64:637–644.

van Steenberghe D, Rosling B, Soder PO, et al. A 15 month evaluation of the effects of repeated subgingival minocycline in chronic adult periodontitis. *J Periodontol.* 1999;70:657–667.

Wennstrom JL, Newman HN, MacNeil SR, et al. Utilization of locally delivered doxycycline in non-surgical treatment of chronic periodontitis. A comparative multi-center trial of 2 treatment approaches. *J Clin Periodontol.* 2001;28:753–761.

Williams RC, Paquette DW, Offenbacher S, et al. Treatment of periodontitis by local administration of minocycline microspheres: a controlled trial. *J Periodontol.* 2001;72:1535–1544.

Host Modulation

Learning Objectives

- Explain the term host modulation.

- Explain the potential importance of host modulation.

- Name some anti-inflammatory mediators.

- Name some proinflammatory mediators.

- List three types of drugs that have been studied for use as possible host modulating agents.

- Explain why low dose doxycyclines are useful as host modulating agents.

- Explain the term sub-antibacterial dose.

- Make a list of treatment strategies for a periodontitis patient that includes host modulation.

Key Terms

Host modulation
Biochemical mediators
Anti-inflammatory mediators
Proinflammatory biochemical
  mediators

Doxycycline
Sub-antibacterial doses
Nonsteroidal anti-inflammatory
  drugs (NSAIDS)
Bisphosphonates

Section 1
Introduction to the Concept of Host Modulation

For several decades the focus of therapy for patients with inflammatory periodontal diseases has been directed toward controlling the microbial etiology of these diseases. Minimizing the bacterial challenge to the periodontium has been a successful strategy for the treatment of many patients with both gingivitis and periodontitis. Beyond any doubt, plaque biofilm control strategies will continue to play a major role in the therapy for patients with periodontal disease.

Based upon current knowledge of the underlying pathology involved in periodontal diseases, additional strategies for therapy can now also be employed for patients with inflammatory periodontal diseases. One of these additional strategies relates to the concept of host modulation. The concept of host modulation focuses on how the body responds to the bacterial challenge rather than simply reducing that bacterial challenge.

1. **Host Modulation**
    A. **The Importance of Host Modulation**
        1. Host modulation in dentistry can be defined as altering the host's (patient's) defense responses to help the body limit damage to the periodontium from infections such as periodontitis.
            a. Host modulation has been a part of medical care of patients with a variety of systemic diseases for many years. An example of a systemic disease for which physicians frequently use host modulation is osteoporosis.
            b. Modulation of host defenses is currently an important focus for periodontal research, and host modulation will undoubtedly play a larger part in periodontal therapy in the future.
        2. The potential importance of host modulation as one strategy in managing periodontitis patients is huge.
            a. As already discussed in other chapters, most adults show signs of periodontal or gingival disease with severe periodontitis affecting approximately 15% of the adult population in the US. Because so many patients have inflammatory periodontal diseases, there is a continuing need for cost-effective strategies for managing periodontitis patients.
            b. As the population in the United States ages, it is reasonable to expect the prevalence of periodontitis to increase, making the need for the most cost-effective therapy even greater.
            c. In addition, there is mounting evidence that periodontal health and several systemic conditions (such as diabetes and cardiovascular disease) are linked, again making it more likely that the demand for periodontal therapy will increase over the upcoming decades.
    B. **Overview of Host Responses That Can Be Modulated**
        1. The fundamental pathologic processes for periodontitis have been outlined in other chapters of this textbook; in those chapters the following issues have been discussed.
            a. Bacteria (and bacterial products) that are a part of the plaque biofilm initiate inflammatory responses in the periodontium. Bacteria stimulate the immune cells to produce biochemical mediators—biologically active compounds—that activate the body's inflammatory response. The inflammatory response is protective and keeps the bacterial infection from doing serious harm to the periodontium in many patients partly through the production of chemicals called anti-inflammatory biochemical mediators.

   b. Anti-inflammatory mediators are biochemical mediators that are protective and keep the bacterial infection from doing serious harm to the periodontium, such as the cytokines interleukin-4 (IL-4) and interleukin-10 (IL-10).

   c. Box 29-1 shows some of the anti-inflammatory biochemical mediators.

   d. If the bacterial challenge is great enough, however, the nature of the protective responses changes, resulting in the production of additional biochemical mediators that can lead to actual damage within the periodontium.

      1) Some biochemical mediators (referred to as proinflammatory biochemical mediators) can damage the periodontium. These proinflammatory mediators include chemicals such as matrix metalloproteinases (MMPs), certain cytokines, prostanoids, and other less well understood mediators.

      2) Specific examples of these proinflammatory mediators include prostaglandin E_2, interleukin-1 alpha (IL-1α), interleukin-1 beta (IL-1β), interleukin-6 (IL-6), and tumor necrosis factor alpha.

      3) For example, one of the MMPs is an enzyme called collagenase that can actually break down collagen. Collagen is one of the major building blocks in the periodontium, and its breakdown is part of the fundamental pathology in periodontitis.

      4) Box 29-2 shows some of the proinflammatory biochemical mediators.

   e. In the periodontium these altered host defense responses can result in both breakdown of connective tissue fibers and resorption of alveolar bone (the precise types of tissue destruction seen in periodontitis).

   f. Much of the destruction of the periodontium that accompanies periodontitis is a result of these altered processes that occur as part of the host defenses (the host inflammatory and immune responses).

2. Fundamentally, the concept of host modulation as a strategy in treating periodontitis patients is to limit the damaging effect of the altered host responses by modifying (or modulating) the effect of these destructive biochemical mediators.

Box 29-1. Examples of Anti-inflammatory Biochemical Mediators. These mediators help the body fight off the effects of the bacterial challenge

- IL-4 (interleukin-4)
- IL-10 (interleukin-10)
- IL-1ra (receptor antagonist)
- Tissue inhibitors of matrix metalloproteinases (TIMPs)

Box 29-2. Examples of Proinflammatory Biochemical Mediators. These mediators can lead to destruction of tissues in the periodontium

- IL-1 (interleukin-1)
- IL-6 (interleukin-6)
- *PGE$_2$* (prostaglandin E$_2$)
- *TNFα* (tumor necrosis factor alpha)
- *MMPs* (matrix metalloproteinases)

2. **Potential Host Modulating Agents**
    A. **Doxycycline**
        1. Doxycycline is an antibiotic drug that is used to treat a variety of infections.
            a. As with other antibiotics, doxycycline must be given in doses high enough to affect the targeted bacteria to help the body fight an infection.
            b. Antibiotic doses high enough to inhibit or kill bacteria are sometimes called antibacterial doses. A typical antibacterial dose for doxycycline would be 50 to 100 mg every 12 hours.
        2. Doxycycline has other effects besides its antibiotic effect that is seen with higher doses.
            a. If this medication is given even at low doses (below that needed for any antibacterial effect), it decreases the effects of the enzyme collagenase (one of the MMPs).
            b. As already discussed, MMPs (such as collagenase) can be released in inflamed periodontal tissues and can cause breakdown of the connective tissue. Prevention of the action of collagenase can inhibit the progress of periodontitis.
            c. Doses of an antibiotic that are below the normal bacterial killing or inhibiting doses are referred to as sub-antibacterial doses.
            d. Since doxycycline at low doses (or sub-antibacterial doses) alters the body defenses by inhibiting part of the destruction that can occur in periodontitis, it is considered one example of a host-modulating agent.
            e. The FDA approves sub-antibacterial doses of doxycycline (20 mg tablets) for use in treating patients with periodontitis.
                1) Low doses of doxycycline must be taken twice daily in tablet form to be effective in periodontitis patients.
                2) No antibacterial effect on the oral bacteria or bacteria in other parts of the body have been found with use of low dose doxycycline.
                3) Studies of this drug have also shown a clinical benefit when used as an adjunct to periodontal instrumentation.
                4) Though tetracyclines used at antibacterial doses can have side effects (including nausea, vomiting, photosensitivity, and hypersensitivity reactions), doxycycline at low doses appears to be accompanied by a very low incidence of adverse effects.
        3. Studies have shown reductions in probing depths and gains in clinical attachment levels as well as the prevention of periodontal disease progression with the use of sub-antibacterial doses of doxycycline in periodontitis patients.
    B. **Nonsteroidal Anti-inflammatory Drugs**
        1. Nonsteroidal anti-inflammatory drugs (referred to as NSAIDs) have been used for many years in medical care to treat pain, acute inflammation, and chronic inflammatory conditions.
        2. Box 29-3 shows examples of drugs included in the group called NSAIDS.
        3. NSAIDs can reduce tissue inflammation by inhibiting prostaglandins including PGE_2.
        4. In periodontal studies systemically administered NSAIDs have been evaluated for their effect on periodontitis (a disease intimately associated with inflammation).
            a. In the periodontium NSAIDs can both reduce inflammation and inhibit osteoclast activity.
            b. Some NSAIDs, when administered daily over 3 years, have been shown to slow the rate of alveolar bone loss associated with periodontitis.

Box 29-3. Examples of NSAIDS Medications

- Salicylates (aspirin)
- Indomethacin
- Ibuprofen
- Flurbiprofen
- Naproxen

---

5. However, long-term use of NSAIDs in periodontitis patients is not recommended because of significant side effects that can develop with the use of these drugs.
   a. Side effects from NSAIDs can include gastrointestinal problems, hemorrhage (bleeding), and kidney or liver impairment.
   b. In addition, when a patient with periodontitis stops taking daily doses of NSAIDs, there can be an acceleration of the bone loss seen prior to taking the drugs.
   c. At present no NSAIDs are approved for the treatment of periodontal disease.
6. Even though NSAIDs are not currently recommended for use in host modulation in periodontitis patients, they have been discussed here because of the extensive dental research that has involved these drugs.
7. In addition to systemically administered NSAIDs, topically applied NSAIDs have been studied for their possible benefits to periodontitis patients.
   a. Topical NSAIDs have also been shown to reduce PGE_2 in gingival crevicular fluid in periodontitis patients.
   b. Topically administered NSAIDs have not been approved for the management of periodontitis, but more study of the possible use of topical NSAIDs is warranted.

C. **Bisphosphonates**
   1. Bisphosphonates are drugs that can inhibit the resorption of bone by altering osteoclastic activity, though the mechanism of action for these drugs is not fully understood.
   2. Early research indicates there may be some benefit to periodontitis patients from the ability of bisphosphonates to alter osteoclastic activity (bone resorption activity).
   3. Some of the bisphosphonates have side effects that may limit their use in periodontitis patients, but they are discussed in this section because of the interest that has been shown in these drugs over the last few years.
   4. One of the possible side effects of these drugs is osteonecrosis of the jaws following their extended use. Osteonecrosis is the destruction and death of bone tissue, in this case the bone tissue of the jaw. Studies are underway to clarify the precise risk and etiology of this serious side effect.
   5. At present there are no bisphosphonate drugs that are approved for the treatment of periodontal disease.

D. **Additional Host Modulation Agents**
   1. Several potential agents have been investigated for use as adjuncts to periodontal surgical procedures.
   2. These drugs do not produce the same types of effects discussed for the other potential host modulating agents, but they are mentioned here because some authors have referred to them as "host modulating agents."

3. These agents are generally applied topically during periodontal surgical procedures and have been suggested for use for possible enhancement to wound healing or possible enhancement of regeneration of periodontal tissues following the surgery.

4. Some agents of this type that have been investigated are enamel matrix proteins, bone morphogenetic proteins (BMP-2, BMP-7), and certain growth factors.

5. Currently the only local host modulation agent approved for adjunctive use during periodontal surgery is an enamel matrix protein called Emdogain, and this agent is under continuing study.

6. Members of the dental team should expect additional host modulation products to be investigated and to appear on the market; careful evaluation of each of the products will be needed.

Section 2
Host Modulation as a Part of Comprehensive Periodontal Management

1. Studies of gingival crevicular fluid content indicate that markers of periodontal disease in patients with periodontitis undergo little change following conventional mechanical periodontal therapy. Thus, it appears that even though conventional periodontal therapy based upon minimizing the bacterial challenge is usually successful, the underlying disease processes may be diminished in severity though they may remain fundamentally unchanged.

2. Employing host modulation in the comprehensive management of periodontitis patients seems to be a promising strategy to employ in selected patients.

   A. *It should be reemphasized that at present the only host modulating agent currently being recommended is the low dose tetracyclines, but investigations have indicated theoretically that other possible host modulations may one day be employed in periodontitis patients.*

   B. When used in periodontitis patients, sound clinical practice would dictate that low dose doxycycline therapy be accompanied by usual treatment strategies such as risk factor reduction (i.e., smoking cessation counseling) and bacterial challenge reduction (i.e., self-care training and periodontal debridement).

3. Box 29-4 lists the array of therapeutic strategies that can be employed when managing a patient with periodontitis, including host modulation.

4. Figure 29-1 shows some theoretical possibilities for host modulation as a part of overall management of periodontitis patients.

Box 29-4. Options for Therapy for a Periodontitis Patient

1. Patient education and motivation in self-care.

2. Reduction of the bacterial challenge by periodontal instrumentation.

3. Use of local delivery systems for antimicrobial agents.

4. Risk factor reduction (such as smoking cessation).

5. Host modulation.

6. Periodontal surgery.

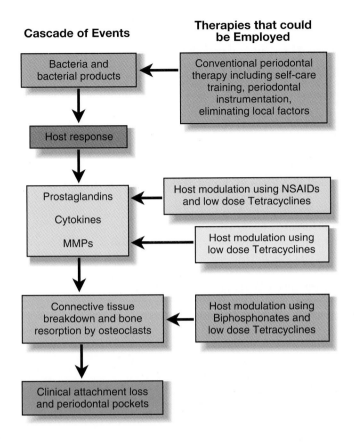

Cascade of Events

Therapies that could be Employed

Bacteria and bacterial products → Conventional periodontal therapy including self-care training, periodontal instrumentation, eliminating local factors

Host response

Prostaglandins / Cytokines / MMPs ← Host modulation using NSAIDs and low dose Tetracyclines

← Host modulation using low dose Tetracyclines

Connective tissue breakdown and bone resorption by osteoclasts ← Host modulation using Biphosphonates and low dose Tetracyclines

Clinical attachment loss and periodontal pockets

Figure 29.1. Theoretical Possibilities for Host Modulation that Could be Employed in Periodontitis Patients.

Chapter Summary Statement

Host modulation (altering the body's defense mechanisms to limit damage from the oral bacterial challenge) is an interesting and ongoing line of investigation. Host modulation has been suggested as an additional therapeutic strategy in periodontitis patients. At this point, low dose doxycycline has been approved for use as a host-modulating agent in humans with periodontitis. When used in sub-antimicrobial doses, this drug can help inhibit the progress of periodontitis. Members of the dental team are likely to see much research activity related to additional host modulating agents over the next several decades.

Section 3
Focus on Patients

Case 1

A new patient in your dental team's office has a periodontal diagnosis of generalized severe chronic periodontitis. Explain how host modulation might be included among other treatment strategies used to help control the damage to the periodontium that normally accompanies periodontitis.

Suggested Readings

Al Shammari KF, Giannobile WV, Aldredge WA, et al. Effect of non–surgical periodontal therapy on C-telopeptide pyridinoline cross-links (ICTP) and interleukin-1 levels. *J Periodontol.* 2001;72:1045–1051.

Birkedal-Hansen H. Role of matrix metalloproteinases in human periodontal diseases. *J Periodontol.* 1993;64:474–484.

Caton JG, Ciancio SG, Blieden TM, et al. Treatment with subantimicrobial dose doxycycline improves the efficacy of scaling and root planing in patients with adult periodontitis. *J Periodontol.* 2000;71:521–532.

Choi DH, Moon IS, Choi BK, et al. Effects of subantimicrobial dose doxycycline therapy on crevicular fluid MMP-8, and gingival tissue MMP-9, TIMP-1 and IL-6 levels in chronic periodontitis. *J Periodontal Res.* 2004;39:20–26.

Crout RJ, Lee HM, Schroeder K, et al. The "cyclic" regimen of low-dose doxycycline for adult periodontitis: a preliminary study. *J Periodontol.* 1996;67:506–514.

Emingil G, Atilla G, Sorsa T, et al. The effect of adjunctive low-dose doxycycline therapy on clinical parameters and gingival crevicular fluid matrix metalloproteinase-8 levels in chronic periodontitis. *J Periodontol.* 2004;75:106–115.

Genco RJ. Host responses in periodontal diseases: current concepts. *J Periodontol.* 1992;63:338–355.

Golub LM, Evans RT, McNamara TF, et al. A non-antimicrobial tetracycline inhibits gingival matrix metalloproteinases and bone loss in *Porphyromonas gingivalis*-induced periodontitis in rats. *Ann NY Acad Sci.* 1994;732:96–111.

Golub LM, Lee HM, Greenwald RA, et al. A matrix metalloproteinase inhibitor reduces bone-type collagen degradation fragments and specific collagenases in gingival crevicular fluid during adult periodontitis. *Inflamm Res.* 1997;46:310–319.

Golub LM, McNamara TF, Ryan ME, et al. Adjunctive treatment with subantimicrobial doses of doxycycline: effects on gingival fluid collagenase activity and attachment loss in adult periodontitis. *J Clin Periodontol.* 2001;28:146–156.

Golub LM, Sorsa T, Lee HM, et al. Doxycycline inhibits neutrophil (PMN)-type matrix metalloproteinases in human adult periodontitis gingiva. *J Clin Periodontol.* 1995;22:100–109.

Golub LM, Suomalainen K, Sorsa T. Host modulation with tetracyclines and their chemically modified analogues. *Curr Opin Dent.* 1992;2:80–90.

Golub LM, Wolff M, Lee HM, et al. Further evidence that tetracyclines inhibit collagenase activity in human crevicular fluid and from other mammalian sources. *J Periodont Res.* 1985;20:12–23.

Grossi SG, Zambon JJ, Ho AW, et al. Assessment of risk for periodontal disease. I. Risk indicators for attachment loss. *J Periodontol.* 1994;65:260–267.

Howell TH, Williams RC. Non-steroidal anti-inflammatory drugs as inhibitors of periodontal disease progression. *Crit Rev Oral Biol Med.* 1993;4:177–196.

Jeffcoat MK, Reddy MS, Haigh S, et al. A comparison of topical ketorolac, systemic flurbiprofen, and placebo for the inhibition of bone loss in adult periodontitis. *J Periodontol.* 1995;66:329–338.

Kornman KS. Host modulation as a therapeutic strategy in the treatment of periodontal disease. *Clin Infect Dis.* 1999;28:520–526.

Lee HM, Golub LM, Chan D, et al. α_1-Proteinase inhibitor in gingival crevicular fluid of humans with adult periodontitis: serpinolytic inhibition by doxycycline. *J Periodontal Res.* 1997;32:9–19.

Nakaya H, Osawa G, Iwasaki N, et al. Effects of bisphosphonate on matrix metalloproteinase enzymes in human periodontal ligament cells. *J Periodontol.* 2000;71:1158–1166.

Novak MJ, Johns LP, Miller RC, Bradshaw MH: Adjunctive benefits of subantimicrobial dose doxycycline in the management of severe, generalized, chronic periodontitis. *J Periodontol.* 2002;73:762–769.

Offenbacher S, Heasman PA, Collins JG. Modulation of host PGE2 secretion as a determinant of periodontal disease expression. *J Periodontol.* 1993;64:432–444.

Offenbacher S. Periodontal diseases: pathogenesis. *Ann Periodontol.* 1996;1:821–878.

Page RC, Kornman KS. The pathogenesis of human periodontitis: an introduction. *Periodontol 2000.* 1997;14:9–11.

Page RC. Milestones in periodontal research and the remaining critical issues. *J Periodontal Res.* 1999;34:331–339.

Preshaw PM, Hefti AF, Bradshaw MH. Adjunctive subantimicrobial dose doxycycline in smokers and non-smokers with chronic periodontitis. *J Clin Periodontol.* 2005;32:610–616.

Preshaw PM, Hefti AF, Novak MJ, et al. Subantimicrobial dose doxycycline enhances the efficacy of scaling and root planing in chronic periodontitis: a multi-center trial. *J Periodontol.* 2004;75:1068–1076.

Reddy MS, Weatherford TW, Smith CA, et al. Alendronate treatment of naturally-occurring periodontitis in beagle dogs. *J Periodontol.* 1995;66:211–217.

Salvi GE, Lawrence HP, Offenbacher S, Beck JD. Influence of risk factors on the pathogenesis of periodontitis. *Periodontol 2000.* 1997;14:173–201.

Shoji K, Horiuchi H, Shinoda H. Inhibitory effects of a bisphosphonate (risedronate) on experimental periodontitis in rats. *J Periodont Res.* 1995;30:277–284.

Thomas JG, Metheny RJ, Karakiozis JM, et al. Long-term sub-antimicrobial doxycycline (Periostat) as adjunctive management in adult periodontitis: effects on subgingival bacterial population dynamics. *Adv Dent Res.* 1998;12:32–39.

Vilcek J, Feldmann M. Historical review: cytokines as therapeutics and targets of therapeutics. *Trends Pharmacol Sci.* 2004;25:201–209.

Walker C, Preshaw PM, Novak J, et al. Long-term treatment with subantimicrobial dose doxycycline has no antibacterial effect on intestinal flora. *J Clin Periodontol.* 2005;32:1163–1169.

Walker C, Thomas J, Nango S, et al. Long-term treatment with subantimicrobial dose doxycycline exerts no antibacterial effect on the subgingival microflora associated with adult periodontitis. *J Periodontol.* 2000;71:1465–1471.

Weinreb M, Quartuccio H, Seedor JG, et al. Histomorphometrical analysis of the effects of the bisphosphonate alendronate on bone loss caused by experimental periodontitis in monkeys. *J Periodontal Res.* 1994;29:35–40.

Williams RC, Jeffcoat MK, Howell TH, et al. Altering the progression of human alveolar bone loss with the non-steroidal anti-inflammatory drug flurbiprofen. *J Periodontol.* 1989;60:485–490.

Williams RC, Jeffcoat MK, Howell TH, et al. Indomethacin or flurbiprofen treatment of periodontitis in beagles: comparison of effect on bone loss. *J Periodontal Res.* 1987;22:403–407.

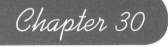

Chapter 30

Periodontal Surgical Concepts for the Dental Hygienist

Learning Objectives

- List objectives for periodontal surgery.
- Explain the term relative contraindications for periodontal surgery.
- Define the terms repair, reattachment, new attachment, and regeneration.
- Explain the difference between healing by primary intention and healing by secondary intention.

- Explain the term elevation of a flap.
- Explain two methods for classification of periodontal flaps.
- Describe two types of incisions used during periodontal flaps.
- Describe healing following flap for access and open flap debridement.
- Describe the typical outcomes for apically positioned flap with osseous surgery.
- Define the terms ostectomy and oteoplasty.
- Define the terms osteoinductive and osteoconductive.
- Explain the terms autograft, allograft, xenograft, and alloplast.
- Name two types of materials available for bone replacement grafts.
- Explain why a barrier material is used during guided tissue regeneration.
- Explain the term periodontal plastic surgery.
- List two types of crown lengthening surgery.
- List some disadvantages of gingivectomy.
- Describe the technique for a gingival curettage.
- Explain what is meant by biological enhancement of periodontal surgical outcomes.
- Name two broad categories of materials used for suturing periodontal wounds.
- Explain the term interrupted interdental suture.
- List general guidelines for suture removal.
- Describe the technique for periodontal dressing placement.
- List general guidelines for periodontal dressing management.
- Explain the important topics that should be covered in postsurgical instructions.
- List steps in a typical postsurgical visit.

Key Terms

Resective
Osseous defect
Relative contraindications
Repair
Reattachment
New attachment
Regeneration
Primary intention
Secondary intention
Periodontal flap
Elevation
Full-thickness flap
Blunt dissection
Partial-thickness flap
Sharp dissection
Nondisplaced flap
Displaced flap
Horizontal incision
Crevicular incision
Internal bevel incision
Vertical incision
Flap for access
Open flap debridement
Osseous resective surgery
Ostectomy
Osteoplasty

Apically positioned flap with osseous
  resective surgery
Bone replacement graft
Osteogenesis
Osteoconductive
Osteoinductive
Autograft
Allograft
Xenograft
Alloplast
Guided tissue regeneration
Periodontal plastic surgery
Mucogingival surgery
Free gingival graft
Subepithelial connective tissue graft
Laterally positioned flap
Coronally positioned flap
Semilunar flap
Frenectomy
Crown lengthening surgery
Functional crown lengthening
Esthetic crown lengthening
Gingivectomy
Gingivoplasty
Gingival curettage
Suture

Section 1
Introduction to Periodontal Surgery

As members of dental teams, dental hygienists must understand fundamental concepts related to periodontal surgery so that they can discuss this important topic with both patients and with other healthcare providers. In addition, hygienists play a primary role in the management of patients following periodontal surgery. A basic understanding of surgical procedures can provide the framework for improved patient care during critical stages of healing of periodontal surgical wounds. The objective of this chapter is to provide the dental hygienist with foundation information about basic concepts associated with periodontal surgery. This first chapter section begins the discussion of periodontal surgery by looking at indications and contraindications for these surgical procedures.

1. **Concepts of Periodontal Surgery**
   A. **Historical Surgical Techniques.** Various types of periodontal surgery have been recommended for dental patients with advanced periodontitis and other periodontal conditions for many years.
      1. Historically, periodontal surgery was recommended mainly to remove what was thought to be dead or infected tissue in the periodontium; thus, these early periodontal surgical procedures were mainly resective. Resective periodontal surgery refers to those procedures that simply cut away and remove damaged periodontal tissues.
      2. Some resective periodontal surgical procedures have limited use in modern periodontal care (i.e., gingivectomy as discussed in subsequent chapter sections), but many modern periodontal surgical procedures have moved away from this early concept of simply resecting tissues.
   B. **Modern Periodontal Surgical Techniques**
      1. During the past few decades, as more research data became available, an evolution of both the goals and techniques for periodontal surgery has taken place.
      2. The emphasis in periodontal surgery has shifted from the resective types of periodontal surgery to periodontal surgical procedures that attempt to rebuild or regenerate lost periodontal tissues.
      3. *Most modern periodontal surgical techniques begin by performing a periodontal flap.* Periodontal flap surgery is discussed later in this chapter.
   C. **Outcomes of Modern Periodontal Therapy**
      1. Outcomes of nonsurgical periodontal therapy are discussed in detail in Chapter 24; those outcomes primarily included readaptation of the soft tissues to the tooth root by the formation of a long junctional epithelium plus resolution of inflammation associated with periodontal pockets.
      2. Figure 30-1 illustrates three possible outcomes that may result from successful periodontal surgery: (1) formation of a long junctional epithelium (as can be seen in response to nonsurgical therapy), (2) resolution of inflammation and the associated periodontal pocket (as can be seen in response to nonsurgical therapy), and (3) regeneration (which is an expectation for some types of periodontal surgery but not expected as a result of nonsurgical therapy alone).

2. **General Indications for Periodontal Surgery.** All busy general dental practices encounter many patients that can benefit from periodontal surgery. One fundamental overreaching goal for most periodontal surgical procedures is to provide an environment in the periodontium that can be maintained in health and comfort throughout the life of the patient. In most instances as the severity of periodontitis increases, controlling the disease with nonsurgical therapy alone becomes more and more difficult, and the need for periodontal surgery as part of comprehensive patient care becomes increasingly likely. In addition, there are numerous specific

indications for periodontal surgery. Examples of indications for periodontal surgery are summarized in Box 30-1.

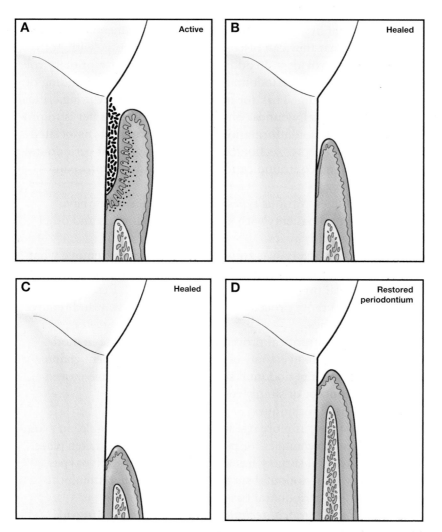

Figure 30.1. **Possible Results Following Periodontal Surgery.** A: The periodontal pocket with bacterial plaque biofilm and inflammation within the tissues prior to therapy. B: Healing in the area of the former pocket at the site by formation of a long junctional epithelium. C: Healing at the site by resolution of the inflammation in the tissues and shrinkage of the tissues. D: Healing at the site by regeneration of the periodontal tissues.

Box 30-1. Indications for Periodontal Surgery

- To provide access for improved periodontal instrumentation of root surfaces
- To reduce pocket depths
- To provide access to periodontal osseous defects
- To resect or remove tissue
- To regenerate the periodontium lost due to disease
- To graft bone or bone-stimulating materials into osseous defects
- To improve the appearance of the periodontium
- To enhance prosthetic dental care
- To allow for the placement of a dental implant

INDICATIONS AND CONTRAINDICATIONS FOR PERIODONTAL SURGERY

1. **Indications for Periodontal Surgery**
   A. **To Provide Access for Improved Periodontal Instrumentation of Root Surfaces**
      1. Periodontal surgery can provide access for more thorough periodontal instrumentation.
      2. Even though clinicians can select from a wide array of hand and ultrasonic instruments, as probing depths in the dentition increase, it becomes more and more difficult to reach root surfaces for thorough periodontal instrumentation.
      3. Periodontal surgery involving carefully planned incisions through the gingiva can allow for temporary lifting of the soft tissue off the tooth surface.
      4. More details about this type of surgery are presented under flaps for access in the following descriptions of periodontal surgery.
   B. **To Reduce Pocket Depths**
      1. As pocket depth increases, it can become too deep to control plaque biofilm effectively with standard daily self-care techniques, and plaque biofilms that thrive in the environment of the deep pocket can make it impossible to stop the progress of periodontitis.
      2. Periodontal surgical procedures can reduce the pocket depths so that a combination of daily self-care and periodic periodontal maintenance increases the chance of maintaining the periodontium in health throughout the life of the patient.
   C. **To Provide Access to Periodontal Osseous Defects**
      1. An osseous defect is a deformity in the tooth supporting alveolar bone usually resulting from periodontitis. Figure 30-2 shows an example of an osseous defect as viewed during a periodontal surgical procedure.
         a. As periodontitis advances, alveolar bone loss results in changes in the normal contour and structure of the alveolar bone.
         b. The pattern of bone loss can vary from one tooth to the next and even on different aspects of the same tooth, creating an array of osseous defects.
      2. Periodontal surgery to modify the alveolar bone level or contour is called periodontal osseous surgery.
         a. Bone defects can be managed surgically through a variety of techniques discussed later in this chapter.
         b. Information about how osseous defects can be managed using periodontal surgery is presented under the topics osseous resective surgery, apically positioned flap with osseous surgery, bone replacement graft, and guided tissue regeneration in other sections of this chapter.

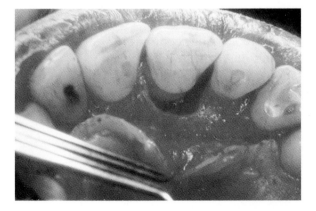

Figure 30.2. Periodontal Osseous Defect Exposed During Surgery. The soft tissues have been incised and moved away from the teeth to reveal the bone contour. Note the extensive alveolar bone loss around one of the central incisor teeth. This type of bone defect would be an ideal site for bone replacement graft discussed later in the chapter.

D. **To Resect or Remove Tissue**
   1. Enlarged gingival tissues can be unsightly and can also interfere with proper self-care; in some patients, enlarged gingiva can even interfere with comfortable mastication.
   2. Even though the focus of most periodontal surgery is not resection of tissues, this surgical approach is still used in some instances.
   3. Periodontal surgery can be used to remove and reshape enlarged gingiva; additional information on this type of periodontal surgery is found in the chapter section that discusses gingivectomy.

E. **To Regenerate the Periodontium Lost due to Disease**
   1. One of the long-range goals in periodontics is to be able to regenerate the periodontium predictably; the term regenerate implies growing back of lost cementum, lost periodontal ligament, and lost alveolar bone to reconstruct the periodontium damaged by periodontitis.
   2. Periodontal regenerative procedures can reconstruct some of the damage by periodontitis through regenerating lost bone and other tissues.
   3. Although it is not possible to regenerate the periodontium in all instances, it is possible to achieve this regeneration in many sites using some sophisticated periodontal surgical techniques; information on periodontal surgery that can be expected to regenerate the periodontium is presented under guided tissue regeneration in another section of this chapter.

F. **To Graft Bone or Bone-Stimulating Materials into Osseous Defects**
   1. Some periodontal osseous defects offer the opportunity for the periodontal surgeon to graft either bone or bone-stimulating materials into the defects.
   2. Although this surgery may seem quite similar to periodontal regeneration surgery, grafting bone does not necessarily imply regeneration of other parts of the periodontium such as cementum and periodontal ligament. More information on this interesting topic is located under bone replacement graft in another section of this chapter.

G. **To Improve the Appearance of the Periodontium**
   1. Some patients have gingival levels or gingival contours that result in an unattractive smile; periodontal surgery also includes a variety of techniques for improving the appearance of the gingiva and improving the quality of a patient's smile.
   2. There are, of course, many restorative techniques for improving the appearance of the teeth themselves, but in many patients alteration of the appearance of the gingiva must be coordinated with restorative dentistry and orthodontics to achieve a truly pleasing appearance. More information on this topic is found in the other sections of this chapter under periodontal plastic surgery and crown lengthening surgery.

H. **To Enhance Prosthetic Dental Care**
   1. Modern prosthetic dental care has created the need for a variety of periodontal surgical procedures such as altering alveolar ridge contours, lengthening tooth crowns, augmenting the amount of gingiva, or augmenting the bone in an edentulous site prior to implant placement.
   2. Modern periodontal surgery includes many procedures directed toward enhancing some aspect of restorative dentistry and enhancing prosthetic dental care. These surgical procedures may involve combinations of all types of periodontal surgery.

I. **To Allow for the Placement of a Dental Implant**
   1. Replacement of missing teeth with a dental implant is an option that must be considered when natural teeth are lost. The topic of dental implants

is discussed in Chapter 32, but is listed here as one of the indications for periodontal surgery for completeness.

2. Periodontal surgery can also be used to prepare sites for dental implants.

   a. One of the basic tenets of dental implant placement is that the implant must be surrounded by sound alveolar bone.

   b. It is not at all unusual for edentulous sites—where implants are to be placed—to be deficient in the amount of alveolar bone needed to surround the implant. Such sites require some type of bone grafting procedure prior to implant placement.

2. **Contraindications for Periodontal Surgery**

   A. **Relative Contraindications.** Most contraindications for periodontal surgery are relative contraindications.

      1. Relative contraindications are conditions that may make periodontal surgery inadvisable for some patients when the conditions or situations are severe or extreme; these same conditions may not be contraindications when the conditions are mild.

      2. An example of this concept of relative contraindications for periodontal surgery might be patients with hypertension (high blood pressure).

         a. A patient with uncontrolled severe hypertension would not be a candidate for periodontal surgery as long as the blood pressure remained severely elevated.

         b. At the same time, a patient with only mildly elevated blood pressure may be a suitable candidate for periodontal surgery.

Box 30-2. Relative Contraindications for Periodontal Surgery

- Patients who have certain systemic diseases or conditions

- Patients who are totally noncompliant with self-care

- Patients who have a high risk for dental caries

- Patients who have unrealistic expectations for surgical outcomes

---

   B. **Common Relative Contraindications.** Box 30-2 outlines a list of the more common *relative contraindications* for periodontal surgery; each of these relative contraindications is discussed briefly below.

      1. Patients who have certain systemic diseases or conditions.

         a. Systemic diseases or conditions that can be relative contraindications for periodontal surgery include conditions such as the following:

            1) Uncontrolled hypertension
            2) Recent history of myocardial infarction (heart attack)
            3) Uncontrolled diabetes
            4) Certain bleeding disorders
            5) Kidney dialysis
            6) History of radiation to the jaws
            7) HIV infection

         b. It should be noted that consultation with a patient's physician is always indicated if there is any doubt about the patient's health status or if there is any doubt about how that status might affect planned periodontal surgical intervention.

   2. Patients who are totally noncompliant with self-care.
     a. The outcomes of many types of periodontal surgery are at least in part dependent upon the level of plaque biofilm control maintained by the patient's daily efforts at self-care following the surgical procedure.
     b. Lack of compliance with self-care instructions can be a relative contraindication for some types of periodontal surgery if that lack of compliance is so poor that it precludes the possibility of acceptable periodontal surgical outcomes.
   3. Patients who have a high risk for dental caries.
     a. Some types of periodontal surgery result in exposure of portions of tooth roots. In a patient with uncontrolled dental caries where the risk for dental caries will remain quite high, it would not be wise to perform the types of periodontal surgery that increase root exposure due to the potentially devastating effect of root caries.
     b. Thus, a high risk for dental caries can be a relative contraindication for some types of periodontal surgery.
   4. Patients who have unrealistic expectations for surgical outcomes.
     a. Periodontitis damages the tissues that support the teeth, and surgical correction of that damage does not always result in a perfectly restored periodontium even when performed by the most skilled periodontal surgeon.
     b. If a patient cannot understand the nature of periodontal surgery and cannot develop realistic expectations for the outcomes of any planned periodontal surgery, it would not be wise to proceed with a plan for periodontal surgery. Thus, patient expectations can also be a relative contraindication for periodontal surgery.

TERMINOLOGY TO DESCRIBE HEALING AFTER PERIODONTAL SURGERY

Terminology used to describe healing following periodontal surgery can be quite confusing. Two sets of terminology are used in most descriptions of healing of periodontal surgical wounds. The dental hygienist needs to have an accurate understanding of both sets of terms. All periodontics textbooks present four terms that are used in describing the types of healing of the periodontium following periodontal surgery: repair, reattachment, new attachment, and regeneration. These terms are used to convey very specific concepts when describing the results of periodontal surgery.

   1. **Terminology Describing Types of Wound Healing**
     A. **Healing by *REPAIR***
       1. Repair is healing of a wound by formation of tissues that do not precisely restore the original architecture or original function of the body part.
         a. An example of healing by repair would be the formation of a scar during the healing of an accidental cut involving a finger.
         b. Certainly the healing of the finger wound is complete following formation of the scar, but the scar tissue is not precisely the same type of tissue in appearance or function that existed on that part of the finger before the cut.
       2. Repair is a perfectly natural type of healing for many wounds, including some wounds created during periodontal surgery.
         a. An example of repair in the periodontium is the healing that occurs following periodontal instrumentation (scaling and root planing).

1) The usual healing of the wound created by periodontal instrumentation results is a close readaptation of epithelium to the tooth root.

2) This readaptation of epithelium has been referred to as formation of a long junctional epithelium and has been discussed and illustrated in Chapter 24.

b. A long junctional epithelium is a perfectly legitimate type of healing, but it does not duplicate the precise periodontal tissues that were originally anatomically close to the tooth root. *With the formation of a long junctional epithelium, there is no formation of new bone, new cementum, or new periodontal ligament during the healing process.*

B. Healing by REATTACHMENT

1. Reattachment is healing of a periodontal wound by the reunion of the connective tissue and roots where these two tissues have been separated by incision or injury but *not by disease.*

2. Frequently it is necessary to move *healthy tissue* away from the tooth root or bone temporarily during some types of periodontal surgery. For example, moving the tissue may be necessary to allow access to damaged parts of the periodontium on adjacent teeth. The expected healing for this type of incision is healing by reattachment.

C. Healing by NEW ATTACHMENT

1. New attachment is a term used to describe the union of a *pathologically exposed root* with connective tissue or epithelium.

2. Healing by new attachment occurs when the epithelium and connective tissues are newly attached to a tooth root *where periodontitis had previously destroyed this attachment* (i.e., where attachment loss has occurred).

3. New attachment differs from reattachment because new attachment only occurs in an area formerly *damaged by disease*, whereas reattachment occurs when tissues are separated in the *absence of disease* (frequently as a result of the surgical procedure).

4. Figure 30-3 illustrates the specific area on a tooth that must have newly attached epithelium and connective tissue for the healing to be called new attachment.

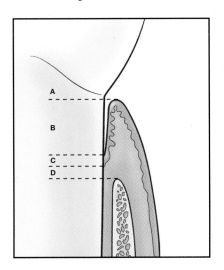

Figure 30.3. Area of the Tooth Root Involved in New Attachment. This drawing shows a site on a tooth where attachment loss has occurred. **A:** Enamel surface. **B:** Area of attachment loss. **C:** Junctional epithelium. **D:** Connective tissue attachment. To be qualified as new attachment the tissues must be attached to the tooth surface in the area labeled **B** in this drawing.

D. Healing by REGENERATION

1. Regeneration is the biologic process by which the architecture and function of lost tissue is *completely* restored.

2. Healing by regeneration results in the regrowth of the precise tissues that were present before the disease or damage occurred.

3. For healing of the periodontium to be described as regeneration, the healing would have to result in the reformation of lost cementum, lost PDL, and lost alveolar bone.

4. Regeneration of the periodontium is indeed possible with modern periodontal surgical procedures, but unfortunately the periodontium *cannot be regenerated predictably* in all sites with current periodontal surgical techniques.

2. **Terminology Describing the Degree of Wound Closure.** A second set of terms has also been used to describe events following periodontal surgery. These terms describe the degree of wound closure (i.e., how the margins or edges of the surgical wound relate to each other following the surgery but prior to the healing). These terms include healing by primary intention, healing by secondary intention, and healing by tertiary intention.

A. **Healing by Primary Intention**

1. Healing by primary intention occurs when the wound margins or edges are closely adapted to each other.

2. An example of primary intention healing would be seen in a small wound in a finger that required stitches. To adapt the margins of the wound closely, a physician places stitches.

3. Healing by primary intention is usually faster than the other types of healing, but it is not always possible to create wounds where the wound margins are closely adapted when performing periodontal surgery.

4. It should be noted that healing by primary intention in the periodontium may pose challenges for the healing that differ from healing by primary intention in other sites in the body—such as, healing of a cut finger.

    a. One edge of a surgical wound in the periodontium may be a tooth root that is, of course, avascular and cannot contribute any living cells to the wound healing process.

    b. This would differ from healing by primary intention for a wound such as a cut finger, because both edges of the wound in finger would be able to contribute living cells to the healing process.

B. **Healing by Secondary Intention**

1. Healing by secondary intention takes place when the margins or edges of the wound are not closely adapted (i.e., the two wound edges are not in close contact with each other).

2. When healing by secondary intention takes place, granulation tissue must form to close the space between the wound margins prior to growth of epithelial cells over the surface of the wound.

3. Healing by secondary intention is generally slower than healing by primary intention, since more vascular and cellular events are required in this type of healing.

4. Ideally all wounds created during periodontal surgery wound be wounds that would be expected to heal by primary intention, but in reality many of the wounds created during this type of surgery involve some wound healing by secondary intention.

C. **Healing by Tertiary Intention**

1. An example of healing by tertiary intention would be healing of a wound that is temporarily left open with the specific intent of surgically closing that wound at a later date.

2. Healing by tertiary intention is not normally a type of healing that applies to healing of periodontal surgical procedures, and is mentioned here only for completeness.

Section 2
Understanding the Periodontal Flap

The periodontal flap is an important step in most periodontal surgical procedures. As periodontitis progresses, it damages the attachment of the connective tissue to tooth roots and it destroys supporting alveolar bone. Treating patients with periodontitis and repairing damage done to the underlying periodontium requires gaining access both to tooth roots and to alveolar bone. As attachment loss associated with periodontitis progresses, access to tooth roots with conventional nonsurgical periodontal therapy becomes difficult if not impossible. Elevating a periodontal flap is the mechanism for gaining access to the underlying periodontal structures and to the tooth roots affected by the disease; any overview of periodontal surgery requires some understanding of the principles involved in performing a periodontal flap. This chapter section discusses the techniques and the associated terminology related to performing the many variations of a periodontal flap.

1. **Introduction to Periodontal Flaps**
   A. **Description of Procedure**
      1. A periodontal flap is a surgical procedure in which incisions are made in the gingiva or mucosa to allow for separation of the surface tissues (epithelium and connective tissue) from the underlying tooth roots and underlying alveolar bone.
      2. Separating the surface tissues from the underlying tooth root and alveolar bone is commonly referred to as elevation or raising of the flap; the term elevation is used to convey the concept of lifting the surface tissues away from the tooth roots and away from the alveolar bone.
      3. Once the surface gingiva or mucosa is elevated off the underlying roots and bone, it can be replaced at its original position or it can be displaced to different locations that will be discussed in upcoming sections under some of the specific types of surgery.
      4. Figure 30-4 shows a series of drawings that illustrate a typical periodontal flap surgical procedure used to gain access to the underlying tooth roots and alveolar bone.

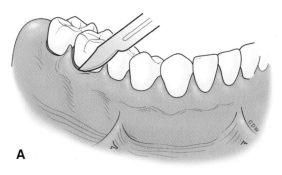

A

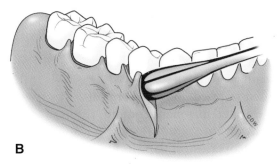

B

Figure 30.4. Drawings Illustrating a Typical Periodontal Flap Surgical Procedure Used to Gain Access to Underlying Tooth Roots and Alveolar Bone. A: Making an incision to allow for separation the soft tissue from the roots and alveolar bone. **B:** Elevating (or lifting) the soft tissue flap from the roots of the teeth and alveolar bone.

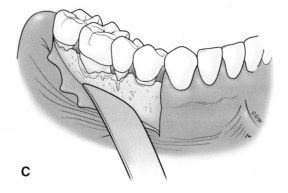

C: Improved visualization of both the tooth roots and alveolar bone contours with the flap elevated.

C

B. **Indications for a Periodontal Flap**
   1. Most modern periodontal surgical procedures require performing periodontal flaps as a part of the procedure.
   2. Basically the flap elevation is done to provide access for some treatment either to tooth roots or to the alveolar bone, or to both of these structures.
      a. Periodontal flaps can be elevated simply to provide access to tooth root surfaces for completion of meticulous periodontal instrumentation (scaling and root planing) that was begun as a part of nonsurgical periodontal therapy. Use of a periodontal flap for improved access to tooth roots is discussed in more detail later in this chapter under the heading flaps for access.
      b. Periodontal flaps may also be used to provide access to reshape or treat alveolar bone defects resulting from periodontitis. In the following sections of this chapter, the topic of apically positioned flaps with osseous resective surgery provides an example of this type of procedure.
2. **Classification of Periodontal Flaps**
   A. **Degree of Bone Exposure.** One method of classification of periodontal flaps is to describe the flap based upon the degree of exposure of bone following flap elevation. Using this method of classification flaps would be described as being either full-thickness or partial-thickness.
   1. A full-thickness flap, or mucoperiosteal flap as it is also called, includes elevation of entire thickness of the soft tissue (including epithelium, connective tissue, and periosteum). The periosteum is a dense membrane composed of fibrous connective tissue that closely wraps the outer surface of the alveolar bone.
      a. The full-thickness flap provides the complete access to underlying bone that might be needed when bone replacement grafting or periodontal regeneration procedures are anticipated.
      b. The full-thickness flap is elevated with what is generally referred to as a blunt dissection.
         1) Blunt dissection means that the tools used to elevate the flap are not sharpened on the edge (i.e., blunted or slightly rounded); blunt dissection minimizes the chance of accidental damage to the flap.
         2) In this type of flap elevation the flap is lifted or pried up using surgical tools called periosteal elevators, and it is elevated in a manner quite similar to lifting the peeling off an orange.
         3) Figure 30-5 illustrates a full-thickness or mucoperiosteal flap elevated during a periodontal surgical procedure.

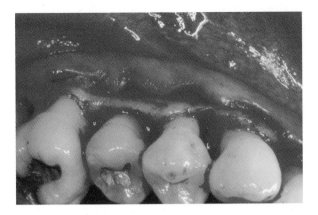

Figure 30.5. Full-Thickness or Mucoperiosteal Flap. This photo taken during a typical periodontal flap surgery shows a full-thickness or mucoperiosteal flap (i.e., a flap of soft tissue that includes epithelium, underlying connective tissue, and the periosteum elevated off the teeth and alveolar bone). Note the exposure of the underlying alveolar bone margin and osseous defects associated with that bone interdentally.

  2. A partial-thickness flap, or split-thickness flap as it is also called, includes elevation of only the epithelium and a thin layer of the underlying connective tissue rather than the entire thickness of the underlying soft tissues.
     a. The partial-thickness flap is elevated with sharp dissection; sharp dissection requires incising the underlying connective tissue in such a manner as to separate the epithelial surface plus a small portion of the connective tissue from the periosteum. Use of this technique would leave the periosteal tissues covering the bone.
     b. To perform the sharp dissection needed in a partial-thickness flap a surgeon must limit this approach to areas of gingiva that are thick; careful inspection of gingiva will reveal that gingiva is quite thin in some patients but relatively thick in others.
     c. Research data indicates that when alveolar bone is exposed during a flap procedure there is a potential loss of a very small surface layer of the bone following the procedure, and this can make using a full-thickness flap inadvisable in certain instances.
B. **Location of the Soft Tissue Margin.** Another method of classifying periodontal flaps is to describe flaps based upon the location of the margin of the soft tissue when it is sutured back in place. Using this method of classification, flaps would be described as being either nondisplaced or displaced.
  1. A nondisplaced flap is a flap that is sutured with the margin of the flap at its original position in relationship to the CEJ on the tooth.
  2. A displaced flap is a flap that is sutured with the margin of the flap placed at a position other than its original position in relationship to the CEJ of the tooth. A displaced flap can be positioned either apically, coronally, or laterally in relationship to its original position.
     a. For a displaced flap to be moved to a new position (such as coronally or laterally), the surgeon must perform the flap elevation in such a manner that the base of the flap extends into the moveable mucosal tissues.
     b. Displaced flaps are generally not possible to perform on the palatal surface of the teeth because of the absence of movable mucosa in this anatomical location.
C. **Common Terminology.** Box 30-3 provides an overview of common terminology used to classify periodontal flaps.

Box 30-3. Classification of Periodontal Flaps

1. Based upon Bone Exposure
  • Full-thickness flap
  • Partial-thickness flap
 	
2. Based on Location of Flap Margin
  • Nondisplaced flap
  • Displaced flap

Box 30-4. Types of Incisions Utilized During Periodontal Flaps

1. Horzontal Incisions
  • Crevicular Incisions
  • Internal Bevel Incisions
 	
2. Vertical Incisions
  • Vertical Releasing Incision

3. **Types of Incisions Used During Periodontal Flap Surgeries.** Most of the incisions made prior to elevation of a periodontal flap are made with surgical scalpel blades, but there are a variety of special periodontal knives that can be used to perform some of these incisions. Several basic types of incisions are utilized during periodontal flap surgery. Some familiarization with terminology related to flap incisions could be useful to the dental hygienist in understanding specific types of periodontal surgery. These incisions can be broadly classified as either horizontal or vertical incisions. Box 30-4 provides an overview of the types of incisions utilized during periodontal flaps.

  A. **Horizontal Incisions.** Horizontal incisions run parallel to the gingival margins in a mesio-distal direction.

    1. One type of horizontal incision commonly employed during flap surgery is the crevicular incision or sulcular incision as it is sometimes called.

    2. In the crevicular incision the surgical scalpel is simply placed into the gingival crevice or sulcus and the tissues are incised apically to bone.

    3. A second type of horizontal incision is the internal bevel incision.

    4. In an internal bevel incision the surgical scalpel enters the marginal gingiva, but is not placed directly into the crevice or sulcus; the scalpel blade enters the gingival margin approximately 0.5- to 1.0-mm away from the margin and follows the general contour of the scalloped marginal gingiva.

    5. Using an internal bevel incision results in leaving a small collar of soft tissue around the tooth root (including the lining of the preexisting periodontal pocket) that is later removed during most periodontal flap procedures.

    6. Terminology related to these incisions can be quite confusing.

      a. The internal bevel incision has also been referred to as a "reverse bevel incision" or the "initial incision" since it is usually made as a first step during a routine periodontal flap procedure.

      b. The sulcular incision has also be referred to as the "second incision," since it is usually made as the second step during a routine flap procedure.

  B. **Vertical Incisions.** Vertical incisions run perpendicular to the gingival margin in an apico-occlusal direction.

    1. Vertical incisions are primarily used to allow elevation of the flap during the surgical procedure without stretching or damaging the soft tissues during flap elevation.

    2. The primary type of vertical incisions have also been referred to as vertical releasing incisions, since once this type of incision passes the mucogingival junction, the flap is "released" or has possibilities for movement in relationship to the underlying bone and adjacent soft tissues.

Section 3
Descriptions of Common Types of Periodontal Surgery

1. **Flap for Access**
   A. **Procedure Description**
      1. Flap for access (or modified Widman flap surgery) is used to provide access to the tooth roots for improved root preparation. In this surgical procedure the gingival tissue is incised and temporarily elevated (lifted away) from the tooth roots.
      2. There are two main advantages of flap for access.
         a. Flap for access surgery provides excellent access to the tooth roots for thorough instrumentation in sites where deep pocket depths hindered periodontal instrumentation during nonsurgical therapy.
         b. Flap for access surgery also provides an intimate adaptation of healthy connective tissues to the debrided tooth roots following suturing of the wound to allow for healing by primary intention.
      3. The tissues are elevated only enough to allow good access for periodontal instrumentation of the tooth roots. Following root treatment, the gingival tissue is replaced at its original position (i.e., a nondisplaced flap) and stabilized with sutures.
   B. **Steps in a Typical Flap for Access.** The usual steps followed during flap for access surgery are outlined below.
      1. An internal bevel incision is begun through the surface of the gingiva surrounding the teeth; the incision is made approximately 0.5 to 1.0 mm away from the gingival margin and follows the scallop of the marginal gingiva.
      2. The internal bevel incision that was begun as the first incision through the surface gingiva is retraced and extended apically all the way to the alveolar bone.
      3. The flap is elevated far enough to provide good access to the tooth roots.
      4. A crevicular incision or sulcular incision is then made from the base of the pocket to the bone to facilitate removal of the small collar of tissue remaining around the necks of the teeth.
      5. If needed, an incision may be made at the base of remaining tissue collar to completely free this tissue, and the tissue collar is removed.
      6. With the flap elevated tooth roots are instrumented to remove remaining plaque biofilm, calculus deposits, root contaminants, and root irregularities. While performing the debridement, residual periodontal ligament fibers adhering to the tooth root near the base of the pocket are left undisturbed. Figure 30-6 shows a flap for access with the flap elevated and partial removal of collar of tissue.

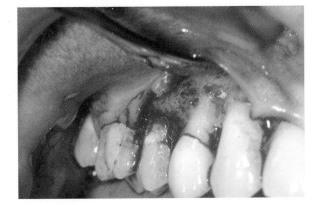

Figure 30.6. Flap for Access in Progress. This photo was taken during a flap for access. In the photo the flap has been incised and elevated. Partial removal of the collar of tissue has been performed.

7. The flaps may be thinned if needed to allow for intimate adaptation of the gingiva to the necks of the teeth; alveolar bone contour is not altered unless minor recontouring is needed to allow for proper adaptation of the flap.

8. The flap is repositioned and sutured at its original position (nondisplaced); special effort is made to insure that the tips of the facial and lingual papillae are in actual contact to promote healing by primary intention at this critical interdental site.

C. Healing After Flap for Access

1. The type of healing expected from flap for access surgery is *healing by repair* and usually involves formation of a *long junctional epithelium*.

2. Research shows that flap for access surgery can result in a stable dentogingival unit that can be maintained in health with periodic periodontal maintenance by the dental team and proper self-care by the patient.

D. Special Considerations for the Dental Hygienist

1. During routine nonsurgical periodontal instrumentation, it may not be possible to perform thorough calculus removal if the pocket depths are deeper than 6 mm. Flap for access surgery provides greatly improved access to root surfaces in areas of deeper pockets where the results of conventional nonsurgical periodontal instrumentation alone would be limited.

2. Even in patients where flap for access surgery is part of the treatment plan, every effort should be made to minimize the inflammation associated with chronic periodontitis by performing complete nonsurgical therapy prior to the surgical intervention.

   a. The dental hygienist plays a critical role in promoting patient understanding of how nonsurgical and surgical treatment are related—first, nonsurgical therapy followed by surgical therapy if needed.

   b. Thorough and meticulous nonsurgical therapy even in areas of deep pockets can reduce the extent of any planned periodontal surgical treatment, and is always an important part of patient care.

2. Open Flap Debridement

A. Procedure Description

1. **Open flap debridement** is a term that describes a periodontal surgical procedure quite similar in concept and execution to flap for access surgery. In the periodontal literature another term has been used interchangeably with open flap debridement is flap curettage.

2. Historically the term open flap debridement was used to describe some of the original flap procedures that were first developed by periodontal surgeons many years ago.

3. Today open flap debridement (or flap curettage) is usually performed with steps quite similar to flap for access with the following exceptions:

   a. Exception no. 1. Open flap debridement usually includes more extensive flap elevation than flap for access—providing access not only to the tooth roots but also to all of the alveolar bone defects. Remember that during flap for access surgery the flap is elevated only far enough to provide good access to the tooth roots.

   b. Exception no. 2. Whereas flap for access includes a nondisplaced flap, open flap debridement may include displacing the flap margin to a new location (i.e., during an open flap debridement the flap margin may be sutured in a position more apical to its original position).

B. **Steps in Typical Open Flap Debridement**
   1. The procedure begins with horizontal incisions that can be either crevicular or internal bevel incisions; vertical releasing incisions can be included as needed to allow for atraumatic flap elevation.
   2. Full-thickness (mucoperiosteal) flaps are elevated to provide access both to tooth roots and to the underlying alveolar bone defects.
   3. Granulation tissue is removed from existing osseous defects and from interdental areas.
   4. Tooth roots are instrumented to remove remaining plaque biofilm, calculus deposits, root contaminants, and root irregularities.
   5. Osteoplasty, which is not normally included in open flap debridement, is performed only if it is needed to allow for readaptation of the tissues to the tooth roots.
   6. Flaps are sutured either at their original level (nondisplaced) or at a level more apical to their original position (displaced).
   7. Figure 30-7 illustrates critical steps in a typical open flap debridement.

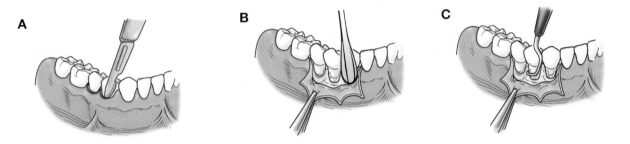

Figure 30.7. **Critical Steps During a Typical Open Flap Debridement.** A: Incisions being made to bone from within the crevice or pocket base. B: Flap elevation to expose tooth roots and alveolar bone. C: Periodontal instrumentation of the roots of the teeth.

C. **Healing Expected After Open Flap Debridement**
   1. Healing from open flap debridement is typically resolution of much of the existing inflammation within the periodontal tissues.
   2. The formation of a long junctional epithelium can occur along with slight remodeling of some of the osseous bone defects caused by periodontitis.
   3. Typically little if any bone regrowth occurs following open flap debridement.
   4. It is common for residual periodontal pockets to remain in some sites following this procedure—thus, complicating both patient self-care and professional periodontal maintenance.

3. **Osseous Resective Surgery.** The word "osseous" is defined as "having to do with bone." Thus, periodontal osseous surgery is surgery involving the alveolar bone.
   A. **Description of Procedure**
      1. Periodontal osseous resective surgery or periodontal osseous surgery is a term used to describe periodontal surgery employed to correct many of the strange deformities of the alveolar bone that often result from advancing periodontitis.
      2. The fundamental goal for this type of periodontal surgery is to eliminate periodontal pockets, and this goal can be achieved when osseous surgery is combined with an apically displaced flap as discussed in the next section.
   B. **Rationale for Periodontal Osseous Surgery**
      1. Gingiva has a tendency to follow its natural architecture with or without the support of underlying alveolar bone; the natural architecture of gingiva

includes a scalloped contour where the gingiva over the facial and lingual surfaces of teeth is apical to the level of the interdental papillae.

2. As periodontitis progresses, the contours of alveolar bone are altered by the formation of osseous defects referred to with names such as osseous craters, one-walled, two-walled, and three-walled osseous defects which have been discussed in other chapters of this textbook. In areas where these osseous defects form, attachment loss accompanies the alveolar bone contour changes and periodontal pockets form.

3. Osseous surgery attempts to reestablish alveolar bone contours that mimic the predictable eventual contours of the gingiva following healing from periodontal surgery. Thus periodontal osseous surgery can be used to minimize the discrepancy between the bone contour and the gingival contour to eliminate periodontal pockets following complete healing.

4. Periodontal osseous resective surgery is commonly performed in patients with moderate periodontitis where the bone defects created by the periodontitis are primarily osseous craters; as discussed in other chapters of this book, osseous craters are the most common type of periodontal osseous defect in periodontitis patients.

C. **Special Terminology Associated with Osseous Surgery—Ostectomy and Osteoplasty.** Osseous surgery is frequently employed in the treatment of patients with moderate periodontitis, and this topic is discussed in detail in all periodontal textbooks. Two terms frequently arise during discussions of osseous surgery (ostectomy and osteoplasty), and these terms can be a bit confusing.

1. One of these terms is ostectomy. Ostectomy or osteoectomy refers to the removal of alveolar bone that is actually attached to the tooth (i.e., it is still providing some support for the tooth).

   a. Ostectomy results in the immediate loss of a small amount of attachment at certain sites, and for that reason ostectomy must be used with appropriate caution by the surgeon.

   b. In spite of the slight attachment loss that occurs during ostectomy, this is an excellent method of eliminating periodontal pockets associated with certain commonly occurring osseous defects such as osseous craters. The removal of small amounts of supporting bone is justified by the attainment of alveolar bone contours that are compatible with the natural contours of the gingiva.

   c. Figure 30-8 illustrates technique for ostectomy that might be performed during periodontal osseous resective surgery.

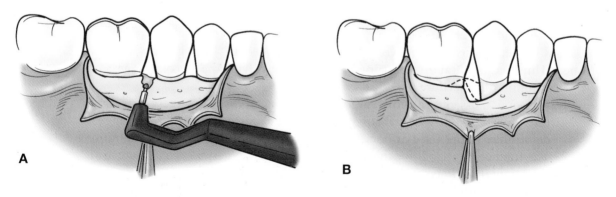

A   **B**

Figure 30.8. Ostecomy Technique. A: Following exposure of the interdental osseous crater, one of the crater walls (facial wall in this illustration) is being removed with a special surgical bur. B: Based upon the newly established bone level at the site, the surrounding bone is contoured in an attempt to reestablish a more natural bone contour.

2. The second of these terms is osteoplasty. Osteoplasty refers to reshaping the surface of alveolar bone without actually removing any of the supporting bone.

3. In reality, most periodontal osseous resective surgery involves both ostectomy and osteoplasty, and when performed with precision, these procedures can result in alveolar bone contours that mimic the contours of the gingiva following complete healing.

4. Box 30-5 outlines the special terminology associated with periodontal osseous surgery.

Box 30-5. Special Terminology Associated with Periodontal Osseous Surgery

- Ostectomy–removal of some tooth-supporting bone
- Osteoplasty–reshaping of the surface bone contours

  D. **Steps in Periodontal Osseous Resective Surgery**
1. Incisions are made and flaps are elevated to provide access to the osseous defects and to the surrounding alveolar bone; these incisions typically are done on both the facial and lingual surfaces of the teeth and typically include both horizontal and vertical releasing incisions.
2. Granulation tissue associated with the osseous defects is thoroughly debrided to allow full visualization to the extent and shape of the osseous defects.
3. All remaining soft tissue tags in the surgical site are identified and removed usually using a combination of hand and ultrasonic instrumentation.
4. Tooth root surfaces are debrided to remove all plaque biofilm, calculus, root contaminants, and root irregularities.
5. Osteoplasty is performed to remove thick bone ledges where they exist on the facial and lingual surfaces of the alveolar bone.
6. Ostectomy is performed to eliminate interproximal osseous defects.
7. Bone contours are refined with hand instruments and surgical burs.
8. The gingiva is sutured into place (usually at a more apical position than the original level as discussed in the next section).

  E. **Healing After Periodontal Osseous Resective Surgery**
1. When periodontal osseous resective surgery is performed in areas of the dentition where osseous craters exist, it is normally possible for the surgeon to recreate a natural contour to the alveolar bone.
2. When this osseous resective surgery is combined with the apically positioned flap as discussed in the next section of this chapter, it is frequently possible to reestablish a normal crevice or sulcus depth without the presence of residual periodontal pockets following the surgery.
3. For most patients with moderate periodontitis once periodontal pockets are eliminated using this type of surgery, with reasonable self-care by the patient and with periodic periodontal maintenance by the dental team it is possible to maintain the dentition in health.

4. **Apically Positioned Flap with Osseous Resective Surgery**
  A. **Procedure Description**
1. An apically positioned flap with osseous resective surgery is a periodontal surgical procedure involving a combination of a displaced flap (displaced in an apical direction) plus resective osseous surgery.

    a. As already discussed, correction of altered alveolar bone contours to mimic the contours of healthy alveolar bone is usually referred to as periodontal osseous resective surgery.

    b. Following contouring of the alveolar bone, the flap in this procedure is sutured at a position that is more apical to its original position in relationship to the tooth CEJs (apically positioned or apically displaced flap).

  2. This periodontal surgical procedure is ideal for minimizing periodontal pocket depths in patients with osseous craters caused by moderate periodontitis.

    a. An apically displaced flap can result in a gingival margin that is apical to the CEJ of the tooth. This new position of the gingival margin means that more of the root of the tooth is visible in the mouth.

    b. The reduced pocket depth can facilitate both self-care by the patient and periodontal maintenance by the dental team.

B. Steps in an Apically Positioned Flap with Osseous Resective Surgery

  1. This procedure normally begins with an internal bevel incision. The internal bevel incision can preserve the width of keratinized tissue that is important to the overall procedure, because this width of keratinized tissue will be displaced apically as a final step.

  2. The internal bevel incision is followed by flap elevation and crevicular incision prior to removal of the collar of tissues around the necks of the teeth.

  3. Vertical releasing incisions are made as needed to avoid damage to the flap.

  4. Granulation tissues are debrided, and osseous defects are exposed as discussed in the previous section.

  5. Periodontal osseous resective surgery is performed to mimic the contours of healthy alveolar bone; this osseous surgery normally includes both ostectomy and osteoplasty.

  6. The flap is sutured at a position apical to its original position (usually near the tooth–bone junction).

  7. The surgical site is covered with periodontal dressing to stabilize the flap at its apical location.

  8. Figure 30-9 illustrates the critical steps in an apically positioned flap with osseous resective surgery.

C. Healing of an Apically Positioned Flap with Osseous Resective Surgery

  1. Final healing of this type of surgery results in a normal attachment (both junctional epithelium and connective tissue attachment) at a position more apical on the tooth root.

  2. It should be emphasized that apically positioned flap with osseous resection cannot eliminate all periodontal osseous defects, especially where the defects are quite severe.

  3. Research has shown that an apically positioned flap combined with periodontal osseous surgery can result in a stable dentogingival junction that can be maintained in health with reasonable self-care by the patient and periodic periodontal maintenance by the dental team.

  4. Figure 30-10 illustrates the results of a healed apically positioned flap used to treat a furcation involvement on a molar tooth.

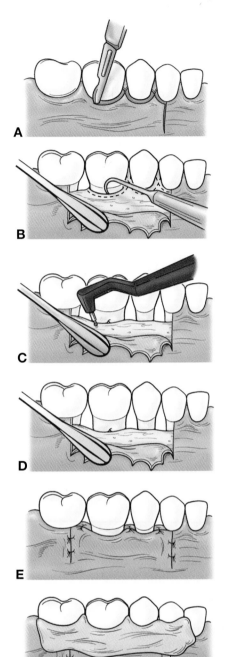

Figure 30.9. **Critical Steps in an Apically Positioned Flap with Osseous Resective Surgery. A:** Internal bevel incision and vertical releasing incision being made around the teeth. **B:** Removal of the collar of soft tissue following flap elevation. **C:** Ostectomy being performed after identification of osseous defects. **D:** Inspection of the final bone contours after ostectomy and osteoplasty. **E:** Suturing of both the flap margins and the vertical releasing incisions. Note that the level of the flap margin is displaced in an apical position compared to its original position. **F:** Placement of periodontal dressing to stabilize the flap at its new position during the early phase of healing.

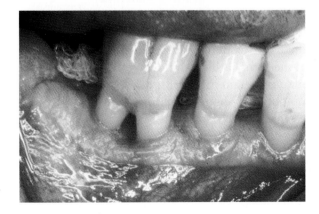

Figure 30.10. **Results of an Apically Positioned Flap.** This apically positioned flap was performed to treat a large furcation involvement on the molar tooth. Note that in this case the healed gingival margin leaves the tooth CEJ coronal to the gingival margin.

D. **Special Considerations for the Dental Hygienist**
1. During surgery to minimize periodontal pockets, it is common for the gingival margin to be positioned at a more apical level to the CEJ than it is originally occupied.
   a. This apical positioning results in exposure of a portion of the root to the oral cavity.
   b. Visiblilty of a portion of the root may be an esthetic concern for the patient.
   c. In patients with a high caries risk, exposure of root surface in the oral cavity can lead to root caries. Therefore, this type of surgery may be contraindicated in patients with a high risk for dental caries.
2. Temporary dentinal hypersensitivity is a frequent patient postsurgical complaint following this type of surgery. As discussed in other chapters, dentinal hypersensitivity usually diminishes over time if the patient maintains good plaque biofilm control.
3. Before surgery, the members of the dental team should inform the patient about anticipated changes in appearance and about the potential for dentinal hypersensitivity. The dental hygienist should also assure the patient that if sensitivity does occur, measures could be taken to minimize the sensitivity.

5. **Bone Replacement Grafts**
   A. **Procedure description**
   1. Bone replacement graft is a surgical procedure used to encourage the body to rebuild alveolar bone that has been lost usually as a result of periodontal disease.
   2. Bone grafting has been commonplace in medicine for many years, but grafting bone replacement materials into the periodontium offers some unique challenges different from bone grafting in medicine.
      a. Bone grafts placed into periodontal defects are subject to constant contamination from bacteria and saliva traveling along existing tooth roots adjacent to the graft site; this constant potential for contamination from bacteria would not be the case in many bone grafts in medicine (such as a bone graft done during a hip replacement).
      b. In addition, the healing of bone grafts in periodontal defects can be disrupted by the growth of epithelium into the wound that can lead to graft failure; this potential disruption by the growth of epithelium would also not be the case in most medical bone grafts.
   B. **Terminology Associated with Bone Replacement Grafts**
   1. Osteogenesis is the term that is used to describe the potential for new bone cells and new bone to form following bone grafting. Bone replacement graft materials frequently are referred to based on their osteogenic potential.
      a. Some grafting materials have been described as osteoconductive. Osteoconductive grafting materials are grafts where the grafting materials form a framework for bone cells existing outside the graft to use to penetrate the graft during the formation of the new bone.
      b. Other grafting materials have been described as osteoinductive. Osteoinductive grafting materials are grafts where the actual cells within the grafting material are converted into bone forming cells, and these cells then form the new bone (i.e., when the material can induce new bone formation).
   2. The ideal bone replacement graft material would be one that is osteoinductive and one that has a high osteogenic potential.
   C. **Broad Categories of Materials Used for Bone Replacement Grafting.** Many potential grafting materials have been studied in relationship to their osteogenic potential. In general these grafting materials can be described as falling into one

of four broad categories: autografts, allografts, xenografts, and alloplasts. These four categories of bone graft material have widely varying osteogenic potentials.

1. Autografts are bone replacement materials taken from the patient that is receiving the graft. Periodontal autografts can be taken from sites in the patient's own jaws or occasionally from other areas of the patient's body.

2. Allografts are bone replacement grafts taken from individuals that are genetically dissimilar to the donor (i.e., another human). Of course when allografts are used, these grafting materials must be modified to eliminate the potential for rejection.

3. Xenografts are bone replacement grafts taken from another species, such as bovine bone replacement graft material which can be placed in a human. Again, these materials must be modified to eliminate the potential for rejection.

4. Alloplasts are bone replacement grafts that are synthetic materials or inert foreign materials.

5. Autografts have the highest osteogenic potential, and alloplasts have the least osteogenic potential with osteogenic potential for allografts and xenografts between those two extremes.

6. Though autografts have the most osteogenic potential, it is not always possible to obtain enough autogenous bone from a patient to fill all of the osseous defects that need grafting. This creates the need during many periodontal surgical procedures for a bone graft material from a source other than the patient being treated.

7. In some instances these grafting materials can be used in combinations such as mixing autogenous bone with an allograft material to obtain the needed volume of grafting material for a particular grafting site.

8. Box 30-6 provides an overview of materials used for bone replacement grafts.

Box 30-6. Materials Used for Bone Replacement Grafts

- Autograft—bone taken from patient's own body
- Allograft—bone taken from another human
- Xenograft—bone taken from another species
- Alloplast—synthetic bone-like material

D. **Examples of Specific Materials Used for Bone Replacement Grafting.** Numerous materials have been studied for possible use for bone replacement grafting over the past several decades. None of the materials is ideal, but many of them have been shown to have some osteogenic potential. The discussion below describes some examples of the types of bone replacement graft materials that have been studied.

1. Autogenous bone grafts from intraoral sites
   a. As already discussed, autografts are graft materials taken from the patient's own body.
   b. Autografts from intraoral sites have been used in periodontics for many years, and currently these autogenous grafts are considered the gold standard when comparing other grafting materials for their osteogenic potential.

   c. It should not be surprising that autogenous bone is the most effective grafting material, since it already contains living bone cells and viable bone growth factors from the patient—in contrast to some of the other grafting materials such as alloplasts which are usually manufactured materials.

   d. Intraoral sources for the autograft material can be from sites such as from bone removed during ostectomy or osteoplasty, from exostoses removed during surgery, from bone removed from edentulous ridges, from bone taken from healing extraction sites, from bone taken from the chin, and from bone harvested from the jaws distal to the teeth in a dental arch.

   e. A variety of techniques for harvesting the graft material and insuring its osteogenic potential have been advocated. These techniques usually include exposing the alveolar bone by elevating a periodontal flap, removing granulation tissue associated with an osseous defect, treating the tooth root adjacent to the defect, placing the graft material into the defect, and closing the flap by suturing it at its original level on the teeth.

   f. In addition to harvesting particles or larger pieces of bone, autogenous bone grafts include the use of materials such as osseous coagulum. Osseous coagulum is a mixture of bone dust and blood taken from the patient made by removing small particles of cortical bone and mixing it with blood from the surgical site.

   g. One technique for collecting autogenous graft material from a patient during a periodontal surgical procedure involves the bone blend technique. This technique involves collecting bone in a plastic capsule and pestle and triturating the material into a workable mass of bone blend that can be grafted into osseous defects.

   h. Though small particles or pieces of cortical bone are usually selected as autogenous grafting material, cancellous bone marrow may also be used. One common intraoral site to harvest bone marrow is from a maxillary tuberosity.

   i. One disadvantage to using autogenous bone grafts is that when they are used, they frequently require a second surgical site for harvesting the graft material, increasing the potential for postsurgical problems.

2. Autogenous bone from extraoral sites

   a. Iliac (or hip) cancellous marrow has been studied as an autogenous bone replacement graft material.

   b. When used in periodontal defects this material does result in bone formation in osseous defects. Today marrow from the hip is rarely used for autogenous grafting into periodontal defects, however, because of the potential for root resorption adjacent to the grafting site, the potential for postoperative problems associated with the donor site, and the difficulty in obtaining this type of donor material.

3. Freeze-dried bone allografts. Bone allografts (taken from another human and processed) are attractive surgical options as bone replacement graft materials. There has been a lot of interest in periodontics in identifying an ideal bone allograft. If the ideal bone allograft could be identified for use in periodontal patients, there would be no need for a second surgical site to obtain an autogenous graft. In addition if the ideal bone allograft could be identified, there would be no worry about limitation of the availability of the amount of graft material needed.

   a. As already discussed, allografts are graft materials taken from another individual of the same species (i.e., another human who is recently deceased).

   b. Freeze-dried bone allografts (both calcified and decalcified) have been used successfully as bone replacement allografts, and bone allograft products have been available commercially for some time.
      1) Bone allograft materials are obtained from the cortical bone of a donor within a few hours of death, defatted, washed in alcohol, and frozen.
      2) The graft material is then demineralized, ground into particles, and stored in sterile vials until used in a clinical setting.
   c. Since allografts are materials that are foreign to the body of the patient receiving the graft and since potential deceased donors may have diseases that could be transmitted to the patient being treated, steps must be taken to maximize the safety of this type of grafting material. These steps usually include
      1) Excluding potential donors that are members of disease high-risk groups,
      2) Testing of cadaver tissues to exclude donors with infection or malignant disease, and
      3) Treating the allograft with chemical agents or with other techniques to inactivate viruses.
   d. Whereas the risk of disease transmission using allograft materials is not zero, the risk of viral transmission by the use of allograft bone replacement material has been described as highly remote.
   e. Allograft products for use in periodontal defects are available in two types based on how they are processed: Freeze-dried bone allographs and decalcified freeze-dried bone allografts.
      1) Freeze-dried bone allografts (FDBA)
         a) Freeze-dried bone allografts or FDBA is an osteoconductive allograft graft material that has been reported to result in some bone fill.
         b) Bone fill from FDBA can be improved if the material is mixed with some autogenous bone at the time of placement.
      2) Decalcified freeze-dried bone allografts (DFDBA)
         a) Decalcified freeze-dried bone allografts or DFDBA is an osteoinductive graft material that has a higher osteogenic potential than FDBA, and DFDBA is preferred by many clinicians.
         b) The osteogenic potential for DFDBA has been shown to vary depending upon several factors such as the extent of demineralization as well as other factors.

4. Bovine-derived bone
   a. Bovine-derived bone is an example of a xenograft material; xenografts are materials taken from another species.
   b. Xenografts such as bovine-derived bone have also been used as bone replacement grafts in periodontal defects.
   c. An anorganic bovine bone has been tested and marketed, and studies have shown successful regrowth of some bone with this material.
      1) Anorganic bovine bone is bovine bone that has been treated to remove all of its organic components to eliminate the risk of rejection.
      2) Removing the organic components from bovine bone leaves a porous structure, similar in structure to human bone.
      3) It has been suggested that the porous structure of anorganic bovine bone can act as scaffolding for new bone and that it can act through this mechanism as an osteoinductive material.

5. Plaster of Paris
    a. Plaster of Paris has been used as an alloplastic bone replacement grafting material.
    b. Plaster of Paris is actually calcium sulfate, which is porous and biocompatible when placed in periodontal wounds; when calcium sulfate is placed in a periodontal wound it resorsorbs within a few weeks.
    c. Though this material has been studied and used in humans as a bone replacement graft material, its efficacy related to osteogenic potential has not been proven.

6. Bioactive glass
    a. Bioactive glass ceramics have been studied and used as alloplastic bone replacement grafting materials.
    b. This ceramic material consists of calcium salts, phosphates, and silicone dioxide; when used as an alloplastic bone replacement graft, bioactive glass is used in particulate form.
    c. When bioactive glass comes in contact with periodontal tissues, the particulate surfaces can incorporate proteins and can attract osteoblasts that can subsequently form bone.

7. Calcium phosphate
    a. Calcium phosphate biomaterials have been used as alloplastic grafting materials for several decades.
    b. Calcium phosphate is osteoconductive and is well tolerated by body tissues.
    c. Two types of calcium phosphate materials have been used: hydroxyapatite and tricalcium phosphate.
    d. Though these materials can result in some clinical repair of periodontal defects, they are either poorly resorbable (tricalcium phosphate) or not resorbable at all (hydroxyapatite) and can remain encapsulated by collagen within the periodontal tissues.

E. **Healing After Bone Replacement Grafting**
    1. Final healing expected from bone replacement grafting usually includes a partial rebuilding of alveolar bone lost because of periodontitis.
        a. It is not known, however, if successful bone grafting always results in the reformation of cementum and periodontal ligament in addition to the alveolar bone.
        b. In spite of what appears to be good radiographic and clinical healing, the reformed bone in some cases may not actually be attached to the cementum by periodontal ligament fibers.
    2. Research has shown that a successful bone graft combined with reasonable self-care by the patient and periodic periodontal maintenance by the dental team can result in retaining a severely compromised tooth over time.

F. **Special Considerations for the Dental Hygienist**
    1. The site of a bone replacement graft should be left undisturbed for many months and should not be probed until an appropriate interval has elapsed. The dental hygienist should consult with the dentist to determine when a grafted site may be probed safely.
    2. Meticulous plaque biofilm control in any grafted site is critical. In the early stages of the healing, the dental team maintains some of the responsibility for plaque biofilm control at the site, because the patient may temporarily be unable to perform adequate self-care.

6. **Guided Tissue Regeneration**
   A. **Procedure Description**
      1. Guided tissue regeneration (GTR) is a periodontal surgical procedure employed to encourage regeneration of lost periodontal structures (i.e., to regrow lost cementum, lost periodontal ligament, and lost alveolar bone).
         a. When a periodontal surgical wound is created such as the elevation of a flap, the healing of the wound may involve cells from several different sources surrounding the wound.
         b. Figure 30-11 illustrates the potential sources of cells that could contribute to healing tissues within a periodontal surgical wound.
         c. GTR techniques involve the use of a barrier membrane to delay the normally rapid ingrowth of epithelium into a healing periodontal wound; the rapid growth of epithelium into the wound can interfere with the slower growth of other cells critical to the healing process.
         d. Figure 30-12 illustrates how a barrier membrane might be placed under a periodontal flap at the time of surgery to delay the ingrowth of unwanted types of cells into the healing of the wound.

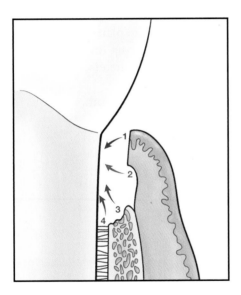

Figure 30.11. Potential Sources of Cells in a Healing Periodontal Surgical Wound. There are four potential sources of cells that can contribute to the healing of a periodontal surgical wound such as a flap: (*1*) Gingival epithelial cells, (*2*) Gingival connective tissue cells, (*3*) Bone cells, and (*4*) PDL cells. Of these four types of cells the most rapidly growing of them all are the gingival epithelial cells.

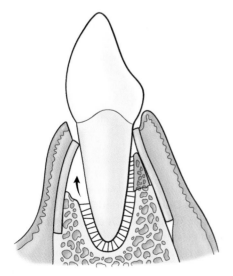

Figure 30.12. Use of Barrier Material to Inhibit the Rapid Growth of the Gingival Epithelial Cells. Note that the barrier has been placed to interfere with the growth of the epithelial cells from the flap margin along the tooth root to give the undifferentiated cells a chance to populate the wound and contribute to the healing.

e. Delay of the ingrowth of epithelium into a healing periodontal wound can allow for undifferentiated cells from the periodontal ligament to populate the root area and differentiate into the tissues that normally comprise the periodontium (i.e., cementum, PDL, and alveolar bone).

f. The barrier membranes used during a GTR procedure can also be used in conjunction with bone graft materials in some instances.

g. As the name implies, guided tissue regeneration can result in a true regeneration of the periodontium.

2. Goal of guided tissue regeneration

a. When the entire array of types of periodontal surgery is viewed, periodontal regeneration is the ultimate goal, and there is much ongoing research related to GTR.

b. Although regeneration of the cementum, periodontal ligament, and alveolar bone is the ultimate goal of periodontal therapy, regeneration of the periodontium is not completely predictable with techniques in use today.

B. Steps in a Typical Guided Tissue Regeneration Procedure

1. The first step in GTR is to make appropriate incisions and elevate a flap. In this procedure the flap usually is elevated 1 to 2 teeth beyond the site of the osseous defects.

2. The osseous defects are thoroughly debrided and the roots in the site are planed.

3. The selected membrane is trimmed to the size needed for the site; during this membrane trimming, the membrane is allowed to extend several millimeters beyond the defect in all directions.

4. The membrane is sutured into place with a sling suture placed around the tooth.

5. The flap is sutured into place (frequently slightly coronally) so that the flap covers the membrane completely.

6. Figure 30-13 illustrates the use of a barrier membrane during a guided tissue regeneration procedure used to treat a furcation involvement in a molar tooth.

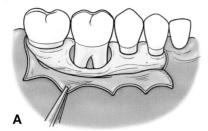

A

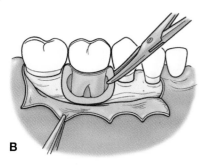

B

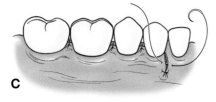

C

Figure 30.13. **Use of Barrier Material During Guided Tissue Regeneration in the Treatment of a Molar Tooth with Deep Furcation Involvement.** A: Flap is incised and elevated prior to debridement of the osseous defect and debridement of the tooth root. B: A barrier is selected, custom trimmed to size, and sutured into place. C: Flap is sutured into place completely covering the barrier material.

C. **Barrier Materials Used During Guided Tissue Regeneration**
  1. Some of the barrier materials in current use require removal following healing of the wound, so their use necessitates a second surgical procedure to remove the barrier material.
     a. Expanded polytetrafluoroethylene (ePTFE) is the most commonly used nonresorbable membrane material.
     b. These nonresorbable membranes are also available commercially with embedded titanium strips to prevent collapse of the membrane into larger osseous defects.
  2. Other barrier materials in current use are resorbable and thus do not require removal at some later date; bioresorbable membranes are preferred by many clinicians for most surgical applications.
     a. There are several types of bioresorbable membranes; these types include ployglycoside synthetic polymers, bovine and porcine collagen, and calcium sulfate.
     b. One disadvantage of bioresorbable membranes are that they lack rigidity that can be provided by titanium reinforcements available in some nonresorbable membranes.

D. **Use of Guided Tissue Regeneration with Bone Replacement Grafts**
  1. The simultaneous use of barrier membranes to promote regeneration along with bone replacement grafts is one clinical option.
  2. At this point, most of the studies have been directed toward the use of barrier materials combined with either decalicified freeze-dried bone allographs or with calcium sulfate.
  3. Available studies suggest that regeneration efforts can be improved by the combined use of both barrier materials and bone replacement grafting.

E. **Healing Following Guided Tissue Regeneration**
  1. The healing expected from guided tissue regeneration is *regeneration* of part or all of the periodontium that was destroyed by periodontitis.
  2. As already mentioned, guided tissue regeneration requires the use of a barrier material.
     a. During surgery, a barrier material is placed under the flap to stop the rapidly growing epithelium from migrating along the root surface and interfering with the connective tissue regrowth on the root. It is the connective tissue components from the periodontal ligament space that actually provide the cells needed to regrow cementum, periodontal ligament, and alveolar bone.
     b. *It is important to remember that if a barrier material were not used, the epithelial tissue would regrow very rapidly, covering the tooth root and blocking access to the root by the slower growing connective tissue and undifferentiated cells. The epithelial growth covering the root blocks the connective tissue cells of the periodontal ligament from making contact with the root surface.*

F. **Special Considerations for the Dental Hygienist**
  1. During the GTR surgical procedure, every effort is made to close the wound to cover the barrier material completely.
     a. If exposure of part of the barrier material is noted at any of the postsurgical visits, measures should be instituted to minimize bacterial contamination of the barrier material.
     b. For example, a patient with exposed barrier materials may need special self-care instructions for the topical application of antimicrobial agents to the surgical site.

2. Sites treated by guided tissue regeneration should not be probed for several months following the procedures. The dental hygienist should consult with the dentist to determine when each individual site can be probed safely.

7. **Periodontal Plastic Surgery**
    A. **Description**
        1. Periodontal plastic surgery is the term most commonly used in modern dentistry to describe periodontal surgery that is directed toward correcting problems with attached gingiva, aberrant frenum, or vestibular depth.
        2. The term periodontal plastic surgery includes an array of periodontal surgical procedures that can be used to improve esthetics of the dentition and to enhance prosthetic dentistry as well as to deal with damage resulting from periodontitis.
        3. Some of these procedures include techniques that have been used in medical plastic surgery for many years. Periodontal plastic surgery can be used to alter the tissues surrounding both natural teeth and dental implants.
    B. **Terminology Relating to Periodontal Plastic Surgery**
        1. Readers of periodontal literature can sometimes be confused by the terminology associated with periodontal plastic surgery, since some other terms have also been used to describe procedures currently included under this term.
        2. The term mucogingival surgery has been used in the past to describe periodontal surgical procedures that alter the relationship between gingiva and mucosa. Some of the periodontal plastic surgical procedures utilized in modern dentistry were previously described as mucogingival surgical procedures and this older terminology can still be encountered.
        3. Another term that has been used to describe some of these types of procedures is reconstructive surgery; the term reconstructive surgery underscores that the goal of some of these procedures is to reconstruct (or rebuild) periodontal tissues such as gingiva.
    C. **Goals of Periodontal Plastic Surgery**
        1. Many periodontal plastic surgical procedures are designed to alter components of the attached gingiva, and that type of procedure can dramatically alter the appearance of the tissues. Most patients want a pleasing smile, and because the gingiva is readily visible in many patients, patients frequently seek improvements in the appearance of the gingiva.
        2. In addition to altering the appearance of the tissues, some periodontal plastic surgical procedures improve function. Function can be compromised when lack of attached gingiva on a tooth limits the options for restoration of a tooth by contraindicating the intracrevicular placement of restoration margins.
        3. This chapter part includes an overview of some of the more common types of procedures included under the heading periodontal plastic surgery. Box 30-7 provides an overview of the types of procedures commonly included in periodontal plastic surgery.

Box 30-7. Overview of Procedures Commonly Included in Periodontal Plastic Surgery

- Free gingival graft
- Subepithelial connective tissue graft
- Laterally positioned flap
- Coronally positioned flap
- Semilunar flap
- Frenectomy
- Crown lengthening surgery

8. **Free Gingival Graft**
    A. **Description of a Free Gingival Graft**
        1. A free gingival graft is a type of periodontal plastic surgery that was one of the first procedures used to augment the width of attached gingiva.
        2. The free gingival graft requires harvesting a donor section of tissue, usually from the palate, so there are two intraoral wounds that are created during this surgery: the donor site and the recipient site.
            a. The donor tissue for a free gingival graft includes both the *surface epithelium and some of the underlying connective tissue.*
            b. Taking the tissue for a free gingival graft from a donor site leaves a wound that is an open connective tissue surface that must be allowed to heal by secondary intention, and this donor wound can be troublesome for the patient.
        3. Figure 30-14 shows a free gingival graft sutured in place on the facial surface of a mandibular incisor tooth root.
        4. The free gingival graft has been used to provide root coverage in areas of recession of the gingival margin but augmentation of the width of attached gingiva can also be performed without the need for obtaining any root coverage.
        5. The free gingival graft is an example of an autograft since the donor tissue is taken from the same individual that is to receive that donor tissue.
        6. One complicating factor for the free gingival graft that is used for root coverage is that the graft is completely severed from its blood supply and at least a portion of the graft is then placed over an avascular root surface; special care is required to encourage diffusion of nutrients to the graft to maintain its viability during the early stages of healing.

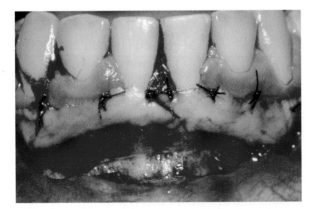

Figure 30.14. Free Gingival Graft Placed on Facial Surface of Tooth Root. The graft is placed over an area of root previously exposed by advanced recession of the gingival margin. Note the sutures that have been placed to immobilize the graft during healing.

    B. **Steps in a Typical Free Gingival Graft**
        1. The root surfaces in the area of recession of the gingival margin are planed to remove plaque biofilm, calculus, root contaminants, and root irregularities.
        2. Horizontal and vertical incisions are made at the recipient site after planning the precise location of the needed graft; surface epithelium is removed to prepare a firm connective tissue bed to receive the graft material.
        3. A template (frequently made from foil) is prepared to provide a pattern for the exact size and shape of the donor graft that will be needed.
        4. Using the template as a guide for the size and shape, the graft is obtained from the donor site (usually the palate) by incising through the epithelium and through a thin layer of connective tissue beneath the epithelium; the graft is removed from the site using sharp dissection.

5. The graft is sutured at the recipient site; during suturing, care is taken to prevent a blood clot from forming between the graft and the recipient vascular bed.

6. Both the donor site and recipient site are protected with periodontal dressing; in some instances the donor site on the palate is covered with a previously prepared acrylic retainer to hold the dressing over the donor site.

C. **Healing Expected with a Typical Free Gingival Graft**

1. Successful healing of a free gingival graft depends upon survival of the connective tissue part of the graft. In most instances the epithelium sloughs off during the healing period, later to be replaced by new epithelium.

2. Survival of the tissues depends initially upon diffusion of nutrient containing fluid from the vascular recipient tissues followed by growth of new blood vessels into the grafted material. Immobilization of the graft during the healing phase is a critical element in allowing the diffusion of nutrients, reconnection of existing blood vessels, and formation of new blood vessels.

3. Successful augmentation of gingiva as well as successful root coverage has been reported following the use of the free gingival graft.

4. Unfortunately, following complete healing of the free gingival graft, there is normally a less than ideal color match between the healed graft and the adjacent gingiva.

9. **Subepithelial Connective Tissue Graft**

A. **Description of Subepithelial Connective Tissue Graft**

1. The subepithelial connective tissue graft is a periodontal plastic surgical procedure that can also be used to augment the width of attached gingiva and to cover areas of recession of the gingival margin.

2. In addition to gingival augmentation, the subepithelial connective tissue graft is used to alter the contour of alveolar ridges to improve the esthetics of some types of dental prostheses.

3. This procedure uses an autograft of connective tissue (without epithelium) that can be harvested from a variety of intraoral sites, but that is usually taken from the patient's palate.

B. **Typical Steps in a Subepithelial Connective Tissue Graft**

1. A partial-thickness flap is elevated at the recipient site using sharp dissection; the flap normally extends one half to one tooth to the mesial and distal of the site of recession to be covered.

2. The exposed tooth root is thoroughly planed to remove plaque biofilm, calculus, root contaminants, and root irregularities.

3. The connective tissue graft is obtained by incising through the epithelium of the palate and lifting a segment of connective tissue from beneath the epithelium using sharp dissection; the surface tissues at the donor site can then be sutured to allow for healing by primary intention.

4. The graft tissue is placed over the denuded tooth root and under the partial-thickness flap at the recipient site.

5. The outer portion of the partial thickness flap is placed over the graft and sutured into place, making sure that at least half of the graft is covered by the outer portion of the flap.

6. Periodontal dressing is placed to protect the grafted site; since the donor site will heal by primary intention, normally no dressing is needed at the donor site.

C. **Healing Expected After a Subepithelial Connective Tissue Graft**
1. When root coverage is attempted with the subepithelial connective tissue graft, it is reasonable to expect coverage, though not all sites result in complete root coverage.
2. The subepithelial connective tissue graft results in excellent esthetics since the color of the healed tissues often mimics the natural preexisting tissue color precisely.

D. **Acellular Dermal Matrix Allograft**
1. As a substitute for autogenous connective tissue, an acellular dermal matrix allograft material is now available.
2. Following harvesting, the allograft is treated to remove cellular components, but it retains blood vessel channels, collagen, elastin, and proteoglycans.
3. This dermal matrix allograft material can be used in some periodontal surgical procedures in place of autogenous connective tissue, but when used it must be completely covered by a partial thickness flap.

10. **Laterally Positioned Flap**
A. **Description of a Laterally Positioned Flap**
1. The laterally positioned flap is a periodontal plastic surgery technique that can be used to cover root surfaces with gingiva in isolated sites of recession of the gingival margin.
2. The laterally positioned flap involves a displaced flap (displaced laterally in this case).
3. Use of this technique requires an adequate donor tissue (gingiva) on a tooth root adjacent to the site of recession.
4. Since the gingiva to be displaced laterally will be taken from an adjacent tooth, the site of the donor tissue must have thick, healthy covering of gingiva to allow the donor tissue to be taken without resulting in harm to the donor site.

B. **Steps in a Typical Laterally Positioned Flap**
1. The recipient site is prepared by thoroughly planing the exposed tooth root and by removing epithelium from the surface of the gingiva surrounding the area of recession, thus exposing some connective tissue to serve as a vascular recipient bed for the displaced flap.
2. A partial thickness flap is elevated from the donor site using a series of carefully planned vertical incisions to provide mobility in the flap after elevation.
3. The elevated flap is rotated laterally so as to cover the recipient site including both the prepared bed of connective tissue and the prepared tooth root.
4. The flap is stabilized at its new location using a combination of interrupted sutures and sling sutures.
5. The surgical site is covered with aluminum foil and periodontal dressing to protect the healing wound.

C. **Healing Expected After a Laterally Positioned Flap**
1. With careful selection of donor sites and skillful manipulation of the tissues, little recession will occur on the donor site.
2. The laterally positioned flap can result in excellent root coverage in many instances since the flap maintains part of its own blood supply (unlike the free gingival graft which is completely severed from its blood supply).

11. **Coronally Positioned Flap**
A. **Description of a Coronally Positioned Flap**
1. The coronally positioned flap is a periodontal plastic surgical procedure that can be used to repair recession of the gingival margin if the recession is not advanced.
2. As the name implies the coronally positioned flap is a displaced flap (displaced in a coronal direction in this case).

3. One advantage to this procedure compared to a free gingival graft or a subepithelial connective tissue graft is that it does not require a second surgical site to provide the donor tissue.

4. One disadvantage to this procedure is that it can be difficult to stabilize the flap with sutures at a more coronal position.

5. In some instances the coronally positioned flap requires a two-stage procedure.

   a. If the thickness of the gingiva at the proposed donor site is inadequate, gingiva must be augmented at the donor site with a surgical procedure prior to advancement of the coronally positioned flap.

   b. When indicated, this gingival augmentation may be accomplished with a free gingival graft prior to the coronal positioning.

B. **Steps in a Typical Coronally Positioned Flap**

   1. Exposed tooth roots are planed to remove plaque biofilm, calculus, root contaminants, and root irregularities.

   2. Internal bevel and vertical releasing incisions are made at the site to be coronally positioned; the vertical releasing incisions extend into the alveolar mucosa to allow for mobility of the flap margin in a coronal direction.

   3. Surface epithelium is removed from the site to create a vascular recipient bed.

   4. The flap is elevated; the elevation can be full-thickness or split-thickness or a combination of the two depending upon the overall thickness of the tissues being elevated.

   5. The flap is advanced in a coronal direction and sutured using a combination of interrupted and sling sutures.

   6. Periodontal dressing is placed to prevent movement of the flap during healing.

C. **Healing Expected with a Typical Coronally Positioned Flap.** The coronally positioned flap can be used successfully to cover areas of recession of the gingival margin when the recession of the gingival margin is not advanced.

12. **Semilunar Flap**

A. **Description of a Semilunar Flap.** The semilunar flap is a periodontal plastic surgical procedure that can be used to cover recession of the gingival margin where the recession is not far advanced and where the keratinized tissues have an adequate thickness. The semilunar flap is a variation of a coronally positioned flap.

B. **Steps in a Typical Semilunar flap**

   1. The level of the alveolar bone is sounded (located) to insure that coronal positioning of the semilunar flap does not inadvertently expose alveolar bone at the base of the flap.

   2. A semilunar, curved incision is made from one interdental area to the adjacent interdental area over the tooth root.

      a. The interdental sites for the incisions are selected to be slightly coronal to the position anticipated for the flap advancement.

      b. This incision begins in the gingiva and arcs into the mucosa and then back into the gingiva.

   3. A split-thickness flap is performed using sharp dissection to free the surface of the flap from the underlying connective tissue.

   4. The semilunar flap is displaced coronally and stabilized with gentle pressure for several minutes; if needed the flap can be stabilized with interrupted sutures, but sometimes suturing is not required.

13. **Frenectomy**
    A. **Description of a Frenectomy**
       1. Frenectomy is a periodontal plastic surgical procedure that results in removal of a frenum, including removal of the attachment of frenum to bone.
          a. Some authors use the term frenotomy to indicate a variation of the frenectomy.
          b. The frenotomy includes only incision of the frenum, but does not remove the attachment of the frenum from the bone surface.
       2. If a frenum is attached too close to the gingival margin, it can result in repeated pulling of the gingival margin away from the tooth surface and can contribute to persistent inflammation in the tissues; in addition, a frenum too close to the gingival margin can interfere with daily self-care.
          a. An aberrant frenum position that requires a frenectomy occurs most often in the frenum between the maxillary and mandibular central incisors.
          b. An aberrant frenum position can also occur in other locations such as on the facial surface of premolar and canine teeth and on the lingual surface of the mandibular central incisors.
    B. **Steps in a Typical Frenectomy**
       1. The frenum is grasped with a hemostat placed to the depth of the vestibule.
       2. Incisions are made through the tissues on both the under surface and the upper surface of the beaks of the hemostat.
       3. The triangular piece of tissue held by the hemostat is removed exposing connective tissue over the surface of the bone.
       4. The connective tissue covering the bone is incised and dissected.
       5. Periodontal dressing is applied to the wound.
    C. **Alternative Techniques for the Frenectomy**
       1. Frequently the frenectomy is performed in conjunction with other types of periodontal surgery, and a variety of techniques have been described.
       2. Other techniques for performing a frenectomy include removing the tissue of the frenum with electrosurgery or with a laser.
    D. **Healing following a Frenectomy.** Expected healing expected following a frenectomy is elimination of the gingival margin movement caused by the frenum.
14. **Crown Lengthening Surgery**
    A. **Description of Procedure.** Crown lengthening surgery refers to periodontal plastic surgery designed to create a longer clinical crown for a tooth by removing some of the gingiva and usually by removing some alveolar bone from the necks of the teeth.
    B. **Terminology.** Two terms frequently used when describing crown lengthening surgery are functional crown lengthening and esthetic crown lengthening
       1. Functional crown lengthening refers to crown lengthening performed on a tooth where the remaining tooth structure is inadequate to support a needed restoration.
          a. Functional crown lengthening surgery can be used to make a restorative dental procedure (such as a crown) possible when the only sensible alternative might be to remove the tooth.
          b. Crown lengthening surgery may be necessary when a tooth is decayed or broken below the gingival margin.
             1) When a badly damaged tooth is to be restored, the dentist will evaluate the tooth and surrounding tissues to determine if the final restoration of the tooth will damage the soft tissue attachment (i.e., encroach upon the biologic width).
             2) If such damage can be expected, crown lengthening surgery is usually indicated prior to the placement of the final restoration.

2. Esthetic crown lengthening refers to crown lengthening performed on teeth to improve the appearance of the teeth where there is excessive gingiva or a "gummy smile" as it is sometimes called.

    a. Crown lengthening surgery can be used to improve the esthetics of the gingiva, especially on anterior teeth with short clinical crowns.

        1) An individual's smile may be unattractive because the height or lack of symmetry of the gingiva surrounding the teeth

        2) In some cases tooth crowns are actually the correct length, but they appear too short in the mouth because there is an excess of gingival tissue covering the teeth.

    b. During esthetic crown lengthening, the gingival tissues are incised and reshaped to expose more of the natural crown of the tooth; frequently some of the alveolar bone must also be removed to insure healing of the tissues at a more apical position.

C. Surgical Procedure. The actual surgical procedure followed during crown lengthening surgery usually involves an apically positioned flap (displaced flap) with osseous resective surgery much like that already discussed.

    1. Unlike the typical apically positioned flap with osseous surgery, crown lengthening surgery may be indicated in the presence of a perfectly healthy periodontium simply to allow for improved esthetics or to allow for exposure of more tooth structure prior to restoration.

    2. Also unlike the typical apically positioned flap with osseous surgery, esthetic crown lengthening frequently requires the use of a template prepared to guide the surgeon in positioning the tissues during the surgery.

    3. Occasionally, esthetic crown lengthening may require only a gingivectomy type procedure to be discussed later in this chapter, but most often esthetic crown lengthening requires some alveolar bone removal, so an apically positioned flap with osseous surgery is most often indicated instead of a gingivectomy.

D. Healing after Crown Lengthening Surgery

    1. Healing of crown lengthening surgery is similar to that described for the apically positioned flap with osseous surgery.

    2. Final healing of crown lengthening surgery results in a normal attachment (both junctional epithelium and connective tissue attachment) at a position more apical on the tooth root.

E. Special Considerations for the Dental Hygienist

    1. Since crown lengthening surgery usually involves exposure of additional tooth surface to the oral environment, temporary dentinal hypersensitivity is also a common result of this type of periodontal surgery; it is imperative for the dental team to warn patients in advance that they may experience temporary dentinal hypersensitivity following crown lengthening surgery.

    2. As already discussed, when dentinal hypersensitivity results, the dental hygienist may need to institute measures to help the patient deal with the sensitivity.

    3. Control of dentinal hypersensitivity requires meticulous plaque biofilm control during the healing phase, and this can be a problem since mechanical plaque biofilm control must be restricted following most surgical procedures.

    4. It is the responsibility of the members of the dental team to aid the patient in plaque biofilm control until healing allows the patient to resume routine self-care.

15. **Gingivectomy**
    A. **Description of a Gingivectomy**
        1. The gingivectomy is a surgical procedure designed to excise and to remove some of the gingival tissue. Historically the gingivectomy was used for many years in periodontics as a primary treatment modality, but it plays a greatly reduced role in modern dentistry.
        2. When a gingivectomy is performed, the tissues are excised (cut away), removing some of the gingiva that would normally be attached to the tooth surface, thus the gingivectomy is a resective procedure.
        3. The gingivectomy results in a more apical position of the marginal gingiva in relationship to the CEJ of the tooth.
        4. Terminology related to gingivectomy can be confusing because of the overlapping use of two terms: gingivectomy and gingivoplasty.
            a. In contrast to the gingivectomy described above, gingivoplasty is a term used to *describe a surgical procedure that simply reshapes the surface of the gingiva to create a natural form and contour to the gingiva.*
            b. *Unlike t*he gingivectomy, gingivoplasty implies reshaping the surface of the gingiva without removing any of the gingiva actually attached to the tooth surface.
            c. In reality during almost all gingivectomy type procedures, a certain amount of gingivoplasty is also performed, so the precise distinction between these two companion terms can be a bit cloudy.
        5. There is still a limited place in modern dentistry for the gingivectomy procedure.
            a. Periodontal diseases can produce deformities of the gingiva including conditions such as gingival enlargements, gingival craters, and gingival clefts.
            b. Occasionally even in the absence of periodontal pockets these deformities occur and need to be altered to allow for improved esthetics, improved mastication, or enhanced ease of patient self-care.
        6. Figure 30-15 illustrates the types of incisions involved when performing a gingivectomy.

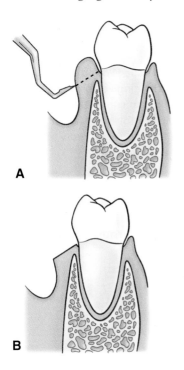

A

B

Figure 30.15. **Gingivectomy Incisions.** A: The placement of a special gingivectomy knife to incise the excess gingival tissue. Note that the direction of the tissue bevel being created is approximately 45 degrees to the tooth surface. B: The excess tissue has been excised and removed creating a more natural level and contour of the gingiva on the tooth surface.

B. **Disadvantages of Gingivectomy**
1. In modern periodontal therapy, the gingivectomy is usually limited to removing enlarged gingiva to improve esthetics or to allow for better access for self-care in isolated sites.
2. Though gingivectomy can be used to reshape more extensive areas of enlarged gingiva as might be seen in gingival overgrowth in response to certain medication use, periodontal surgeons have other more effective surgical options today.
3. As a surgical technique, gingivectomy has several *disadvantages*:
   a. One disadvantage to gingivectomy is that it leaves a large open connective tissue wound that results in a somewhat slower surface healing than most other periodontal surgical procedures; this generally results in the expectation of more discomfort for the patient during the healing phase.
   b. Figure 30-16 illustrates the type of connective tissue wound that occurs following a gingivectomy.
   c. Another disadvantage of gingivectomy is that following healing it invariably results in a longer appearing tooth because of the excision of some of the gingiva.
   d. A third disadvantage to the gingivectomy is that it does not provide access to the underlying alveolar bone, so when access to the alveolar bone is needed, the surgeon must select another type of surgical approach.
   e. A fourth disadvantage to the gingivectomy is that is does not conserve keratinized tissue (gingiva); in many surgical sites it is unwise to remove keratinized tissue since it may already be minimal in width.
   f. In spite of these disadvantages, the gingivectomy can be a useful surgical procedure in selected sites.

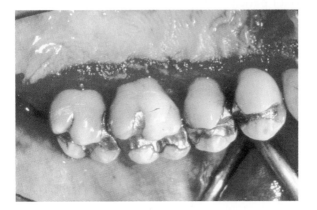

Figure 30.16. **Connective Tissue Wound Created by Gingivectomy**. Note that the gingivectomy results in a rather large wound that exposes connective tissue. This large wound usually results in protracted healing since the healing requires that the epithelium grow across the wound created by the gingivectomy.

C. **Steps in Performing a Typical Gingivectomy**
1. Existing periodontal pockets are explored and the levels of the bases of the pockets are marked on the surface of the gingiva by punching a hole through the surface of the gingiva.
2. Using special gingivectomy knives (both broad bladed and narrow bladed), gingiva is excised at the levels of the bases of the pockets.
3. As the incision is made, care is taken to produce a 45-degree bevel of the gingiva against the tooth to mimic the natural contour of the surface of the gingiva in relationship to the tooth.

4. The excised portion of the gingiva is removed (which also removes the soft tissue wall of existing periodontal pockets).

5. The wound surface is inspected, remaining tissue tags are removed, and gingival contours are refined as needed.

6. The tooth surfaces are inspected and debrided to remove plaque biofilm, calculus, root contaminants, and root irregularities.

7. The surgical wound is covered with periodontal dressing.

D. **Healing Expected After a Gingivectomy**

1. Healing of the gingivectomy requires healing by secondary intention since the gingivectomy incisions invariably leave an exposed connective tissue surface.

2. The approximate rate that gingiva grows across a connective tissue wound in the oral cavity is 0.5 mm each day; since the gingivectomy normally leaves many millimeters of connective tissue exposed, the healing time can be protracted.

3. The final healing of the wound created by a gingivectomy is a normal attachment of the epithelium and connective tissues to the tooth root at a level that is more apical in position than the original gingival level.

4. Following a gingivectomy, the teeth in the surgical area will appear to be longer since more of the root is exposed where the tissue was excised.

   a. Of course, if more tooth exposure is the desired result of the procedure, this procedure can result in an acceptable outcome.

   b. However, if the exposure of more root structure is not esthetically desirable in a particular site in the oral cavity, another surgical approach would be selected by the surgeon.

E. **Special Considerations for the Dental Hygienist**

1. As already mentioned, the gingivectomy wound leaves a broad connective tissue surface exposed that can be very uncomfortable for the patient during the healing phase.

2. Postsurgical discomfort can be managed by placing a periodontal dressing over the wound to provide protection and by prescribing analgesics (pain medications) for use following surgery.

3. At the time of the dressing removal at the first postsurgical visit following a gingivectomy, the dental hygienist will frequently need to replace the periodontal dressing to enhance wound comfort until total epithelialization of the wound has occurred.

4. Healing of the wound created by a gingivectomy procedure progresses in a predictable manner.

   a. As already discussed, research studies have shown that oral epithelium grows across the exposed connective tissue at an approximate rate of 0.5 mm/day.

   b. Thus it is possible for the clinical team to predict approximate healing times by estimating the wound size; this of course is useful when counseling patients about what to expect during the postsurgical phase.

16. **Gingival Curettage**

A. **Procedure Description**

1. Gingival curettage is an older type of periodontal surgical procedure that involves an attempt to scrape away the lining of the periodontal pocket usually using a periodontal curet, often a Gracey curet.

   a. During periodontal instrumentation, some unintentional curettage of the gingiva always occurs, but the term gingival curettage refers a separate surgical procedure performed after routine periodontal instrumentation has removed most of the plaque biofilm, calculus, and root contaminants.

b. *Research has demonstrated that normally the same benefits from gingival curettage can be derived from thorough periodontal instrumentation by the clinician plus meticulous self-care by the patient. Thus, curettage is rarely needed as a separate periodontal surgical procedure in modern dentistry.*

2. Variations of the gingival curettage. Although the gingival curettage is no longer routinely recommended as a separate periodontal surgical procedure, some clinicians have advocated variations on this technique.

   a. One variation is performing gingival curettage with caustic chemicals.
      1) Examples of some chemicals that have been used for a chemical curettage include sodium hypochlorite and phenol.
      2) The extent of tissue destruction that follows the use of caustic chemicals cannot be controlled, and studies have failed to show any efficacy for this type of curettage.

   b. Another variation is performing gingival curettage with ultrasonic devices.
      1) In this technique ultrasound is used to debride the epithelial lining of periodontal pockets.
      2) Some authors have found the use of ultrasound as effective as manual curets in removing the pocket linings, but since the fundamental premise for gingival curettage is not sound, this technique is not advocated today either.

   c. A third variation of the gingival curettage is the excisional new attachment procedure (known as ENAP).
      1) The excisional new attachment procedure was developed as a definitive curettage performed with a surgical scalpel.
      2) During an ENAP, a surgical scalpel is used to incise away the lining of a periodontal pocket, including the linings of interproximal pockets.
      3) Sutures are placed only if the tissues do not rest against the necks of the teeth passively.

B. **Indications for Gingival Curettage in Modern Dentistry**

   1. Studies have shown that healing of soft tissues following periodontal instrumentation is not normally improved by subsequent gingival curettage, so the indications for this procedure today are quite limited.

   2. Though gingival curettage is not normally recommended as part of modern periodontal therapy, a few indications for this procedure still exist; these indications include the following.

      a. Gingival curettage can be performed in lieu of more definitive types of surgery when the more definitive procedures are contraindicated because of health concerns in the patient.

      b. Gingival curettage can be performed during periodontal maintenance in sites of persistent inflammation where definitive periodontal surgery has already been performed.

C. **Steps in a Typical Gingival Curettage**

   1. Curettes are used to scrape away the lining of the soft tissue wall of the periodontal pockets.

   2. Care is taken to place the cutting edge of the curet in direct contact with the soft tissue rather than away from the soft tissue as might be done during routine periodontal instrumentation.

3. A horizontal stroke with the curet is used to engage the lining of the pocket.
4. Light finger pressure can be used against the surface of the gingiva to stabilize the tissue during the scraping motion.

D. **Healing Following Gingival Curettage**
   1. Healing expected following gingival curettage would be healing by repair and the formation of a long junctional epithelium.
   2. This is the same type of healing you would expect following thorough periodontal instrumentation.
   3. Figure 30-17 illustrates the type of healing that would be expected following a gingival curettage.

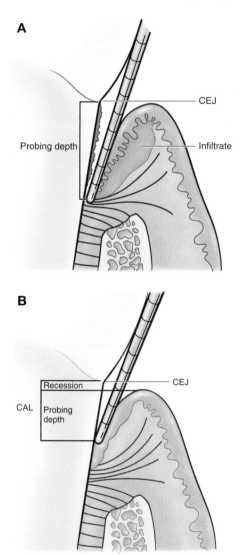

Figure 30.17. **Healing Following Gingival Curettage. A:** Periodontal pocket prior to treatment showing inflammation and calculus on the roots. **B:** Healing following gingival curettage and root instrumentation. Healing includes resolution of inflammation and readaptation of some junctional epithelium.

17. **Dental Implant Placement.** Dental implants are discussed in Chapter 32, but they are briefly mentioned in this section to underscore that the placement of dental implants can utilize many periodontal surgical techniques. The planning and surgical placement of dental implants is quite complex and the interested reader is directed toward the many excellent textbooks devoted to that topic. In addition to the surgery involved in placing dental implants, periodontal surgical procedures can help prepare sites for the placement of dental implants.

A. Description of Dental Implant Placement
1. As discussed in Chapter 32, a dental implant is an artificial tooth root that is placed into the alveolar bone to hold a replacement crown or prosthesis (denture or bridge).
2. Most dental implants in current use are endosseous implants that are placed in alveolar bone and protrude through the mucoperiosteum.
    a. Dental implant placement usually requires exposure of alveolar bone using the principles of periodontal flap surgery, drilling a precise hole in the alveolar bone, insertion of a metallic implant into the site, and suturing of the wound created.
    b. There are a variety of dental implants in current use including various lengths, diameters, and designs; most types of dental implants have threads much like a screw has threads.
3. Some dental implants are designed to be covered with gingiva during healing, and others are designed to leave a portion of the implant exposed in the oral cavity during healing. Those that are covered require a second surgical procedure following healing to expose the top of the implant.
4. When preparing a site to receive a dental implant and during dental implant placement, any of the periodontal surgical procedures already discussed may be employed.

B. Healing Expected Following Dental Implant Placement
1. Healing following placement of a dental implant results in bone growth in such close proximity to the implant surface that the implant is stable enough to support a tooth shaped restoration or a dental prosthetic appliance.
2. It should be noted that though dental implants are not surrounded by cementum and PDL (as are natural teeth), these implants are subject to periodontal disease that can result in the loss of supporting bone just like the natural tooth.

C. Special Considerations for the Dental Hygienist
1. Patient self-care following placement of a dental implant is as critical as it is following every periodontal surgical procedure, and the members of the dental team must assume responsibility for helping the patient with plaque biofilm control during the critical healing period.
2. Once an implant site heals, the gingiva surrounding the implant can be maintained in health using self-care techniques similar to what is required to keep tissues around a natural tooth healthy.
3. Implant maintenance and the role played by the dental hygienist are discussed in detail in Chapter 32.

18. **Periodontal Microsurgery.** Periodontal microsurgery is a term used to describe periodontal surgery performed with the aid of a surgical microscope. Principles of microsurgery have had a good deal of influence in medicine and will continue to influence the performance of certain periodontal surgical procedures, especially periodontal plastic surgery. Periodontal surgery performed using microsurgery techniques can result in procedures performed with increased precision on the part of the surgeon.

Section 4
Biological Enhancement of Surgical Outcomes

Many attempts have been made to enhance the outcomes of periodontal surgery by using chemical or biologic mediators to influence the healing following periodontal surgical procedures. This chapter section provides a brief overview of some of the biologic mediators that have been studied to date. There is much ongoing research into this topic, and it is reasonable to expect that this ongoing research will reveal fundamental mechanisms for enhancing periodontal surgical outcomes that will prove useful in a clinical setting.

1. **Root Surface Modification**
   A. **Mechanical Root Preparation**
      1. Many years of observation of the healing of periodontal surgical wounds demonstrates that gingival tissues adjacent to tooth roots—that have previously been exposed because of attachment loss—heal better when the roots are free of plaque biofilm, calculus, and root contaminants.
      2. These observations have lead to the incorporation of mechanical root preparation as a routine part of most periodontal surgical procedures. Hand and ultrasonic instruments have been used extensively for this purpose.
   B. **Chemical and Biologic Mediators.** Chemical and biologic mediators also have been used in attempts to enhance the healing of the gingiva adjacent to the tooth roots beyond what can be achieved by periodontal instrumentation alone. Several chemical mediators have been studied for possible benefits to the gingival healing process.
      1. Ethylenediamine tetraacetic acid (EDTA) has been used to decalcify the surface of the root following mechanical root preparation.
         a. Possible benefits of using EDTA on roots include removal of the dentin smear layer, exposure of ends of embedded collagen fibers in remaining cemental surface, and removal of endotoxin buried deeper below the root surface.
         b. Though some clinicians have used this chemical to enhance root preparation, most of the evidence indicates that there is very little positive effect on the outcomes of any surgery by the use of this chemical to prepare tooth roots.
      2. A second chemical agent that has been referred to as a biologic mediator, again to enhance the outcomes of periodontal root preparation, is tetracycline.
         a. Tetracyclines are a family of antibiotics with varied properties in addition to their antibiotic effects. It has been suggested that tetracyclines applied to roots during surgery may enhance the migration of fibroblasts to the root surfaces during healing in addition to slightly decalcifying the surfaces of the roots.
         b. Most studies indicate that using this biologic mediator on root surfaces during surgery has little effect on the outcomes of the surgical procedures.
2. **Growth Factors.** Growth factors are naturally occurring proteins that regulate both cell growth and development. Several growth factors are being studied for their effect in enhancing the predictability of periodontal regeneration and studies of these potential biologic mediators are continuing. These growth factors include platelet-derived growth factor (PDGF) and insulin-derived growth factor (IGF). It is reasonable to expect that continued research into the use of growth factors to improve periodontal surgical outcomes might lead to clinical application of some of these factors in the future.

3. **Enamel Matrix Derivative (EMD)**
   A. **Periodontal Regeneration Factors**
      1. It is clear that periodontal regeneration depends upon the type of cells that first populate the periodontal surgical wound.
      2. As already discussed, using barrier materials to insure that the correct cells enter the healing surgical wound without the early interference of epithelium can result in more predictable periodontal regeneration. The use of barriers to insure periodontal regeneration, however, has not been very successful in all sites of more advanced osseous defects.
   B. **Protein Preparations.** Research into using protein preparations and growth factors to enhance periodontal regeneration by mimicking natural healing processes has shown some promising results.
      1. Enamel matrix derivative (EMD) has been used to enhance periodontal regeneration.
      2. Enamel matrix derivative (EMD) is a preparation of proteins extracted from porcine tooth buds; EMD is the tooth bud extract mixed with a propylene glycol alginate carrier.
      3. The major constituents of this extract appear to be proteins called amelogenins and enamelin.
      4. At this point it appears that EMD may indeed enhance periodontal regeneration and that the safety of this material is quite high when used in conjunction with periodontal surgery.
      5. EMD is currently being used by clinicians in an attempt to improve outcomes of some types of periodontal surgery.
      6. Studies into the precise constituents in this protein extract that can enhance healing are continuing.
4. **Platelet Rich Plasma (PRP).** Another example of a biologic mediator is platelet rich plasma (PRP). Using PRP requires obtaining a sample of the patient's blood and separating the blood sample into three separate fractions: platelet rich plasma (PRP), red blood cells, and platelet poor plasma. The PRP fraction of blood contains high numbers of platelets plus platelet derived growth factor (PDGF), TGF-β (tumor derived growth factor-beta), and fibrinogen. Clinically both calcium and thrombin are added to the PRP to activate the production of fibrin before the preparation is applied in the surgical site. Though some studies indicate some enhancement of the healing process following the use of this preparation, it is not clear that the growth factors are present in high enough concentrations to have much effect on the actual surgical outcomes, and additional studies of this material are underway.
5. **Bone Morphogenetic Proteins (BMPs).** Bone morphogenetic proteins (BMPs) are a group of regulatory glycoproteins that have been studied for possible use in the field of periodontal regeneration because of their known osteoinductive effects. Both purified and recombinant BMPs are currently being studied, and early results indicate possible enhancement of regeneration in some treated sites. Unfortunately using BMP to enhance surgical outcomes has resulted in tooth ankylosis and much futher study of this material is indicated. Investigations into the use of bone morphogenetic proteins to enhance periodontal regeneration are continuing.

Section 5
Patient Management Following Periodontal Surgery

The dental hygienist plays a major role in supporting the management of patients following periodontal surgery. This chapter section discusses components of postsurgical management including use of sutures, use of periodontal dressings, delivery of postsurgical instructions, and organizing postsurgical visits. It is important to realize that the management of the patient during the healing phase following periodontal surgery can be as important to the surgical outcomes as the skill of the surgeon performing the surgery.

USE OF SUTURES IN PERIODONTAL SURGICAL WOUNDS

1. **Overview of the Use of Sutures in Periodontal Wounds.** Many periodontal surgical procedures such as periodontal flaps require the placement of sutures to stabilize the position of the soft tissues during the early phases of healing; a suture, or stitch as it is sometimes called, is a device placed by a surgeon to hold tissues together during healing.
   A. **Characteristics of Suture Material**
      1. To be useful in periodontal wounds suture materials need to be nontoxic, flexible, and strong.
      2. Some suture materials have been reported to have a "wicking" effect (i.e., they can allow bacteria to travel down the suture and contaminate the surgical wound); this wicking effect is believed to have a negative effect on the surgical outcomes.
      3. When placing sutures, periodontal surgeons take great care not to put tension on a flap with sutures (i.e., to insure that the flap lies passively at the intended position prior to suturing); sutures are used to stabilize the flap in its passive position.
      4. If a suture places tension on a flap, the suture material will pull out of the tissues during healing and will fail to serve the purpose of stabilizing the tissues.
   B. **Types of Suture Material.** In general two types of suture material are used: nonabsorbable and absorbable. Box 30-8 provides an overview of some of the suture materials available for use in periodontal wounds.
      1. Nonabsorbable suture is a suture made from a material that does not dissolve in body fluids. A clinician must remove the nonabsorbable sutures after some healing of the wound has occurred.
      2. Absorbable suture is a suture made from a material designed to dissolve harmlessly in body fluids over time; though absorbable sutures do not normally require removal by the dental team, some absorbable sutures do not dissolve particularly well in saliva.

Box 30-8. Examples of Suture Materials

Nonabsorbable:
- Braided silk
- Monofilament nylon
- Expanded polytetrafluoroethylene (ePTFE)
- Braided polyester

Absorbable:
- Plain and chromic gut
- Polyglactin 910
- Polyglecaprone 25

Box 30-9. Overview of General Indications for Common Suture Techniques

1. Interrupted suture: closure of vertical incisions, closure of nondisplaced flaps
2. Sling suture: closure of displaced flaps
3. Continuous sling suture: closure of displaced flaps, closure of nondisplaced flaps

2. **Suture Placement Techniques.** Familiarity with some general techniques for suturing can guide the hygienist assigned the task of suture removal at a postsurgical appointment. Box 30-9 provides an overview of general indications for some of the more common suturing techniques for periodontal surgical wounds. Three of the most common suture placement techniques are discussed and illustrated below.

A. **Interrupted Interdental Suture**
   1. During most periodontal flap surgery, flaps are elevated on both the facial and lingual (or palatal) surfaces of the teeth; an interrupted interdental suture usually involves suturing the facial and lingual papillae together, but this technique is also ideal for closing vertical incisions
   2. When interrupted interdental sutures are placed to close a periodontal flap procedure, a separate suture is placed and tied in each of the interdental sites.
   3. An interrupted interdental suture that might be utilized during a periodontal flap for access procedure is illustrated in Figures 30-18 and 30-19.
   4. When removing interrupted interdental sutures, the clinician must cut each of the interdental sutures prior to pulling out the suture material.

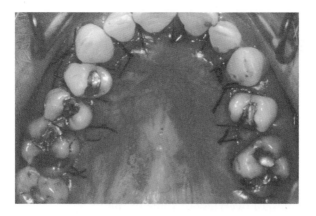

Figure 30.18. **Interrupted Interdental Sutures.** Interrupted interdental sutures have been placed in each interdental site on the maxillary arch. Note that there is a knot associated with each of these interrupted sutures that would need to be cut prior to removal. (Courtesy of Dr John S. Dozier, Tallahassee, Florida.)

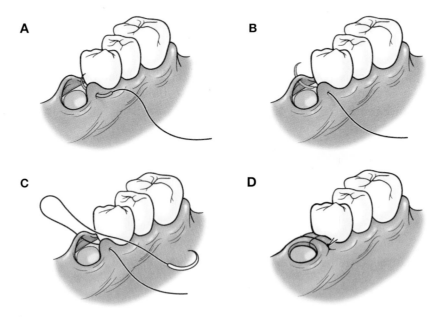

Figure 30.19. **Interrupted Interdental Suture.** In these drawings the most mesial tooth has been removed to allow for visualization of the path of the interrupted interdental suture. A: Suture placed through papilla on the facial. B: Suture placed through the papilla on the lingual. C: Suture returned to facial surface. D: Knot tied in suture on the facial.

B. Continuous Loop Suture

1. The continuous loop suture is preferred by many clinicians for suturing many types of periodontal flaps.
2. When continuous loop sutures are used, following placing the suture material through two interdental papillae, the end of the suture is looped around the teeth to reach the next interdental site rather than being tied at each interdental site; the suture is tied following placement of the loop around the terminal tooth.
3. A continuous loop suture that might be utilized during an apically positioned flap is illustrated in Figures 30-20 and 30-21.
4. Removal of a continuous loop suture can frequently be accomplished with a single cut through the suture near the knot prior to pulling out the suture material.

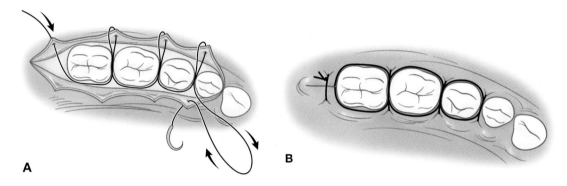

A   **B**

Figure 30.20. **Continuous Loop Suture.** Note that the suture is looped around each of the cervical areas of the teeth and passed through the tissues associated with each interdental area, but that it is tied only at the end of the continuous loop.

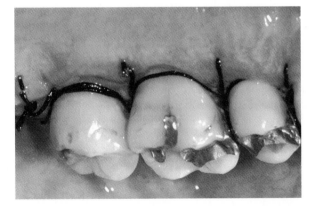

Figure 30.21. **Continuous Loop Suture.** Continuous loop suture has been placed on the segment of teeth in maxillary arch. Note that the only knot visible is associated with the most distal tooth. (Courtesy of Dr Don Rolfs Periodontal Foundations, Wenatchee, Washington.)

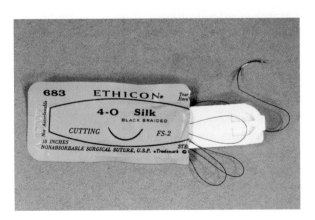

Figure 30.22. **Typical Suture Material Used for Periodontal Surgery.** Note that the suture comes sterilized in a sealed packet. On the packet face the type of suture material and the size (here 4-0) are identified along with some other information useful to the surgeon.

C. **Sling Suture**
1. Some periodontal surgical wounds require the placement of a sling suture; the sling suture is used to sling or suspend the tissues around the cervical area of a tooth rather than to tie soft tissue to other soft tissue.
2. The sling suture is frequently used when a flap is displaced in an apical direction. Figure 30-23 illustrates a sling suture.
3. It should be noted that when facial and lingual flaps are sutured using the sling suture technique, a separate sling suture must be placed on both the facial and lingual surfaces.
4. Removal of the sling suture only requires locating the individual knots, cutting the suture near the knot, and careful extraction of the suture.

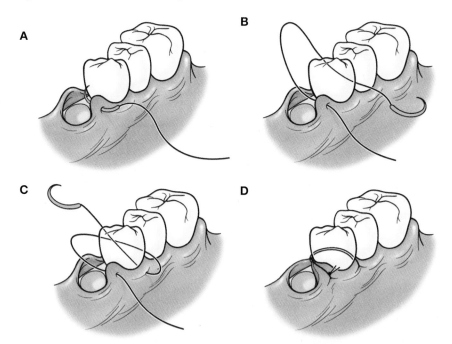

Figure 30.23. **Sling Suture.** In these drawings the most mesial tooth has been removed to allow for visualization of the path of the sling suture. A: Suture placed through the facial papilla. B: Suture looped around the lingual surface of the tooth without engaging the lingual soft tissues. C: Suture continues back to the facial surface under the contact and engages the facial papilla on the distal of the tooth. D: Suture continues back on same path and is tied on the surface where it first penetrated the facial papilla.

3. **Suture Removal**
A. **Removal of Nonabsorbable Sutures**
1. Nonabsorbable sutures placed during surgical procedures are removed as part of routine postsurgical visits. Frequently remnants of absorbable sutures can also be removed at the routine postsurgical visits to avoid unnecessary tissue inflammation that can be caused by retained absorbable suture material which does not dissolve in a timely manner.
2. Guidelines for timing of removal vary, but in general, sutures should be removed when wound healing has progressed to the point at which the sutures are no longer needed to stabilize the tissues. Many sutures are loose and no longer needed to stabilize the tissues at the time of the 1-week postsurgical visit.
3. Most periodontal sutures should not be left in place longer than 2 weeks because they can act as irritants if the suture material remains in the tissues too long. It should be noted that sutures in some periodontal wounds are routinely left in place for much longer periods.

BOX 30-10. General Guidelines for Suture Removal
Guideline 1: Remove sutures in a timely manner.
Guideline 2: Read the surgical note in the patient's chart.
Guideline 3: Understand the typical sizing system for sutures.
Guideline 4: Nerver allow the knot to be pulled through the tissues.
Guideline 5: Always confirm that all of the sutures have been removed

TABLE 30-1. Typical Designations for Suture Sizes Used in Periodontal Surgery

Suture Size	Approximate Diameter of Suture (mm)
3-0	0.20
4-0	0.15
5-0	0.10

4. Each periodontal surgical procedure is unique, and suture removal procedures can vary, but some general guidelines for suture removal are outlined below and in Box 30-10.

B. General Guidelines for Suture Removal

1. Guideline 1: Remove sutures in a timely manner. Nonabsorbable sutures are generally removed after 1 week of healing; most absorbable sutures can be left in place 1 to 3 weeks.

2. Guideline 2: Read the surgical note in the patient's chart prior to suture removal.

   a. The number and type of sutures placed should be a routine part of the chart entry recorded for each periodontal surgery.

   b. Knowing the number of sutures placed during the actual surgical procedure can help the dental hygienist confirm that all sutures have been located and removed during a postsurgical visit.

3. Guideline 3: Understand the typical sizing system used for periodontal sutures.

   a. Though there are numerous sizes of sutures used in a medical setting, typical designations for suture sizes used in periodontal surgery are sizes 3-0, 4-0, and 5-0.

      1) In this sizing system, the 3-0 size is larger than the 4-0 size, and 4-0 is larger than 5-0.

      2) In the mouth, 5-0 can be more difficult to locate than a 4-0 size, especially in the posterior part of the mouth.

   b. The dental hygienist should learn the precise abbreviations used in the chart entries in the individual clinical setting. A typical example of an abbreviation would be "4-0 BSS." This would mean the size of the suture is 4-0, and BSS stands for black silk suture, a commonly used nonabsorbable suture material.

   c. Table 30-1 outlines designations for typical suture sizes used during periodontal surgery as they might appear in a patient's chart.

4. Guideline 4: Never allow the knot to be pulled through the tissues.
   a. Sutures should be removed by cutting the suture material near the knot and grasping the knot with sterile cotton pliers.
   b. When the suture is gently pulled from the tissue, care should be taken not to force the knot itself through the tissue. This technique is illustrated in Figure 30-24.
   c. It should be noted that suture removal is rarely painful for the patient if care is taken not to create unnecessary tissue movement.
5. Guideline 5: Always confirm that all of the sutures have been removed.
   a. Following suture removal, it is imperative to inspect the wound with care to insure that all of the sutures have indeed been located and removed.
   b. Remember that the patient chart entry made on the day of the surgery usually will contain information about how many sutures were actually placed.

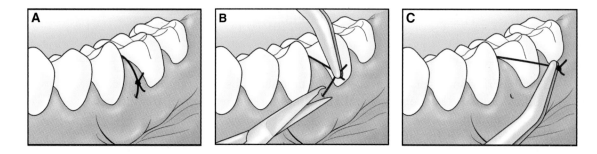

Figure 30.24. **Suture Removal.** A: Suture in place. B: Grasp the suture material and cut it near the knot. C: Gently pull the suture material from the tissue taking care not to pull the knot through the tissue.

USE OF PERIODONTAL DRESSING

1. **Purpose of Periodontal Dressing**
   A. Periodontal dressing, or periodontal pack as it sometimes called, is a protective material applied over a periodontal surgical wound. Periodontal dressings are used somewhat like using a bandage to cover a finger wound.
   B. Though the placement of periodontal dressings following periodontal surgery used to be routine, modern surgical techniques may or may not require placement of a periodontal dressing.
      1. The surgical wound created by the gingivectomy procedure leaves a raw connective tissue surface exposed that always requires a periodontal dressing.
      2. Periodontal flaps that are well adapted to the alveolar bone and tooth roots may not always require a periodontal dressing.
      3. Periodontal dressings can be placed to facilitate flap adaptation and are frequently indicated when the surgical procedures have created varying tissue levels or when displaced flaps are used.
      4. The periodontal surgeon will determine the need for dressing placement at the time of the surgical procedure.

2. **General Guidelines for Management of Periodontal Dressings**
   A. **Proper Placement**
      1. Remember that the periodontal dressing does not normally adhere to the teeth or gingiva and is retained primarily by pushing some of the material into the embrasure spaces to lock the dressing around the necks of the teeth mechanically.
      2. The use of less periodontal dressing is better than more dressing during placement; the proper amount of dressing is only enough to cover the wound.
      3. The dressing should be placed so that there is no contact between the dressing and the teeth in the opposing arch when the patient bites down; occlusal contact with teeth in the opposing arch will quickly dislodge the dressing.
      4. Figure 30-25 illustrates the proper placement of a periodontal dressing.
      5. It should be noted that suture material could accidentally become trapped within the periodontal dressing. When removing dressings, it may be necessary to loosen the dressing slightly and cut the suture before completely removing the dressing from the necks of the teeth.
      6. Periodontal dressings should be replaced every 5 to 7 days until the surgical wound is healed enough to be exposed.

A

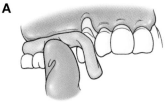

B   **C**

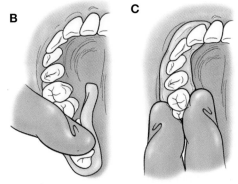

D

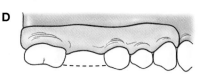

E

Figure 30.25. **Periodontal Dressing Placement.** A: Dressing is pressed into the interdental spaces with gentle finger pressure on the facial. B: Dressing is looped around the most distal tooth and pressed into the interdental spaces on the palatal. C: Gentle finger pressure is continued to join the dressing interdentally on the facial and on the palatal aspects. D: Dressing can be bridged across edentulous areas. E: Dressing amount should be minimal to avoid contact of the dressing with the teeth in the opposite arch.

3. **Types of Periodontal Dressing.** There are two types of modern periodontal dressings commonly available for use today. Both types of periodontal dressing are held in place primarily by mechanical retention around the necks of the teeth.

   A. **Chemical Cure Paste.** One type is a two-paste chemical cure material that requires the mixing of paste from two tubes to form a dressing with a putty-like consistency.

      1. This type usually contains zinc oxide, mineral oils, and rosin plus a bacteriostatic or fungicidal agent.

      2. Mixing of these two-paste dressings is either by hand or in an auto-mix cartridge.

      3. Examples of two-paste dressings are Coe-Pak manufactured by GC America, Inc. and PerioCare manufactured by Pulpdent Corp.

   B. **Light-Cured Paste.** A second type is a light-cured gel that contains polyether urethane dimethacrylate resin.

      1. The dental hygienist must study the manufacturer's instructions with care and must practice placement of the dressing on a typodont (model) before using it in a patient's mouth.

      2. This type of dressing is available as a clear, translucent material that is preferred for use by some clinicians in esthetic areas of the dentition.

      3. An example of a light-cured gel periodontal dressing is Barricaid VLC periodontal surgical dressing manufactured by Dentsply Caulk Co.

POSTSURGICAL INSTRUCTIONS AND FOLLOW UP VISITS

A member of the dental team should provide postsurgical instructions to the patient following periodontal surgery. Usually the patient is provided with both written and verbal instructions to minimize confusion and to maximize compliance. Typical postsurgical instructions are outlined in Box 30-11. For patients where sedation was required, the companion who accompanied the patient to the office is included when postsurgical instructions are given.

Box 30-11. Typical Postsurgical Instructions

1. If you have questions or concerns, call the office or the office emergency number right away. Office: 555–1111; emergency 555–2222.

2. *Do* take medications as prescribed. Report any problems with the medications immediately.

3. *Do* take it easy for several days. Limit your activity to mild physical exertion.

4. *Expect* some bleeding following the procedure. If heavy bleeding persists, call the office emergency number.

5. *Expect* some swelling. Use of an ice pack on the face in the area of the surgery during the first 8 to 10 hours following surgery can minimize swelling.

6. Diet Recommendations:

   a. Soft food only on the day of the surgery

   b. No hot beverages on the day of surgery

   c. Avoid chewing on the surgical site

7. Oral Self-care:

   a. Rinse with recommended mouth rinse starting the day after surgery

   b. If dressing was placed, it may also be brushed lightly

1. **Postsurgical Instructions to the Patient**
   A. **Restrictions on Self-Care.** Most periodontal surgical procedures require some restrictions on self-care during the early phase of healing.
      1. It is common practice to prescribe 0.12% chlorhexidine mouthrinse to be used twice daily to aid with self-care until the patient can safely resume mechanical plaque biofilm control.
      2. In most cases following routine flap surgery and gingivectomy, manual self-care can be resumed by the patient in 10 to 14 days.
      3. For selected surgical procedures (such as guided tissue regeneration or bone grafting procedures) the surgical sites should not be cleaned with routine mechanical plaque biofilm control for up to 4 to 6 weeks.
      4. Areas of the dentition not involved by the periodontal surgery may be cleaned with routine self-care techniques.
   B. **Postsurgical Medications.** Patients should be encouraged to take medications as prescribed.
      1. If systemic antibiotics are prescribed, it is particularly important for the patient to understand that all of these prescribed antibiotic medications should be taken.
      2. Common postsurgical medications include either nonsteroidal or narcotic pain medications, but usually, these pain medications should only be taken as long as needed.
   C. **Dietary Changes.** Chewing frequently must be limited to areas not involved by the surgery until healing has progressed to an acceptable level.
      1. Many of these periodontal procedures require that the surgical site be undisturbed for an extended period of time.
      2. Recommendations for a soft or liquid diet for 24 to 48 hours are routine following most periodontal surgical procedures.
      3. Chewing should be limited to the side of the mouth not involved by the surgery, especially during the early phases of healing.
2. **Postsurgical Complications**
   A. **Facial Swelling:** It is common for the patient to experience some facial swelling following most types of periodontal surgery.
      1. Swelling can arise from the tissue trauma incurred during the procedure and can even occur during the second and third day following the surgery.
      2. Although this swelling can be disconcerting to the patient, it is usually not a sign that healing is compromised.
      3. Swelling can be minimized by the intermittent use of ice packs for the first 8 to 10 hours following the surgery.
   B. **Postsurgical Bleeding:** Some bleeding following periodontal surgery is to be expected.
      1. Patients should be reassured that minor bleeding is not a cause for alarm.
      2. Postsurgical instructions should be clear, however, that if excessive bleeding occurs the emergency number should be contacted immediately.
   C. **Smoking.** Surgical patients, who have elected to continue smoking, should be cautioned to refrain during the healing phase.
3. **Organizing Postsurgical Visits.** It is the dentist's responsibility to manage postsurgical problems, such as extreme pain or infection. The dental hygienist, however, can perform much of the routine postsurgical patient management. Following periodontal flap surgery, the patient is most often reappointed in 5 to 7 days for the first postsurgical visit. Postsurgical care for the various types of periodontal surgery varies; however, steps to be followed at a typical postsurgical visit are outlined below.

A. Steps Involved in a Typical Postsurgical Visit

1. Step 1. Patient interview: An interview is conducted with the patient to determine what the patient experienced during the days following the surgery. The patient interview should be detailed enough to provide the dental hygienist with an overview of possible problems to investigate and solve at the postsurgical visit. The following are some of the items that would normally be included in this interview. It is imperative that the dental hygienist alerts the dentist if any unusual conditions are reported by the patient or are observed during the postsurgical visit.

   a. Analgesics: Following periodontal surgery, analgesics (pain control medications) are used to control patient discomfort. The patient should be asked about the current level of discomfort and if another prescription is needed.

   b. Antibiotics: If antibiotics were needed following a surgical procedure, remind the patient that all of the antibiotic tablets should be taken. It is also important to find out if the patient experienced any unusual reactions to the antibiotic.

   c. Antimicrobial mouth rinse: An antimicrobial mouth rinse such as 0.12% chlorhexidine gluconate may have been prescribed for the patient to use during healing, since mechanical plaque biofilm control must be restricted at the surgical site following periodontal surgery. Ask about the amount of mouth rinse remaining. During the course of the visit, it may be necessary to provide the patient another prescription for this mouth rinse.

   d. Swelling: Following periodontal surgery, it is common for the patient to experience some facial swelling. Remember that although this swelling can be disconcerting to the patient, it is common and usually not a sign that healing is compromised.

   e. Postsurgical bleeding: Inquire about postsurgical bleeding. It is common for patients to experience a little bleeding following periodontal surgery, but heavy bleeding should not have occurred following the procedure. If abnormal bleeding is suspected, the dentist should be alerted prior to planning any additional periodontal surgical intervention.

   f. Sensitivity to cold: Sensitivity to cold following root exposure during many types of periodontal surgery is quite common. Although this is an annoying postsurgical occurrence, the sensitivity normally disappears within the first few weeks following the surgery if excellent plaque biofilm control is maintained. Dentinal hypersensitivity is discussed in other chapters in this textbook.

2. Step 2. Vital signs: The patient's vital signs including blood pressure, pulse, and temperature are assessed. An elevated temperature at the first postsurgical visit can indicate a developing infection.

3. Step 3. Periodontal dressing: Any periodontal dressing placed at the time of surgery is removed so that the surgical site can be examined. The surgical site is rinsed with warm sterile saline and cotton-tipped applicators are used to remove any debris adherent to the teeth, soft tissues, or sutures. Suture material can become trapped within the periodontal dressing. When removing dressings, it might be necessary to loosen the dressing slightly and cut the suture before completely removing the dressing from the necks of the teeth. Figure 30-26 shows interrupted interdental sutures ready for removal at the 1-week postsurgical visit.

4. Step 4. Examination of surgical site: Examine the surgical site with care. Tissue swelling or exudate such as pus can indicate a developing infection. Excessive granulation tissue that occasionally forms in the surgical site should be removed with a sharp curet.

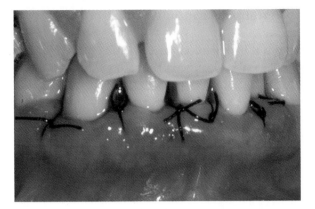

Figure 30.26. Interrupted Interdental Sutures Ready for Removal. At the 1-week postsurgical visit the periodontal dressing has been removed, the sutures have been cleaned with sterile saline, and the sutures are ready for removal.

5. Step 5. Suture removal: The sutures are cut and removed using sterile scissors and cotton pliers. Remember to pull the suture out of the tissue without drawing the knot through the tissue.
6. Step 6. Plaque biofilm removal: All plaque biofilm on the teeth in the area of the surgery is removed. It is usual that patients cannot perform perfect plaque biofilm control during the days following periodontal surgery, so plaque biofilm accumulation is likely. Part of the responsibility of the dental team is to help the patient with plaque biofilm control during the critical stages of healing.
7. Step 7. Replacement of periodontal dressing: If indicated, the periodontal dressing is replaced. For most surgical procedures, the periodontal dressing should be discontinued as soon as the patient can resume some mechanical plaque biofilm control. In a few instances the tissues will not be well adapted to the necks of the teeth, and replacement of the periodontal dressing should be considered to protect the continuing healing of the wound for at least another week.
8. Step 8. Self-care instructions: The patient is instructed in self-care. Mechanical plaque biofilm control should be resumed as soon as possible following periodontal surgery, but special instructions may be necessary during the first few weeks following the surgery.
   a. Special tools such as brushes with very flexible bristles may be required during early stages of healing.
   b. During postsurgical healing, it is frequently necessary to continue to modify the patient's plaque biofilm control techniques as the tissues heal and mature. Gingival margin contours usually are altered to some degree by the surgery, and this may necessitate the introduction of additional self-care aids that were not necessary prior to the surgery. Monitoring and modification of the patient's self-care efforts during the healing phase is one of the most important responsibilities of the dental team and can help assure success of the surgical procedure.
9. Step 9. Reappointment: The patient is reappointed for the second postsurgical visit. This second visit should occur 2 to 3 weeks following the surgery.

B. **Follow-up Visits**
1. Following the initial postsurgical visit, additional postsurgical visits must be scheduled based upon the extent of healing of the surgical wound.
2. Professional tooth polishing should be performed every 2 weeks until the patient can safely resume routine self-care.

3. When healing is deemed complete by the dental team, the patient is always placed on a program of periodontal maintenance.

4. Attachment of the flap back to the alveolar bone is usually complete within 3 weeks following the surgery, and for many surgical procedures it is safe to proceed with restorative care in the surgical site after at least 6 weeks of healing. Note that some periodontal surgical procedures (such as bone replacement graft and periodontal regeneration) will require much longer periods of healing prior to restoration placement.

5. Remodeling of the soft tissue can continue, however, for up to 6 months, so the dentist may wait quite a while prior to final restoration placements in esthetic zones such as on anterior teeth.

Chapter Summary Statement

Periodontal surgery is a critical element in the care of most patients with moderate to severe periodontitis and a critical element in the care of many patients in need of restorative dental procedures. The periodontal flap is a fundamental part of most periodontal surgical procedures, and a basic understanding of the principles of periodontal flap surgery is important to the dental hygienist. The healing of periodontal surgical wounds is a complex process, and the terminology that has been used to describe the various types of healing that can occur in the periodontium can be confusing. A variety of specific types of periodontal surgery are being used; these techniques include procedures such as flap for access, osseous resective surgery, bone replacement grafting, periodontal regeneration, and periodontal plastic surgery among others; the dental hygienist should be familiar with the common types of periodontal surgery employed. Current research into enhancing the outcomes of periodontal surgery by using biologic mediators is ongoing. Postsurgical care following periodontal surgery is vital to successful surgical outcomes, and dental hygienists play a key role in the management of patients following periodontal surgery.

Section 6
Focus on Patients

Case 1

You are assigned the task of providing nonsurgical therapy for a periodontitis patient. During routine nonsurgical periodontal therapy, you encounter multiple sites where the probing depths exceed 6 mm. During periodontal instrumentation, you are unable to instrument the root surfaces thoroughly in the areas of the deepest pockets. What should you tell the patient related to this clinical observation?

Case 2

During nonsurgical periodontal therapy, a patient with chronic periodontitis informs you that the dentist had previously discussed the possibility of periodontal surgery. The patient expresses deep concern and fear over the thought of agreeing to any periodontal surgery. The patient tells you about an aunt who had periodontal surgery many years ago and had many problems following the surgery. How should you proceed?

Case 3

At the time of the first-week postsurgical visit, you note that a patient who had undergone flap for access surgery has a temperature of 101.5°F and a pulse rate of 70 beats/min. Clinical examination of the surgical site reveals that the sutures are in place, but there appears to be a good deal of swelling in one part of flap. How should you proceed?

Case 4

You are assigned the task of managing the first-week postsurgical visit for a patient who had an apically positioned flap with osseous resective surgery. Following removal of the periodontal dressing and removal of the sutures, you note that there are several areas where the healing is progressing by secondary intention because the flap could not be adapted to the teeth perfectly at the time of surgery. Though healing is progressing satisfactorily, it is apparent that not all of the connective tissue wound around the teeth is completely covered by epithelium yet. How should you proceed?

Suggested Readings

American Academy of Periodontology. Position Paper: the potential role of growth and differentiation factors in periodontal regeneration. *J Periodontol.* 1996;67:545–553.

Anson D. Using calcium sulfate in guided tissue regeneration. *Compend Contin Educ Dent.* 2000;21:365–370.

Barnett JD, Mellonig JT, Gray JL, Towle HT. Comparison of freeze-dried bone allograft and porous hydroxylapatite in human periodontal defects, *J Periodontol* 60:231–237, 1989.

Becker BE. Crown lengthening: the periodontal-restorative connection. *Compend Contin Educ Dent.* 1998;19:239–240.

Bier SJ, Sienensky MC. The versatility of calcium sulfate: resolving periodontal challenges. *Compend Contin Educ Dent.* 1999;20:655–661.

Bowen JA, Mellonig JT, Gray JL, Towle HT. Comparison of decalcified freeze-dried bone allograft and porous particulate hydroxyapatite in human periodontal defects. *J Periodontol.* 1989;60: 647–654.

Bragger U, Lauchenauer D, Lang NP. Surgical lengthening of the clinical crown. *J Clin Periodontol.* 1992;19(1):58–63.

Camargo PM, Melnick PR, Kenney EG. The use of free gingival grafts for aesthetic purposes. *Periodontol 2000.* 2001;27:72–96.

Caton J, Nyman S. Histometric evaluation of periodontal surgery. I. The Modified Widman flap procedure. *J Clin Periodontol.* 1980;7:212–223.

Caton J, Nyman S. Histometric evaluation of periodontal surgery. II. Connective tissue attachment level after four regenerative procedures. *J Clin Periodontol.* 1980;7:224–231.

Caton J, Nyman S. Histometric evaluation of periodontal surgery. III. The effect of bone resection on the connective tissue attachment level. *J Periodontol.* 1981;52:405–409.

Christgau M, Schmalz G, Wenzel A, Hiller KA. Periodontal regeneration of intrabony defects with resorbable and nonresorbable membranes: 30-month results. *J Clin Periodontol.* 1997;24:17–27.

Cochran DL, Jones AA, Lilly LC, et al. Evaluation of recombinant human bone morphogenetic protein-2 in oral applications including the use of endosseous implants: 3-year results of a pilot study in humans. *J Periodontol.* 2000;71:1241–1257.

Cochran DL, Wozney JM. Biological mediators for periodontal regeneration. *Periodontol 2000.* 1999;19:40–58.

Cole R, Crigger M, Bogle G, et al. Connective tissue regeneration to periodontally diseased teeth. A histologic study. *J Periodont Res.* 1980;15:1–9.

Cortellini P, Pini Prato G, Baldi C, Clauser C. Guided tissue regeneration with different materials. *Int J Periodontics Restorative Dent.* 1990;10:136–151.

Cortellini P, Pini Prato G, Tonetti MS. Periodontal regeneration of human intrabony defects with titanium reinforced membranes. A controlled clinical trial. *J Periodontol.* 1995;66:797–803.

Coverly L, Toto P, Gargiulo A. Osseous coagulum: a histologic evaluation. *J Periodontol.* 1975;46:596–602.

Demirel K, Baer P, McNamara T. Topical application of doxycycline on periodontally involved root surfaces in vitro: comparative analysis of substantivity on cementum and dentin. *J Periodontol.* 1991;62:312–316.

Eickholz P, Hausmann E. Evidence for healing of interproximal intrabony defects after conventional and regenerative therapy: digital radiography and clinical measurements. *J Periodont Res.* 1998;33:156–165.

Froum SJ, Weinberg MA, Tarnow D. Comparison of bioactive glass synthetic bone graft particles and open debridement in the treatment of human periodontal defects. A clinical study. *J Periodontol.* 1998;69:698–709.

Gantes BG, Garrett S. Coronally displaced flaps in reconstructive periodontal therapy. *Dent Clin North Am.* 1991;35:495–504.

Garrett S. Periodontal regeneration around natural teeth. *Ann Periodontol* 1996;1:621–666.

Genco RJ, Newman MG, eds. Consensus report—mucogingival therapy. *Ann Periodontol.* 1996;1:702–706.

Giannobile WV, Ryan S, Shih MS, et al. Recombinant human osteogenic protein-1 (OP-1) promotes periodontal wound healing in class III furcation defects. *J Periodontol.* 1998;69:129–137.

Gottlow J, Nyman S, Lindhe J, et al. New attachment formation in the human periodontium by guided tissue regeneration. *J Clin Periodonol.* 1986;13:604–616.

Gottlow J. Guided tissue regeneration using bioresorbable and non-resorbable devices: initial healing and long-term results. *J Periodontol*. 1993;64:1157–1165.

Guillemin MR, Mellonig JT, Brusvold MA, et al. Healing in periodontal defects treated by decalcified freeze-dried bone allografts in combination with ePTFE membranes. Assessment by computerized densitometric analysis. *J Clin Periodontol*. 1993;20:520–527.

Guillemin MR, Mellonig JT, Brusvold MA. Healing in periodontal defects treated by decalcified freeze-dried bone allografts in combination with ePTFE membranes. I. Clinical and scanning electron microscope analysis. *J Clin Periodontol*. 1993;20:528–536.

Hammarstrom L. Enamel matrix and cementum development, repair and regeneration. *J Clin Periodontol*. 1997;24:658–668.

Harris R. Root coverage with connective tissue grafts: an evaluation of short- and long-term results. *J Periodontol*. 2002;73:1054–1059.

Heijl L, Heden G, Svardstrom G, Ostgren A. Enamel matrix derivative (EMDOGAIN) in the treatment of intrabony periodontal defects. *J Clin Periodontol*. 1997;24:705–714.

Jorgensen MG, Nowzari H. Aesthetic crown lengthening. *Periodontol 2000*. 2001;27:47–58.

Laney J, Saunders V, Garnick J. A comparison of two techniques for attaining root coverage. *J Periodontol*. 1992;63:19–23.

Langer B, Langer L. Subepithelial connective tissue graft technique for root coverage. *J Periodontol*. 1985;56:715–720.

Levin MP, Getter L, Adrian J, et al. Healing of periodontal defects with ceramic implants. *J Clin Periodontol*. 1974;1:197–205.

Levine RA, McGuire M. The diagnosis and treatment of the gummy smile. *Compend Contin Educ Dent*. 1997;18:757–764.

Lovelace TB, Mellonig JT, Meffert RM, et al. Clinical evaluation of bioactive glass in the treatment of periodontal osseous defects in humans. *J Periodontol*. 1998;69:1027–1035.

Low SB, King CJ, Krieger J. An evaluation of bioactive ceramic in the treatment of periodontal osseous defects. *Int J Periodontics Restorative Dent*. 1997;17:358–367.

Lynch SE, Williams RC, Polson AM, et al. A combination of platelet-derived and insulin-like growth factors enhanced periodontal regeneration. *J Clin Periodontol*. 1989;16:545–548.

Mariotti A. Efficacy of chemical root surface modifiers in the treatment of periodontal disease. A systematic review. *Ann Periodontol*. 2003;8:205–226.

Marx RE, Carlson ER, Eichstaedt RM, et al. Platelet-rich plasma: growth factor enhancement for bone grafts. *Oral Surg Oral Med Oral Pathol Oral Radiol Endod*. 1998;85:638–646.

McClain PK, Schallhorn RG. Long-term assessment of combined osseous composite grafting, root conditioning, and guided tissue regeneration. *Int J Periodontics Restorative Dent*. 1993;13:9–27.

Mellonig JT. Enamel matrix derivative for periodontal reconstructive surgery: technique and clinical and histologic case report. *Int J Periodont Restor Dent*. 1999;19:8–19.

Mellonig JT. Freeze-dried bone allografts in periodontal reconstructive surgery. *Dent Clin North Am*. 1991;35:505–520.

Mellonig JT. Human histologic evaluation of a bovine-derived bone xenograft in the treatment of periodontal osseous defects. *Int J Periodont Restor Dent*. 2000;20:19–29.

Miller PD Jr, Allen EP. The development of periodontal plastic surgery. *Periodontol 2000*. 1996;2:7–17.

Miller PD Jr. Regenerative and reconstructive periodontal plastic surgery. *Dent Clin North Am*. 1988;32:287–306.

Murphy KG, Gunsolley JC. Guided tissue regeneration for the treatment of periodontal intrabony and furcation defects. A systematic review. *Ann Periodontol*. 2003;8:266–302.

Nyman S, Lindhe J, Karring T, et al. New attachment following surgical treatment of human periodontal disease. *J Clin Periodontol*. 1982;9:290–296.

Ochsenbein C. A primer for osseous surgery. *Int J Periodont Restor Dent*. 1986;6:8–47.

Okuda K, Momose M, Miyazaki A, et al. Enamel matrix derivative in the treatment of human intrabony osseous defects. *J Periodontol*. 2000;71:1821–1828.

Oreamuno S, Lekovic V, Kenney EB, et al. Comparative clinical study of porous hydroxyapatite and decalcified freeze-dried bone in human periodontal defects. *J Periodontol*. 1990;61:399–404.

Palcanis KG. Surgical pocket therapy. *Ann Periodontol*. 1996;1:589–617.

Papapanou PN, Tonetti MS. Diagnosis and epidemiology of periodontal osseous lesions. *Periodontol 2000*. 2000;22:8–21.

Polson A, Ladenheim S, Hanes P. Cell and fiber attachment to demineralized dentin from periodontitis-affected root surfaces. *J Periodontol*. 1986;57:235–246.

Ramfjord SP, Nissle RR. The modified Widman flap. *J Periodontol*. 1974;45:601–607.

Reynolds MA, Aichelmann-Reddy ME, Branch-Mays, Gunsolley JC. The efficacy of bone replacement grafts in the treatment of periodontal osseous effects: A systematic review. *Ann Periodontol*. 2003;8:227–265.

Rosenberg ES, Garber DA, Evian CI. Tooth lengthening procedures. *Compend Contin Educ Dent*. 1980;1:161–172.

Rummelhart JM, Mellonig JT, Gray JL, Towle HJ. A comparison of freeze-dried bone allograft and demineralized freeze-dried bone allograft in human periodontal osseous defects. *J Periodontol*. 1989;60:655–663.

Sachs HA, Farnoush A, Checchi L, Joseph CE. Current status of periodontal dressings. *J Periodontol*. 1984;55:689–696.

Sanders JJ, Sepe WW, Bowers GM, et al. Clinical evaluation of freeze-dried bone allograft in periodontal osseous defects. Part III. Composite freeze-dried bone allografts with and without autogenous bone grafts. *J Periodontol*. 1983;54:1–8.

Sanz M, Newman MG, Anderson L, et al. Clinical enhancement of post-periodontal surgical therapy by a 0.12 per cent chlorhexidine gluconate mouthrinse. *J Periodontol*. 1989;60:570–576.

Schallhorn RG, McClain PK. Combined osseous grafting, root conditioning and guided tissue regeneration. *Int J Periodontics Restorative Dent*. 1988;4:8–31.

Scheyer ET, Velasquez-Plata D, Brunsvold MA, et al. A clinical comparison of a bovine-derived xenograft used alone and in combination with enamel matrix derivative for the treatment of periodontal osseous defects in humans. *J Periodontol*. 2002;73:423–432.

Schwartz Z, Mellonig JT, Carnes DL, et al. Ability of commercial demineralized freeze-dried bone allograft to induce new bone formation. *J Periodontol*. 1996;67:918–926.

Sculean A, Barbe G, Chiantella GC, et al. Clinical evaluation of an enamel matrix protein derivative combined with a bioactive glass for the treatment of intrabony periodontal defects in humans. *J Periodontol*. 2002;73:401–408.

Sculean A, Donos N, Blaes A, et al. Comparison of enamel matrix proteins and bioabsorbable membranes in the treatment of intrabony periodontal defects. A split-mouth study. *J Periodontol*. 1999;70:255–262.

Sepe WW, Bowers GM, Lawrence JJ, et al. Clinical evaluation of freeze-dried bone allografts in periodontal osseous defects-Part II. *J Periodontol*. 1978;49:9–14.

Shaffer CD, App G. The use of plaster of Paris in treating infrabony periodontal defects in humans. *J Periodontol*. 1971;42:685–690.

Shigeyama Y, D'Errico JA, Stone R, Somerman MJ. Commercially prepared allograft material has biological activity in vitro. *J Periodontol*. 1995;66:478–487.

Simion M, Trisi P, Maglione M, Piettelli A. Bacterial penetration in vitro through GTAM membrane with and without topical chlorhexidine application. A light and scanning election microscopic study. *J Clin Periodontol*. 1995;22:321–331.

Smith BA, Echeverri M. The removal of pocket epithelium: a review. *J West Soc Periodontol*. 1984;32:45–59.

Smith DH, Ammons WF, Van Belle G. A longitudinal study of periodontal status comparing osseous recontouring with flap curettage. 1. Results after six months. *J Periodontol*. 1980;51:367–375.

Snyder AJ, Levin MP, Cutright DE. Alloplastic implants of tricalcium phosphate ceramic in human periodontal osseous defects. *J Periodontol*. 1984;55:273–277.

Sottosanti JS. Calcium sulfate: a biodegradable and a biocompatible barrier for guided tissue regeneration. *Compend Contin Educ Dent*. 1992;13:226–228.

Stahl SS, Froum SJ. Histologic healing responses in human vertical lesions following the osseous allografts and barrier membranes. *J Clin Periodontol*. 1991;18:149–152.

Tal H, Moses O, Zohar R, et al. Root coverage of advanced gingival recession: A comparative study between acellular dermal matrix allograft and subepithelial connective tissue grafts. *J Periodontol*. 2002;73:1404–1411.

Tarnow DP. Semilunar coronally positioned flap. *J Clin Periodontol*. 1986;13:182–185.

Tibbetts LS, Shanelec D. Periodontal microsurgery. *Dent Clin North Am*. 1998;42(2):339–359.

Trejo PM, Weltman R, Caffesse RG. Guided tissue regeneration. A status report for the American Journal of Dentistry. *Am J Dentistry*. 1995;8:313–319.

Urist MR, Sato K, Brownell TI, et al. Human bone morphogenetic protein (hBMP). *Proc Soc Exp Biol Med*. 1983;173:194–199.

Wagenberg BD, Eskow RN, Langer B. Exposing adequate tooth structure for restorative dentistry. *Int J Periodontics Restorative Dent*. 1989;9:323–331.

Weltman R, Trojo PM, Morrison E, Caffesse R. Assessment of guided tissue regeneration procedures in intrabony defects with bioabsorbable and non-reabsorbable barriers. *J Periodontol.* 1997;68:582–590.

Wennstrom J. Regeneration of gingiva following surgical excision. A clinical study. *J Clin Periodontol.* 1983;10:287–297.

Wennstrom JL. Mucogingival therapy. *Ann Periodontol.* 1996;1:671–701.

Wylam JM, Mealey BL, Mills MP, et al. The clinical effectiveness of open versus closed scaling and root planing on multi-rooted teeth. *J Periodontol.* 1993;64:1023–1028.

Yukna RA, Mellonig JT. Histologic evaluation of periodontal healing in humans following regenerative therapy with enamel matrix derivative. *J Periodontol.* 2000;71:752–759.

Zhang M, Powers RM, Wolfinbarger L. A quantitative assessment of osteoinductivity of human demineralized bone matrix. *J Periodontol.* 1997;68:1085–1092.

Chapter 31

Maintenance for the Periodontal Patient

Learning Objectives

- Explain the term periodontal maintenance.

- List three objectives of periodontal maintenance.

- Describe how periodontal maintenance relates to other phases of periodontal treatment.

- Name usual procedures performed during a patient appointment for periodontal maintenance.

- Define the term baseline data.

- Describe guidelines for determining whether the general practice office or the periodontal office should provide periodontal maintenance for a particular patient.

- Describe how to establish an appropriate maintenance interval.

- Define the term recurrence of periodontitis.

- List clinical signs of recurrence of periodontitis.

- List reasons for recurrence of periodontitis.

- Explain the term compliance.

- Define the terms compliant patient and noncompliant patient

- List reasons for noncompliance with periodontal maintenance recommendations.

- List strategies that can be used to improve patient compliance.

- Explain the term root caries.

- List recommendations for use of fluorides in the prevention of root caries.

Key Terms

Periodontal maintenance
Baseline data
Recurrence of periodontitis
Refractory periodontitis
Compliance

Compliant patient
Noncompliant patient
Root caries
Caries management by risk assessment
   (CAMBRA)

Section 1
Introduction to Periodontal Maintenance

1. **Overview and Objectives of Periodontal Maintenance**
   A. **Definition.** Periodontal maintenance refers to continuing patient care provided by the dental team to help the periodontitis patient maintain periodontal health following complete nonsurgical or surgical periodontal therapy.
      1. Though periodontal maintenance is the preferred term, other terms that have been used for the periodontal maintenance phase of treatment are supportive periodontal therapy (SPT) and periodontal recall.
      2. Periodontal maintenance is performed on both natural teeth and dental implants and occurs at specific intervals throughout the life of the dentition or implants.
   B. **Importance of Periodontal Maintenance**
      1. Periodontal maintenance is one of the most important phases of periodontal treatment.
         a. With good periodontal maintenance, most periodontitis patients can retain their teeth and implants in function and comfort throughout their lives.
         b. In the absence of periodontal maintenance, patients usually exhibit a decrease in self-care and a recurrence of periodontitis.
         c. Periodontal maintenance can be successful regardless of the specific type of periodontal surgical treatment needed by the patient.
      2. The success of periodontal maintenance in reducing tooth loss is well documented in the literature. Figure 31-1 illustrates some of the outcomes possible with periodontal maintenance.
         a. Periodontitis is a chronic disease that *cannot be totally cured with the therapies currently available* to the dental team. Periodontitis can be *controlled*, however, in the vast majority of patients with this condition.
         b. Unfortunately among those patients treated for periodontitis, the disease tends to recur, and constant vigilance is needed on the part of the dental team to keep periodontitis under control.
         c. In most dental teams the dental hygienist is the primary healthcare provider for much of the maintenance phase of treatment.

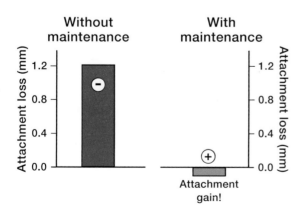

Figure 31.1. Attachment Loss With and Without Maintenance. A study by Axelsson and Lindhe assessed the efficacy of a periodontal maintenance care program to prevent the recurrence of disease in patients treated for advanced periodontitis. Patients who were not in a periodontal maintenance program had progressive attachment loss over a 6-year period. Similar patients in the study who were placed on maintenance care every 2 to 3 months over the 6-year period exhibited some attachment gain. (Data from Axelsson P, Lindhe L. The significance of maintenance care in the treatment of periodontal disease. *J Clin Periodontol.* 1981;8:281–294.)

C. **Objectives of Periodontal Maintenance.** There are several overlapping objectives of periodontal maintenance in the treated periodontitis patient; examples of these objectives are discussed below and are summarized in Box 31-1.

1. One objective for periodontal maintenance is to control inflammation in the periodontium by controlling etiologic risk factors.

   a. Of course, the primary risk factor for inflammatory periodontal disease is bacterial plaque biofilm.

      1) In spite of a patient's best self-care efforts, it is common for plaque biofilms to form in some sites and for some calculus to reform. Periodic professional plaque biofilm and calculus removal is an important part of periodontal maintenance.

      2) It is common for a patient's self-care efforts to become less effective over time. Reinforcement or improvement of self-care techniques is also an important part of periodontal maintenance.

   b. Secondary risk factors for inflammatory periodontal diseases include plaque biofilm–retentive areas (such as restorations with overhangs), smoking, and certain systemic factors.

      1) Whereas these secondary risk factors are always addressed as part of nonsurgical periodontal therapy, the condition of most patients changes over time. For example, restorative dental procedures can alter plaque biofilm–retentive sites or a patient's systemic condition can change over time.

      2) Continuing reassessment of the impact of secondary risk factors is also an important part of periodontal maintenance.

2. A second objective for periodontal maintenance is to preserve attachment levels over time. Attachment loss is the hallmark feature of periodontitis, and stabilizing attachment levels in most treated periodontitis patients requires ongoing periodontal maintenance.

3. A third objective for periodontal maintenance is to preserve alveolar bone levels. This objective overlaps with the objective of stabilizing attachment levels, but it is listed here for completeness.

4. *It should be noted that the term periodontal maintenance applies specifically to treated periodontitis patients. It is normally not appropriate to use the term periodontal maintenance for patients treated for other conditions such as those treated for the various types of gingivitis.*

Box 31-1. Objectives of Periodontal Maintenance

- Control inflammation in the periodontium
- Preserve tooth attachment levels
- Maintain alveolar bone levels

The expected outcome of achieving these objectives is to maintain the dentition throughout the life of the patient

D. Patient-Clinician Roles in Periodontal Maintenance

1. Periodontal maintenance is a team effort that requires commitment from everyone involved. The periodontal maintenance team includes the members of the dental team plus the patient and occasionally other healthcare providers such as the patient's physician.

2. Periodontal maintenance requires considerable effort from the patient in sustaining meticulous self-care and cooperating with regular ongoing professional periodontal maintenance care. Patients must be made aware of the need for this ongoing effort even prior to receiving nonsurgical periodontal therapy.

3. In addition, periodontal maintenance requires considerable effort on the part of the dental health team for professional care at regular intervals, renewal of patient motivation, instruction in self-care techniques, and elimination or reduction of primary and secondary risk factors.

2. **Relationship of Periodontal Maintenance to Other Phases of Therapy.** It is important for a clinician to understand how periodontal maintenance for a periodontitis patient relates to the other phases of comprehensive periodontal therapy; these phases are outlined below and are summarized in Figure 31-2.

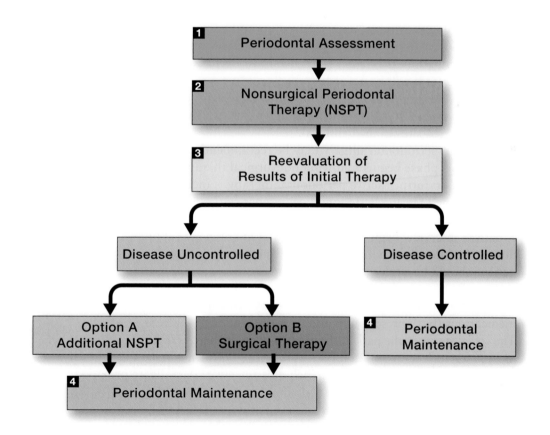

Figure 31.2. Relationship of Periodontal Maintenance to Other Phases of Periodontal Therapy. This flow chart outlines the normal sequence of periodontal therapy for a patient and illustrates where periodontal maintenance falls in the sequence.

Section 2
Procedures and Planning for Periodontal Maintenance

1. **Overview of Periodontal Maintenance Procedures.** Successful periodontal maintenance requires the active participation of the patient as well as all members of the dental team. In most dental offices the dental hygienist plays a major role in procedures performed during periodontal maintenance. A typical patient office visit for periodontal maintenance includes procedures discussed below and outlined in TABLE 31-1.
   A. **Assessment and Nonsurgical Periodontal Therapy**
      1. Comprehensive periodontal therapy always begins with a thorough clinical periodontal assessment. This assessment includes gathering data that results in a periodontal diagnosis and a plan for nonsurgical periodontal therapy.
      2. The second major phase in comprehensive periodontal therapy is nonsurgical periodontal therapy. During this phase of treatment, the dental team performs all the necessary nonsurgical measures to bring the existing periodontitis under control.
   B. **Reevaluation Following Nonsurgical Therapy.** Following nonsurgical periodontal therapy, a reevaluation of the patient's status is performed with a particular emphasis on the results obtained from nonsurgical therapy.
      1. As discussed in previous chapters, based upon the findings of this reevaluation, additional therapy such as periodontal surgery might be recommended.
      2. At the reevaluation, the dental team also must decide what periodontal maintenance care will be needed.
      3. For most patients periodontal maintenance will begin following this reevaluation since in many patients no further active therapy is needed at least in selected sites in the dentition.
      4. Even though periodontal surgery may be recommended in some sites, the maintenance phase begins following nonsurgical therapy at least for those sites where no further active periodontal therapy is indicated.
2. **Procedures Performed During Periodontal Maintenance**
   A. **Patient Interview**
      1. A patient interview begins each periodontal maintenance appointment; during the interview changes in the medical, social, or dental status of the patient should be explored and documented.
      2. During the update of the medical status, new illnesses or changes in the medical status must be identified. It is always critical to identify current medications (both prescription and over-the-counter).
      3. The social status of the patient should be updated; changes in lifestyle, bereavement, and work status are examples of important elements in the social history.
      4. The patient interview should also include a review of dental care provided by other clinicians since the previous maintenance visit.
      5. In addition, the patient interview should clarify the patient's perception of her/his oral status including the patient's thoughts about problems encountered during self-care efforts.
   B. **Clinical Assessment**
      1. Following the patient interview, a thorough clinical assessment should be performed. Results of the clinical assessment should then be compared with previous baseline data. The term baseline data refers to clinical data gathered at the beginning of the periodontal treatment that is subsequently used for comparison. Baseline values are first established during the initial assessment phase and again following initial periodontal therapy.

TABLE 31-1. Procedures Performed During Periodontal Maintenance

Procedure	Indicators or Risk Factors for Disease
Patient interview	New illnesses such as diabetes
	Change in medical status
	Changes in medications
	Smoking
Clinical assessment	Tooth loss since last charting
	Oral lesions
	Overhangs, poorly contoured restorations
	Tissue damage from removable prosthesis
	Radiographic evidence of progressing bone loss
	Inflammation in periodontium
	Deepening probing depths
	Increased loss of attachment
	Presence of bleeding on probing
	Presence of furcation involvement
	Increasing mobility
	Progressive recession of the gingival margin
	Minimal keratinized gingiva
	Occlusal contributing factors
Evaluation of effectiveness of self-care	Lack of manual dexterity
	Discontinued use of self-care methods
	Open embrasure spaces
Identification of treatment needs	
Periodontal instrumentation	
Patient counseling	
Application of fluorides	

2. The actual clinical assessment usually includes steps such as those listed below.
   a. Extraoral and intraoral examination
   b. Dental examination
   c. Radiographic examination if indicated
   d. Periodontal examination including the following features:
      1) Probing depths
         a) Probing depths should be recorded with the same attention to detail that was employed during the initial examination.
         b) Disease progression (continuing attachment loss) should be suspected when a 2-mm increase in probing depth is noted at a site.
      2) Bleeding on probing
         a) When present, bleeding on probing is generally visible within 10 seconds after gentle periodontal probing.
         b) Research suggests that after a few years of maintenance, a high frequency of bleeding on probing is a predictor of increased risk for progressive attachment loss.
         c) Bleeding sites should be charted because these sites may need more attention during periodontal instrumentation.

3) Attachment level
  a) Attachment levels should be recorded at critical sites in the dentition.
  b) *The most reliable way to evaluate periodontal disease control is by sequential comparison of clinical attachment level measurements.*
  c) Disease progression is indicated by a 2-mm increase in clinical attachment loss at a specific site as measured with a manual periodontal probe.

4) Tooth mobility
  a) In the assessment of tooth mobility, mobility can be stable or increasing. Increasing mobility over time is one of the important clinical features to note.
  b) The more severe the mobility measured in a tooth, the greater the risk of eventual tooth loss.

5) Furcation involvement
  a) Periodontal disease control is more difficult in areas of furcation involvement.
  b) The more advanced the furcation involvement, the greater the risk of tooth loss over time.

6) Mucogingival involvement
7) Levels of plaque biofilm and calculus

C. **Evaluation of Effectiveness of Patient Self-Care Efforts**
  1. Patients often spend considerable time on self-care and justifiably expect to be informed about the effectiveness of their efforts.
    a. Plaque scores recorded after using a disclosing solution are good indications of the patient's level of self-care compliance, and disclosing solution can be used to allow patients to see bacterial plaque biofilm accumulation.
    b. Plaque scores may reveal that the patient is in need of renewed instruction in plaque biofilm control methods.
    c. Plaque scores should be documented to provide an objective record of the level of self-care at a particular time and to permit comparison over time.
  2. Plaque biofilm accumulation can be related to many factors; examples of these factors are listed below.
    a. Patients may lack the manual dexterity needed to carry out the self-care regimen that was recommended previously. When manual dexterity is a problem, alternative self-care techniques should be considered. Older patients can loose skills that they were perfectly capable of performing at a previous maintenance visit.
    b. It is common for patients to discontinue the use of one or more of the self-care methods recommended previously.
    c. Gingival recession or shrinkage may have occurred following periodontal surgery; introduction of new interdental aids may be indicated for plaque biofilm removal on proximal root surfaces.
  3. Special microbial monitoring may be indicated for selected high-risk patients.
    a. Occasionally microbial monitoring may be used to determine the specific periodontal pathogens before antimicrobial or other therapy is initiated.
    b. Examples of the types of microbial monitoring that have been used include bacterial culture and DNA analysis.

D. **Identification of Treatment Needs**
   1. It is a routine part of periodontal maintenance to perform thorough periodontal instrumentation to remove plaque biofilm and calculus, but other treatment needs can also be identified.
   2. Examples of other treatment needs can include local delivery of antimicrobials, restoration of dental caries, and reinstitution of active periodontal therapy (as discussed in a subsequent section of this chapter).
   3. Selective tooth polishing may be indicated for removal of tooth stains that are visible when the patient smiles.

E. **Periodontal Instrumentation**
   1. Periodic deplaquing and removal of calculus is one of the most important steps for periodontal disease control; the goal of periodontal debridement is to disrupt the subgingival biofilm and create an environment that is biologically acceptable to the tissues of the periodontium.
   2. Root instrumentation is accepted as the most important means of disrupting the subgingival biofilm.
      a. Following periodontal therapy, some patients will present for periodontal maintenance with little or no subgingival calculus deposits. In these patients, firm stroke pressure with the instrument against the tooth is not necessary and should be avoided.
      b. Conservation of root substance is an important goal during periodontal instrumentation.
         1) Ultrasonic instrumentation with a precision-thin tip has been shown to remove less root substance than hand instrumentation and offers the added benefit of the antimicrobial effect created by the vibrating ultrasonic tip.
         2) Plastic curets (such as those used to debride dental implants) can be effective for deplaquing root surfaces and minimize trauma to the root during maintenance care when no calculus is present.

F. **Patient Counseling**
   1. As already discussed, maintenance patients should always be counseled related to the effectiveness of self-care efforts since plaque biofilm control by the patient is a critical element in preventing recurrence of periodontitis.
      a. Failure to provide this information may give a patient the impression that the clinician is not truly interested in the patient's dental health status.
      b. Most patients will need some reinforcement of motivation for plaque biofilm control in addition to retraining in the complex skills involved.
      c. Pointing out areas where there is less redness, reduced bleeding, or decreased plaque biofilm accumulation is a positive way to motivate the patient to continue with his or her self-care.
   2. It is also wise to include counseling that explains the need for compliance with the periodontal maintenance regimen. Patient compliance with the periodontal maintenance regimen will always remain a problem area.
   3. Other counseling may be indicated for specific patients. Examples of counseling that may be needed are caries prevention counseling, smoking cessation, or dietary changes.

G. **Application of Fluorides**
   1. Routine professional application of fluoride treatments during periodontal maintenance care is normally indicated to promote remineralization, aid in the prevention of root caries, and aid in the control of dentinal hypersensitivity.

2. Research studies suggest that high concentrations of topical fluorides may also have some antimicrobial properties and may be of some benefit in decreasing plaque biofilm accumulation.

3. **Planning Related to Periodontal Maintenance**
    A. **Office Guidelines for Provision of Periodontal Maintenance.** A thoughtful dental team will discuss guidelines for how periodontal maintenance should be provided: either in the general dental practice office or by referral to a periodontal practice. This decision is of course dependent in part on the experience and comfort levels of the members of the dental team, but some general guidelines are outlined below.
        1. Patients who have been treated for mild chronic periodontitis can usually receive periodontal maintenance in a general dental practice.
        2. Patients who have been treated for moderate chronic periodontitis can usually be managed by alternating periodontal maintenance visits between the general dental practice and the periodontal practice.
        3. Patients with severe chronic periodontitis should receive periodontal maintenance in a periodontal practice. In addition, annual or semiannual visits should be scheduled with a general dentist who will provide restorative and other general dental care.
        4. Patients who have been treated for aggressive periodontitis should receive all periodontal therapy including periodontal maintenance in a periodontal practice. In addition, annual or semiannual visits should be scheduled with a general dentist who will provide restorative and other general dental care.
    B. **Establishing Appropriate Periodontal Maintenance Intervals**
        1. Establishing a periodontal maintenance interval that is appropriate for the patient is always challenging. The frequency of periodontal maintenance visits must be determined on an individual basis. Some factors to consider in determining the interval between maintenance visits include the following:
            a. Severity of Periodontitis. In general the more severe the periodontitis, the shorter the intervals should be between periodontal maintenance visits.
            b. Adequacy of Patient Self-Care. In general the more effective the patient's self-care, the less frequently the patient needs to be seen. For patients with less than optimal self-care the intervals between maintenance visits should be shorter.
            c. Host Response. Systemic or genetic factors may negatively affect the host response. For example, a patient who continues to smoke or one with poorly controlled diabetes should be seen at shorter intervals.
        2. An important guide for determining the frequency of maintenance care is based on the time interval for the repopulation of periodontal pathogens following thorough periodontal debridement.
            a. Studies indicate that following periodontal instrumentation the subgingival pathogens return to predebridement levels in 9 to 11 weeks in most patients.
            b. *Research evidence shows that periodontal maintenance should be performed at least every 3 months or less for the removal and disruption of subgingival periodontal pathogens.* This 3-month interval is the one most frequently recommended.
            c. Patients who receive frequent periodontal maintenance will experience less attachment loss and tooth loss than patients who have less frequent maintenance care.

C. **Recurrence of Periodontitis.** The members of the dental team should be alert for the need for re-treatment that may be identified at any time during periodontal maintenance. When periodontitis recurrence is identified, planning of the needed re-treatment can include several options.
   1. If inadequate patient self-care appears to be the fundamental cause of the disease recurrence, then nonsurgical therapy should be reinstituted followed by a reevaluation of the patient's periodontal status after an appropriate healing time.
   2. If there appears to be disease recurrence in limited individual sites in the presence of adequate patient self-care, treatment options include localized periodontal instrumentation, local delivery of antimicrobial agents, or localized surgical therapy.
   3. If there appears to be disease recurrence in multiple sites in the presence of adequate patient self-care, periodontal surgical therapy is frequently indicated.
   4. If generalized attachment loss has recurred, the systemic condition of the patient should be reassessed with emphasis on the possible need for periodontal surgical intervention.

Section 3
Disease Recurrence and Patient Compliance

1. **Recurrence of Periodontitis**
   A. **Introduction to Disease Recurrence.** The term recurrence of periodontitis refers to the return of the disease in a patient that has been previously, successfully treated for periodontitis.
      1. The term recurrence implies that the periodontitis was brought under control during nonsurgical periodontal therapy (or nonsurgical periodontal therapy plus periodontal surgery) and that the periodontitis is once again resulting in progressive attachment loss.
      2. Recurrence of periodontitis can occur at specific sites only. For example, it would be possible for a patient treated for periodontitis to experience disease recurrence on the mesial surface of a single premolar tooth and for all other teeth in the dentition to continue to show good disease control.
      3. In spite of having received excellent treatment, treated periodontitis patients are at risk for recurrence of periodontitis for the rest of their lives.
      4. One of the sites in a dentition that has been reported to be most susceptible to recurrence of periodontitis is in areas of furcation involvement.
   B. **Identification of Recurrence.** At present the most effective way to identify sites of recurrence of periodontitis (i.e., sites of progressive attachment loss) is through thorough periodic clinical assessments. Clinical signs of recurrence of periodontitis are listed in Box 31-2.

Box 31-2. Clinical Signs of Recurrence

- Progressive clinical attachment loss
- Pockets that get deeper over time
- Pockets that bleed upon probing

- Pockets that exhibit exudate
- Radiographic evidence of progressing bone loss
- Increasing tooth mobility

C. **Reasons for Disease Recurrence.** Periodontitis recurs in patients for a variety of reasons, and the dental team should be aware that it is not always possible to determine a specific reason for disease recurrence. However, the most common reasons for recurrence of periodontitis are:
1. Inadequate self-care by the patient
2. Incomplete professional treatment
   a. Incomplete periodontal instrumentation
   b. Failure to control all local risk factors
3. Failure to control systemic factors
4. Inadequate control of occlusal contributing factors
5. Improper periodontal surgical technique
6. Attempting to treat teeth with a poor prognosis

D. **Refractory Disease.** Unfortunately periodontitis in certain patients is difficult or impossible to control with current therapies in spite of the efforts of the most skilled clinicians.
1. The term refractory periodontitis refers to periodontitis that is resistant to control even with what appears to be appropriate therapy.
2. Referral to a periodontal practice is indicated when refractory periodontitis is suspected.

2. **Patient Compliance with Periodontal Maintenance Programs**
   A. **Overview of Patient Compliance.** Compliance is defined as the extent to which a person's behavior coincides with medical or health advice; compliance has also been called adherence or therapeutic alliance, but compliance is the most common term used in the literature.
   1. Patients are described as being compliant patients if the patients follow recommendations for healthcare advice. Examples of compliant patients would be a patient who faithfully takes antihypertensive medications as prescribed by a physician or a patient who cooperates in meeting regularly scheduled periodontal maintenance appointments as recommended by the dental team.
   2. Patients are described as being noncompliant patients if they do not follow recommendations for healthcare advice. Examples of noncompliant patients would be a patient that does not take medications daily to control diabetes as prescribed by a physician or a patient that does not follow instructions for performing daily self-care.
   B. **Patient Compliance with Periodontal Maintenance.** Periodontal maintenance requires that the patient faithfully adhere to a strict program of dental recall appointments several times each year and follow very specific recommendations for meticulous daily self-care.
   1. Patient compliance with most medical advice is poor, and it should not be surprising that patient compliance with periodontal maintenance is also poor.
   2. In one study involving an 8-year retrospective study of compliance exhibited by periodontal maintenance patients only 16% of the patients were classified as being fully compliant while 49% of the patients were classified as being erratic in their compliance. In the same study 34% of the patients never even participated in the periodontal maintenance recommended.
   3. Reasons for patient noncompliance with periodontal maintenance are complex, and those reasons can be different for each patient and for the same patient at different times.

4. Examples of some reasons that have been suggested for noncompliance with recommended programs of periodontal maintenance include the following.
   a. Patient fear of receiving any dental treatment
   b. The expense of the dental treatment involved in multiple dental appointments each year
   c. The low priority for dental care for some patients in the face of competing demands for time or financial resources
   d. Denial on the part of some patients related to the periodontal challenges they face
   e. Failure for some patients to understand the implications of noncompliance
   f. Perceived indifference on the part of dental healthcare providers

C. **Strategies of Improving Compliance.** The thoughtful dental team will adopt strategies for improving compliance with periodontal maintenance. Strategies for improving compliance are discussed below and outlined in Figure 31-3.
   1. Give patients printed self-care instructions that they can refer to at home.
      a. Place the instruction sheet in a plastic sheet protector, like those available for use in three-ring notebooks. These sheet protectors are readily available in office supply stores and are priced economically.
      b. Note the next periodontal maintenance appointment at the bottom of the instruction sheet.
      c. Supply instruction sheets that are translated into the patient's native language.
   2. Simplify self-care recommendations as much as possible.
      a. Patients often perceive self-care instructions as being difficult to follow and as time-consuming.
      b. Plaque biofilm control instructions should be as clear and as simple as possible while addressing the specific needs of the patient. The use of dental terminology should be avoided in patient discussions and replaced by words that are easily understood by the patient.
      c. A limited number of self-care aids should be recommended. Studies indicate that patients are less likely to comply with self-care when they are instructed to use multiple aids on a daily basis.
      d. Where possible, alternatives to traditional dental floss should be considered since compliance with flossing is poor.
   3. Vary the office approach to patient education and self-care instructions. Patients often complain about having to listen to the "same old lecture" from the dental hygienist at each periodontal maintenance appointment.
   4. Seek out patient concerns and provide opportunities for communication by asking patients open-ended questions. Examples of open-ended questions appear below.
      a. "What are your concerns about this suggestion or treatment?"
      b. "How do you think you will fit this self-care recommendation into your daily schedule?"
      c. "How would you compare using this powered flossing device to using traditional dental floss?"
   5. Accommodate the patient's needs whenever possible. A satisfied patient is more likely to comply with self-care and maintenance appointments.
   6. Keep patients fully informed about their periodontal condition.
      a. At each visit counsel the patients about their periodontal health status.
      b. Explain the benefits of having regularly scheduled periodontal maintenance visits and the risks of infrequent professional care.

7. Monitor compliance with the maintenance appointments and contact patients promptly when compliance seems to become a problem.
   a. Use a postcard or telephone call to remind the patient of upcoming appointments.
   b. Contact the patient when an appointment is missed. The sooner the patient is contacted after missing an appointment, the more likely he or she is to reschedule.
8. Provide positive feedback to patients as frequently as possible. Positive reinforcement can help improve compliance.
   a. Areas of improvement should be pointed out to the patient, such as less plaque biofilm, fewer bleeding sites, or less inflamed tissue.
   b. The patient should be complimented in front of other members of the dental team by describing how the patient's efforts have led to improved periodontal health.
   c. Positive reinforcement should be used to convey a motivational message rather than criticism.

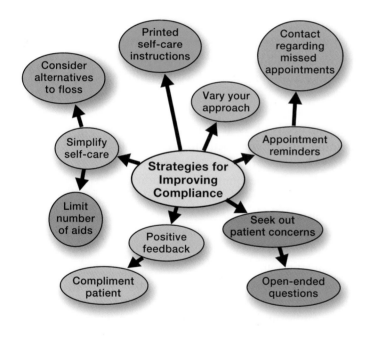

Figure 31.3. Suggestions for Improving Patient Compliance. An idea map of various strategies for improving patient compliance.

Section 4
Root Caries as a Complication During Maintenance

1. **Introduction to Root Caries**
   A. **Occurrence of Root Caries in Patients with Periodontitis**
      1. Whereas dental caries frequently occurs on enamel surfaces, the term root caries refers to tooth decay that occurs on the tooth root surfaces.
      2. According to the 1985–1986 United States Public Health Service (USPHS) survey of adults
         a. About half of the adults in the United States are afflicted with root surface caries by age 50.
         b. The percentage increases to 70% by age 60, with an average prevalence of about three lesions by age 70 [1].
      3. A 2004 systematic review on root caries incidence found that 23.7% of older adults *develop at least one new lesion annually* [2].
      4. Root caries occurs only if the root surface is exposed to the oral environment due to loss of attachment [3].
         a. In health, the root surface is protected by the periodontal attachment apparatus and is not exposed to the oral environment.
         b. The root may be exposed to the oral environment due to gingival recession or within a periodontal pocket.
   B. **Clinical Appearance**
      1. New root caries usually is seen as a shallow, softened area on the tooth root that is yellow to light brown in color. As the root caries progresses, it may develop a leather-like consistency. Older root caries lesions can appear brown to black. Figure 31-4 shows the typical clinical appearance of root caries.
      2. Root caries usually begins at or slightly coronal to the free gingival margin; the carious lesions can spread laterally and can even extend circumferentially around the root surface [4].
   C. **Etiology of Root Caries**
      1. No specific microorganisms have been proven to cause root caries.
         a. Root caries is most likely a mixed infection or a succession of bacterial populations.
         b. Mutans streptococci and *Lactobacillus* are associated with root caries.
         c. Recent studies, with few exceptions, fail to find association between *Actinomyces* and root caries [5].

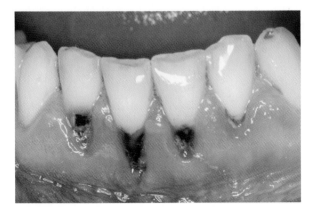

Figure 31.4. **Root Caries.** Root caries on the mandibular incisors of an individual with periodontitis. (Courtesy of Dr Richard J. Foster, Guilford Technical Community College, Jamestown, NC).

2. Like enamel caries, root caries requires a susceptible tooth surface, dental plaque biofilm, and time to initiate and progress. However, root caries differs from enamel caries in some aspects:
   a. Root surfaces are more vulnerable to demineralization than enamel surfaces. Root surfaces demineralize at a pH of 6.2 to 6.7 [6].
   b. Mineral loss for the root surface during the process of demineralization is up to 2.5 times greater than enamel [7].
3. Risk factors that have been reported for the development of root caries include attachment loss, inadequate patient self-care, cariogenic diet, infrequent dental visits, past caries experience, inadequate salivary flow, lack of fluoride exposure, and removable partial dentures.
4. In addition, individuals who have coronal caries are 2 to 3.5 times more likely to develop root caries [8].

2. **General Recommendations for the Prevention of Root Caries.** Root caries is a common problem in patients with periodontitis. Managing root caries from a restorative standpoint can be quite difficult, and the best strategy for managing root caries is to prevent the root caries from forming.

   A. **Prevention of Periodontitis.** The prevention of periodontitis and its associated attachment loss is the most effective way to prevent root caries. In patients with existing periodontal disease, prevention of further attachment loss will reduce the surface area susceptible to decay.

   B. **Fluoride for the Prevention of Root Caries**
   1. Root lesions can be arrested by remineralization. A 2007 systematic review of fluoride interventions for root caries concluded that fluoride appears to be a preventive and therapeutic treatment for root caries [9, 10].
   2. A variety of fluoride products can be helpful in preventing root caries. Figure 31-5 depicts some of these products.
      a. Fluoridated Drinking Water. Several studies have demonstrated that the presence of fluoridated drinking water throughout the lifetime of an individual reduces the development of root surface caries [11].
      b. Toothpaste
         1) The use of an 1,100 ppm sodium fluoride (NaF) dentifrice results in a significant decrease in root surface caries of 67% [12].
         2) A recent clinical trial demonstrated that prescription strength fluoride toothpaste, containing 5,000 ppm NaF, was effective in reversing root caries. About 57% of patients using the high strength dentifrice had reversal of root caries.
         3) Patients should avoid rinsing with large volumes of water after the use of fluoride toothpaste [13].
      c. Mouth rinses. Fluoride mouthrinses containing 0.05% NaF have been shown to significantly reduce root caries incidence [14].

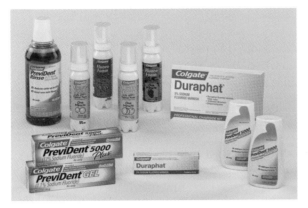

Figure 31.5. **Fluoride Products.** There are a variety of fluoride products for professional or home use that are helpful in the control of root caries. These include toothpastes, gels, foams, rinses, and varnishes. (Courtesy of Colgate-Palmolive Company.)

  d. Professional Application of Fluoride
    1) A large long-term clinical study showed that semiannual applications of 1.23% APF gel significantly reduced the formation of new root caries and the number of remineralized lesions was significantly increased by daily rinsing with a 0.05% NaF rinse [15].
    2) Fluoride varnish applied every 3 months has been shown to reduce new root caries formation by over 50% [16].
  C. **Antimicrobial and Supplemental Remineralization Therapies**
    1. Chlorhexidine has been shown to reduce dental caries and is effective in controlling mutans streptococci [17]. High and extreme caries risk adults should rinse with 10 mL of 0.12% chlorhexidine once daily for 1 week/month.
    2. Xylitol containing gums and mints are recommended for high and extreme caries risk patients. The therapeutic dose of xylitol is 6 to 10 g spread throughout the day.
    3. Casein phosphopeptide-amorphous calcium phosphate (CPP-ACP) pastes are recommended for extreme caries risk patients.
      a. The paste can be applied with a fingertip on a daily basis.
      b. Most research on CPP-ACP is laboratory based rather than in vivo. However, CPP-ACP may promote remineralization in patients with low salivary flow.
      c. A 2008 systematic review concluded that there is insufficient evidence to make conclusions regarding the effectiveness of CPP-ACP in preventing caries [18].
3. **Caries Management by Risk Assessment (CAMBRA)**
  A. **Caries Risk Assessment**
    1. Recent research clearly demonstrates that assigning caries risk assessment levels facilitates the effective management of patients for dental caries [19].
    2. Subsequent to this research, protocols for clinical management of caries risk factor level were developed and employed at a number of dental schools [20]. While complete consensus on these protocols continues to develop, there is strong agreement about treating patients for dental caries based on risk level [21].
    3. These protocols for clinical management of caries risk, known as "Caries Management by Risk Assessment (CAMBRA)" were published in the journal of the California Dental Association in 2007 [19,21].
    4. The CAMBRA protocols seek to provide practical clinical guidelines for managing dental caries based upon risk group assessment. The protocols are based upon the best evidence at this time and can be used in planning effective caries management for any patient.
    5. Caries experts and members of CAMBRA coalitions support implementation of the guidelines presented in Table 31-2 [19,21].

B. CAMBRA Treatment Recommendations

  1. A Caries Risk Assessment Form

   a. In 2002, a group of experts from across the United States produced a caries risk assessment form [22].

   b. In 2006, outcomes research based upon the use of the form in a large cohort of patients was published, validating the form [23]. The results from this study are the basis for the current version of the caries risk assessment form shown in Figure 31-6.

  2. Caries Risk Determination. Assigning a patient to a caries risk level is the first step in managing the disease process. Table 31-2 presents the four risk level groups (low, moderate, high, and extreme) and the recommendations for caries management procedures for each level.

   a. High caries risk is signified by the presence of any one of the following: visible cavities or radiographic penetration of the dentin, radiographic interproximal enamel lesions, white spots on smooth surfaces, or restorations in the last 3 years.

   b. Extreme caries risk is high caries risk and severe salivary gland hypofunction (salivary flow rate of <0.5 mL/min).

   c. Low or moderate caries risk is assigned based on clinical judgment following an evaluation of the risk factors and protective factors of the patient.

  3. Evidence-Based Treatment Plan. The next step is to develop an evidence-based treatment plan based upon the patient's risk level.

   a. Low risk patients should use fluoride toothpaste twice daily and professional topical fluoride applications are optional. Bacterial and salivary tests are not necessary. Most periodontal maintenance patients are not considered low risk because exposed roots is a primary risk factor for root caries.

   b. Moderate caries risk patients should use fluoride toothpaste twice daily, rinse with a 0.05% sodium fluoride mouthrinse, and receive fluoride varnish applications at maintenance appointments. Bacterial and salivary test are optional.

   c. High caries risk patients should use a prescription 1.1% sodium fluoride toothpaste twice daily and receive 1 to 3 fluoride varnish applications during initial therapy. Fluoride varnish should be applied at 3-month intervals. Bacterial and salivary tests are recommended.

   d. Extreme caries risk patients receive the same CAMBRA therapies as high risk. In addition baking soda rinses, 0.5% sodium fluoride rinses and calcium/phosphate pastes may be recommended.

Caries Risk Assessment Form - Children Age 6 and Over/Adults

Patient Name: _____ Chart #: _____ Date: _____

Assessment Date: Is this (please circle) base line   or   recall

Disease Indicators (Any one "YES" signifies likely "High Risk" and to do a bacteria test**)	YES = CIRCLE	YES = CIRCLE	YES = CIRCLE
Visible cavities or radiographic penetration of the dentin	YES		
Radiographic approximal enamel lesions (not in dentin)	YES		
White spots on smooth surfaces	YES		
Restorations last 3 years	YES		
Risk Factors (Biological or predisposing factors)			
MS and LB both medium or high (by culture**)		YES	
Visible heavy plaque on teeth		YES	
Frequent snack (>3x daily between meals)		YES	
Deep pits and fissures		YES	
Recreational drug use		YES	
Inadequate saliva flow by observation or measurement (***If measured, note the flow rate below)		YES	
Saliva reducing factors (medications/radiation/systemic)		YES	
Exposed roots		YES	
Orthodontic appliances		YES	
Protective Factors			
Lives/work/school flouridated community			YES
Fluoride toothpaste at least once daily			YES
Fluoride toothpaste at least 2x daily			YES
Fluoride mouthrinse (0.05% NaF) daily			YES
5,000 ppm F fluoride toothpaste daily			YES
Flouride varnish in last 6 months			YES
Office F topical in last 6 months			YES
Chlorhexidine prescribed/used one week each of last 6 months			YES
Xylitol gum/lozenges 4x daily last 6 months			YES
Calcium and phosphate paste during last 6 months			YES
Adequate saliva flow (>1ml/min stimulated)			YES
Bacteria/Saliva Test Results: MS: LB: Flow Rate: ml/min. Date:			

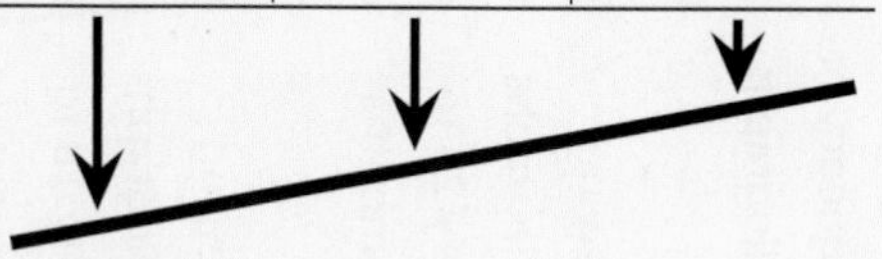

VISUALIZE CARIES BALANCE
(Use circled indicators/factors above)
(EXTREME RISK = HIGH RISK + SEVERE SALIVARY GLAND HYPOFUNCTION)
CARIES RISK ASSESSMENT (CIRCLE): EXTREME   HIGH   MODERATE   LOW

Signature: _____ Date: _____

Figure 31.6. Caries Risk Assessment Form. (Used with permission from Featherstone JD, et al. Caries risk assessment in practice for age 6 through adult. *J Calif Dent Assoc.* 2007;35(10); Table 1, p. 704.)

TABLE 31-2. CAMBRA: Clinical Guidelines

Risk Level[a,b]	Frequency of Radiographs	Frequency of Caries Recall	Saliva Test (Saliva Flow and Bacterial Culture)	Antibacterials Chlorhexidine Xylitol[c]	Fluoride	pH Control	Calcium Phosphate Topical Supplements
Low risk	Bitewing radiographs every 24 to 36 months	Every 6 to 12 months to reevaluate caries risk	May be done as a base line reference for new patients	Per saliva test if done	OTC fluoride-containing toothpaste twice daily; Optional NaF varnish if excessive root exposure or sensitivity	Not required	Not required; Optional for excessive root exposure or sensitivity
Moderate risk	Bitewing radiographs every 18 to 24 months	Every 4 to 6 months to reevaluate caries risk	May be done as a base line reference for new patients or if there is a suspicion of high bacterial challenge	Per saliva test if done; Xylitol (6 to 10g/day) of gum or candies	OTC fluoride-containing toothpaste twice daily plus 0.05% NaF rinse daily. Initially 1 to 2 applications of NaF varnish; 1 application at 4 to 6 month recall	Not required	Not required; Optional for excessive root exposure or sensitivity
High risk[d]	Bitewing radiographs every 6 to 18 months or until no cavitated lesions are evident	Every 3 to 4 months to reevaluate caries risk and apply fluoride varnish	Saliva flow test and bacterial culture initially and at every caries recall application to assess efficacy and patient cooperation	Chlorhexidine gluconate 0.12%; 10mL rinse for 1 minute daily for 1 week each month. Xylitol (6 to 10g/day)	1.1% NaF toothpaste twice daily instead of regular fluoride toothpaste; Optional 0.2% NaF rinse daily (One bottle) then OTC 0.05% NaF rinse 2× daily. Initially 1 to 3 applications of NaF varnish; 1 application at 3 to 4 month recall	Not required	Optional: apply calcium/phosphate paste several times daily
Extreme risk[e] (High risk plus dry mouth or special needs	Bitewing radiographs every 6 months or until no cavitated lesions are evident	Every 3 months to reevaluate caries risk and apply fluoride varnish	Saliva flow test and bacterial culture initially and at every caries recall appt. to assess efficacy and patient cooperation	Chlorhexidine gluconate 0.12% (preferably CHX in water base rinse) 10mL rinse for 1 minute daily for 1 week daily for 1 week each month. Xylitol (6 to 10g/day)	1.1% NaF toothpaste twice daily instead of regular fluoride toothpaste. OTC 0.05% NaF rinse when mouth feels dry, after snacking, breakfast, and lunch. Initially 1 to 3 applications NaF varnish; 1 application at 3 month recall	Acid neutralizing rinses as needed if mouth feels dry, after snacking, bedtime, and after breakfast. Baking soda gum as needed	Required. Apply calcium/phosphate paste twice daily

[a] For all risk levels: Patients must maintain good self-care and a diet low in frequency of fermentable carbohydrates.

[b] All restorative work to be done with minimally invasive philosophy in mind.

[c] Xylitol is not good for pets (especially dogs).

[d] Patients with one (or more) cavitated lesion(s) are high-risk patients.

[e] Patients with one (or more) cavitated lesion(s) and severe hyposalivation are extreme-risk patients. (Used with permission from Jenson L, et al. Clinical protocols for caries management by risk assessment. J Calif Dent Assoc. 2007;35(10); Table 1, p. 716.)

Chapter Summary Statement

Periodontal maintenance refers to continuing patient care provided by the dental team to help the periodontitis patient maintain periodontal health following complete nonsurgical or surgical periodontal therapy. In most dental offices the dental hygienist plays a major role in procedures performed during periodontal maintenance visits. Procedures in a typical office visit for periodontal maintenance include patient interview, clinical assessment, evaluation of effectiveness of self-care, identification of treatment needs, periodontal instrumentation, patient counseling, and application of fluorides. Currently the most frequently recommended interval for periodontal maintenance is every 3 months. Recurrence of periodontitis in treated patients with the need for additional active periodontal treatment is always a possibility. Patient compliance with periodontal maintenance recommendations is poor, but strategies can be employed to improve compliance. Root caries is a complication in many treated periodontitis patients.

Section 5
Focus On Patients

Case 1

Your dental team has just completed a reevaluation of the results of nonsurgical therapy for a patient with generalized slight chronic periodontitis. The findings of the reevaluation reveal that the periodontitis is under control and that periodontal maintenance is the next logical step. When should the first maintenance appointment be scheduled and what factors should be considered when assigning this maintenance interval?

Case 2

One of your dental team's chronic periodontitis patients has recently undergone periodontal surgery and now has several sites of gingival recession exposing tooth roots. Unfortunately, this patient has had a high incidence of both coronal and root caries over the past few years. What measures might your team take to minimize the risk of further root caries in this patient?

Case 3

A patient who has been treated for chronic periodontitis by your team has been followed for periodontal maintenance for more than 3 years. During each maintenance visit, there have been no indications of recurrence of the periodontitis. The patient calls you before her next maintenance visit to inform you that she has just been diagnosed with diabetes mellitus. She looked up diabetes on the internet and now wants to know if this will affect her periodontal condition. How should your dental team respond to the patient's concern?

References

1. Oral health of US adults: NIDR 1985 national survey. *J Public Health Dent*. 1987;47(4): 198–205.
2. Griffin SO, Griffin AM, Swann JL, et al. Estimating rates of new root caries in older adults. *J Dent Res*. 2004;83(8):634–638.
3. Brown LJ, Brunelle JA, Kingman A. Periodontal status in the United States, 1988–1991: prevalence, extent, and demographic variation. *J Dent Res*. 1996;75 Spec No:672–683.
4. Berry TG, Summitt JB, Sift Jr EJ. Root caries. *Oper Dent*. 2004;29(6):601–607.
5. Zambon JJ, Kasprzak SA. The microbiology and histopathology of human root caries. *Am J Dent*. 1995;8(6):323–328.
6. Atkinson JC, Wu AJ. Salivary gland dysfunction: causes, symptoms, treatment. *J Am Dent Assoc*. 1994;125(4):409–416.
7. Ogaard B, Arends J, Rolla G. Action of fluoride on initiation of early root surface caries in vivo. *Caries Res*. 1990;24(2):142–144.
8. Papas A, Joshi A, Giunta J. Prevalence and intraoral distribution of coronal and root caries in middle-aged and older adults. *Caries Res*. 1992;26(6):459–465.
9. Heijnsbroek M, Paraskevas S, Van der Weijden GA. Fluoride interventions for root caries: a review. *Oral Health Prev Dent*. 2007;5(2):145–152.
10. Griffin SO, Regnier E, Griffin PM, Huntley V. Effectiveness of fluoride in preventing caries in adults. *J Dent Res*. 2007;86(5):410–415.
11. Brustman BA. Impact of exposure to fluoride-adequate water on root surface caries in elderly. *Gerodontics*. 1986;2(6):203–207.
12. Jensen ME, Kohout F. The effect of a fluoridated dentifrice on root and coronal caries in an older adult population. *J Am Dent Assoc*. 1988;117(7):829–832.
13. Sjogren K, Birkhed D. Factors related to fluoride retention after toothbrushing and possible connection to caries activity. *Caries Res*. 1993;27(6):474–477.
14. Ripa LW, Leske GS, Forte F, Varma A. Effect of a 0.05% neutral NaF mouthrinse on coronal and root caries of adults. *Gerodontology*. 1987;6(4):131–136.
15. Wallace MC, Retief DH, Bradley EL. The 48-month increment of root caries in an urban population of older adults participating in a preventive dental program. *J Public Health Dent*. 1993;53(3):133–137.
16. Schaeken MJ, Keltjens HM, Van Der Hoeven JS. Effects of fluoride and chlorhexidine on the microflora of dental root surfaces and progression of root-surface caries. *J Dent Res*. 1991;70(2):150–153.
17. Anderson MH. A review of the efficacy of chlorhexidine on dental caries and the caries infection. *J Calif Dent Assoc*. 2003;31(3):211–214.
18. Azarpazhooh A, Limeback H. Clinical efficacy of casein derivatives: a systematic review of the literature. *J Am Dent Assoc*. 2008;139(7):915–924; quiz 994–995.
19. Featherstone JD, et al. Caries risk assessment in practice for age 6 through adult. *J Calif Dent Assoc*. 2007;35(10):703–707, 710–713.
20. Young DA, Featherstone JD, Roth JR. Curing the silent epidemic: caries management in the 21st century and beyond. *J Calif Dent Assoc*. 2007;35(10):681–685.
21. Jenson L, Budenz AW, Featherstone JD, Ramos-Gomez FJ, et al. Clinical protocols for caries management by risk assessment. *J Calif Dent Assoc*. 2007;35(10):714–723.
22. Featherstone JD, Adair SM, Anderson MH, Berkowitz RJ, et al. Caries management by risk assessment: consensus statement, April 2002. *J Calif Dent Assoc*. 2003;31(3):257–269.
23. Domejean-Orliaguet S, Gansky SA, Featherstone JD. Caries risk assessment in an educational environment. *J Dent Educ*. 2006;70(12):1346–1354.

Suggested Readings

Ainamo J, Ainamo A. Risk assessment of recurrence of disease during supportive periodontal care. *J Clin Periodontol*. 1996;23:232–239.

American Academy of Periodontology. Position paper: Periodontal maintenance. *J Periodontol*. 2003;74:1395–1401.

Atkinson JC, Wu AJ. Salivary gland dysfunction: causes, symptoms, treatment. *J Am Dent Assoc*. 1994;125:409–416.

Axelsson P, Lindhe L. The significance of maintenance care in the treatment of periodontal disease. *J Clin Periodontol*. 1981;8:281–294.

Bardet P, Suvan J, Lang NP. Clinical effects of root instrumentation using conventional steel or non-tooth substance removing plastic curettes during supportive periodontal therapy (SPT). *J Clin Periodontol.* 1999;26:724–742.

Berry TG, Summitt JP, Sift EJ Jr, et al. Root caries. *Oper Dent.* 2004;29:601–607.

Brambilla E. Fluoride—is it capable of fighting old and new dental diseases? An overview of existing fluoride compounds and their clinical applications. *Caries Res.* 2001;35(Suppl 1):6–9.

Brown LJ, Brunelle JA, Kingman A. Periodontal status in the United States 1988–1991: prevalence, extent and demographic variation. *J Dent Res.* 1996;75(Special Issue):672–683.

Brustman BA. Impact of exposure to fluoride-adequate water on root surface caries in elderly. *Gerodontics.* 1986;2:203–207.

Claffey N, Nylund K, Keger R, et al. Diagnostic predictability of scores of plaque, bleeding, suppuration and probing depth for probing attachment loss. 3½ years of observation following initial periodontal therapy. *J Clin Periodontol.* 1990;17:108–114.

Dahlen G, Lindhe J, Sato K, et al. The effect of supragingival plaque control on the subgingival microbiota in subjects with periodontal disease. *J Clin Periodontol.* 1992;19:802–809.

De Vore CH, Duckworth JE, Beck FM, et al. Bone loss following periodontal therapy in subjects without frequent periodontal maintenance. *J Periodontol.* 1986;57:354–359.

Greenstein G. Periodontal response to mechanical non-surgical therapy: a review. *J Periodontol.* 1992;63:118–130.

Griffin SO, Griffin AM, Swann JL, et al. Estimating rates of new root caries in older adults. *J Dent Res.* 2004;83:634–638.

Haffajee AD, Socransky SS, Smith C, et al. Relation of baseline microbial parameters to future periodontal attachment loss. *J Clin Periodontol.* 1991;18:744–750.

Jensen ME, Kohout F. The effect of a fluoridated dentifrice on root and coronal caries in an older adult population. *J Am Dent Assoc.* 1988;117:829–832.

Lang NP, Joss A, Tonetti MS. Monitoring disease during supportive periodontal treatment by bleeding on probing. *Periodontol 2000.* 1996;12:44–48.

Lang NP, Nyman SR. Supportive maintenance care for patients with implants and advanced restorative therapy, *Periodontol 2000.* 1994;4:119–226.

Mazza JE, Newman MG, Sims TN. Clinical and antimicrobial effect of stannous fluoride on periodontitis. *J Clin Periodontol.* 1981;8:203–212.

McGuire MK. Prognosis versus actual outcome: a long-term survey of 100 treated periodontal patients under maintenance care. *J Periodontol.* 1991;62:51–58.

Mendoza AR, Newcomb GM, Nixon KC. Compliance with supportive periodontal therapy. *J Periodontol.* 1991;62:731–736.

National Institute of Dental Research (U.S.). *Epidemiology and Oral Disease Prevention Program, Oral health of United States adults: the National Survey of Oral Health in US. Employed Adults and Seniors, 1985–1986: National Findings.* NIH publication no. 87-2868. Bethesda: U.S. Department of Health and Human Services Public Service National Institutes of Health; 1987.

Øgaard B, Arends J, Rolla G. Action of fluoride on initiation of early root surface caries in vivo. *Caries Res.* 1990;24:142–144.

Pappas A, Koski A, Giunta J. Prevalence and intraoral distribution of coronal and root caries in middle-aged and older adults. *Caries Res.* 1992;26:459–465.

American Academy of Periodontology. Parameters of care. *J Periodontol.* 2000;71(5 Suppl):i–ii, 847–883.

Ripa LJ, Leske GS, Forte F, et al. Effect of a 0.05% neutral NaF mouthrinse on coronal and root caries in adults. *Gerodontology.* 1987;6:131–136.

Ryan RJ. The accuracy of clinical parameters in detecting periodontal disease activity. *J Am Dent Assoc.* 1985;111:753–760.

Schaeken MJM, Keltjens HMAM, van der Hoeven JS. Effect of fluoride and chlorhexidine on the microflora of dental root surfaces. *J Dent Res.* 1991;70:150–153.

Shiloah J, Patters MR. Repopulation of periodontal pockets by microbial pathogens in the absence of supportive therapy. *J Periodontol.* 1996;67:130–139.

Sjogren K, Birkhed D. Factors related to fluoride retention after use of fluoride. *Caries Res.* 1993;27:474–477.

Slots J. Subgingival microflora and periodontal disease. *J Clin Periodontol.* 1979;6:351–382.

ten Cate JM. Consensus statements on fluoride usage and associated research questions. *Caries Res.* 2001;35(Suppl):71–73.

Wallace MC, Retief DH, Bradley EL. The 48-month increment of root caries in an population of older adults participating in a preventive dental program. *J Public Health Dent.* 1993;53:133–137.

Wilson TG Jr, Glover ME, Schoen J, et al. Compliance with maintenance therapy in a private periodontal practice. *J Periodontol.* 1984;55:468–473.

Wilson TG Jr, Glover ME, Malik AK, et al. Tooth loss in maintenance patients in a private periodontal practice. *J Periodontol.* 1987;58:231–235.

Wilson TG Jr. Compliance: a review of the literature with possible applications to periodontics. *J Periodontol.* 1987;58:706–714.

Wilson TG, Kornman KS. Retreatment. *Periodontol 2000.* 1996;12:119–121.

Wilson TG: Maintaining periodontal treatment. *J Am Dent Assoc.* 1990;121:491–494.

Zambon JJ, Kasprzak SA. The microbiology and histopathology of human root caries. *Am J Dent.* 1995;8:323–328.

Zero DT, Raubertas RF, Fu J, et al. Fluoride concentrations in plaque, whole saliva, and ductal saliva after application of home-use topical fluorides. *J Dent Res.* 1992;71:1768–1775.

Chapter 32

Maintenance of the Dental Implant Patient

Learning Objectives

- Define the term dental implant and describe the components of a typical dental implant and restoration.

- Define the term peri-implant tissues.

- Compare and contrast the periodontium of a natural tooth with the peri-implant tissues that surround a dental implant.

- Define the terms osseointegration and biomechanical forces as they apply to dental implants.

- Compare and contrast the terms peri-implant mucositis and peri-implantitis.

- Discuss the special considerations for periodontal instrumentation of a dental implant.

- Describe an appropriate maintenance interval for a patient with dental implants.

- In the clinical setting, select appropriate self-care aids for a patient with dental implants.

Key Terms

Dental implant
Implant body
Implant abutment
Biocompatible
Peri-implant tissues

Biological seal
Osseointegration
Peri-implant mucositis
Peri-implantitis
Biomechanical forces

Section 1
Anatomy of the Dental Implant

A **dental implant** is a nonbiologic (artificial) device surgically inserted into the jawbone to (1) replace a missing tooth or (2) provide support for a prosthetic denture. Over the past 30 years, research has validated the success of implant placement as a feasible option to replace missing teeth in partially or fully edentulous patients [1–7]. The dental hygienist plays an important role in patient education and professional maintenance of the dental implant. Understanding the basic concepts of implantology and the anatomy of the peri-implant tissues is a prerequisite to understanding the maintenance of dental implants.

1. **The Dental Implant System**
   A. **Introduction to Dental Implant Systems.** Dental implant systems are used to replace individual teeth or support a fixed bridge or removable denture (FIG. 32-1). The components of a dental implant system are the (1) implant body, (2) abutment, and (3) a prosthetic crown or prosthesis (FIG. 32-2).
   B. **The Implant Body**
      1. An **implant body** is the portion of the implant system that is surgically placed into the living alveolar bone (FIG. 32-3, 32-4, 32-5). This is sometimes referred to as the implant fixture or implant.
      2. The implant body acts as the "root" of the implant restoration. The implant body usually is threaded like a screw. These threads provide a greater surface area for contact with the alveolar bone.
         a. The metal used for dental implants is titanium. Titanium is an ideal material for dental implants because it is a bone-friendly metal that is biocompatible and because it is a poor conductor of heat and electricity.
         b. The major disadvantage of titanium is that it is softer than other dental restorative metals and thus it scratches easily.
   C. **The Abutment**
      1. The **implant abutment** is a titanium post that attaches to the implant body and protrudes partially or completely through the gingival tissue into the mouth (FIG. 32-4).
      2. The abutment supports the restorative prosthesis (crown or denture).
      3. The titanium abutment is extremely **biocompatible** (not rejected by the body) and allows tissue healing around the abutment.

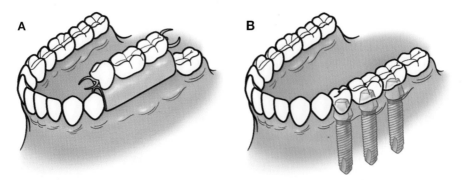

Figure 32.1. Replacement of Missing Teeth. A: Extracted teeth replaced by a traditional removable partial denture. B: Missing teeth replaced by three individual dental implants.

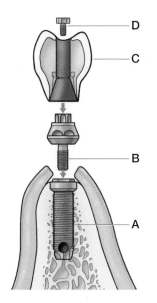

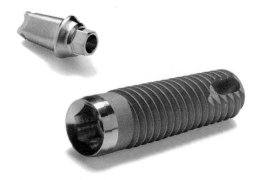

Figure 32.2. **The Dental Implant System**. The components of a dental implant system are the implant body (A) and the abutment (B). The implant body is placed into living alveolar bone. The abutment extends into or through living gingival tissue into the mouth. A crown (C) or prosthesis is connected to the abutment either by a screw (D) or by dental cement.

Figure 32.3. **Implants and Components**. An example of a titanium implant screw and abutment. (Used with permission ©2009 Zimmer Dental Inc. All rights reserved.)

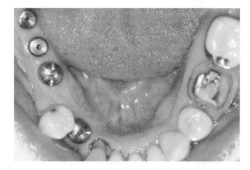

Figure 32.4. **Abutments**. This photograph shows the healing abutments for four implants. (Courtesy of Dr John S. Dozier, DMD, MSD, Tallahassee, FL.)

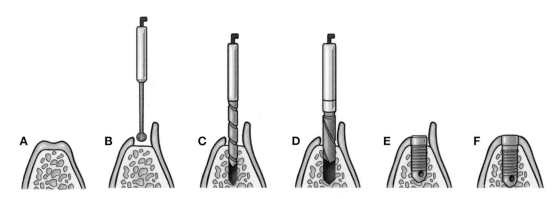

Figure 32.5. **Surgical Placement of Dental Implants**. A: Edentulous alveolar ridge. B: Initial osteotomy site established. C, D: Drills of increasing diameters used to prepare osteotomy to the size of the planned implant. E: Implant body seated in the osteotomy. The top of the implant body may be slightly above, level with, or slightly below the crest of the bone. F: Implant body seated in bone with cover screw attached. At the end of placement surgery, the implant can be covered with gingiva or left exposed to the oral cavity, as shown here. A healing time of several weeks to months is allowed so that osseointegration can occur.

2. The Peri-implant Tissues. The peri-implant tissues are the tissues that surround the dental implant (FIG. 32-6). The peri-implant tissues are similar in many ways to the periodontium of a natural tooth, but there are some important differences (TABLE 32-1).

   A. Implant-to-Epithelial Tissue Interface

      1. The epithelium adapts to the titanium abutment post, creating a biological seal. The union of the epithelial cells to the implant surface is very similar to that of the epithelial cells to the natural tooth surface.

      2. The biological seal functions as a barrier between the implant and the oral cavity.

      3. As with a natural tooth, a sulcus lined by sulcular epithelium and junctional epithelium surrounds the abutment or in some cases, the top of the implant body.

   B. Implant-to-Connective Tissue Interface

      1. *The implant-to-connective tissue interface is significantly different from that of connective tissue of a natural tooth.*

      2. The implant surface lacks cementum, so the gingival fibers and the periodontal ligament cannot insert into the titanium surface as they do into the cementum of a natural tooth.

         a. On a natural tooth:

            1) The supragingival fibers brace the gingival margin against the tooth and strengthen the attachment of the junctional epithelium to the tooth. The supragingival fibers insert into the cementum.

            2) The periodontal ligament suspends and maintains the tooth in its socket.

            3) The periodontal ligament fibers also serve as a physical barrier to bacterial invasion.

         b. On an implant:

            1) The connective tissue fiber bundles support the healthy gingiva against the abutment. The connective tissue fiber bundles in the gingiva around an implant have been shown to be either (1) oriented parallel to the implant surface or (2) encircling the implant abutment [8]. The fibers do not attach to the dental implant.

            2) There are no periodontal ligament fibers to provide protection for the dental implant. *Therefore, periodontal pathogens can destroy bone much more rapidly along a dental implant than along a natural tooth with its protective barrier of periodontal ligament fibers* [9–12].

      3. Keratinized gingival tissue may or may not be present around the dental implant.

   C. Implant-to-Bone Interface

      1. Osseointegration is the direct contact of the living bone with the surface of the implant body (with no intervening periodontal ligament). Osseointegration is a major requirement for implant success.

      2. Clinically, osseointegration is regarded as successful if there is

         a. An absence of clinical mobility of the implant

         b. An absence of gingival inflammation of peri-implant tissues

         c. No discomfort or pain when the implant is in function

         d. No increased bone loss or radiolucency surrounding the dental implant on a radiograph

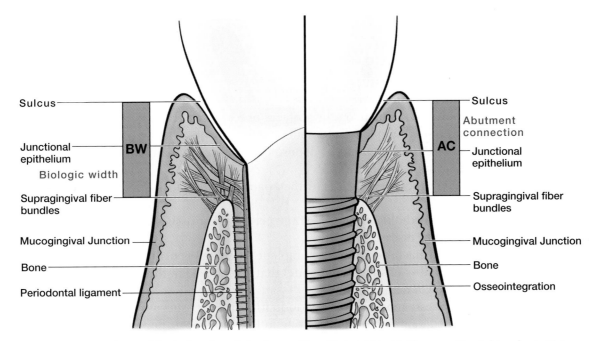

Figure 32.6. Comparison of Periodontium Interface with a Natural Tooth Versus a Dental Implant. Note that the interface between a tooth and the periodontium differs from the interface between an implant and the periodontium. The implant lacks the periodontal ligament connection to the alveolar bone and the gingival fibers do not insert into the titanium.

TABLE 32-1. Tissues Surrounding a Dental Implant	
Tissues	**Peri-implant Tissues**
Junctional epithelium	Attaches to the implant surface or abutment surface (biologic seal)
Connective tissue fibers	Run parallel to or encircle the implant and abutment surface
Periodontal ligament	No periodontal ligament
Cementum	No cementum
Alveolar bone	In direct contact with the implant surface (osseointegration)

Section 2
Peri-implant Disease

1. **Pathologic Changes in Implant Tissues**
   A. **Peri-implant Tissue Inflammation**
      1. Plaque biofilm can accumulate on the surfaces of teeth, restorations, oral appliances, and also on implants and abutments.
      2. The continuous presence of bacterial deposits can result in inflammation of the soft tissues around the implant.
      3. When the disease process progresses further, partial or total loss of osseointegration can occur.
   B. **Peri-implant Disease.** Pathologic changes of the peri-implant tissues can be referred as peri-implant disease (FIG. 32-7).
      1. Peri-implant mucositis (also called peri-implant gingivitis) is plaque-induced gingivitis (with no loss of supporting bone) that is localized in the gingival tissues surrounding a dental implant.
      2. Peri-implantitis is essentially chronic periodontitis in the tissues surrounding an osseointegrated dental implant, resulting in loss of alveolar bone.
         a. Peri-implantitis begins at the coronal portion of the implant, while the apical portion continues to be osseointegrated.
         b. An advanced peri-implantitis lesion can be diagnosed by the detection of radiographic bone loss around the implant (FIG. 32-8).
            1) The implant does not become mobile until the final stages of peri-implantitis.
            2) Implants that show mobility and signs of loss of osseointegration should be removed [13].
2. **Etiology of Peri-implant Disease.** The major etiological factors associated with peri-implant disease are bacterial infection and biomechanical factors. Smoking is an additional factor that has been implicated in implant failure.
   A. **Bacterial Infection**
      1. The pathogenesis of periodontal disease—in natural teeth and dental implants—requires the presence of bacterial plaque biofilm and the host inflammatory response.
      2. It appears that periodontal disease in both the peri-implant tissues and periodontium in natural teeth progresses in a similar fashion. *The rate of tissue destruction, however, tends to be more rapid in peri-implant tissues than in periodontal tissues.*
      3. The same bacteria that are pathogenic to natural teeth can be detrimental to dental implants [14–17].
      4. Peri-implantitis is characterized by complex bacterial microcolonies with a high proportion of *Porphyromonas gingivalis, Prevotella intermedia,* and *Fusobacterium nucleatum* [18].
         a. It is theorized that the natural teeth in a partially edentulous mouth act as a reservoir of periodontal pathogens that colonize the implants.
         b. This finding makes meticulous self-care of dental implants even more critical for the partially edentulous patient than for the fully edentulous patient.
   B. **Biomechanical Factors**
      1. Collectively, the forces placed on an implant have been called "biomechanical forces" to underscore the importance of both "biological" and "mechanical" aspects of controlling those forces to achieve long term success with implants.
      2. Biomechanical forces on implants are influenced by a variety of factors that must be assessed by the clinician. Factors that influence the biomechanical forces include how much the occlusion is placed on the implant(s), the position

of the implant, the number of implants supporting a prosthesis; and the distribution of the occlusal forces among the implants and remaining teeth.

3. Since dental implants do not have a periodontal ligament, forces placed on an implant are transmitted directly to the alveolar bone. It is critical to minimize forces placed on an implant to avoid damage to the surrounding alveolar bone.

   a. Around a natural tooth the periodontal ligament helps absorb some of the forces placed on the tooth. These forces placed on natural teeth can arise from chewing food, supporting a dental appliance, or perhaps from habits such as bruxing.

   b. Dental implants lack the protective structure of the periodontal ligament that is found on natural teeth. For all practical purposes, the dental implant is in direct contact with the alveolar bone that completely supports it.

4. Both plaque biofilm–related causes and excess biomechanical forces can contribute to the development of peri-implant disease.

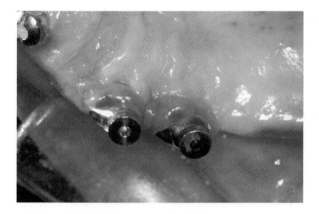

Figure 32.7. Peri-implant Disease. Inflammatory enlargement of peri-implant tissue resulting from poor daily self-care of the abutments and implant supported removable denture.

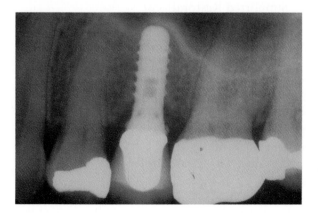

Figure 32.8. Peri-implantitis. This radiograph shows a titanium implant supporting a single crown. Note the residual cement near the crown margin. This has become a contributing factor for peri-implantitis since bone loss is evident on the radiograph.

Section 3
Maintenance of Dental Implants

One of the most important factors in the long-term success of dental implants is the maintenance of the health of the peri-implant tissues. Successful maintenance requires the active participation of the patient and the dental team.

1. **Considerations for Implant Maintenance**
   A. **Goals of Maintenance Therapy for Dental Implants**
      1. Maintenance of Alveolar Bone Support
         a. Alveolar bone support is evaluated by use of good-quality radiographs taken with a long-cone paralleling technique at specific time intervals.
         b. The bone height and density around the implants is compared with previous radiographs of the site.
      2. Control of inflammation
         a. Patient and professional plaque biofilm control is important for proper gingival health.
         b. Patient self-care must be reevaluated and, if necessary, reinforced each time the patient is seen for maintenance. The better the patient self-care, the better the possibilities of maintaining stable results.
      3. Maintenance of a Healthy and Functional implant
         a. Implant components should be checked for prosthesis integrity (such as loose screws, cement washout, material wear); implant, screw, or abutment fracture; unseating of attachments and proper adaptation of all components.
         b. *Any mobility of an implant or its restorative components requires immediate consultation with a dentist or specialist.*
   B. **Patient-Provided Information.** Before beginning an examination, it is helpful to obtain information from the patient related to implant-supported restorations or prostheses. The patient can often identify problems for clinicians that are otherwise difficult to find. Implant patients should be encouraged to share their perceptions of any changes in the fit, tightness, or feel of the implant restoration including the occlusion. Helpful questions to ask the patient are as follows:
      1. Questions About Daily Self-Care of Implant-Supported Restorations/Prosthesis
         a. Are you able to easily clean around the neck portions of your implants?
         b. Do you still have enough cleaning aids to perform daily oral self-care?
      2. Questions Concerning Patient Satisfaction. General questions regarding the patient's satisfaction with the implant-supported restorations/prosthesis are part of a quality management concept for maintenance.
         a. Are you satisfied with the way your implants function?
         b. Are you satisfied with the appearance of your implants?
      3. Questions Regarding Patient-Perceived Changes Since Last Appointment
         a. Do you think any part of the implant is loose?
         b. Do the gums around your implants bleed?
         c. Do you notice a bad taste coming from your implants?
         d. Have you noticed any changes in your implants?
   C. **The Dental Implant Maintenance Visit**
      1. Modern dental implants may be difficult to recognize intraorally since their restorations often have the same appearance as the crowns and fixed bridges used to restore natural teeth (Fig. 32-9). *For this reason, dental implants should be clearly noted in the chart so that all dental team members are alerted to the fact that this is a dental implant patient.*

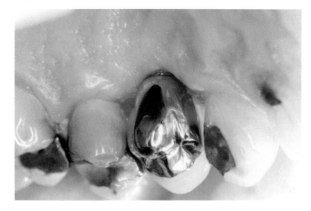

Figure 32.9. Fixed Prosthetic Crown. The first premolar in this photo is a prosthetic crown supported by a dental implant. During an intraoral examination, it would be difficult to distinguish between a crown that is supported by a natural tooth and a crown supported by a dental implant.

TABLE 32-2. Assessment of Dental Implants	
Characteristics of a Healthy Implant Site	**Characteristics of a Diseased Implant Site**
Firm, pink tissue	Red, swollen tissue
No bleeding on probing	Bleeding on probing or just after tissue manipulation
No purulence (pus) noted when tissue is compressed	Purulence in peri-implant tissues
No mobility	Mobility may be present
Radiographic evidence of bone in close contact with the implant	Radiographic evidence of bone loss at the crest next to the implant or radiolucency around the implant
Radiographic bone levels with minimal or no change from previous observations	Radiographic bone loss evident and/or getting worse

2. Assessment and maintenance therapy for dental implants is similar to periodontal maintenance for a patient who has been treated for periodontitis (TABLE 32-2).
3. The following may be included in a maintenance visit; however, each maintenance visit should be individualized based on previous examinations, history, and judgment of the clinician: evaluation of peri-implant tissue health, examination of prosthesis/abutment components, evaluation of implant's stability, occlusal examination, assessment of patient's self-care, radiographic examination, and treatment (e.g., periodontal instrumentation).

D. **Radiographic Examination**
   1. Maintenance of bone levels around dental implants is an important criterion for determining treatment success. Radiographic evaluation of bone height and topography is necessary for the longitudinal monitoring of peri-implant stability [10,12,19,20].
      a. Vertical bone loss of less than 0.2 mm annually following the implant's first year of function is a criterion utilized to determine treatment success.

   b. Radiographs also allow for the evaluation of the fit of the prosthesis and the integrity and adaptation of the different implant components.

2. Dental implants should be evaluated radiographically at least once a year and should be checked more often in patients in whom periodontal breakdown around an implant was noted at a previous visit.

E. **Implant Mobility**

1. Absence of mobility is a very important clinical criterion for dental implants. The presence of mobility presently is the best indicator for diagnosis of implant failure [12].

   a. Implants should not move if osseointegrated and healthy [21,22].

   b. Mobility of an implant indicates a lack of osseointegration.

   c. Mobility of an implant restoration could indicate the presence of a loose abutment or the rupture of the cement seal on cemented restorations.

   d. Mobility also can result from a loosening of the internal screw that attaches the abutment to the implant or the restoration to the abutment and thus not be the result of peri-implant disease.

   e. Severe mobility accompanied with discomfort also might indicate fracture of the implant itself.

   f. Long-term mobility or misfit between the prosthetic components (e.g., screws between the crown and implant) may lead to persistent inflammation, bone loss, and the eventual complete failure of the implant.

2. The technique for assessing mobility of a dental implant is similar to that used to assess a natural tooth. Two instrument handles are used to grasp the *implant restoration* and apply force back and forth in the facial and lingual direction. The use of two instruments with plastic handles is recommended if the implant itself must be touched.

3. Radiographic evaluation is recommended when any mobility is noted. Loose internal screws or components will often be seen as a gap between the implant components on a radiograph.

F. **Periodontal Instrumentation of Dental Implants**

1. The use of traditional metal curets is contraindicated around implant components [23–25]. Implant components are made of titanium, a soft metal, that can be permanently damaged (grooved, scratched) if treated with metal instruments (FIG. 32-10).

   a. There is an increased likelihood of plaque biofilm retention and peri-implantitis if the titanium is scratched.

   b. Metal instruments can also disturb the surface coating of the implant, reducing the biocompatibility with the peri-implant tissues.

   c. The use of ultrasonic or sonic devices with standard metal tips is also contraindicated on titanium surfaces. Several manufacturers, however, offer specialized ultrasonic tips for use on titanium surfaces (Box 32-1).

2. Instruments used for assessment and periodontal instrumentation of implants and other titanium surfaces should be made of a material that is softer than the implant. Plastic instruments are most commonly used (FIG. 32-11).

   a. Plastic instruments are safe for use on all types of implants, abutments, and components and will not cause damage to the surface.

   b. Standard dental restorative materials, for example, gold and porcelain, can be cleaned with conventional periodontal instruments. Care must be taken, however, not to use these instruments apical to the margin of the prosthetic crown where titanium might be contacted.

    c. Usually calculus deposits are removed readily from smooth titanium surfaces because there is no interlocking or penetration of the deposit with the surface. Light lateral pressure with a plastic instrument is recommended.

3. Implants, abutments, and components do not require routine polishing.

    a. When indicated, polishing of the implant restoration can be accomplished with rubber cups and nonabrasive polishing paste [12,26–29].

    b. Polishing has been shown to improve titanium surfaces *that have previously been roughened or scratched. However, if no surface alterations are noted, the titanium surfaces should not be polished.*

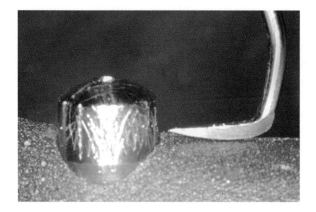

Figure 32.10. Surface Damage From Improper Instrumentation. Metal instruments can scratch the surface of the implant. (Courtesy of Drs Mota and Baumhammers, University of Pittsburgh School of Dental Medicine.)

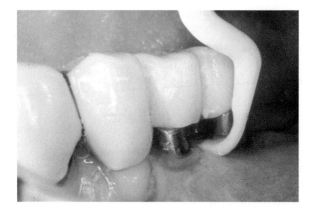

Figure 32.11. Plastic Curet. Plastic instruments are safe for use on dental implants.

Box 32-1. Sources of Specialized Ultrasonic Tips for Titanium Surfaces

- Cavitron SofTip: www.dentsply.com
- GentleCLEAN www.parkell.com
- Periosoft Tips: www.acteongroup.com
- GentleCLEAN www.parkell.com
- Titanium implant scaler (T.I.S.) www.tonyriso.com

G. Peri-implant Probing
1. *Routine periodontal probing of dental implants is not recommended. No probing is necessary if the peri-implant tissue is healthy.*
   a. Probing could damage the weak epithelial attachment, possibly allowing entry of periodontal pathogens [10,19,20].
   b. Probing is indicated only in implants where signs of infection are present such as bleeding, inflamed peri-implant tissue, or if exudate is present [12].
2. When a dental implant shows signs of either radiographic or clinical changes, clinical attachment levels can be used to monitor peri-implant health.
   a. To interpret probe readings, the clinician must have baseline data relating to the implant such as abutment type, size, prosthetic design, baseline probed levels of attachment, and a fixed reference point for repeatable probing comparisons.
   b. Probing measurements should be made from a fixed reference point on the implant, abutment, or prosthetic implant crown.
      1) Due to variation in the depth of surgical placement, as well as different lengths of the abutments and the connective tissue interface with the abutment, probing depths may be deeper than the 1- to 3-mm depths that are considered normal in natural teeth.
      2) A healthy peri-implant sulcus has been reported to range from 1.3 to 3.8 mm [30].
3. Probing should be avoided until postoperative healing is complete, approximately 3 months after abutment connection.
   a. Commercially available plastic probes should be used when investigating the depth of the peri-implant sulcus [12].
   b. Only a light probing technique should be used since the biological seal is weakly adherent to the titanium surface. Heavy probing force will be invasive since the probe easily can penetrate through the biological seal and introduce bacteria into the peri-implant environment.
   c. Penetration of the plastic probe tip also is dependent on the health (or inflammatory stage of the peri-implant tissues) and the thickness of the tissue around the abutment.
4. Peri-implant probing depth measurements vary from site-to-site and patient-to-patient.
   a. Successful implants generally allow probe penetration of approximately 3 to 4 mm. Deeper sites appear to be more susceptible to breakdown.
   b. Bleeding on probing should also be assessed and considered along with the probing depths to determine areas of inflammation.

H. Maintenance Frequency
1. Maintenance intervals should be determined on an individual basis because there is a lack of data detailing precise intervals [2].
   a. A 3-month maintenance interval is usually appropriate for the first year following restoration of the implant [12]. However, the clinician must determine the best interval for each specific case.
   b. After the initial 12-month period, a 3- to 6-month maintenance interval may be used [12,26]. Periodontal maintenance appointments should be scheduled as frequently as necessary to keep the periodontium and peri-implant tissues healthy.
2. The following are indications for more frequent maintenance intervals.
   a. Reduced Bone Support Around Implants. Reduced bone support indicates that close monitoring of bone support is needed or the dental implant might be lost.

    b. Inflammation. A patient who has signs of inflammation around implants, even in the presence of good plaque biofilm control, needs more frequent maintenance visits.

    c. Host Response. Systemic conditions or diseases may affect the host-bacterial interaction. A shorter maintenance interval is needed for these patients.

2. Patient Self-Care of Dental Implants

  A. Considerations

    1. Meticulous self-care is of the utmost importance in preventing peri-implant disease. *An individualized self-care routine should be developed for each patient.*

    2. Some patients undergoing implant therapy may have had a long history of dental neglect and/or poor plaque biofilm control.

    3. The dental hygienist can assist the patient in maintaining dental implants by providing self-care education appropriate for implants and home care devices that are effective and simple to use.

  B. Care of Fixed Prosthetic Crown(s)

    1. A fixed prosthetic crown is an artificial tooth that fits over the abutment. These are made from a variety of routinely encountered restorative materials.

    2. Self-Care Challenges

      a. The single tooth prosthesis (crown) can present a challenge for plaque biofilm control in that the patient may quickly begin to regard it to be just the same shape and anatomy as a natural tooth.

        1) In fact, these restorations often have different designs and unusual contours that require special self-care attention.

        2) Self-care practices must be modified to include aids that can effectively clean the altered morphology of the peri-implant region.

      b. The crown covering the implant abutment is larger in circumference than the abutment and will have contours added to it to make it look and function like a natural tooth.

        1) The "bulky" contours of the crown may contact the tissue and then "dip in" to meet the abutment at or below the gingival margin.

        2) Dental floss or tufted dental floss should be adapted along the margin of the crown and then pulled gently back and forth to direct it into the sulcus and around the abutment (Fig. 32-12).

      c. In some cases, the restoration may be similar to a fixed bridge (e.g., a pontic supported by two dental implants). Tufted dental floss, specially designed interdental brushes, end-tuff brushes, and a toothpick in a holder are effective cleaning devices for deplaquing the large embrasure spaces and into the sulci of these fixed bridge-type restorations.

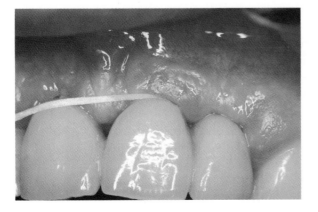

Figure 32.12. Implant Self-Care. Dental floss is used to clean a single implant with a prosthetic crown. The "bulky" contours of the crown may contact the tissue and then "dip in" to meet the abutment at or below the gingival margin.

    d. Restoration of multiple tooth replacement situations can involve complex, denture-like prostheses which are attached to multiple implants and which are not removable by the patient.

        1) These prostheses are removable by the dentist or specialist at which time cleaning access is optimal.

        2) Daily care by the patient requires an individualized plan and a combination of devices to overcome the limited access often encountered. Oral irrigators can be used cautiously. Antimicrobial mouth rinses are helpful.

  3. Techniques, and Devices

    a. Standard multitufted, soft nylon bristle, manual toothbrushes can be used effectively by patients having sufficient dexterity and understanding of the task.

    b. Powered toothbrushes are safe for titanium surfaces and these devices are particularly helpful for implant patients in general.

    c. Interdental brushes can be effective in plaque biofilm removal and may effectively clean the peri-implant sulcus [31].

        1) *Note that interdental brushes used to clean implants and components should have a soft protective coating on the twisted wire that secures the bristles.*

        2) The use a standard interdental brush (that does not have a plastic or nylon coating on the twisted wire) should be avoided since the exposed wire could scratch titanium.

    d. Patients must be instructed to use cleaning devices carefully, especially around anterior implant sites that are visible and esthetically important.

    e. Daily use of an antimicrobial mouth rinse is beneficial for many patients [32,33]. The entire mouth can be rinsed twice daily after brushing. Or, if that is not acceptable to the patient, the mouth rinse can be applied topically to each implant area twice daily with a cotton-tipped applicator or with gauze.

C. Care of a Removable Prosthesis

  1. An implant supported removable prosthesis is similar to a traditional full denture except that in the case of implants, it is attached to the abutments by devices such as o-rings, magnets, or clips (FIG. 32-13).

    a. This type of prosthesis can also be designed as an implant and tissue supported prosthesis or as an overdenture.

    b. The patient can remove the prosthesis to clean it, the attachment devices, the abutments and the remainder of the mouth.

  2. Techniques and Tools

    a. Selection of cleaning devices for implants and abutments should be based on the knowledge that implant components are made from titanium, which is a relatively soft metal.

        1) Tools for plaque biofilm removal around the abutments may include soft bristle manual toothbrushes, single-tufted manual toothbrushes, and interdental brushes.

        2) Tufted dental floss or implant floss sometimes can easily be wrapped around the abutment for plaque biofilm removal.

        3) Powered toothbrushes are safe for titanium surfaces. These devices are particularly helpful for implant patients, especially for those patients having multiple implant sites to clean and for those patients who have any limitations of dexterity.

    b. Cleaning devices must be selected for ease of use by each individual patient, and the recommendation of fewer, rather than more, devices is best. The cleaning aids that are recommended should be demonstrated for the patient and then evaluated by the hygienist to verify their effective use by the patient.

    c. In some cases, a metal bar connects the abutments and is used to attach the prosthetic denture in the mouth. Tufted dental floss or an unfolded 2 × 2 gauze square can be useful in cleaning underneath the metal bar and around the abutments (Fig. 32-14).

    d. Patients who have limited ability or poor success with mechanical plaque biofilm removal will benefit from the daily use of an antimicrobial mouth rinse [32,33]. The entire mouth can be rinsed twice daily after brushing.

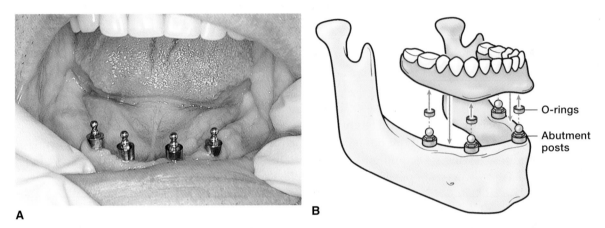

A   **B**

Figure 32.13. Implant Supported Removable Prosthesis. A: Abutment posts on the mandibular arch. **B:** An implant supported removable prosthesis is attached to the abutment posts by o-rings, magnets, or clips.

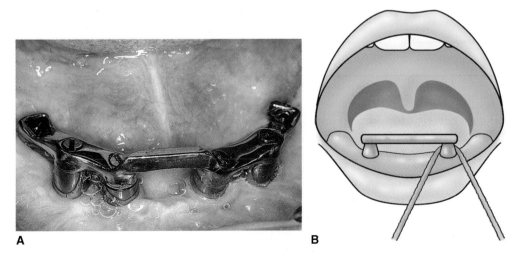

A   **B**

Figure 32.14. Abutments Joined by Metal Bar. Tufted dental floss is useful in cleaning the implant abutments and underneath the connecting metal bar.

Chapter Summary Statement

As dental implant therapy becomes more common, dental hygienists will care for increasing numbers of patients needing implant maintenance. An important role of the dental hygienist is the education of patients about the importance of meticulous self-care and frequent maintenance visits. Implant restorations necessitate customized self-care instructions and devices. Implant maintenance appointments should include monitoring of plaque biofilm levels, examination of soft tissues, assessment of the restorative integrity, reinforcement of patient plaque biofilm control measures, periodontal instrumentation of implant abutments and prostheses, and radiographic examination.

Section 4
Focus on Patients

Case 1

While you are performing nonsurgical therapy on a chronic periodontitis patient, the patient tells you that he is thinking about having all of his teeth removed, since they are not healthy anyway, and just having some implants placed. He tells you that this would be easier, since he would not have to worry about the implants like he does his teeth. How should you respond?

Case 2

You are scheduled to record the information needed to make a periodontal diagnosis for a patient new to your dental team. Radiographs have not yet been ordered for the patient. As you begin your probing, the patient informs you that she has two dental implants. Visual examination of the patient's dentition does not immediately reveal which teeth are replaced by the implants. How should you proceed?

Case 3

At a maintenance visit for one of your team's patients you note obvious mobility of a crown supported by an implant. How should you proceed?

References

1. Cochran DL, Nummikoski PV, Schoolfield JD, Jones AA, et al. A prospective multicenter 5-year radiographic evaluation of crestal bone levels over time in 596 dental implants placed in 192 patients. *J Periodontol.* 2009;80(5):725–733.
2. Iacono VJ. Dental implants in periodontal therapy. *J Periodontol.* 2000;71(12):1934–1942.
3. Albrektsson T, Dahl E, Enbom L, Engevall S, et al. Osseointegrated oral implants. A Swedish multicenter study of 8139 consecutively inserted Nobelpharma implants. *J Periodontol.* 1988; 59(5):287–296.
4. Fugazzotto PA, Gulbransen HJ, Wheeler SL, Lindsay JA. The use of IMZ osseointegrated implants in partially and completely edentulous patients: success and failure rates of 2,023 implant cylinders up to 60+ months in function. *Int J Oral Maxillofac Implants.* 1993;8(6): 617–621.
5. Patrick D, Zosky J, Lubar R, Buchs A. Longitudinal clinical efficacy of Core-Vent dental implants: a five-year report. *J Oral Implantol.* 1989;15(2):95–103.
6. Sbordone L, Barone A, Ciaglia RN, Ramaglia L, et al. Longitudinal study of dental implants in a periodontally compromised population. *J Periodontol.* 1999;70(11):1322–1329.
7. Spiekermann H, Jansen VK, Richter EJ. A 10-year follow-up study of IMZ and TPS implants in the edentulous mandible using bar-retained overdentures. *Int J Oral Maxillofac Implants.* 1995;10(2):231–243.
8. Lang NP, Karring T; British Society of Periodontology. *Proceedings of the 1st European Workshop on Periodontology, Charter House at Ittingen, Thurgau, Switzerland, February 1–4, 1993.* London; Chicago: Quintessence Pub. Co.; 1994:478.
9. Lang NP, Karring T, Lindhe J, et al. *Proceedings of the 3rd European Workshop on Periodontology: implant dentistry: Charter House at Ittingen, Thurgau, Switzerland, January 30-February 3, 1999.* Berlin; Chicago: Quintessenz Pub. Co.; 1999:615.
10. Bader H. Implant maintenance: a chairside test for real-time monitoring. *Dent Econ.* 1995;85(6):66–67.
11. Nevins M, Langer B. The successful use of osseointegrated implants for the treatment of the recalcitrant periodontal patient. *J Periodontol.* 1995;66(2):150–157.
12. Silverstein L, Garg A, Callan D, Shatz P. The key to success: maintaining the long-term health of implants. *Dent Today.* 1998;17(2):104, 106, 108–111.
13. Esposito M, Hirsch J, Lekholm U, Thomsen P. Differential diagnosis and treatment strategies for biologic complications and failing oral implants: a review of the literature. *Int J Oral Maxillofac Implants.* 1999;14(4):473–490.
14. Quirynen M, De Soete M, van Steenberghe D. Infectious risks for oral implants: a review of the literature. *Clin Oral Implants Res.* 2002;13(1):1–19.
15. Renvert S, Roos-Jansaker AM, Lindahl C, Renvert H, et al. Infection at titanium implants with or without a clinical diagnosis of inflammation. *Clin Oral Implants Res.* 2007;18(4):509–516.
16. Shibli JA, Martins MC, Lotufo RF, Marcantonio E, Jr. Microbiologic and radiographic analysis of ligature-induced peri-implantitis with different dental implant surfaces. *Int J Oral Maxillofac Implants.* 2003;18(3):383–390.
17. Shibli JA, Melo L, Ferrari DS, Figueiredo LC, et al. Composition of supra- and subgingival biofilm of subjects with healthy and diseased implants. *Clin Oral Implants Res.* 2008;19(10):975–982.
18. Sbordone L, Barone A, Ramaglia L, Ciaglia RN, et al. Antimicrobial susceptibility of periodontopathic bacteria associated with failing implants. *J Periodontol.* 1995;66(1):69–74.
19. Ericsson I, Lindhe J. Probing depth at implants and teeth. An experimental study in the dog. *J Clin Periodontol.* 1993;20(9):623–627.
20. Lang NP, Wetzel AC, Stich H, Caffesse RG. Histologic probe penetration in healthy and inflamed peri-implant tissues. *Clin Oral Implants Res.* 1994;5(4):191–201.
21. Cochran D. Implant therapy I. *Ann Periodontol.* 1996;1(1):707–791.
22. Papaioannou W, Quirynen M, Nys M, van Steenberghe D. The effect of periodontal parameters on the subgingival microbiota around implants. *Clin Oral Implants Res.* 1995;6(4):197–204.
23. The American Academy of Periodontology. Guidelines for periodontal therapy. *J Periodontol.* 1998;69(3):405–408.
24. Supportive periodontal therapy (SPT). *J Periodontol.* 1998;69(4):502–506.
25. Speelman JA, Collaert B, Klinge B. Evaluation of different methods to clean titanium abutments. A scanning electron microscopic study. *Clin Oral Implants Res.* 1992;3(3):120–127.

26. Eskow RN, Smith VS. Preventive periimplant protocol. *Compend Contin Educ Dent.* 1999;20(2):137–142, 144, 146 passim; quiz 154.

27. Huband ML. Problems associated with implant maintenance. *Va Dent J.* 1996;73(2):8–11.

28. Jovanovic SA. Peri-implant tissue response to pathological insults. *Adv Dent Res.* 1999;13: 82–86.

29. Matarasso S, Quaremba G, Coraggio F, Vaia E, et al. Maintenance of implants: an in vitro study of titanium implant surface modifications subsequent to the application of different prophylaxis procedures. *Clin Oral Implants Res.* 1996;7(1):64–72.

30. van Steenberghe D, Klinge B, Linden U, Quirynen M, et al. Periodontal indices around natural and titanium abutments: a longitudinal multicenter study. *J Periodontol.* 1993;64(6):538–541.

31. Balshi TJ. Hygiene maintenance procedures for patients treated with the tissue integrated prosthesis (osseointegration). *Quintessence Int.* 1986;17(2):95–102.

32. Ciancio SG, Lauciello F, Shibly O, Vitello M, et al. The effect of an antiseptic mouthrinse on implant maintenance: plaque and peri-implant gingival tissues. *J Periodontol.* 1995; 66(11):962–965.

33. Mombelli A, Lang NP. Antimicrobial treatment of peri-implant infections. *Clin Oral Implants Res.* 1992;3(4):162–168.

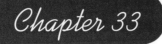

Periodontal Emergencies

Learning Objectives

- Name and describe the three types of abscesses of the periodontium.
- Define the terms acute and circumscribed.
- List the possible causes of abscesses of the periodontium.
- Compare and contrast the abscess of the periodontium and the endodontic abscess.
- Outline the typical treatment steps for a gingival abscess and a periodontal abscess.
- Describe the clinical situation that can result in a pericoronal abscess.
- Outline the typical treatment for a pericoronal abscess (pericoronitis).
- List the two types of necrotizing periodontal diseases.
- Describe the characteristics of necrotizing ulcerative gingivitis.
- Outline the typical treatment steps for necrotizing ulcerative gingivitis.
- Describe the symptoms of primary herpetic gingivostomatitis.

Key Terms

Acute periodontal conditions
Abscess of the periodontium
Pus
Circumscribed
Pulpal abscess
Gingival abscess
Periodontal abscess
Pericoronal abscess

Pericoronitis
Operculum
Necrosis
Ulceration
Punched out papillae
Pseudomembrane
Sequestrum
Primary herpetic gingivostomatitis

INTRODUCTION TO ACUTE PERIODONTAL CONDITIONS

Most periodontal diseases are chronic, progressing slowly and taking years or decades to destroy the periodontium, but there are several periodontal conditions that can bring patients to the dental office for emergency care. The emergency conditions described in this chapter are examples of acute periodontal conditions. The term acute periodontal conditions refers to conditions that are commonly characterized by a rapid onset and rapid course, that are frequently accompanied by pain and discomfort, and that may be unrelated to the presence of preexisting gingivitis or periodontitis.

The characteristics of acute periodontal conditions are summarized in Box 33-1. It is imperative that all members of the dental team be alert for these conditions because their recognition and early intervention can limit subsequent permanent damage to the periodontium. Some of these conditions can be encountered in their earliest stages by the dental hygienist during routine treatment and recall appointments. This chapter outlines the more common periodontal emergency conditions and briefly describes the treatment that may be recommended and performed by the dentist or the dental hygienist.

Box 33-1. Characteristics of Acute Periodontal Conditions

- Rapid onset and rapid course
- Accompanied by pain and discomfort
- May be unrelated to existing gingivitis or periodontitis

Section 1
Abscesses of the Periodontium

1. Overview of Abscesses of the Periodontium
    A. Introduction to Abscesses of the Periodontium
        1. An abscess of the periodontium may be defined as an acute infection involving a circumscribed collection of pus in the periodontium.
        2. Abscesses of the periodontium are collections of pus. Pus consists primarily of dead white blood cells that can result when body defense mechanisms are involved in attempting to control an infection.
        3. In its earliest stages, the abscess of the periodontium can be discovered by the dental hygienist during an oral inspection at a routine treatment visit, but in more advanced stages the abscess of the periodontium can bring the patient to the dental office for relief of pain.
        4. Abscesses of the periodontium are described as being circumscribed. The term circumscribed means that the abscess is localized or confined to a specific site (i.e., the facial surface of a single tooth). Figure 33-1 illustrates a typical example of an abscess of the periodontium.
        5. The precise bacterial etiology of the abscess of the periodontium is not clear, but it is known that most of these lesions contain microflora that are predominantly gram negative and anaerobic. Most studies indicate that the bacteria seen in these abscesses are similar to bacteria seen in periodontitis patients with deeper pockets.

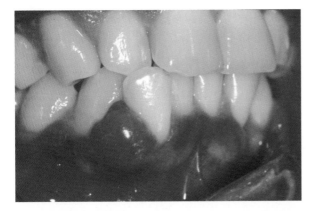

Figure 33.1. Abscess of the Periodontium. Note that the localized swelling between the mandibular right canine and first premolar. Palpation of the swelling would reveal what feels like a fluid-filled sack.

Box 33-2. Characteristics of an Abscess of the Periodontium

- Pain that is constant and localized
- Circumscribed swelling in the periodontium
- Possible increase in tooth mobility
- Radiographic loss of alveolar bone not involving the tooth apex
- Tooth has a vital pulp

B. Characteristics of an Abscess of the Periodontium

1. Typical patient complaints related to an abscess of the periodontium include dental pain and swelling in the gingiva (Box 33-2).
   a. Pain resulting from an abscess of the periodontium is usually described by the patient as a constant pain. Patients frequently report that the pain is easy for them to localize (i.e., the patient can point to the exact spot that hurts).
   b. In addition to pain and swelling, the patient may report difficulty in mastication and may report a bad taste in the mouth.
2. Oral examination will usually reveal the presence of a circumscribed swelling of the soft tissue. This swelling may involve the gingiva only, or it may involve both the gingiva and the mucosa.
3. Many teeth with an abscess of the periodontium also exhibit a temporary increase in mobility.
4. Dental radiographs of a tooth with an abscess of the periodontium frequently reveal alveolar bone loss in the area of the abscess but not involving the tooth apex. Figure 33-2 is a radiograph of a tooth with an abscess of the periodontium.
   a. Alveolar bone loss resulting from an abscess of the periodontium can occur extremely rapidly when compared with the rate of alveolar bone loss usually associated with all forms of periodontitis.
   b. Although a dental radiograph of an abscess of the periodontium may reveal alveolar bone loss, in a periodontitis patient it is not possible to tell what part of the missing bone resulted from the acute infection and what part of the missing bone was caused by chronic periodontitis that was present before the abscess formed.

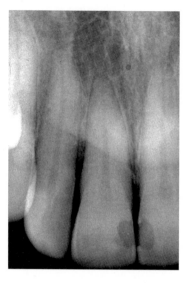

Figure 33.2. **Radiographic Evidence of an Abscess of the Periodontium**. This radiograph shows bone loss around the right central but not involving the apex of the tooth. Radiographic findings must always be correlated with the clinical findings to confirm the diagnosis.

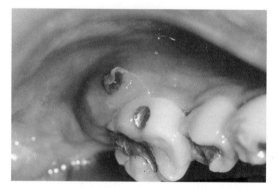

Figure 33.3. **Path of Drainage.** The abscess of the periodontium shown here has broken through the surface tissues, establishing a path of drainage on its own.

5. Teeth affected by an abscess of the periodontium are usually vital (have healthy pulp tissue).

6. Another clinical sign of an abscess of the periodontium can be an elevated body temperature; an elevated body temperature would not normally be present unless the abscess of the periodontium is spreading, so this would represent a serious sign if present.

7. When there is delay in treating an abscess of the periodontium, there can be additional oral changes. The collection of pus can break through the surface tissues, thus establishing a path of drainage on its own. Figure 33-3 illustrates an abscess of the periodontium that has drained spontaneously.

C. **Causes of Abscesses of the Periodontium.** Several causes of abscesses of the periodontium have been reported. Theories about the origin of the abscess of the periodontium vary, but most investigators attribute formation of this type of abscess to one of the following.

1. Blockage of the orifice (or opening) of an existing periodontal pocket has been suggested as a cause of some abscesses of the periodontium. Most periodontal pockets have readily accessible openings that give easy access to a periodontal probe. Some authors have theorized that in certain instances the opening of a periodontal pocket can become restricted in size because of temporary improvement of the surface tissue tone. This improvement of tissue tone can result in trapping bacteria and fluids in a pocket, leading to an abscess that begins within the existing periodontal pocket.

2. It has also been suggested that an abscess of periodontium can be caused by forcing a foreign object into the supporting tissues of a tooth.
   a. A variety of foreign objects have been implicated in the formation of some abscesses of the periodontium. For example, an abscess could result when a patient accidentally punctures the gingiva with a toothpick, forcing bacteria into the tissue.
   b. Another common event that can result in an abscess of the periodontium is accidentally forcing some food product like a husk from a kernel of popcorn or a peanut skin into a periodontal pocket.
3. Incomplete calculus removal in a periodontal pocket has also been suggested as one cause of an abscess of the periodontium.
   a. When this occurs, it is usually in a site with a very deep probing depth where the calculus deposits are removed only in the most coronal aspects of the pocket near the gingival margin, but calculus deposits deeper in the pocket are not removed because of difficulty of access.
   b. It is theorized that removal of the more coronal deposits allows the gingival margin to heal somewhat and to tighten around the tooth, like a drawstring of a pouch, preventing drainage of bacterial toxins and other waste products from the pocket. Bacteria remaining in the deeper aspects of the periodontal pocket can result in the formation of an abscess of the periodontium.

D. Clinical Recognition and Diagnosis. The clinical recognition and diagnosis of an abscess of the periodontium can be complicated because of the overlap of signs of an abscess of the periodontium with the signs of a pulpal abscess.
1. Abscesses affecting the tissues around a tooth can result from two separate sources: (1) the periodontium itself or (2) the pulpal tissues of the tooth.
   a. It is helpful for the dental hygienist to be familiar with the characteristics of these two types of abscesses, since abscess of the periodontium and the pulpal abscess sometimes appear to have somewhat similar clinical characteristics.
   b. The characteristics of each of these types of abscesses are outlined in TABLE 33-1.
2. As already discussed, an abscess of the periodontium is an abscess that results from an acute infection of the periodontium.
3. On the other hand, a pulpal abscess is an abscess that results from an infection of the tooth pulp.
   a. A pulpal abscess can be caused by death of the tooth pulp from trauma to the tooth or from deep dental decay; a dead tooth pulp is frequently referred to as a nonvital pulp.
   b. Management of a patient with a pulpal abscess usually requires root canal treatment and is not discussed in this chapter.

TABLE 33-1. Differentiation of the Types of Abscess

Characteristic	Abscess of the Periodontium	Endodontic Abscess
Vitality test results	Vital pulp	Usually nonvital pulp
Radiographic	Bone loss present	Bone loss at root apex
Symptoms	Localized, constant pain	Difficult to localize, intermittent pain

2. **Types of Abscesses of the Periodontium.** Authors generally describe three types of abscesses of the periodontium: (1) the gingival abscess, (2) the periodontal abscess, and (3) the pericoronal abscess, but there is considerable overlap in this loose classification system.

A. **Gingival Abscess.** The gingival abscess refers to an abscess of the periodontium that is primarily limited to the gingival margin or interdental papilla without involvement of the deeper structures of the periodontium.

1. The gingival abscess can occur in a previously periodontally healthy mouth when some foreign object is forced into a healthy gingival sulcus. An abscess of the periodontium that is limited to the gingival margin area can follow this traumatic event.

2. Figure 33-4 illustrates a typical gingival abscess where the swelling is limited to the marginal gingiva.

B. **Periodontal Abscess.** The periodontal abscess refers to an abscess of the periodontium that affects the deeper structures of the periodontium as well as the gingival tissues.

1. The periodontal abscess usually occurs in a site with preexisting periodontal disease including preexisting periodontal pockets.

2. The periodontal abscess usually affects the deeper structures of the periodontium and is not limited to the gingiva only.

C. **Pericoronal Abscess.** The pericoronal abscess refers to an abscess of the periodontium that involves tissues around the crown of a partially erupted tooth. The pericoronal abscess is also referred to as pericoronitis.

1. This type of abscess is seen in teeth where some of the soft tissues surrounding the teeth actually cover part of the occlusal surface of the teeth. Figure 33-5 illustrates a patient with a pericoronal abscess under a soft tissue flap on a third molar tooth.

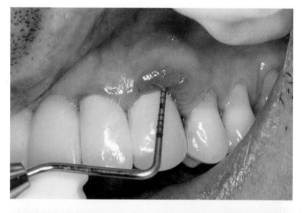

Figure 33.4. **An Abscess of the Periodontium Limited to Gingival Tissues or Gingival Abscess.** Note that this abscess is limited to the gingival margin on the facial surface of this maxillary canine. (Courtesy of Dr Richard Foster, Guilford Technical Community College, Jamestown, NC.)

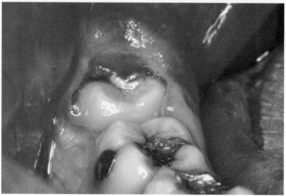

Figure 33.5. **Pericoronitis.** A patient with pericoronitis under a soft tissue flap on a third molar. The tissues of the flap are red and swollen. Manipulation of the flap causes discomfort for the patient.

Box 33-3. Signs and Symptoms of a Pericoronal Abscess

- Pain at the site
- Swelling of operculum
- Possible trismus (limited mouth opening)

- Possible elevated body temperature
- Possible lymphadenopathy

---

2. The pericoronal abscess (or pericoronitis) is most frequently seen around mandibular third molar teeth. Since many third molar teeth do not have space to erupt fully, these teeth can have a flap of tissue covering part of the occlusal surface.

3. The flap of gingival tissue that covers a portion of the crown of a partially erupted tooth can become infected, and it is this type of infection under this flap of tissue that is referred to as a pericoronal abscess.

4. This flap of soft tissue is called an operculum, and some authors also refer to the pericoronal abscess as an operculitis.

5. The signs and symptoms of the pericoronal abscess are discussed below and outlined in Box 33-3.

6. Pain is common with the pericoronal abscess. The pain can arise from the tissue swelling itself, but pain can also arise when an opposing tooth occludes with the infected, swollen operculum.

7. Soft tissue swelling (edema) and redness (erythema) also usually accompany the pericoronal abscess.

8. As damage to tissue covering the partially erupted tooth progresses and the tissue swelling increases, the opposing tooth can frequently be seen to impinge (press) on the swollen tissue, creating additional tissue damage and additional patient discomfort.

9. Limited mouth opening is also seen in some cases of advanced pericoronal abscess; limited mouth opening is referred to as trismus.

10. Elevated body temperature (fever) and swollen lymph nodes (lymphadenopathy) also can be seen in advanced cases of pericoronitis.

3. **Management of Patients with Abscesses of the Periodontium**
   A. **Treatment of a Gingival or Periodontal Abscess.** The treatment of a patient with either a gingival or a periodontal abscess is similar.
   1. Fundamental treatment steps include (1) establishment of a path of drainage for the pus and (2) thorough periodontal debridement of the tooth surfaces in the area of the abscess, and (3) relief of pain.
   2. Steps commonly followed in treatment of patients with a gingival or a periodontal abscess are outlined below and are outlined in Box 33-4.
      a. It is normally necessary to anesthetize the site to be treated, since manipulation of the tissues involved by an abscess can be quite uncomfortable.
      b. Drainage of the pus from the abscess is critical. The abscess can be drained either through the pocket itself or by performing periodontal surgery (as discussed in Chapter 30). When drainage is established through the pocket, the toe of a sterile curet is used to puncture the soft tissue wall of the pocket to allow drainage. In some cases, drainage can be accomplished by incising through the surface tissues.
      c. Thorough periodontal instrumentation of the tooth surfaces in the site of the abscess is important in bringing this type of abscess under control.

d. Some adjustment of the tooth occlusion is usually also indicated since inflammation resulting from the abscess can force a tooth to extrude slightly from its socket, leading to trauma from occlusion and pain when masticating.

e. In more advanced cases of abscesses antibiotics may be needed, as with any other serious oral infection.

f. Some clinicians recommend using warm saline (saltwater) rinses several times each day to help keep the abscess draining until it has healed completely.

g. A prescription for pain medication should always be considered, but over-the-counter pain medications can be adequate in many patients once the abscess has been drained.

h. Following emergency treatment of a patient with any abscess of the periodontium, the dental team should appoint the patient for a thorough periodontal assessment, since the abscess of the periodontium frequently occurs in a patient with existing untreated periodontal disease, and routine periodontal therapy may be needed.

B. **Treatment of a Pericoronal Abscess.** Treatment of patients with pericoronal abscess differs slightly from treatment of patients with other types of abscesses of the periodontium because of the difference in the anatomical location of these abscesses.

1. Fundamental treatment steps for a patient with pericoronitis include (1) establishment of a path of drainage for the pus, (2) irrigation of the undersurface of the operculum, (3) thorough periodontal debridement of the tooth surfaces in the area of the abscess, and (4) relief of pain.

2. Steps commonly followed in treatment of patients with a pericoronal abscess are discussed below and outlined in Box 33-5.

   a. It is normally necessary to anesthetize the tooth to be treated, since manipulation of the tissues involved by an abscess can be quite uncomfortable.

   b. Drainage of the pus from the abscess is critical. The abscess can be drained either through the pocket itself or by performing periodontal surgery (as discussed in Chapter 30). When drainage is established through the pocket, the toe of a sterile curet is used to puncture the soft tissue wall of the pocket to allow drainage. Abscesses around the crown of a partially erupted third molar tooth may be difficult to drain because of the anatomy of the region.

   c. Thorough periodontal instrumentation of the tooth surfaces in the site of the abscess is important in bringing this type of abscess under control.

   d. The area under the operculum that partially covers the tooth crown should be irrigated thoroughly. This irrigation can be done with sterile saline.

   e. In more advanced cases of abscesses antibiotics may be needed, as with any other serious oral infection.

   f. Some clinicians recommend using warm saline (saltwater) rinses several times each day to help keep the abscess draining until it has healed completely.

   g. A prescription for pain medication should always be considered, but over-the-counter pain medications can be adequate in many patients once the abscess is drained.

   h. Following emergency treatment of a patient with any abscess of the periodontium, the dental team should appoint the patient for a thorough periodontal assessment, since the abscess of the periodontium frequently occurs in a patient with existing untreated periodontal disease.

i. In some cases following resolution of the abscess, it is wise to excise the operculum that was involved in the pericoronal abscess. This removal can prevent recurrence of the abscess. In some cases following resolution of the abscess, the dentist may recommend extraction of malposed third molar teeth if there is inadequate jaw space for the third molar teeth to fully erupt.

Box 33-4. Steps in Treatment of a Gingival or Periodontal Abscess

- Administer local anesthesia
- Drain pus
- Thorough periodontal instrumentation
- Adjust occlusion if needed
- Prescribe antibiotics if needed
- Recommend warm saline rinses
- Prescribe pain medications if needed
- Follow-up appointments

Box 33-5. Common Steps in Treatment of Patient with Pericoronal Abscess

- Administer local anesthesia
- Drain pus
- Thorough periodontal instrumentation
- Irrigate under operculum
- Prescribe antibiotics if needed
- Recommend warm saline rinses
- Prescribe pain medications if needed
- Establish follow-up appointments

Section 2
Necrotizing Periodontal Diseases

Necrotizing periodontal diseases include necrotizing ulcerative gingivitis (NUG) and necrotizing ulcerative periodontitis (NUP). NUG and NUP also are discussed in "Other Periodontal Conditions," Chapter 17. Both of these diseases are acute infections of the periodontium that can bring patients to the dental office for emergency treatment. NUG is an acute infection affecting the gingival tissues only. NUP is an acute infection that mimics NUG but can also affect the deeper structures of the periodontium such as the alveolar bone. Both conditions have been reported to occur in patients with compromised immune systems who therefore have limited host defense mechanisms.

1. **Necrotizing Ulcerative Gingivitis (NUG)**
   A. **Overview of Necrotizing Ulcerative Gingivitis**
      1. NUG is an acute infection of the periodontium that is limited to gingival tissues. Other names for this condition are Vincent's infection, trench mouth, ulceromembranous gingivitis, and acute necrotizing ulcerative gingivitis (ANUG). As the name necrotizing ulcerative gingivitis implies, patients with NUG exhibit necrosis and ulceration of the gingiva.
         a. The term necrosis refers to cell death, in this instance referring to the death of the cells comprising the gingival epithelium.
         b. The term ulceration refers to the loss of the epithelium normally covering underlying connective tissue. In NUG, ulceration results from death of the epithelial cells and the subsequent loss of the epithelium that normally covers the underlying gingival connective tissue.
      2. An impaired host response appears to be associated with the development of NUG in many patients. This impaired response may be related to any of several factors such as poor nutrition, fatigue, psychosocial factors, systemic disease, alcohol abuse, or drug abuse. It should be noted that NUG also may be associated with the immunosuppression seen in HIV infection.
      3. It is not known if bacteria are the primary cause of NUG, but studies indicate that certain bacteria including spirochetal organisms and fusiform bacilli are always associated with the disease. Other organisms have also been reported to be present in NUG.
      4. NUG occurs in patients of all ages, but the highest incidence of NUG is seen in patients between 20 and 30 years of age. In the United States NUG in children is not common, but it has been reported in children in underdeveloped countries.
      5. There are several clinical signs that distinguish NUG from other forms of gingivitis.
         a. One of those clinical signs is the presence of punched out papillae (FIG. 33-6). In NUG the necrosis associated with this condition can destroy the papillae between the teeth, resulting in the clinical appearance that the papillae are missing or "punched out." The term punched out papillae is used to underscore the crater-like appearance left by the absence of the papillae.
         b. Another clinical sign is the formation of a pseudomembrane. The necrotic areas of gingiva are covered with a gray-white layer referred to as a pseudomembrane.
            1) This pseudomembrane actually consists of dead cells, bacteria, and oral debris, and underlying this pseudomembrane is raw connective tissue.
            2) Patients with NUG usually exhibit bleeding with the slightest manipulation of the gingival tissues. This bleeding results from breakage of some of the tiny blood vessels in the connective tissues exposed under the pseudomembrane.

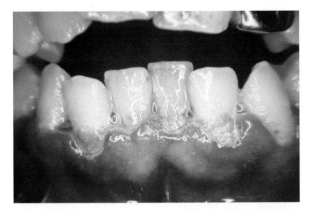

Figure 33.6. **Necrotizing Ulcerative Gingivitis.** Note that the necrotic areas have extended from the papillae onto the facial surfaces. The necrotic areas of the gingiva are covered with gray-white layer called the pseudomembrane.

Box 33-6. Characteristics of NUG

- Oral pain
- Necrotic or punched out gingival papillae
- Gingival bleeding with even slight manipulation of the gingival tissues
- Presence of pseudomembrane on affected sites
- Swollen lymph nodes (lymphadenopathy)
- Vague feeling of discomfort (malaise)
- Elevated body temperature
- Extreme halitosis

B. **Characteristics of Necrotizing Ulcerative Gingivitis.** The characteristics of NUG are described below and outlined in Box 33-6.
1. Patients with NUG experience oral pain and frequently seek emergency care for that oral pain; the ulceration associated with the infection results in exposure of connective tissue, which can be quite uncomfortable for the patients. Because of the exposure of connective tissue, bleeding from the area can appear to be spontaneous.
2. The tissue necrosis can lead to destruction of the interdental papillae resulting in punched out papillae; areas are normally covered with a collection of dead tissue cells and debris called a pseudomembrane.
3. Patients with NUG can display swollen lymph nodes (lymphadenopathy), a vague feeling of discomfort (malaise), and an elevated body temperature.
4. Because of the necrosis or death of cells involved with this disease there is usually noticeable halitosis or bad breath in NUG patients. Some authors have described this halitosis as a fetid breath.
5. Certain associated behaviors or conditions are frequently present in patients who develop NUG; these include a history of smoking, a history of poor nutrition, and a history of severe stress.
6. It has also been reported that some patients that develop NUG have a human immunodeficiency virus (HIV)-positive status. NUG has also been reported to occur in some patients with HIV infection.

C. **Typical Treatment Steps for NUG.** The treatment of patients with NUG is summarized below and outlined in Box 33-7.

1. At the first appointment.
   a. The pseudomembrane should be removed carefully with irrigation and moist cotton.
   b. Supragingival periodontal instrumentation is performed. Instrumentation is limited because of the discomfort elicited by tissue manipulation.
   c. The patient is instructed regarding a gentle self-care regimen. Toothbrushing may need to be restricted to removal of debris with soft brushes.
   d. Patients may need to use standard regimens of twice daily rinses of chlorhexidine. Some authors have suggested using three percent hydrogen peroxide with equal parts of warm water every 2 to 3 hours.

2. At first follow-up appointment 2 days after initial visit.
   a. Subgingival periodontal instrumentation usually can be begun at this appointment.
   b. Further instruction in self-care should be included at this visit.

3. At second follow-up appointment approximately 5 days after initial visit, subgingival instrumentation usually can be completed.

4. In more advanced cases of NUG antibiotics may be needed as in any other severe oral infection.

5. Following the resolution of the infection. The patient should be appointed for a comprehensive clinical assessment to identify any underlying chronic periodontal disease. Figure 33-7 illustrates before and after treatment photographs of a typical patient with early stages of NUG. Some NUG patients require periodontal surgery to reestablish natural gingival contours.

2. **Necrotizing Ulcerative Periodontitis**
   A. **Overview of Necrotizing Ulcerative Periodontitis (NUP)**
      1. Symptoms of NUP are similar to those of NUG but necrotizing ulcerative periodontitis also affects the deeper structures of the periodontium such as the alveolar bone. Necrotizing ulcerative periodontitis can occur in patients with NUG who go untreated.
      2. One unusual finding in NUP is that it can be accompanied by the formation of bone sequestra. A sequestrum is a fragment of necrotic (dead) alveolar bone.
      3. Figure 33-8 illustrates a patient with NUP.
   B. **Typical Treatment of Necrotizing Ulcerative periodontitis.** Treatment of patients with NUP is complex and may require medical consultation since the patients that develop this condition can have serious underlying medical compromising conditions that must be managed simultaneously with dental therapy. When patients with NUP are encountered in a general dental office, immediate referral to a periodontist is indicated.

Box 33-7. Typical Treatment Steps for a Patient with NUG

1. At the first appointment.

   • The pseudomembrane should be removed carefully.

   • Supragingival periodontal instrumentation is performed. Instrumentation is limited because of the discomfort elicited by tissue manipulation.

   • The patient is instructed regarding a gentle self-care regimen.

2. At first follow-up appointment 2 days after initial visit.

   • Subgingival periodontal instrumentation usually can be begun at this appointment.

   • Further instruction in self-care should be included at this visit.

3. At second follow-up appointment approximately 5 days after initial visit.

   • Subgingival instrumentation usually can be completed.

4. Following the resolution of the infection. The patient should be appointed for a comprehensive clinical assessment to identify any underlying chronic periodontal disease.

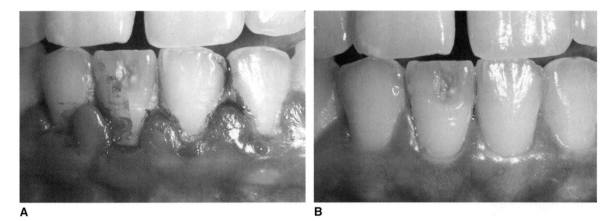

A **B**

Figure 33.7. Necrotizing Ulcerative Gingivitis: Before and After Treatment. A: Necrotizing ulcerative gingivitis before treatment. **B:** The same patient after treatment. (Courtesy of Dr Don Rolfs, Periodontal Foundations, Wachatee, WA.)

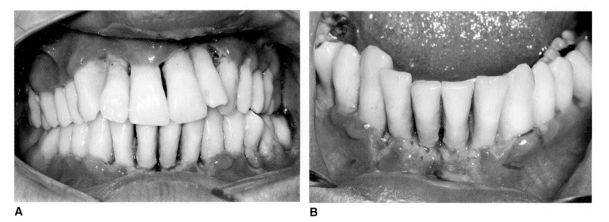

A **B**

Figure 33.8. Necrotizing Ulcerative Periodontitis. A: A patient with NUP. **B:** Close-up of the mandibular arch. (Courtesy of Dr Don Rolfs, Periodontal Foundations, Wachatee, WA.)

Section 3
Primary Herpetic Gingivostomatitis

1. **Overview of Primary Herpetic Gingivostomatitis (PHG)**
   A. **Etiology of PHG.** PHG is actually a medical condition resulting from a viral infection. It is listed here as a periodontal emergency condition since patients with this condition can first seek care in a dental office because of the nature of the oral symptoms that may develop.
   B. **Characteristics of PHG**
      1. Primary herpetic gingivostomatitis is a painful oral condition that results from the initial infection with the herpes simplex virus (HSV).
         a. There are two types of herpes simplex virus, oral herpes virus (HSVI) and genital herpes virus (HSVII). PHG is usually caused by initial infection with HSVI but can also be caused by initial infection with HSVII.
         b. In the majority of patients, the initial infection with these viruses produces no noticeable clinical signs and can go undetected clinically. In other patients, however, the oral symptoms resulting from this initial infection can be quite severe, and it is these severe oral symptoms that are known as primary herpetic gingivostomatitis (FIG. 33-9).

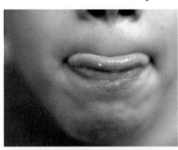

A

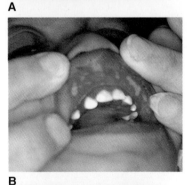

B

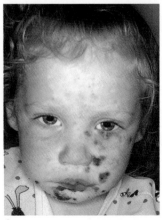

C

Figure 33.9. Primary Oral Infection with Herpes Simplex Virus. These three children demonstrate the spectrum of primary oral infection with the HSV, which ranges from asymptomatic to severe. **A:** The first patient has a single vesicle on his tongue. **B:** The second patient manifests widespread labial lesions. The parent's fingers are shown in the photograph; however, touching the infected area with bare fingers is not recommended. The dental hygienist should advise parents that contact with open sores or saliva can spread the virus. **C:** The third patient shows a severe infection with lesions on the face. (From Fleisher GR, Ludwig W, Baskin MN. *Atlas of Pediatric Emergency Medicine.* Philadelphia: Lippincott Williams & Wilkins; 2004.)

2. *Primary herpetic gingivostomatitis is contagious and requires careful attention to prevent its spread.*
   a. Infections caused by HSV are contagious during the vesicular stage as the virus is contained in the clear fluid in the vesicles.
   b. HSV-1 is primarily spread by direct contact through kissing and contact with open sores or by contact with infected saliva (FIG. 33-10).
   c. HSV-1 can also spread from one part of the body to another, such as from saliva to the fingers, then to the eye. Touching the eye can result in a painful and dangerous herpetic infection of the cornea (herpes keratitis).
3. The initial infection with HSV-I usually occurs in children or in young adults, but it can occur at any age.
4. Once a patient is infected with this virus, the infection can recur periodically throughout the life of the patient in the form of herpes labialis (fever blisters or cold sores).

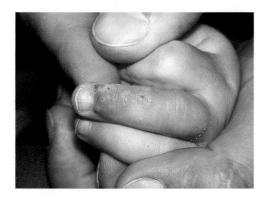

Figure 33.10. Primary Herpes Simplex Virus Infection in Infancy. Finger sucking likely caused the spread of the infection from the mouth to the hand of the infant. The parent's fingers are shown in the photograph; however, touching the infected area with bare fingers is not recommended. (From Goodheart HP. *Goodheart's Photoguide of Common Skin Disorders.* 2nd ed. Philadelphia: Lippincott Williams & Wilkins; 2003.)

2. **Clinical Signs and Treatment of PHG**
   A. **Clinical Signs.** As already mentioned, the clinical signs of primary herpetic gingivostomatitis can range from subclinical (no noticeable signs) to rather severe; the severe clinical signs are discussed below and outlined in Box 33-8.
      1. Severe oral pain can be associated with primary herpetic gingivostomatitis, and this discomfort results in difficulty in eating and drinking.
      2. The gingival tissues appear swollen (edematous), red (erythematous), and bleed quite easily when disturbed.
      3. PHG is accompanied by painful oral ulcers. Careful inspection of the gingival tissue can reveal small clusters of blisters (vesicles) on the tissues that burst, leaving numerous, painful oral ulcers. The ulcers are surrounded by a red halo.
         a. The ulcers can occur on lips, palate, and tongue as well as the gingival tissue.
         b. Pain caused by these ulcers can be such a major problem that eating and drinking can be impaired. Restricting fluids can even lead to dehydration, and dehydration in a child can be a serious medical emergency.
      4. In the more severe clinical manifestation, this infection is associated with signs and symptoms such as elevated body temperature, a vague feeling of discomfort (malaise), headache, and swollen lymph nodes (lymphadenopathy).

B. **Treatment.** Treatment of patients with primary herpetic gingivostomatitis is primarily supportive (i.e., designed to keep the patient as comfortable as possible until the viral infection runs its course). Typical steps in the management of a patient with primary herpetic gingivostomatitis are discussed below and outlined in Box 33-9.

1. The dental hygienist should keep in mind that primary herpetic gingivostomatitis is contagious, and any plan for periodontal debridement of the teeth should be postponed until the initial infection regresses.

2. Primary herpetic gingivostomatitis usually regresses spontaneously (goes away without treatment) in approximately 2 weeks. Controlling discomfort and ensuring fluid intake are the main focus for supportive treatment.

3. Topical oral anesthetics can be used to control oral discomfort temporarily to allow the patient to eat or to drink fluids. Examples of topical anesthetics that can be used are (1) 2% Lidocaine viscous and (2) Orabase with benzocaine.

4. In some patients, treatment will include antiviral medications, medications to reduce fever (antipyretics), and systemic medications to control pain (analgesics).

Box 33-8. Clinical Signs of Primary Herpetic Gingivostomatitis

- Oral pain with difficulty in eating and drinking

- Edematous gingival tissues (swollen gingival tissue)

- Bleeding from gingival tissue

- Vesicles (blisters) and ulceration of the gingival tissue and sometimes the lips, tongue, and palate; ulcerations surrounded by red halo

- Elevated body temperature

- Malaise (vague feeling of discomfort)

- Swollen lymph nodes

Box 33-9. Typical Steps in Management of Primary Herpetic Gingivostomatitis

1. Keep in mind that this disease is highly contagious.

2. Primary Herpetic Gingivostomatitis regresses spontaneously in about 2 weeks.

3. Control oral discomfort. Topical oral anesthetics can be used for temporary relief of oral discomfort so that the patient can eat and drink fluids.

4. Recommend frequent fluid intake to avoid dehydration.

5. Refer the patient to a physician if systemic symptoms are severe or if the patient is unable to tolerate fluid intake.

Chapter Summary Statement

This chapter discussed some acute periodontal conditions that can bring patients to the office for an emergency visit. All members of the dental team should be on alert for these conditions. The dental hygienist may encounter some of these conditions in their earliest stages during routine treatment visits. Acute periodontal conditions include abscesses of the periodontium, necrotizing periodontal diseases, and primary herpetic gingivostomatitis.

Section 4
Focus On Patients

Case 1

During a routine patient visit for periodontal maintenance, you note that there is swelling in the interdental papilla between a patient's two central incisors. The swelling is quite localized to the area between the incisors. As you manipulate the tissues, you note pus coming from the sulcus of one of the central incisors. You also note some mobility of one of the incisor teeth. When questioned, the patient informs you that she is aware that these tissues are swollen and that she has been flossing more in hope that the swelling would go down. In view of these clinical findings how should you proceed at this maintenance visit?

Case 2

A concerned parent, who is one of your maintenance patients, calls you to tell you that her 6-year-old daughter has something wrong with her gums. She reports that her daughter's gums appear swollen and that there appears to be some raw, red areas on the gums. Her child has been complaining of pain in her mouth and has an elevated temperature. How should you respond to the parent's concerns?

Case 3

A patient with necrotizing ulcerative gingivitis (NUG) is referred to you by the dentist for calculus removal. Your examination of the patient reveals ulceration of most interdental papillae with the typical punched out papillae often seen with this disease. The necrotic tissue pseudomembrane is present covering the ulcerations, and heavy calculus deposits are evident. The patient is quite uncomfortable. How should you proceed with the calculus removal?

Suggested Readings

Ahl DR, Hilgeman JL, Synder JD. Periodontal emergencies. *Dent Clin North Am.*1986;30:459–472.

American Academy of Periodontology. Parameter on acute periodontal diseases. *J Periodontol.* 2000;71(5 Suppl):863–866.

Antonelli JR. Acute dental pain, Part 1: Diagnosis and emergency treatment. *Compendium.* 1990;11:492, 494–496, 498–500.

Antonelli JR. Acute dental pain, Part II: Diagnosis and emergency treatment. *Compendium.* 1990;11:526, 528, 530–533.

Barr CB, Robbins MR. Clinical and radiographic presentations of HIV-1 necrotizing ulcerative periodontitis. *Spec Care Dentist.* 1996;16:237–241.

Blakey GH, White RP Jr, Offenbacher S, et al. Clinical/biological outcomes of treatment for pericoronitis. *J Oral Maxillofac Surg.* 1996;54:1150–1160.

Cohen-Cole SA, Cogen RB, Stevens AW, Jr., Kirk K, et al. Psychiatric, psychosocial and endocrine correlates of acute necrotizing ulcerative gingivitis (trench mouth): a preliminary report. *Psychiatr Med.* 1983;1:215–225.

Formicola A, Witte E, Curran P. A study of personality traits and acute necrotizing ulcerative gingivitis. *J Periodontol.* 1970;41:36–38.

Gowdey G, Alijanian A. Necrotizing ulcerative periodontitis in an HIV patient. *J Calif Dent Assoc.* 1995;23:57–59.

Gray JL, Flanary DB, Newell DH. The prevalence of periodontal abscess. *J Indiana Dent Assoc.* 1994;73:18–23.

Haber J, Wattles J, Crowlery M, et al. Evidence for cigarette smoking, bacterial pathogens, and periodontal status. *J Periodontol.* 1993;64:16–23.

Herrera D, Roldán S, González I, Sanz M. The periodontal abscess (1). Clinical and microbiological findings. *J Clin Periodontol.* 2000;27:387–394.

Homing GM, Cohen ME. Necrotizing ulcerative gingivitis, periodontitis, and stomatitis: Clinical staging and predisposing factors. *J Periodontol.* 1995;66:990–998.

Hooper PA, Seymour GJ. The histopathogenesis of acute ulcerative gingivitis, *J Periodontol.* 1997;50:419–423.

Horning GM, Cohen ME. Necrotizing ulcerative gingivitis, periodontitis and stomatitis: Clinical staging and predisposing factors, *J Periodontol.* 1995;66:990–998.

McLeod DE, Lainson PA, Spivey JD. Tooth loss due to periodontal abscess: A retrospective study. *J Periodontol.* 1997;68:963–966.

Minsk L. Diagnosis and treatment of acute periodontal conditions. *Compend Contin Educ Dent.* 2006;27(1):8–11.

Novak MJ. Necrotizing ulcerative periodontitis. *Ann Periodontol.* 1999;4:74–78.

Peltroche-Llacsahuanga H, Reichhart E, Schmitt W, et al. Investigation of infectious organisms causing pericoronitis of the mandibular third molar. *J Oral Maxillofac Surg.* 2000;58:611–616.

Rowland R. Necrotizing ulcerative gingivitis. *Ann Periodontol.* 1999;4:65–73.

Topoll HH, Lange DE, Muller RF. Multiple periodontal abscesses after systemic antibiotic therapy. *J Clin Periodontol.* 1990;17:268–272.

Wade DN, Kerns DG. Acute necrotizing ulcerative gingivitis-periodontitis: A literature review. *Mil Med.* 1998;163:337–342.

Chapter 34

Documentation and Insurance Reporting of Periodontal Care

Learning Objectives

- Understand the foundations of tort law and how it applies to the profession of dentistry.

- Define the term liability as it applies to provision of periodontal care.

- Identify situations in the dental office that trigger liability for dental hygienists.

- Define the terms intentional torts and negligence and give examples of each.

- In the clinical setting, thoroughly document all periodontal treatment including treatment options, cancellations, patient noncompliance, refusal of treatment, and follow-up telephone calls.

- Define the terms insurance codes and insurance form and explain their use in periodontal care.

Key Terms

Liability
Malpractice
Tort
Intentional torts

Negligence
Computer-based patient record
Insurance codes
Dental insurance claim form

Section 1
Legal Issues in the Provision and Documentation of Care

It is important for every dental hygienist to practice to the highest established standards of care, not only to insure the safety of the patient receiving treatment but also to avoid costly malpractice litigation. Potential liability is a reality for every healthcare provider. While patients can sue a dentist or dental hygienist for many reasons, the success of such a suit often depends on the quality of the chart notes. The dental hygienist has a moral and ethical obligation to deliver high quality care and maintain thorough chart notes for each patient visit to protect the practice against liability.

CONCEPTS OF MALPRACTICE AND TORT LAW

1. **Liability.** In the context of healthcare, liability is a healthcare provider's obligation or responsibility to provide services to another person (the patient). The healthcare provider's liability entails the possibility of being sued if the person receiving the services feels as if he has been treated improperly or negligently.
2. **Malpractice.** Malpractice is the improper or negligent treatment by a healthcare provider that results in injury or damage to the patient.
3. **Tort.** The legal basis for most lawsuits in dental and dental hygiene practice is founded on tort law. A tort is a civil wrong where a person has breached a duty to another. A tort is the law that permits an injured person to recover compensation from the person who caused the injury.
   A. **Intentional Torts.** Intentional torts are actions designed to injure another person or that person's property. There are many specific types of intentional torts, including the following:
      1. Battery is the unlawful and unwanted touching or striking of one person by another, with the intention of bringing about a harmful or offensive contact. Forceful discipline of unruly children in the dental chair could be construed as battery.
      2. Assault is an unlawful threat or attempt to do bodily injury to another. A doctor who treats a minor patient without proper parental or guardian informed consent could be charged with assault or battery.
      3. Infliction of emotional distress. An example is talking in a loud or harsh voice to an unruly child.
      4. Fraud is deception carried out for the purpose of achieving personal gain while causing injury to another party.
      5. Misrepresentation occurs when a healthcare provider deliberately deceives a patient about possible outcomes.
      6. Defamation is communication to third parties of false statements about a person that injure the reputation of or deter others from associating with that person. For example, a dental hygienist learns that another hygienist has been making disparaging comments about the quality of care that he provides. The hygienist being disparaged could sue for defamation.
      7. Trespass is to infringe on the privacy, time, or attention of another. An example is discussing a patient's personal information with someone without the patient's permission.
      8. Defamation by computer. Email correspondence and other written documents are discoverable in court, so avoid disparaging remarks in email communications.

B. **Negligence.** Negligence is a failure to exercise reasonable care to avoid injuring others. It is the failure to do something that a reasonable person would do under the same circumstances, or the doing of something a reasonable person would not do. Negligence is characterized by carelessness, inattentiveness, and neglectfulness rather than by a positive intent to cause injury.

1. Negligence is different from an intentional tort in that negligence *does not require* the intent to commit a wrongful action; instead, the wrongful action itself is sufficient to constitute negligence.

2. Examples of negligence include accidentally spilling a chemical on a patient, not updating the patient's health history resulting in the patient's health being jeopardized, and incorrect treatment of periodontal disease. Professional liability insurance typically covers only unintentional torts or negligence.

AREAS OF POTENTIAL LIABILITY

In judging whether a professional has been negligent, the courts use a standard called the *reasonable prudent person or professional*. This means the court compares what a reasonably prudent person or professional would have done in a similar situation. Thus, providing periodontal care that meets or exceeds the standard of care is extremely important for dental hygienists. Failure to include a procedure or step in treatment because the dental hygienist claims to be unaware of the current standard will not hold up in court. The top 10 areas of potential liability for dental hygienists are summarized below in Box 34-1.

The standard of care for periodontal charting is that every adult patient will have a six-point periodontal charting with all numbers recorded a minimum of once per year. Other types of periodontal screening systems, such as PSR recording, do not take the place of the once yearly full-mouth probing and recording.

Box 34-1. Top 10 Areas of Potential Liability for Dental Hygienists

1. Failure to ask and document whether the patient has taken his or her premedication.

2. Failure to detect and document oral cancer.

3. Failure to update the patient's medical history.

4. Failure to detect and thoroughly document the presence of periodontal disease.

5. Injuring a patient.

6. Failure to thoroughly document treatment in the patient chart or computerized record.

7. Failure to protect patient privacy or divulging confidential patient information.

8. Failure to inform the patient about treatment options and the consequences of nontreatment.

9. Practicing outside the legal scope of practice. All dental hygienists should be well informed about the state practice act and follow the rules and regulations explicitly.

10. Failure to provide care that meets the established standards of care.

Section 2
Documentation of Periodontal Care

The dental chart is a legal document. It is the first line of defense in a malpractice suit. *When a patient decides to file a lawsuit, the dental chart becomes the single most important piece of information relative to the suit. Faulty records can be the most important reason for the loss of a lawsuit.* All periodontal assessment, educational, and treatment services should be documented in the patient chart or computerized record. Recommendations for thorough documentation are summarized in TABLE 34-1.

TABLE 34-1. Documentation Guidelines

Action	Why It Is Recommended
Format: • Write on the proper form or computer document. • Write or print legibly in blue or black ink. • Use correct grammar, spelling, and standard dental terminology. • Date each entry correctly.	• It is important to write or print legibly to avoid miscommunication (some lawyers infer sloppy care from sloppy entries or charting). • The date that actions occurred or observations were made is an important element of the dental record, which is a legal account of care provided.

Content:
 	
 • Only record care that you have given or observations that you have made. Do not make entries for another care provider.
 • Enter information in a complete, accurate, concise, and factual manner.
 • Entries may include the
  ○ Reason for today's appointment
  ○ Thorough documentation of medical and dental history
  ○ Patient's chief complaint
  ○ Symptoms reported by the patient
  ○ Findings from the clinical periodontal assessment
  ○ Treatment options and recommendations
  ○ Patient treatment choices
  ○ All assessment, educational, and treatment services
  ○ Items given to patient, such as educational materials or home care aids
  ○ Date or interval of next appointment
 • Remember that in a liability situation, care or recommendations not recorded was not provided.
	• By making an entry in a dental record, you accept legal responsibility for that entry.
	 • Use only commonly accepted dental terminology and standard abbreviations and symbols. Do not create your own abbreviations. Using correct terminology and abbreviations will prevent others from having to second-guess your meaning.
	 • Proper and conscientious recording protects the patient, your employer, and you.

(continued)

TABLE 34-1. Documentation Guidelines (*continued*)

Action	Why It Is Recommended
Accountability: • Check the patient's name on the dental record and on the form where you are recording. • Always sign your first initial, last name and title to each entry. • All entries should be written on the lines. No entries should be made in the margins or below the last line on the page. No lines should be skipped. • Do not use dittos, erasures, or correcting fluids. A single line should be drawn through an incorrect entry and words "mistaken entry" or "error in charting" should be printed above or beside the entry and signed. The entry should then be rewritten correctly. • Identify each page of the record with the patient's name and chart identification number. • Recognize that a patient record (chart) is permanent.	• By verifying the patient's identification information, you ensure that you are recording the person's information on the correct record. • By signing your entry, you indicate that you are the person who needs to be consulted if further clarification of the information is needed. Additionally, signing your entry indicates that you accept legal responsibility for what you have written. • All lines should be used so that there is no opportunity for anyone to add information after a lawsuit is initiated. Making entries in the margins or below the last line on a page can cause juries to wonder if the entry was made at a later date. • Striking through an error is the only legal way to indicate a change in the dental record. Erasing or using correction fluid could be seen as an attempt to hide or change existing information.
Timing: • Record information in a timely manner. • Document care as closely as possible to the time of providing treatment. • Do not record care as given before you have provided the care.	• If you wait until the end of the day to record, you may forget important information. • Something may occur that prevents you from providing the anticipated care (the patient may become ill halfway through the appointment; the patient may refuse a fluoride treatment). If you record care as "provided" in the dental record, but then do not actually complete this care, you will have committed fraud.
Confidentiality: • Clinicians using patient records are bound professionally and ethically to keep in strict confidence all information they learn by reading patient records.	• Individuals have a moral and legal right to expect that the information contained in their patient dental record will be kept private.

1. **Principles for Thorough Documentation.** Jeffery J. Tonner, J.D. [1] recommends several principles that every dental professional should follow when documenting periodontal treatment in the patient chart or computerized record.

   A. **General Guidelines for Chart Entries**

      1. All entries should be complete and accurate using accepted dental terminology and abbreviations. Chart Entry-1 is an example of a complete chart entry.

      2. It is helpful to organize the services documented in sequential order so that no information is omitted.

      3. If handwritten, entries should be legible and in ink.

      4. The healthcare provider making the entry should sign the entry with his or her first initial, last name, and title. Since many different people write in the patient chart, it is important that each entry be signed. If there are multiple dentists in the practice, the dentist that examines the hygienist's patient should be identified also.

      5. Thorough chart entries provide valuable information for the next clinician that treats this patient.

      6. The patient should be thoroughly interviewed regarding his or her medical status at each visit. Patients do not usually volunteer information when they are taking a new medicine or if there has been a change in their medical history. The medical status should be thoroughly documented at each visit.

   B. **Treatment Options.** The healthcare provider should document all treatment options presented to the patient.

   C. **Appointment Schedule and Chart Entries**

      1. Chart entries should be consistent with the appointment schedule.

         a. With most dental software and computer scheduling, the patient's name must be on the schedule in order to make a chart entry.

         b. With manual appointment books, however, entries can be erased and changed.

      2. In the event of a lawsuit, doubt may be cast on the reliability of the office's records if the treatment dates in the chart do not match the appointment book entries.

      3. If the patient is being seen as an emergency patient this circumstance should be recorded in the chart.

   D. **Cancellations and Missed Appointments.** All cancellations and missed appointments should be written in the patient chart. Infrequent periodontal maintenance appointments can lead to a recurrence and progression of periodontal disease. Chart Entry-2 and Chart Entry-3 provide examples of how to document missed and cancelled appointments.

Date	Treatment Rendered
1/10/10	Reason for visit: 3-month periodontal maintenance. Medical history update: patient now taking
	one aspirin a day per his physician's recommendation. Chief complaint: none. Oral cancer exam:
	normal. Periodontal probing: changes noted in charting. Plaque biofilm: light, calculus: light,
	bleeding areas noted on periodontal chart. Perio maintenance: perio instrumentation of all four
	quads; ultrasonic and hand instrumentation. Plaque biofilm removal by patient using toothbrush
	and interdental brush. Patient tolerated all procedures well. Patient education: reviewed use of
	tufted dental floss around distal surfaces of maxillary and mandibular molars. Tray fluoride application
	1.23% APF gel for sensitivity. Four bitewing radiographs. Next maintenance visit in 3 months.
	R. Zimmer, RDH

Chart Entry-1. Complete Chart Entry. This chart entry is an example of a thorough chart entry that documents all the events of the patient's appointment.

E. Patient Noncompliance and Refusal of Treatment
1. Patient noncompliance with recommendations, such as (1) inadequate self-care, (2) continued smoking, (3) failure to regulate diabetes, or (4) failure to follow specific instructions, can lead to disease progression. Noncompliance should be noted in the chart (Chart Entry-4). Chart Entry-5 provides an example of documentation of inadequate self-care.
2. Instances when a patient opts not to have recommended treatment or declines a referral to a specialist should be documented. Further, when a patient is referred to a specialist, it is recommended that a copy of the referral letter be kept in the patient chart.

F. Follow-up Telephone Calls. Patients appreciate a follow-up telephone call from the dentist or hygienist following a long or difficult treatment procedure. For hygienists, a good rule of thumb is to call any patient that required anesthesia for periodontal instrumentation. Follow-up telephone calls should be documented (Chart Entry-6).

Date	Treatment Rendered
1/10/10	Patient missed maintenance appointment because of illness. *R. Zimmer, RDH*

Chart Entry-2. Missed Appointment. This chart entry is an example of documentation of a missed appointment due to illness.

Date	Treatment Rendered
1/10/10	Telephoned patient to confirm her 3-month maintenance appt. Patient cancelled and said that
	she would call to reschedule later. I reminded her of the importance of regular maintenance.
	R. Zimmer, RDH

Chart Entry-3. Cancelled Maintenance Appointment. This chart entry provides an example of the documentation for a cancelled periodontal maintenance appointment.

Date	Treatment Rendered
1/10/10	Discussed options for smoking cessation. Patient stated that "he is not interested in quitting
	smoking." *R. Zimmer, RDH*

Chart Entry-4. Patient Noncompliance. This chart entry provides an example of the documentation for patient noncompliance with recommendations.

Date	Treatment Rendered
1/10/10	Patient reports brushing twice daily but "does not have time to use an interdental brush."
	Showed patient signs of periodontal inflammation in the interdental areas. Explained benefits
	of interdental plaque biofilm removal and several alternatives for interdental self-care. Patient
	decided that he was not interested and stated that "he only wants to brush." *R. Zimmer, RDH*

Chart Entry-5. Inadequate Self-Care. This chart entry is an example of documentation of inadequate self-care by a patient.

Date	Treatment Rendered
1/10/10	Telephoned patient at home this evening to check on her. Patient reports that she "has no
	bleeding and rates her pain as a 2, on a scale of 1 to 10." Reminded her to use warm saltwater
	rinse before bedtime. *R. Zimmer, RDH*

Chart Entry-6. Follow-up Telephone Call. This chart entry is an example of documentation of a follow-up telephone call after a long or difficult treatment procedure.

2. **Pitfalls in Documentation.** Jeffery J. Tonner, J.D. [1] outlines four common pitfalls in documentation.

   A. **Making Entries in Haste.** Chart Entry-7 is an example of an *inadequate* chart entry. For example, in her haste to stay on schedule, the dental hygienist simply forgets to record that she did a periodontal charting and evaluation. Later, if the patient develops periodontal disease, he may accuse the doctor of failure to diagnose. The dentist or hygienist may state to a jury that a periodontal evaluation is done on every patient. *In the eyes of a jury, however, if a procedure is not written in the chart, it was not done.*

   B. **Skipping Lines Between Entries or Writing in Margins**
      1. Keeping in the lines or skipping lines.
         a. Chart entries should be written with small enough strokes to be contained within the space provided.
         b. No lines should be skipped on a treatment record form. All lines should be used so that there is no opportunity for anyone to add information *after* a lawsuit is initiated.
      2. Writing in margins or below the last line. All entries should be written on the lines, and no entries should be written in the margins or below the last line on the page. Doing so can cause juries to wonder if the entry was made at a later date.

   C. **Altering Chart Entries.** *The single most common cause of punitive damages in a dental malpractice suit is altering the chart.*
      1. Correction fluid should never be used to correct an entry. If an error is made, a single line should be drawn through the incorrect entry so that it can still be read, the words *charting error or mistaken entry* written above it, and the correct entry made on the next available line. The revised entry should be signed.
      2. Additional information should never be added to an entry from a previous appointment. Juries perceive such added entries to be fraudulent and deceptive.
      3. Forensic ink dating analysis allows an expert to determine the date that ink was used on a particular document. Therefore, it is foolhardy to add things at a later date to a patient chart in an attempt to avoid or win a lawsuit.

   D. **Not Clearly Indicating Patient Comments.** Quotation marks should be used to indicate patient comments. This is especially important when making follow-up telephone calls after a difficult or invasive procedure. A sample chart entry is shown in Chart Entry-8.

Date	Treatment Rendered
1/10/10	Px, Ex

Chart Entry-7. Incomplete Chart Entry. Although this hygienist may have been quite thorough in delivering care, the chart does not reflect that.

Date	Treatment Rendered
1/10/10	Patient reports that his "gums no longer bleed during brushing." Tissue color, tone, and
	texture are much improved from 3 weeks ago. *R. Zimmer, RDH*

Chart Entry-8. Patient Comments. This chart entry is an example of how to include a patient's comments at a periodontal maintenance visit.

Section 3
Computer-Based Patient Records

1. **Advantages of Computerized Patient Records.** The objective of a computer-based patient record is to improve the uniformity, accuracy, and ease of retrieval of data about patient care. Advantages of computerized records include
   A. **Organization and Data Gathering**
      1. *Standardization of clinical data* where all staff members use the same templates for gathering data and the same abbreviations.
      2. *Greater legibility.* Handwriting can often be illegible, which increases liability risk for the clinician.
      3. *Easier and faster access to information.* Information is only a few keystrokes away. *Patient information is accessible across the network simultaneously.*
      4. *Enhanced use of clinical images and radiographs.* Before and after digital photographs and digital radiographs can be included in the computerized patient record.
      5. *Provision of new ways to analyze clinical information.* Digital radiography allows the clinician to view radiographs with digital tools designed to enhance the image and visualize bone levels around teeth.
      6. *Potential for greater security of patient data.* Paper records are vulnerable to fire, earthquake, and water damage from flooding. Computer-based patient records can be backed up offsite to preserve data. Note that computerized data is more secure only if it is continuously backed up to an offsite location.
   B. **Processing of Information**
      1. *Patient information is accessible across the network simultaneously.* Business assistants can read input from clinicians and be ready for patient checkout before the patient reaches the business office.
      2. *Facilitates submission of insurance claims.* Computerized information facilitates submission of dental insurance claim forms to insurance companies.
   C. **Communication**
      1. *Faster and better multidisciplinary interaction with specialists.* Successful treatment of periodontitis requires a team approach involving the primary care (general) dental team, the periodontal dental team, and often, other dental specialists or physicians.
      2. Continuous communication among healthcare providers is critical to the success of diagnosis, treatment, and maintenance. Ongoing communication is needed because it is common for the patient to be treated in phases, going back and forth between the primary care dental practice and the periodontal practice. A computer-based patient record can greatly increase the effectiveness of communication among dental healthcare providers (FIG. 34-1).
2. **Cautions Regarding Computerized Records.** Even with advancing technologies, practitioners and staff must realize that the transition to computer-based patient records is not seamless, totally safe, or problem-free.
   A. **Data Backup.** Anyone who has ever used a computer recognizes that computers crash, freeze-up, and frequently loose data. Computer-based patient records can be backed up offsite to preserve data. Data should be continuously backed up to a secure offsite location.
   B. **State Regulations.** In some states, computerized records may not eliminate the need to keep paper records due to legal requirements in those states. In such cases, the dental office may need to maintain patient data on paper and in computerized versions.

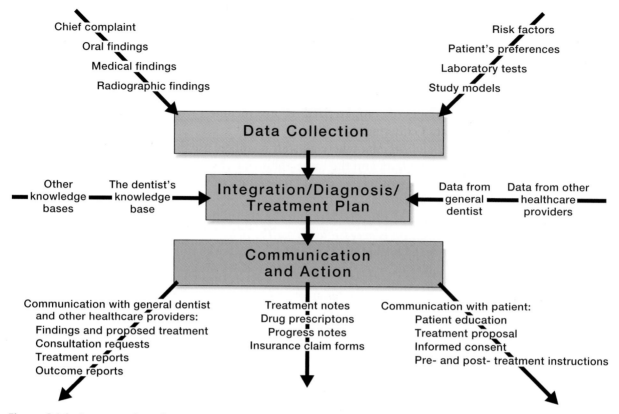

Figure 34.1. Computer-based patient records (CPR) can enhance data gathering, organization, processing, and communication.

Section 4
Insurance Codes for Periodontal Treatment

INSURANCE CODING

1. Insurance codes are numeric codes used by insurance companies and the government to classify different dental procedures. For example, periodontal maintenance procedures are designated by the insurance code D4910. Dental insurance codes are revised frequently and should be reviewed carefully before specific periodontal care is coded.
2. Insurance coding was developed to speed and simplify the reporting of dental treatments to third parties such as insurance companies and the government.
3. The most important use of codes is for insurance billing purposes. Insurance codes are entered on a dental insurance claim form. Dental treatment is listed under the appropriate procedure number. An example of a completed dental insurance claim form is shown in Figure 34-2.
4. In the United States, insurance codes are published in the *American Dental Association Current Dental Terminology* [2]. These codes are very specific and should be reviewed carefully before specific dental treatment is coded.

INSURANCE CODES FOR NONSURGICAL PERIODONTAL SERVICES

1. **Evolution of Dental Terminology**
   A. Members of the dental team should be aware that there is a continuous evolution of terminology used in dentistry and medicine.
      1. Changes in terminology occur as a natural result of scientific advances and improved understanding of disease pathogenesis.
      2. Terminology related to nonsurgical therapy is currently undergoing one such change.
   B. Traditionally in the dental literature, two terms have been used to describe the therapies employed to remove deposits from tooth surfaces. These terms are (1) *dental prophylaxis* and (2) *scaling and root planing*.
   C. Recently in the dental hygiene literature, increasing numbers of authors are using new terminology to describe periodontal instrumentation.
      1. The term periodontal debridement is suggested to replace the older terms dental prophylaxis and scaling and root planing.
      2. *In dental hygiene literature, periodontal debridement is defined as the removal or disruption of bacterial plaque biofilm, its by-products, and plaque biofilm–retentive calculus deposits from coronal surfaces, root surfaces, and within the pocket space and tissue wall, as indicated, for periodontal healing and repair.*
2. **Codes for Insurance Reporting.** The ADA Current Dental Terminology continues to use the terms "prophylaxis" and "scaling and root planing" to describe periodontal instrumentation. *Dental team members will have to use the currently accepted insurance codes when filling out insurance forms and in communications with insurance companies or other third-party payers.*
   A. **Codes for Periodontal Examination**
      1. D0120—Periodic Oral Evaluation. An evaluation performed on a patient of record to determine any changes in the patient's dental and medical health status since a previous comprehensive or periodic evaluation. This includes periodontal screening and may require interpretation of information acquired through additional diagnostic procedures.

DENTAL CLAIM FORM

Check One:
☐ Dentist's pre-treatment estimate
☐ Dentist's statement of actual services

If the cost of treatment is expected to exceed $300, a pre-treatment estimate should be completed. The physician or dentist must indicate: A list of every recommended dental procedure; and the charge for each procedure and provide supporting pre-treatment radiographs.

1. Patient name & address: **Mr. Boyd Bogus** **22 S. Green St. Ardendale, NC 28759**	2. Relationship to employee ☒ Self ☐ Spouse ☐ Child	3. Sex Ⓜ/ F	4. Patient birthdate **05 / 14 / 50**	5. Is dependent a full time Student? ___ Yes ___ No

6. Employee's name (Last, First, Middle Initial) **UUP Benefit Trust Fund**	7. Employee's SSN **001-00-1-1000**	7. Group number/Name **3214192**	

9. Employee'smiling address **22 S. Green Street**	10. City, State, Zip **Ardendale, NC 28759**

11. Other family members employed? If yes, member's name **Brenda Bogus**	SSN# **002-02-0000**	Spouse Birthdate: **09 / 05 / 53**	12. Name and address of employer **22 S. Green Street Ardendale, NC 28759**

11. Is patient covered by another dental plan? ___ Yes **X** No	Dental plan name	Group number	14. Name and address of employer

I have reviewed the following treatment plan, I authorize release of any information relating to this claim.

_____ _____
Signed (patient or parent if minor)   Date

I authorize direct **payment** of benefits to the dentist or supplier.

_____ _____
Signed (employee)   Date

14. Dentist's name **Harry M. Montigue**	22. Is treatment result of Occupational illness or injury? ___ Yes **X** No If **yes**, give brief description and dates

15. Dentist's address **1212 Upward Avenue** **Ardendale, NC 28759**	23. Is treatment result of Auto Accident? ___ Yes **X** No Other accident? ___ Yes ___ No 24. If **yes**, give brief description and dates

16. Dentist's SSN or TIN 17. License# 18. Phone#	25. If Prosthesis, is this initial placement? ___ Yes **X** No If **no**, reason for placement 28. Date of placement

19. First visit date Current series	20. Place of treatment ☐ Office ☐ Hospital ☐ ECF ☐ Other _____	21. Radiographs or models enclosed? ___ Yes ___ No How many? _____	27. Is treatment for Orthodontics? ___ Yes **X** No 28. If services already commenced: Date appliances applied: Months of treatment remaining: _____ _____

19. Identify missing teeth with "X"

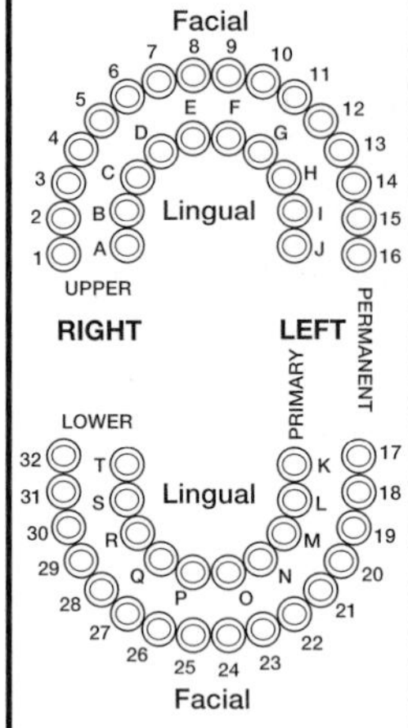

30. EXAMINATION & TREATMENT PLAN. LIST IN ORDER FROM TOOTH NO. 1 THROUGH TOOTH NO. 32 USE CHARTING SYSTEM SHOWN

TOOTH No. or Letter	SURFACE	DESCRIPTION OF SERVICE (Including X-rays, prophylaxis, materials used, etc.)	Date service performed Mo. Day Year	Procedure Code	FEE
		Complete intraoral radiographic series	3 / 28 / 10	D0210	
		Periodontal maintenance	3 / 28 / 10	D4910	
31	D	Localized delivery antimicrobial agent	3 / 28 / 10	D4381	
		Tropical fluoride treatment	3 / 28 / 10	D1204	
		Oral hygiene instructions	3 / 28 / 10	D1330	
			/ /		
			/ /		
			/ /		
			/ /		

I hereby certify that the procedures as indicated by Date ☐ Will be   completed
                                                      ☐ Have been

_____ _____
Signed   Date

TOTAL FEE CHARGED	
MAXIMUM ALLOWABLE	
DEDUCTIBLE	
PLAN %	
PLAN PAYS	
PATIENT PAYS	

REMARKS:

Figure 34.2. Dental Insurance Claim Form. An example of a completed dental insurance claim form.

2. D0180—Comprehensive Periodontal Evaluation—New or Established Patient. This code is used for patients showing signs or symptoms of periodontal disease and for patients with risk factors such as smoking or diabetes. This examination code may be used when the hygienist performs a comprehensive periodontal evaluation including full-mouth, six-point probing and recording, charting of recession, furcations, tooth mobility, or tissue abnormalities once per year.

B. **Currently Accepted Insurance Codes Pertaining to Periodontal Instrumentation**

1. D1110—adult prophylaxis (four quadrants). A dental prophylaxis includes scaling and polishing procedures to remove coronal plaque biofilm, calculus, and stains. *This code usually is used for healthy patients and patients with gingivitis.* Scaling on this type of patient usually can be completed in a single appointment.

2. D4341—Periodontal Scaling and Root Planing—Four or More Teeth Per Quadrant. This procedure involves instrumentation of the crown and root surfaces to remove plaque biofilm and calculus from these surfaces. *It is indicated for patients with periodontal disease and is therapeutic, not preventive in nature.* This procedure may be used as a definitive treatment in some stages of periodontal disease and/or as a part of presurgical procedures in others.

3. D4342—Periodontal Scaling and Root Planing—One to three teeth per Quadrant. This code is essentially the same as the D4341 code, the difference being the number of teeth present in a quadrant.

4. D4910—Periodontal Maintenance. *This procedure is instituted following periodontal therapy and continues at varying intervals for the life of the dentition or implant replacements.* It includes the removal of the bacterial plaque biofilm and calculus from supragingival and subgingival regions, site-specific scaling and root planing where indicated, and polishing of the teeth.

5. D4381—Localized Delivery of Antimicrobial Agents via a Controlled Release Vehicle. Synthetic fibers or other approved delivery devices containing controlled-release chemotherapeutic agents are inserted into a periodontal pocket.

6. D4355—Full-Mouth Debridement to Enable Comprehensive Evaluation and Diagnosis. *This code should not be confused with the term "periodontal debridement" as used in dental hygiene literature.* Full-mouth debridement is the gross removal of plaque biofilm and calculus that interfere with the ability of the dentist to perform a comprehensive oral evaluation. Full-mouth debridement refers to an **incomplete** **removal** of heavy calculus deposits only. This preliminary procedure will necessitate the need for additional periodontal instrumentation.

C. **Codes for Radiographs.** The most common codes for dental radiographs are
   1. D0210—a complete intraoral radiographic series including bitewings
   2. D0220—an intraoral periapical (first film)
   3. D0230—an intraoral periapical film (each additional film)
   4. D0240—an intraoral occlusal film
   5. D0250—an extraoral first film, such as a cephalometric film
   6. D0260—an extraoral film (each additional film)
   7. D0270—a single bitewing film
   8. D0272—two bitewing films
   9. D0274—four bitewing films
   10. D0330—a panoramic film
   11. D0277—vertical bitewings—seven to eight films
   12. D0350—oral/facial images. The oral/facial image code includes traditional photographs or digital images obtained by intraoral cameras.

D. Codes for Topical Fluoride
1. D1204—topical fluoride treatment-adult (prophylaxis not included)
2. D1205—topical fluoride treatment-adult (including prophylaxis). This code is used to report combined procedures of a prophylaxis and fluoride treatment.

E. Codes for Patient Counseling
1. D1310—nutritional counseling for control of dental disease. Counseling on food selection and dietary habits as a part of treatment and control of periodontal disease and caries.
2. D1320—tobacco cessation counseling for control and prevention of oral disease.
3. D1330—oral hygiene (self-care) instructions. Examples include tooth brushing technique, flossing, and the use of special oral hygiene aids.

Chapter Summary Statement

In judging whether a professional has been negligent, the courts use a standard called the *reasonable prudent person or professional*. Thus, providing and documenting periodontal care that meets or exceeds the standard of care is extremely important for dental hygienists.

The dental chart is a legal document. All periodontal assessment, educational, and treatment services should be documented in the patient chart or computerized record. When a patient decides to file a lawsuit, the dental chart becomes the single most important piece of information relative to the suit.

Insurance coding was developed to speed and simplify the reporting of dental treatments to third parties such as insurance companies and the government. These codes are very specific, revised frequently, and should be reviewed carefully before specific dental treatment is coded.

Section 5
Focus On Patients

Case 1

During a social gathering one evening, a dental hygienist tells her friend about an HIV-positive patient she had treated that day. As the news traveled down the grapevine and the patient learned that the hygienist had revealed his HIV status, he sued her. What specific charge could he bring against the hygienist? Would she be covered under the dentist/employer's malpractice coverage or her own personal malpractice coverage?

Case 2

The dental hygienist performed an oral cancer screening on every patient, but she never wrote it in her progress notes. When a patient found out he had oral cancer, he sued his dentist and the dental hygienist. The patient had been seen for a prophylaxis and restorative care 6 months before his diagnosis of oral cancer, and the basis for his suit was that he felt the hygienist and dentist had been negligent in failing to detect the lesion. How could this suit have been avoided?

Case 3

During the informed consent process, the patient is informed of (1) his diagnosis; (2) purpose, description, benefits, and risks of the proposed treatment; (3) alternative treatment options; (4) prognosis of no treatment; and (5) costs. The patient asks questions and demonstrates that he understands all information presented during the discussion. Then the patient refuses any treatment. What, if anything, should the dental hygienist do?

References

1. Tonner J. *Malpractice: What They Don't Teach You in Dental School.* PennWell Publishing; 1996.
2. American Dental Association. *CDT-2009/2010: Current Dental Terminology.* Chicago: American Dental Association; 2008:287; vi.

Suggested Readings

American Dental Association. *The CDT Companion: Your Guide to Dental Coding: CDT 2009–2010.* Chicago: American Dental Association; 2008.

Baxter C. A survey of 242 dental negligence cases with a breakdown as to the sex of the defendent dentist. *Woman Dentist J.* 2004. (http:www.dentistryiq.com; accessed 7/2010).

Hapcook CP Sr. Dental malpractice claims: percentages and procedures. *J Am Dent Assoc.* 2006;137(10):1444–1445.

Lopez-Nicolas M, Falcon M, Perez-Carceles MD, et al. Informed consent in dental malpractice claims. A retrospective study. *Int Dent J.* 2007;57(3):168–172.

Morse D. Dealing with dental malpractice, Part 2. Malpractice prevention. *Dent Today.* 2004;23(3):116–121.

Morse DR. Dealing with dental malpractice, Part 1. *Dent Today.* 2004;23(2):140–143.

Napier RH, Bruelheide LS, et al. Insurance billing and coding. *Dent Clin North Am.* 2008;52(3):507–527; viii.

Pollack B. *Risk Management in Dental Practice.* Carol Stream: Quintessence; 2002.

Rossein KD. Online medical and dental history submission for patients. *Dent Today.* 2008;27(9):136–138.

Stephenson BA. Beyond paperless dentistry: the expanding role of computers in modem dental practice. *Dent Today.* 2008;27(6):122, 124–125.

Tonner J. Are your dental charts working against you? *DentalTown Mag.* 2003. (dentaltown.com; accessed 7/2010.)

Walker P. *Dentistry and North Carolina Law.* (self-publish) Chapel Hill; 2005.

Wilder R. Understanding your legal liability. *Dimen Dental Hyg.* 2005.

Chapter 35

Future Directions for Management of Periodontal Patients

Learning Objective

• Describe some strategies in the management of periodontal patients that may evolve in the future.

There are not many absolutes in periodontics, but there is undoubtedly one—the simple fact that strategies for management of periodontal patients will continue to evolve and change over time. Dental hygienists should expect changes in recommendations for management of periodontal patients as study of these diseases continues. This chapter offers an overview of a few of the possibilities for directions in the management of periodontal patients.

Section 1
Diagnostic Technology for Periodontal Diseases

1. **Probing Depths and Attachment Levels**
    A. The diagnosis and monitoring of patients with periodontal diseases has been based on traditional clinical assessment methods for many years; one of these traditional clinical assessments is the use of manual periodontal probes to measure probing depths and attachment levels.
    B. An experienced clinician can record probing depths fairly rapidly and in many patients probing depths provide a reasonable assessment of periodontal health.
    C. On the other hand, attachment levels provide a more accurate assessment of the precise condition of the periodontium but are difficult to measure and record using manual periodontal probes.
    D. Computer-linked, controlled-force electronic periodontal probes are already available to clinicians.
        1. These computer-linked probes can make it possible to measure both probing depths and attachment levels quickly, as well as provide automatic data entry features.
        2. Unfortunately, most of the computer-linked periodontal probes currently in use have a tendency to underestimate measurements of probing depths and attachment levels in patients when subgingival calculus deposits are present.
        3. This technology of computer-linked periodontal probes will improve. As this technology improves, the use of these computer-linked probes in dental offices will undoubtedly become widespread, making it much easier for clinicians to measure and record attachment levels.
2. **Digital Radiographs**
    A. Another traditional clinical periodontal assessment has been the evaluation of radiographic images, and advances in diagnostic technology also include advances in radiograph techniques.
    B. Digital (filmless) radiographic techniques have been developed to the stage where they are already being used by most clinicians.
        1. Digital radiographic techniques allow members of the dental team to collect radiographic information using special sensors instead of printing the radiographic information on a film.
        2. These digital images are then stored on a computer and can be viewed on a computer screen or even printed when needed.
        3. Modern technology for viewing these images on computer screens has substantial advantages over the traditional use of radiographic film.
        4. Software for viewing these digitized images can eliminate distortion that is seen with traditional film, can allow for easy magnification of details, and can provide precise, anatomically correct measurements.
        5. The same software can also allow for enhancing aspects of a digitized image, providing members of the dental team with more details of the actual status of a tooth or of the periodontium.

      6. In addition, these digital images can be shared with other healthcare providers quite readily—as might be indicated during a patient referral or during consultation with a specialist.

  3. Computed Tomographic Techniques

    A. Another interesting area of technology related to radiographic techniques is the use of computed tomographic techniques. Computed tomographic techniques provide clinicians with the ability to study minute details and precise dimensions of the jaws in a three-dimensional mode on a computer screen.

      1. These details can be so precise that they can include a three-dimensional radiographic image of a thin slice made through the jaws at any specific location.

      2. Computed tomographic techniques are currently in use by many clinicians when planning for the placement of dental implants.

      3. As these computed tomographic techniques become more accessible to the general dentist, treatment planning for many conditions, including periodontal diseases, will improve.

    B. Digital radiographic techniques and computed tomographic techniques are only two examples of enhanced radiographic diagnostic technology.

      1. As radiographic imaging technology improves, the improvements will come into widespread use by members of dental teams.

      2. This enhanced radiographic technology will provide a greater ease in assessing clinical parameters such as measuring alveolar bone loss or documenting healing of a site affected by periodontitis following therapy by the dental hygienist or the dentist.

Section 2
Periodontal Disease/Systemic Disease Connection

Dental and medical researchers have been interested in studying the connection between periodontitis and certain systemic diseases for some time. Research into this critical topic is ongoing and continues to offer insights into these connections. Review of the dental literature will reveal many studies about how systemic conditions are linked to periodontal diseases, but all of these areas require further scientific study.

1. Systemic Diseases with a Link to Periodontal Disease

    A. Some examples of systemic diseases or conditions that have a connection to periodontitis are listed in Box 35-1.

    B. Discussion of these systemic conditions has been included in other chapters of this book, but it is of interest to review some of the relationships between one specific condition, diabetes mellitus, and periodontal disease.

Box 35-1. Examples of Systemic Diseases or Conditions that Have a Connection to Periodontitis

- Bacterial endocarditis
- Cardiovascular disease
- Diabetes mellitus
- Low birth weight for newborns
- Lung abscesses
- Osteoporosis
- Smoking

2. **Diabetes Mellitus in Periodontal Patients**
   A. **Need for Additional Research.** It is clear that additional research into the connection between diabetes and periodontal disease will indeed impact the practice of dental hygiene.
      1. As discussed in other chapters of this book, research has demonstrated that patients with poorly controlled diabetes have an increased risk for periodontitis.
      2. Since periodontitis is a type of infection, and since diabetes can lower the body's resistance to infections in general, it is not surprising that there is a connection between poorly controlled diabetes and periodontitis in some patients.
      3. In addition, research suggests that periodontal infection and the elimination of the periodontal infection through proper periodontal therapy have the potential for altering the body's control of blood sugar levels.
      4. It has even been suggested that thorough treatment of periodontitis in a diabetic patient may make it easier for a patient's physician to control the diabetes.
      5. There are many, many research questions that need to be answered related to the periodontitis/diabetes connection, but a few of those questions that can have a direct impact on the practice of dental hygiene are outlined below.
         a. Are the measures used to prevent or control periodontitis in the patient without diabetes adequate for the patient with diabetes mellitus?
         b. Since wound healing appears altered in patients with diabetes, are there adjustments clinicians need to make in dental hygiene therapy to maximize the potential for healing in these patients?
         c. What precise periodontal maintenance protocols are the most effective for periodontal patients with diabetes?
         d. When a dental hygienist treats a patient with diabetes, what communication protocols can be most effective in insuring that the patient's physician is aware of the patient's periodontal status so that adjustments in the therapy for diabetes can be made where needed?
   B. **Use of Intensive Therapies for Diabetes Mellitus.** In examining the periodontitis/diabetes connection there is another line of inquiry that will also affect dental hygiene practice.
      1. In medicine there have been dramatic improvements in the treatment regimens for patients with diabetes, and these regimens now frequently include intensive treatment with oral agents and with insulin.
      2. Unfortunately, some of these medical treatments have increased the risk for medical emergencies (such as hypoglycemia) during dental office treatment of a patient with diabetes.
      3. This medical trend in intensive therapies for patients with diabetes will continue.
      4. As physicians use more intensive therapies to manage patients with diabetes, the dental hygienist of the future will need to have more knowledge about these therapies, about how to manage these patients in a dental setting, and about how to respond when a medical emergency arises.

Section 3
Protocols For Maintaining Dental Implants

Dental implants are a viable option as one alternative for replacing most missing teeth and dental implants available today have a remarkable success rate. Even though dental implantology has been intensively studied for several decades, there are still many unanswered questions related to this field, and research will continue. Much additional investigation is needed in the area of dental implantology, and some examples of questions related to dental hygiene that are in need of further study are listed below. Answering these types of questions with appropriate scientific investigation is quite likely to have a substantial impact on clinical care delivered by the dental hygienist.

- What self-care measures can best prevent peri-implant infections?
- What are the most effective protocols for effective maintenance of implants?
- Should clinicians recommend the same techniques for minimizing the bacterial challenge to an implant that we apply to a natural tooth?
- When treating dental implants what types of instruments provide the greatest chance of maintaining periodontal health?

Section 4
Treatment Modalities in Periodontal Care

1. Lasers in Periodontal Care
   A. Lasers have been widely used in many fields of medicine since the early 1960s. Lasers produce a narrow beam of light with a single wavelength that can produce intense energy at precise locations.
      1. In dentistry these intense light beams can be passed down narrow optical tubing and can be focused on a small area of tissue within the mouth.
      2. Some laser beams are so intense that they can actually be used to remove oral soft tissue or to cut tissues in the mouth.
      3. There are different types of lasers that have been studied for use in dentistry, and each type has a different effect on soft tissue, enamel, dentin, pulp, and bone.
   B. Lasers have been suggested for use in dentistry for a variety of applications. Some of these devices even have Food and Drug Administration (FDA) safety clearance for some intraoral soft tissue procedures.
      1. More study is needed, however, to clarify how these devices can be used appropriately in subgingival applications.
      2. Some preliminary investigations have suggested a possible use for these devices as part of periodontal therapies such as root debridement, and investigations into these issues are ongoing.
   C. The routine use of lasers in treating patients with chronic periodontitis does not appear to be supported by the available scientific studies at this time.
      1. Additional research will clarify appropriate uses for these devices in periodontal patients and may impact some of the therapy provided for patients with periodontitis.
      2. To clarify any possible advantage in using lasers in periodontal patients there will need to be randomized, blinded, controlled, longitudinal clinical trials, cohort or longitudinal studies, or case-controlled studies indicating that these devices offer advantages not achieved by traditional periodontal therapy.

3. If further study of these devices shows that periodontal patients do benefit from their use, they may one day be a routine part of the care of patients with periodontitis and perhaps even a part of the practice of dental hygiene.

2. **Genetic Technology in Periodontal Care**
    A. Clinicians have known for a long time that there are many factors that can increase the risk of developing periodontitis in their patients.
        1. One factor that is known to increase the risk of developing periodontitis is failure to control bacterial plaque biofilm growth on the teeth, thereby increasing the bacterial challenge to the periodontium.
        2. Scientific studies also indicate that certain genetic factors determine how an individual patient's host defenses actually react to an increased bacterial challenge.
        3. Based upon the current research literature available, it now appears that a key factor in determining whether a patient develops periodontitis in response to the bacterial challenge appears to be how the body reacts to that bacterial challenge.
        4. One major determinant of how the body reacts to the bacterial challenge is genetics (or inherited characteristics).
    B. Much more study into the genetic factors that increase the risk for periodontitis is needed, but it is already possible to use some types of genetic information to guide clinical decision making in a small group of selected patients.
        1. Genetic testing can identify patients carrying gene mutations for several rare syndromes that are often accompanied by a form of periodontal disease.
        2. In addition to identifying patients with rare syndromes, there is already a commercially available genetic susceptibility test for severe chronic periodontitis.
        3. In this test specific gene polymorphisms (forms) that have been associated with the development of periodontitis can be detected.
        4. Ongoing scientific investigations will undoubtedly clarify how such genetic testing can be used in periodontitis patient management.
    C. As more and more scientific information about identifying genetic control of host defenses becomes available, it is quite likely that this information will impact how we manage patients with periodontal diseases and will impact the practice of dental hygiene.

3. **Local Delivery Mechanisms in Periodontal Care**
    A. As already discussed in other chapters of this book, research has demonstrated that using local delivery mechanisms for antimicrobial chemicals in periodontal patients has a small but measurable impact upon clinical parameters such as attachment levels.
    B. There are several areas of research investigation that are needed related to these local delivery mechanisms, and some examples of research questions about this topic that need to be answered are listed below.
        1. Can local delivery mechanisms be designed that have a greater clinical impact than those currently available for clinical use?
        2. What specific local delivery treatment protocols should be followed to produce the most benefit for individual patients?
        3. Are there additional antimicrobial agents that can be delivered safely using the local delivery concept?
        4. Can other therapy provided by the dental hygienist be enhanced by using some of these local delivery mechanisms?
    C. Research into the use of local delivery mechanisms for antimicrobial agents continues. It is entirely possible that as this modality improves in clinical effectiveness, using local delivery mechanisms may become more and more useful in the care of the periodontal patient by the dental hygienist.

4. **Host Modulation Therapies in Periodontal Care**
   A. As already discussed, research has demonstrated that host defenses can play a significant role in the actual development of attachment loss and alveolar bone loss in periodontitis patients.
      1. A variety of host modulation therapies have been investigated that could be used as adjunctive (supplemental) treatment in periodontitis patients.
      2. Host modulation therapies usually involve using medications that can alter biochemical pathways in a manner that will (1) slow attachment loss, (2) slow alveolar bone loss, or (3) decrease inflammation in periodontal patients.
   B. Investigations into possible host modulation therapies have already resulted in one commercially available medication (low dose doxycycline hyclate) that can be used as adjunctive treatment in patients with chronic periodontitis.
      1. This medication can be used to lower levels of collagenase, an enzyme involved in the destruction of collagen.
      2. Collagen is one of the components of many of the structures that make up the periodontium, and lowering the levels of collagenase can slow the progress of periodontitis.
      3. Investigations are ongoing into a number of other possible host modulation therapies that include studies into (1) modulation of cytokines (chemicals involved in periodontitis that can result in increased periodontal disease progression), (2) reduction of prostaglandins (chemicals that enhance inflammation in the gingiva and in the periodontium), and (3) slowing alveolar bone loss with chemical agents.
   C. As further scientific investigations improve our understanding of host modulation therapies in the management of periodontitis patients, there are likely to be a variety of new therapeutic options for members of the dental team to use in patient management.
5. **Disease Risk Assessment of Periodontal Care**
   A. Recently there has been increased interest in identifying clinical tools that can be used to quantify a patient's risk for developing periodontitis.
      1. Traditionally clinicians have assessed the risk of developing periodontitis subjectively, but studies have shown that subjective risk assessment is surprisingly variable even among clinicians who are experts.
      2. Objective periodontal disease risk assessment tools would be quite useful to members of the dental team if they provided a method of risk assessment that could accurately predict which patients are most likely to develop periodontitis.
      3. Examples of risk factors that have been suggested to be predictive of periodontal disease activity are listed in Box 35-2.
      4. Using risk assessment tools to identify the patients with the highest risk for developing periodontitis would allow members of the dental team to provide more aggressive treatment for those patients.
      5. In addition, these tools might identify which periodontal patients should be referred to a specialist early in their treatment and which patients can best be managed in a general dental setting.
   B. Studies have already been published that document that some of these risk assessment tools are predictors of alveolar bone loss and loss of periodontally affected teeth.
      1. It is likely that some of these tools for quantifying a patient's risk will be in widespread use in dental offices in the near future.
      2. Guidelines from the American Academy of Periodontology indicate that periodontal disease risk assessment should be part of every comprehensive dental and periodontal evaluation.

3. The American Academy of Periodontology has even developed a simplified form of risk assessment for use by patients. This web-based patient self-assessment can be viewed at www.perio.org.

4. These risk assessment tools would be useful to the dental hygienist and the dentist in planning therapy and in identifying patients in need of immediate referral.

Box 35-2. Examples of Factors the May Help Predict Periodontal Disease Activity

- Smoking
- Poorly controlled diabetes
- Poor patient self-care
- Severity of alveolar bone loss
- Positive family history
- Presence of pocket depths >6 mm

- Age
- Gender
- Gingival bleeding
- Number of missing teeth
- Presence of periodontal pathogens

Chapter Summary Statement

Dental hygienists should expect many changes to take place in recommendations for management of patients with periodontal diseases as study of these diseases continues. This chapter presented a brief overview of a few of the possibilities for future directions in the management of periodontal patients by dental hygienists.

Suggested Readings

American Academy of Periodontology Statement. American Academy of Periodontology Statement on Risk Assessment. *J Periodontol.* 2008;79:202.

American Academy of Periodontology. Parameter on Systemic Conditions Affected by Periodontal Diseases. *J Periodontol.* 2000(Suppl);71:880–883.

American Academy of Periodontology. Position Paper. Diagnosis of Periodontal Diseases. *J Periodontol.* 2003;74:1237–1247.

American Academy of Periodontology. Position Paper. Implications of Genetic Technology for the Management of Periodontal Diseases. *J Periodontol.* 2005;76:850–857.

American Academy of Periodontology. Position Paper. Modulation of the Host Response in Periodontal Therapy. *J Periodontol.* 2002;73:460–470.

Armitage GC. Clinical evaluation of periodontal diseases. *Periodontol 2000.* 1995;7:39–53.

Benn DK. A review of the reliability of radiographic measurements in estimating alveolar bone changes. *J Clin Periodontol.* 1990;17:14–21.

Cobb CM. Lasers in periodontics: a review of the literature. *J Periodontol.* 2006;77:545–564.

Eickholz P, Kim TS, Benn DK, et al. Validity of radiographic measurement of interproximal bone loss. *Oral Surg Oral Med Oral Pathol Oral Radiol Endod.* 1998;85:99–106.

Goodson JM, Haffajee AD, Socransky SS. The relationship between attachment level loss and alveolar bone loss. *J Clin Periodontol.* 1984;11:348–359.

Goodson JM. Clinical measurements of periodontitis. *J Clin Periodontol.* 1986;13:446–455.

Hausmann E. A contemporary perspective on techniques for the clinical assessment of alveolar bone. *J Periodontol.* 1990;61:149–156.

Jeffcoat MK, Reddy MS. Digital subtraction radiography for longitudinal assessment of peri-implant bone change: method and validation. *Adv Dent Res.* 1993;7:196–201.

Jeffcoat MK, Wang IC, Reddy MS. Radiographic diagnosis in periodontics. *Periodontol 2000.* 1995;7:54–68.

Jeffcoat MK. Osteoporosis: a possible modifying factor in oral bone loss. *Ann Periodontol.* 1998;3:312–321.

Kircos LT, Misch CE. Diagnostic and imaging techniques. In: Misch CE, ed. *Contemporary Implant Dentistry.* St. Louis: Mosby; 1999:73–87.

Loe H. Periodontal disease. The sixth complication of diabetes mellitus. *Diabetes Care.* 1993;16(Suppl 1):329–334.

Mealey BL, Oates, TW. Diabetes mellitus and periodontal diseases. *J Periodontol.* 2006;77: 1289–1303.

Mealey BL. Diabetes mellitus. In: Rose LF, Genco RJ, Mealey BL, Cohen DW, eds. *Periodontal Medicine.* Toronto: BC Decker Publishers; 2000:121–151.

Mealey BL. Periodontal implications: medically compromised patients. *Ann Periodontol.* 1996;1: 256–321.

Mullally BH, Linden GJ. Comparative reproducibility of proximal probing depth using electronic pressure-controlled and hand probing. *J Clin Periodontol.* 1994;21:284–288.

Offenbacher S. Periodontal diseases: pathogenesis. *Ann Periodontol.* 1996;1:821–878.

Page RC, Martin J, Krall EA, et al. Longitudinal validation of a risk calculator for periodontal disease. *J Clin Periodontol.* 2003;30:819–827.

Persson GR, Mancl LA, Martin J, et al. Assessing periodontal disease risk. *J Am Dent Assoc.* 2003;134:575–582.

Rees TD, Biggs NL, Collings CK. Radiographic interpretation of periodontal osseous lesions. *Oral Surg Oral Med Oral Pathol.* 1971;32:141–153.

Ritchey TR, Orban BJ. Three-dimensional roentgenographic interpretation in periodontal diagnosis. *J Periodontol.* 1960;31:275–282.

Rosenfeld AL, Mecall RA. Using computerized tomography to develop realistic treatment objectives for the implant team. In: Nevins M, Mellonig JT, Fiorellini JP, eds. *Implant Therapy: Clinical Approaches and Evidence of Success.* Chicago: Quintessence; 1998.

Smith RA, Berger R, Dodson TB. Risk factors associated with dental implants in healthy and medically compromised patients. *Int J Oral Maxillofac Implants.* 1992;7:367–372.

Taylor GW. Bidirectional interrelationships between diabetes and periodontal diseases: an epidemiological perspective. *Ann Periodontol.* 2001;6:99–112.

Tupta-Veselicky L, Famili P, Ceravolo FJ, et al. A clinical study of an electronic constant force periodontal probe. *J Periodontol.* 1994;65:616–622.

Wang S-F, Leknes KN, Zimmerman GJ, et al. Reproducibility of periodontal probing using a conventional manual and automated force-controlled electronic probe. *J Periodontol.* 1995;66:38–46.

Chapter 36

Comprehensive Patient Cases

Learning Objective

- Apply content from the chapters in this book to the decision-making questions for fictitious Patient Cases 1, 2, and 3.

Section 1
Fictitious Patient Case 1—Mr. Karn

PATIENT PROFILE

Mr. Karn is a 47-year-old high school administrator who has recently moved to your city. He came to the dental office because he would like to know if it is possible to replace his missing upper right first molar tooth with a dental implant.

During Mr. Karn's first office visit, he informs you that he has been too busy lately to get a dental check-up and that he has not seen a dentist for quite a few years. Mr. Karn states that he brushes his teeth twice daily when he has time and that he does not floss regularly even though he knows that he should. He also uses an over-the-counter mouth rinse occasionally.

PATIENT HEALTH HISTORY

- On the day of his first visit to your dental office Mr. Karn's blood pressure is 130/80 mm Hg and his pulse is 62 beats/min.
- A review of Mr. Karn's health history reveals that he takes two medications: Zocor and Nifedipine.
- Mr. Karn also states that he smokes between one-half and one pack of cigarettes each day.

CLINICAL PHOTOGRAPHS FOR MR. KARN

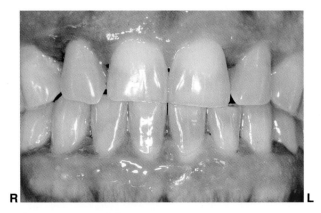

Figure 36.1. Karn: Anterior Teeth, Facial View.

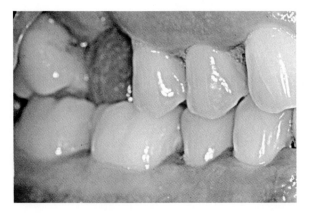

Figure 36.2. Karn: Right Side, Facial View.

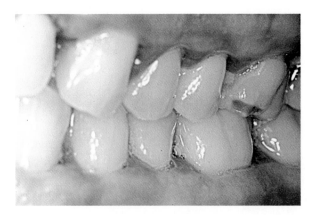

Figure 36.3. Karn: Left Side, Facial View.

CLINICAL PHOTOGRAPHS FOR MR. KARN

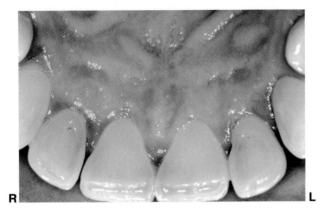

Figure 36.4. Karn: Maxillary Anterior, Lingual View.

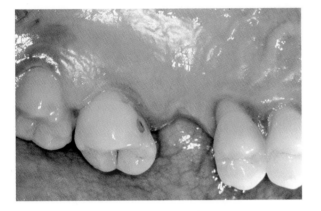

Figure 36.5. Karn: Maxillary Right, Lingual View.

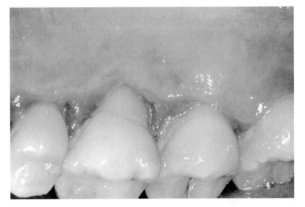

Figure 36.6. Karn: Maxillary Left, Lingual View.

CLINICAL PHOTOGRAPHS FOR MR. KARN

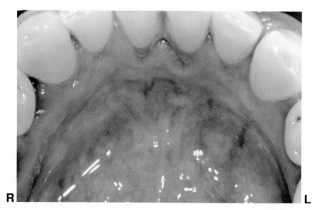

Figure 36.7. Karn: Mandibular Anterior, Lingual View.

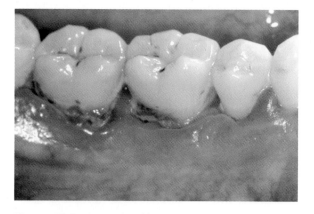

Figure 36.8. Karn: Mandibular Right, Lingual View.

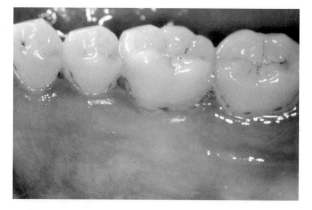

Figure 36.9. Karn: Mandibular Left, Lingual View.

CASE #1

1	2	3	4	5	6	7	8	9	10	11	12	13	14	15	16	**Maxilla**
					I	I						I			I	Mobility (I, II, III)
+	+		+	+	+	+			+	+	+	+	+	+	+	Bleeding/Purulence (+)
646	647		535	536	415	322	322	334	425	435	536	626	638	846	746	Attachment Level (CEJ to BP)
646	635		325	536	525	435	433	334	425	435	536	626	638	846	746	Probing Depth (FGM to BP)

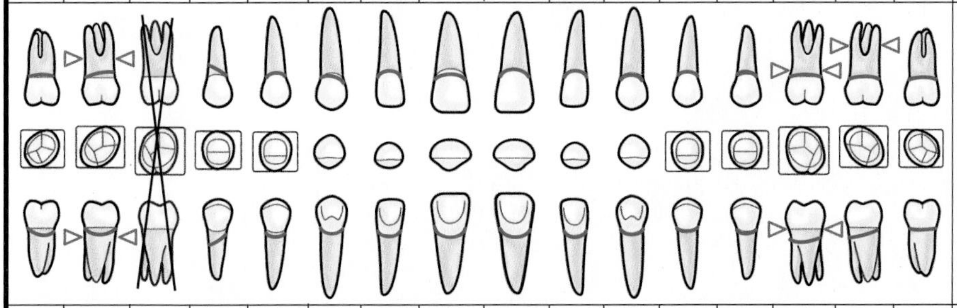

Facial

Palatal

1	2	3	4	5	6	7	8	9	10	11	12	13	14	15	16	
+	+		+	+	+	+	+	+	+	+	+	+	+	+	+	Bleeding/Purulence (+)
646	646		546	526	536	425	443	324	424	525	535	626	859	937	736	Attachment Level (CEJ to BP)
636	525		335	526	536	425	443	324	424	525	535	626	627	827	736	Probing Depth (FGM to BP)
																^F_PPlaque
	✓		✓	✓				✓	✓			✓	✓	✓		Supragingival Calculus
✓	✓		✓	✓	✓	✓	✓	✓	✓	✓	✓	✓	✓	✓	✓	Subgingival Calculus
		4					3					4				PSR Code

Right *Left*

32	31	30	29	28	27	26	25	24	23	22	21	20	19	18	17	**Mandible**
			I			I	I									Mobility (I, II, III)
+		+	+	+	+	+		+		+	+	+		+	+	Bleeding/Purulence (+)
546	746	736	635	435	534	324	534	434	324	324	434	435	536	746	635	Attachment Level (CEJ to BP)
546	736	626	635	535	534	324	423	323	324	324	434	435	536	746	635	Probing Depth (FGM to BP)

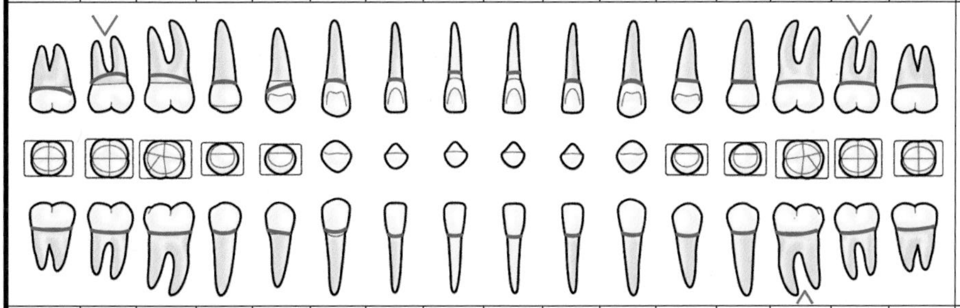

Lingual

Facial

32	31	30	29	28	27	26	25	24	23	22	21	20	19	18	17	
+	+	+	+	+		+	+	+		+		+		+	+	Bleeding/Purulence (+)
546	736	625	535	635	534	324	423	323	324	324	434	435	526	736	625	Attachment Level (CEJ to BP)
546	736	625	535	635	534	324	423	323	324	324	434	435	526	736	625	Probing Depth (FGM to BP)
																^L_FPlaque
					✓	✓	✓	✓	✓			✓	✓			Supragingival Calculus
✓	✓	✓	✓	✓	✓	✓	✓	✓	✓	✓	✓	✓	✓	✓	✓	Subgingival Calculus
		4					3					4				PSR Code

Figure 36.10. Mr. Karn's Periodontal Chart.

RADIOGRAPHIC SERIES FOR MR. KARN

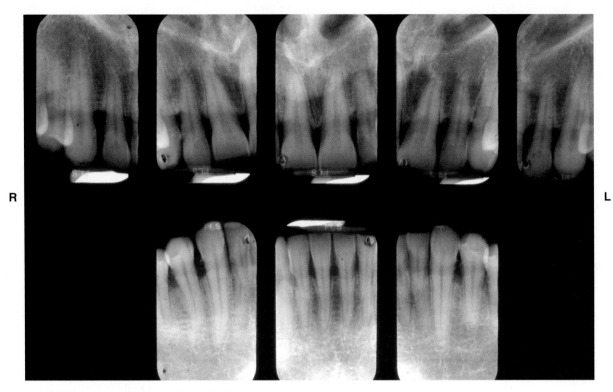

R   L

Figure 36.11A. Karn's Radiographs: Anterior Teeth.

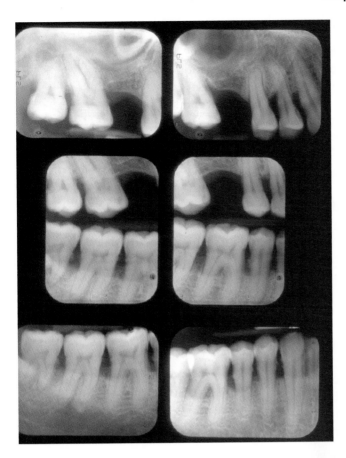

Figure 36.11B. Karn's Radiographs: Right Posterior Teeth.

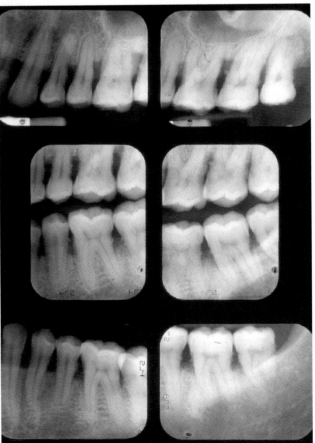

Figure 36.11C. Karn's Radiographs: Left Posterior Teeth.

DECISION-MAKING QUESTIONS FOR CASE 1: MR. KARN

1. What should Mr. Karn be told about the possibility of replacing his maxillary right first molar tooth with a dental implant? Note that this question was what prompted Mr. Karn to make an appointment in your dental office.

2. What factors in Mr. Karn's profile indicate that achieving an acceptable level of patient self-care may be a problem for the dental team?

3. What factors revealed in Mr. Karn's health history will be critical for the dental team to consider during treatment?

4. What signs of gingival inflammation are evident in Mr. Karn's clinical photographs?

5. What etiologic risk factors for gingival and periodontal diseases are evident in Mr. Karn's clinical photographs?

6. How might the presence of the furcation involvements found during Mr. Karn's periodontal evaluation affect his periodontal treatment?

7. Does Mr. Karn's periodontal evaluation indicate that he has attachment loss present on some teeth?

8. What etiologic factors for gingival and periodontal diseases are evident in Mr. Karn's dental radiographs?

9. On Mr. Karn's radiographs what specific findings indicate that he has alveolar bone loss present?

10. How would you characterize Mr. Karn's periodontal condition? Do you think that he has gingivitis, periodontitis, neither, or both? What clinical or radiographic findings did you use to reach your conclusion?

11. Develop a suggested step-by-step plan for nonsurgical periodontal therapy for Mr. Karn.

12. What information should your team give Mr. Karn about his periodontal condition?

13. What should Mr. Karn be told about the possible need for periodontal surgery later in the treatment?

14. What should Mr. Karn be told about the need for continuing treatment such as periodontal maintenance?

Section 2
Fictitious Patient Case 2—Mr. Wilton

PATIENT PROFILE

Mr. Wilton is a 52-year-old manager of a local gardening store who has come to your dental office for an initial visit. During his patient interview, Mr. Wilton informs you that he made this appointment at his wife's insistence. He states that his wife wants to know if there is anything that can be done about his bad breath. Mr. Wilton informs you that he cannot seem to get his bad breath under control using mouth rinses.

PATIENT HEALTH HISTORY

- At the time of his initial visit, Mr. Wilton's blood pressure is 164/100 mm Hg and his pulse rate is 74 beats/min.
- Mr. Wilton informs you that he is taking Amoxicillin prescribed by his physician for an ear infection.
- Mr. Wilton tells you that he had high blood pressure once and that he did take a prescribed medication a few years ago for that condition. He tells you that he was feeling just fine so he stopped taking the prescribed blood pressure medication.

CLINICAL PHOTOGRAPHS FOR MR. WILTON

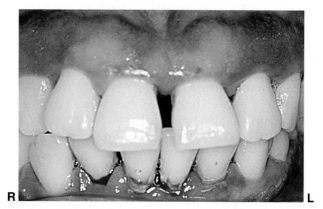

Figure 36.12. Wilton: Anterior Teeth, Facial View.

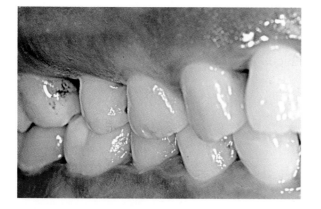

Figure 36.13. Wilton: Right Side, Facial View.

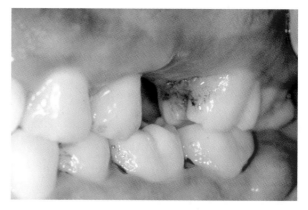

Figure 36.14. Wilton: Left Side, Facial View.

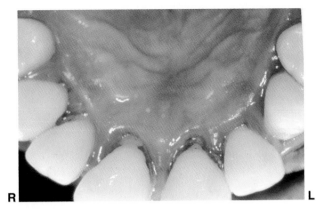

Figure 36.15. Wilton: Maxillary Anteriors, Lingual View.

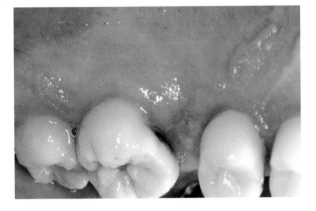

Figure 36.16. Wilton: Maxillary Right, Lingual View.

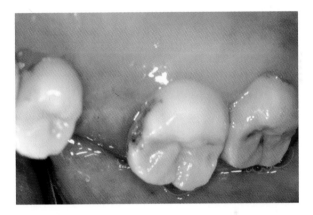

Figure 36.17. Wilton: Maxillary Left, Lingual View.

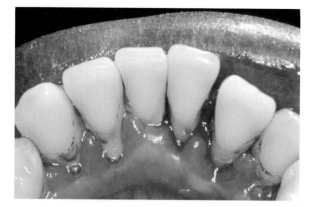

Figure 36.18. Wilton: Mandibular Anteriors, Lingual View.

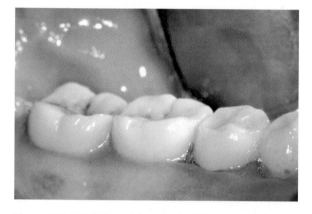

Figure 36.19. Wilton: Mandibular Right, Lingual View.

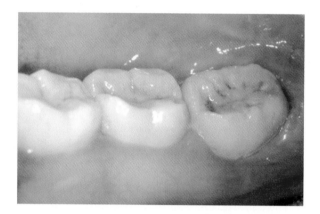

Figure 36.20. Wilton: Mandibular Left, Lingual View.

CASE #2

1	2	3	4	5	6	7	8	9	10	11	12	13	14	15	16	Maxilla
			I			I	I	II	I		I					Mobility (I, II, III)
+	+		+			+	+	+		+	+	+		+	+	Bleeding/Purulence (+)
635	634		338	535	537	626	736	537	625	536	725	524		435	535	Attachment Level (CEJ to BP)
635	634		338	535	537	626	625	537	625	536	725	524		435	535	Probing Depth (FGM to BP)

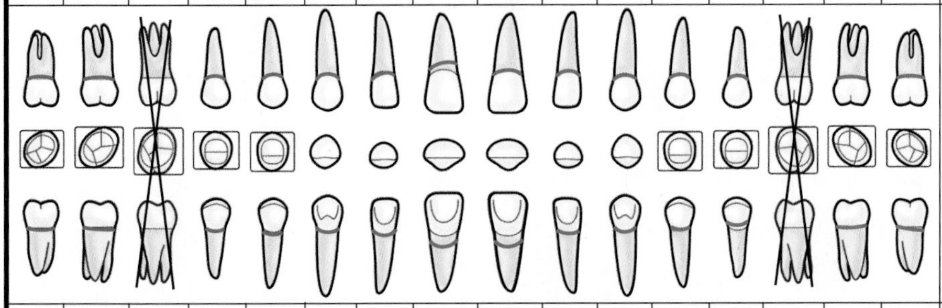

Facial / Palatal

1	2	3	4	5	6	7	8	9	10	11	12	13	14	15	16	
+	+		+	+	+		+	+		+	+	+		+		Bleeding/Purulence (+)
535	634		438	534	636	536	646	746	535	536	726	423		426	535	Attachment Level (CEJ to BP)
535	634		438	534	636	536	535	635	535	536	726	534		426	535	Probing Depth (FGM to BP)
																ᶠ/ₚ Plaque
	✓				✓	✓	✓	✓	✓	✓		✓		✓	✓	Supragingival Calculus
✓	✓		✓	✓	✓	✓	✓	✓	✓	✓	✓	✓		✓	✓	Subgingival Calculus
		4				4						4				PSR Code

Right   Left

32	31	30	29	28	27	26	25	24	23	22	21	20	19	18	17	Mandible
			I			II	II	II	II							Mobility (I, II, III)
	+	+	+		+	+	+	+	+	+	+	+	+		+	Bleeding/Purulence (+)
	435	536	545	524	535	746	656	647	748	635	524	535	535	636	645	Attachment Level (CEJ to BP)
	535	536	545	524	535	635	545	536	637	635	524	535	635	636	635	Probing Depth (FGM to BP)

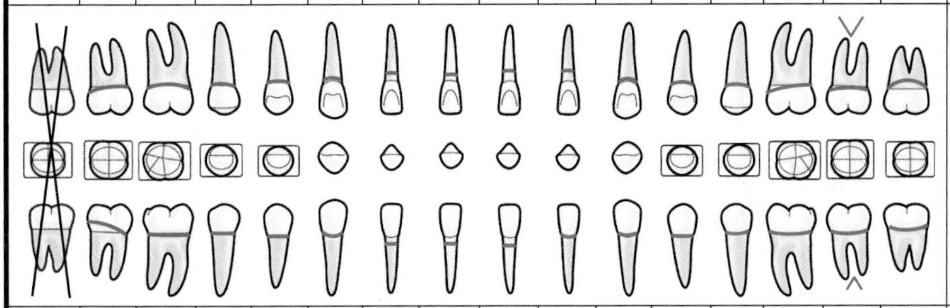

Lingual / Facial

32	31	30	29	28	27	26	25	24	23	22	21	20	19	18	17	
	+	+		+	+	+	+	+	+	+	+		+	+	+	Bleeding/Purulence (+)
	435	526	535	424	535	735	646	636	536	524	525	425	525	526	625	Attachment Level (CEJ to BP)
	535	526	535	424	535	624	535	525	536	524	525	425	525	526	625	Probing Depth (FGM to BP)
																ᴸ/ꜰ Plaque
					✓	✓	✓	✓	✓	✓					✓	Supragingival Calculus
	✓	✓	✓	✓	✓	✓	✓	✓	✓	✓	✓	✓	✓	✓	✓	Subgingival Calculus
			4				4					4				PSR Code

Figure 36.21. Mr. Wilton's Periodontal Chart.

RADIOGRAPHIC SERIES FOR MR. WILTON

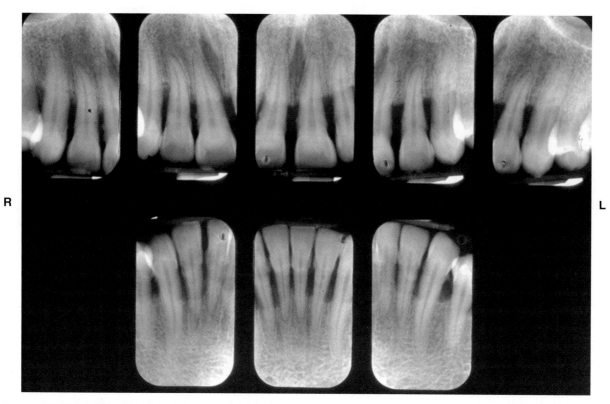

Figure 36.22A. Wilton's Radiographs: Anterior Teeth.

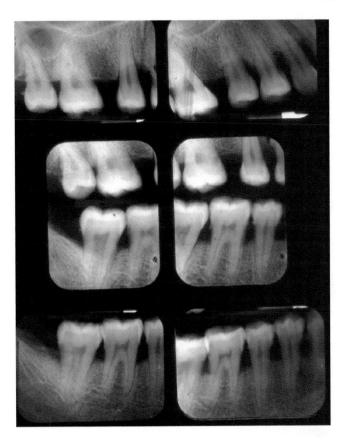

Figure 36.22B. Wilton's Radiographs: Right Posterior Teeth.

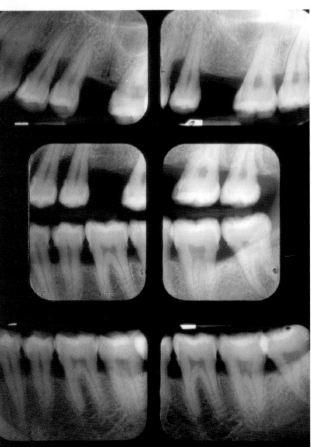

Figure 36.22C. Wilton's Radiographs: Left Posterior Teeth.

DECISION-MAKING QUESTIONS FOR CASE 2: MR. WILTON

1. What information should your team give Mr. Wilton regarding his wife's concern about his bad breath? Note that this was the complaint that prompted Mr. Wilton to make an appointment in your office.

2. What factors in Mr. Wilton's profile indicate that achieving an acceptable level of patient self-care may be a problem for the dental team?

3. What factors revealed in Mr. Wilton's health history will be critical for the dental team to consider during periodontal evaluation or treatment?

4. What signs of gingival inflammation are evident in Mr. Wilton's clinical photographs?

5. What etiologic risk factors for gingival and periodontal diseases are evident in Mr. Wilton's clinical photographs?

6. Does Mr. Wilton's periodontal evaluation indicate that he has attachment loss present on some teeth?

7. In response to your questions, Mr. Wilton informs you that the spaces between his front teeth were not there a few years ago. What do you think may be causing these spaces between his teeth to appear?

8. What etiologic factors for gingival and periodontal diseases are evident in Mr. Wilton's dental radiographs?

9. On Mr. Wilton's radiographs, what specific findings indicate that he has alveolar bone loss present?

10. How would you characterize Mr. Wilton's periodontal condition? Do you think that he has gingivitis, periodontitis, neither, or both? What clinical or radiographic findings did you use to reach your conclusion?

11. Write a suggested step-by-step plan for nonsurgical periodontal therapy for Mr. Wilton.

12. What information should your team give Mr. Wilton about his periodontal condition?

13. What should Mr. Wilton be told about the possible need for periodontal surgery later in the treatment?

14. What should Mr. Wilton be told about the need for continuing treatment such as periodontal maintenance?

15. What should your team tell Mr. Wilton if he refuses your team's recommendations for periodontal therapy?

Section 3
Fictitious Patient Case 3—Mrs. Sandsky

PATIENT PROFILE

Mrs. Sandsky is a 42-year-old department store manager who has come to your dental office to get her dental condition in order. She states that she has neglected her dental care because she has been taking care of the dental needs of her children for many years, but now she is ready to take care of herself.

She informs your dental team that some years ago she was told that she had a gum disease, but elected not to receive any care for that condition at the time. She states that she brushes and flosses daily now in hopes that these actions can help her keep her teeth.

PATIENT HEALTH HISTORY

- At the time of Mrs. Sandsky's initial dental visit her blood pressure measures 130/83 mm Hg and her pulse is 75 beats/min.
- She explains that she has problems with gastroesophageal reflux disease and elevated cholesterol level.
- She reports that currently she is taking Omeprazole and Simvastatin prescribed by her physician and that she is also taking multivitamin tablets because she thinks she needs them.
- Mrs. Sandsky informs you that she smoked one pack of cigarettes daily for about 8 years when she was younger, but that she quit smoking 10 years ago and has not smoked since that time.

CLINICAL PHOTOGRAPHS FOR MRS. SANDSKY

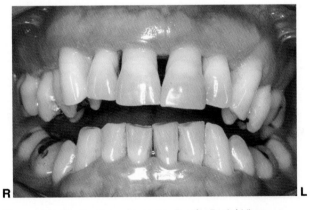

Figure 36.23. Sandsky: Anterior Teeth, Facial View.

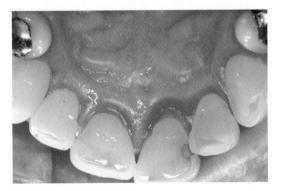

Figure 36.24. Sandsky: Maxillary Anterior Teeth, Lingual View.

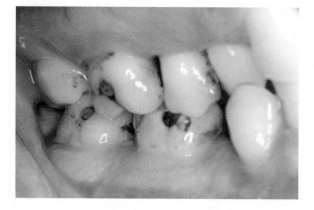

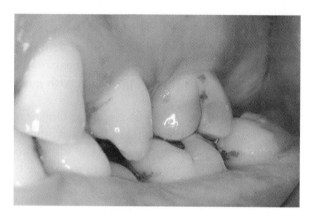

Figure 36.25. Sandsky: Right Side, Facial View.

Figure 36.26. Sandsky: Left Side, Facial View.

CASE #3

	1	2	3	4	5	6	7	8	9	10	11	12	13	14	15	16	Maxilla
Mobility (I, II, III)								I	I			I					
Bleeding/Purulence (+)		+	+	+	+		+	+	+		+	+		+			
Attachment Level (CEJ to BP)		646	544	535	545	646	656	656	656	756	655	646		545			
Probing Depth (FGM to BP)		646	545	535	545	535	545	545	545	645	545	635		545			

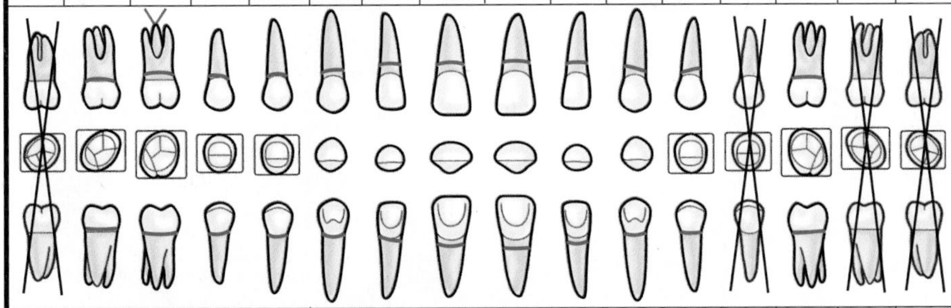

Facial

Palatal

Bleeding/Purulence (+)		+	+	+	+	+	+	+	+	+	+	+		+			
Attachment Level (CEJ to BP)		645	545	543	545	545	645	656	656	666	545	535		545			
Probing Depth (FGM to BP)		645	545	545	545	545	645	545	545	555	545	535		545			
F/P Plaque	☒	☒	☒	☒	☒	☒	☒	☒	☒	☒	☒	☒	☒	☒	☒	☒	
Supragingival Calculus		✓	✓	✓	✓		✓			✓	✓			✓			
Subgingival Calculus		✓	✓	✓	✓	✓	✓	✓	✓		✓	✓		✓			
PSR Code																	

Right   *Left*

	32	31	30	29	28	27	26	25	24	23	22	21	20	19	18	17	Mandible
Mobility (I, II, III)																	
Bleeding/Purulence (+)		+	+	+	+	+	+	+	+	+	+	+	+	+	+		
Attachment Level (CEJ to BP)		455	545		545	545	544	444	544	545	543	543	434	545	545		
Probing Depth (FGM to BP)		455	545		545	545	544	444	544	545	545	434	434	545	545		

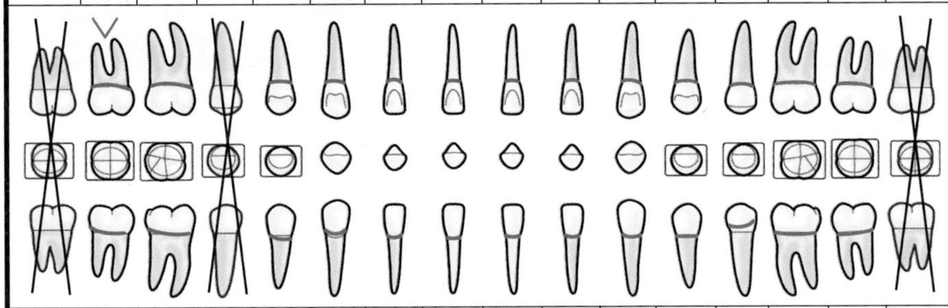

Lingual

Facial

Bleeding/Purulence (+)												I					
Attachment Level (CEJ to BP)		355	545		545	544	444	444	445	545	545	535	525	545	545		
Probing Depth (FGM to BP)		455	545		544	544	444	444	445	545	545	535	646	545	545		
L/F Plaque	☒	☒	☒	☒	☒	☒	☒	☒	☒	☒	☒	☒	☒	☒	☒	☒	
Supragingival Calculus		✓	✓		✓	✓	✓	✓	✓	✓	✓	✓	✓	✓	✓		
Subgingival Calculus		✓	✓		✓	✓	✓	✓	✓	✓	✓	✓	✓	✓	✓		
PSR Code																	

Figure 36.27. Mrs. Sandsky's Periodontal Chart.

RADIOGRAPHIC SERIES FOR MRS. SANDSKY

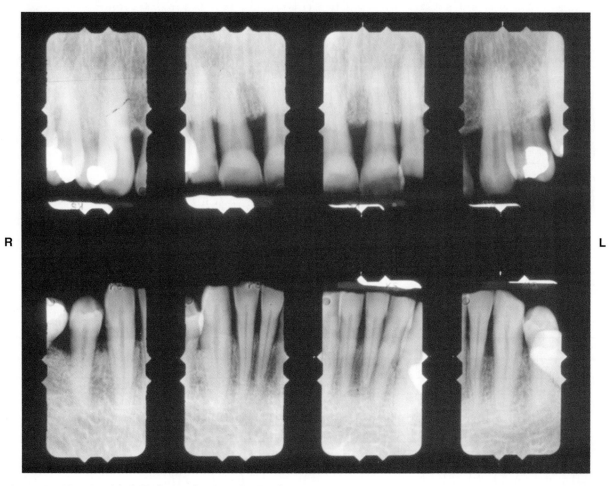

R   L

Figure 36.28A. Sandsky's Radiographs: Anterior Teeth.

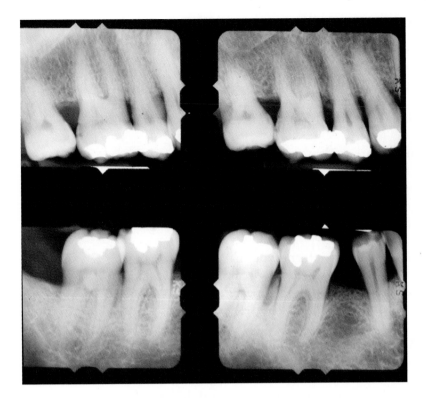

Figure 36.28B. Sandsky's Radiographs: Right Posterior Teeth.

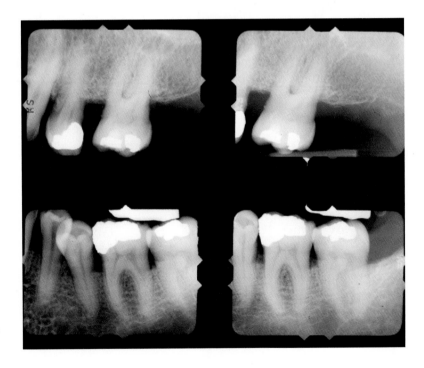

Figure 36.28C. Sandsky's Radiographs: Left Posterior Teeth.

DECISION-MAKING QUESTIONS FOR CASE 3: MRS. SANDSKY

1. What factors in Mrs. Sandsky's profile indicate that achieving an acceptable level of patient self-care may *not* be as difficult for her as it is for many patients?

2. Will the medications being taken by Mrs. Sandsky require any special precautions during treatment by the members of the dental team?

3. How might the history of smoking relate to Mrs. Sandsky's past and current risk for periodontal disease?

4. What signs of gingival inflammation are evident in Mrs. Sandsky's clinical photographs?

5. What etiologic risk factors for gingival and periodontal diseases are evident in Mrs. Sandsky's clinical photographs?

6. Does Mrs. Sandsky's periodontal evaluation indicate that she has attachment loss present on some teeth?

7. In response to your questions, Mrs. Sandsky informs you that the open triangular space between her upper front teeth was not there a few years ago. What do you think may be causing this space between her teeth to appear?

8. What etiologic factors for gingival and periodontal diseases are evident in Mrs. Sandsky's dental radiographs?

9. How would you characterize Mrs. Sandsky's periodontal condition? Do you think that she has gingivitis, periodontitis, neither, or both? What clinical or radiographic findings did you use to reach your conclusion?

10. Develop a suggested step-by-step plan for nonsurgical periodontal therapy for Mrs. Sandsky.

11. What information should your team give Mrs. Sandsky about her periodontal condition?

12. What should Mrs. Sandsky be told about the possible need for periodontal surgery later in the treatment?

13. What should Mrs. Sandsky be told about the need for continuing treatment such as periodontal maintenance?

Glossary

A

Abscess of the periodontium—an acute infection involving a circumscribed collection of pus in the periodontium. Also see gingival abscess, periodontal abscess, pericoronal abscess.

Absorbable suture—a suture made from a material designed to dissolve harmlessly in body fluids over time; though absorbable sutures do not normally require removal by the dental team, some absorbable sutures do not dissolve particularly well in saliva. Also see nonabsorbable suture.

Abutment—a component of a dental implant; the titanium post that attaches to the implant body and protrudes partially or completely through the gingival tissue into the mouth. Also see implant abutment.

"Ask. Advise. Refer."—the American Dental Hygiene Association's national Smoking Cessation Initiative designed to promote smoking cessation intervention by dental hygienists.

Acquired immunodeficiency syndrome (AIDS)—a communicable disease caused by human immunodeficiency virus (HIV). People with acquired immunodeficiency syndrome are at an increased risk for developing certain cancers and for infections that usually occur only in individuals with a weak immune system.

Acquired pellicle—a film composed of a variety of salivary glycoproteins and antibodies that forms within minutes after cleaning a tooth surface; its purpose is to protect the enamel from acidic activity.

Aggregatibacter actinomycetemcomitans—an important periodontal pathogen.

Active disease site—an area of tissue destruction that shows continued apical migration of the junctional epithelium over time.

Acute gingivitis—gingivitis of a short duration, after which professional care and patient self-care return the gingiva to a healthy state. Also see gingivitis and chronic gingivitis.

Acute inflammation—a short-term, normal inflammatory response that protects and heals the body following physical injury or infection. Also see inflammation and chronic inflammation.

Acute periodontal conditions—periodontal conditions that are commonly characterized by a rapid onset and rapid course, that are frequently accompanied by pain and discomfort, and that may be unrelated to the presence of preexisting gingivitis or periodontitis. One example is an abscess of the periodontium.

Adult periodontitis—see chronic periodontitis.

Aerobic bacteria—bacteria that require oxygen to live. Also see facultative bacteria and anaerobic bacteria.

Aggressive periodontitis (AgP)—a bacterial infection of the periodontium characterized by a rapid destruction of the periodontal ligament, rapid loss of supporting bone, high risk for tooth loss, and a poor response to periodontal therapy. Also see chronic periodontitis.

AIDS—see acquired immunodeficiency syndrome.

Allografts—bone replacement grafts taken from individuals that are genetically dissimilar to the donor (i.e., another human donor); these grafting materials must be modified to eliminate the potential for rejection. Also see autographs, xenografts, and alloplasts.

Alloplasts—bone replacement grafts that are synthetic materials or inert foreign materials. Also see autografts, allografts, and xenografts.

Alveolar bone loss—the resorption of alveolar bone as a result of periodontitis. Also see horizontal bone loss and vertical bone loss.

Alveolar bone proper—the thin layer of bone that lines the socket to surround the root of the tooth (also called the cribriform plate); the ends of the periodontal ligament fibers are embedded in the alveolar bone proper.

Alveolar bone—the bone that surrounds the roots of the teeth. It forms the bony sockets that support and protect the roots of the teeth.

Alveolar crest—the most coronal portion of the alveolar process. In health, the alveolar crest is located 1–2 mm apical to (below) the cementoenamel junctions (CEJ) of the teeth.

Alveolar mucosa—the apical boundary, or lower edge, of the gingiva; it can be distinguished easily from the gingiva by its dark red color and smooth, shiny surface.

Alveolar process—the bone of the upper or lower jaw that surrounds and supports the roots of the teeth.

Alveolus—the bony socket; a cavity in the alveolar bone that houses the root of a tooth.

Ambivalence—having mixed feelings and attitudes about something, such as a behavior change.

American Academy of Periodontology (AAP)—an association of dental professionals specializing in the prevention, diagnosis, and treatment of diseases affecting the periodontium.

Anaerobic bacteria—bacteria that cannot live in the presence of oxygen. Also see aerobic bacteria and facultative bacteria.

Anastomose—to join together; in the periodontium, a complex system of blood vessels supplies blood to the periodontal tissues.

Antibiotic resistance—the ability of a bacterium to withstand the effects of an antibiotic by developing mechanisms to protect the bacterium from the killing or inhibiting effects of the antibiotic.

Antibiotics—medications used to help fight infections either because they kill bacteria or because they can inhibit the growth of bacteria. Also see antibiotic resistance.

Antibodies—Y-shaped proteins; one end of the Y binds to the outside of the B cell and the other end binds to a microorganism and helps to kill it. Antibodies are known collectively as immunoglobulins.

Anti-inflammatory biochemical mediators—biologically active compounds secreted by immune cells that are protective and keep the bacterial infection from doing serious harm to the periodontium, such as the cytokines interleukin-4 (IL-4) and interleukin-10 (IL-10).

Antioxidants—substances that occur naturally in the body and in certain foods; antioxidants can inhibit oxidation and thereby block damage to cells by free radicals.

Apical migration—the movement of the cells of the junctional epithelium from their normal position to a position apical to the CEJ.

Apically positioned flap with osseous resective surgery—a periodontal surgical procedure involving a combination of a displaced flap (displaced in an apical direction) plus resective osseous surgery; this procedure is ideal for minimizing periodontal pocket depths in patients with osseous craters caused by moderate periodontitis. Also see displaced flap.

Ascorbic acid-deficiency gingivitis—an inflammatory response of the gingiva caused by dental plaque biofilm that is aggravated by chronically low vitamin C (ascorbic acid) levels; manifests clinically as bright red, swollen, ulcerated gingival tissue that bleeds with the slightest provocation.

Atherosclerosis—a process characterized by a thickening of artery walls.

Attached gingiva—the part of the gingiva that is firm, dense, and tightly connected to the cementum on the cervical third of the root or to the periosteum (connective tissue cover) of the alveolar bone.

Attachment loss—the destruction of the tooth-supporting structures that have been destroyed around a tooth; characterized by relocation of the junctional epithelium to the tooth root, destruction of the fibers of the gingiva, destruction of the periodontal ligament fibers, and loss of alveolar bone support from around the tooth. Also see clinical attachment loss.

Autografts—bone replacement materials taken from the patient who is receiving the graft; periodontal autografts can be taken from sites in the patient's own jaws or occasionally from other areas of the patient's body. Also see allografts, xenografts, and alloplasts.

Autonomy—freedom to determine one's own actions, behaviors, etc.; placing responsibility for behavior change or treatment decisions with the patient.

B

Bacterial blooms—periods when specific species or groups of species grow at rapidly accelerated rates with in a dental plaque biofilm.

Bacterial enzymes—agents that are harmful or destructive to host cells; a variety of enzymes produced by periodontal pathogens are important in tissue destruction.

Bacteria—the simplest organisms that can be seen only through a microscope. Also see innocuous and pathogenic.

Basal lamina—a thin, tough sheet that separates the epithelial cells from the underlying connective tissue. Also see external basal lamina and internal basal lamina.

Baseline data—clinical data gathered at the beginning of the periodontal treatment that is subsequently used for comparison to clinical information gathered at subsequent appointments.

B cells—see B lymphocytes.

Best evidence—the highest level of evidence available for a specific clinical question. Also see best practices and levels of evidence.

Best practices—are clinical practices, treatments, and interventions that result in the best possible outcome for the patient. Also see best evidence and levels of evidence.

Biochemical mediators—biologically active compounds secreted by immune cells that activate the body's inflammatory response; inflammatory mediators of importance in periodontitis are the cytokines, prostaglandins, and matrix metalloproteinases. Also see anti-inflammatory biochemical mediators and proinflammatory biochemical mediators.

Biocompatible—a nonbiologic material that is not rejected by the body. Titanium is a biocompatible metal that allows tissue healing around an implant abutment.

Biofilm—a well-organized community of bacteria that adheres to a surface and is embedded in an extracellular slime layer; forms rapidly on almost any surface that is wet. See extracellular slime layer and fluid channels.

Biologic equilibrium—a state of balance in the internal environment of the body.

Biologic width—the space on the tooth surface occupied by the junctional epithelium and the connective tissue attachment fibers immediately apical to the junctional epithelium.

Biological seal—the union of the epithelial cells to the surface of a dental implant.

Biomechanical forces—the biological and mechanical forces placed on an osseointegrated dental implant; controlling these forces is vital to achieve long-term success with implants.

Bisphosphonates—drugs that can inhibit the resorption of bone by altering osteoclastic activity. One of the possible side effects of these drugs is osteonecrosis of the jaws following their extended use.

Blunt dissection—elevation of a flap during periodontal surgery using tools that are not sharpened on the edge (i.e., blunted or slightly rounded); blunt dissection minimizes the chance of accidental damage to the flap. In this type of flap elevation, the flap is lifted or pried up using surgical tools called periosteal elevators, and it is elevated in a manner quite similar to lifting the peeling off an orange. Also see sharp dissection.

Blunted papilla—a papilla is flat and does not fill the interproximal space.

B lymphocytes—small leukocytes that help in the defense against bacteria, viruses, and fungi; principal function is to make antibodies. B lymphocytes can further differentiate into one of the two types of cells: plasma B cells and memory B cells.

Bone morphogenetic proteins (BMP)—a group of regulatory glycoproteins that have been studied for possible use in the field of periodontal regeneration.

Bone replacement graft—a periodontal surgical procedure used to encourage the body to rebuild alveolar bone that has been lost usually as a result of periodontal disease.

Bruxism—the forceful grinding of the teeth.

Bulbous papilla—an enlarged papilla that appears to bulge out of the interproximal space.

C

Calcium channel blocker—a class of drugs that block the influx of calcium ions through cardiac and vascular smooth muscle cell membranes resulting in the dilation of the main coronary and systemic arteries.

CAMBRA (Caries Management by Risk Assessment)—protocols that seek to provide practical clinical guidelines for managing dental caries based upon risk group assessment. The protocols are based upon the best evidence at this time and can be used in planning effective caries management for any patient.

Cancellous bone—the lattice-like bone that fills the interior portion of the alveolar process between the cortical bone and the alveolar bone proper; cancellous bone is oriented around the tooth to form support for the alveolar bone proper.

Caries Management by Risk Assessment—see CAMBRA.

Cell junctions—cellular structures that mechanically attach a cell and its cytoskeleton to its neighboring cells or to the basal lamina. Also see desmosome and hemidesmosome.

Cells—the smallest structural unit of living matter capable of functioning independently: cells group together to form a tissue.

Cementum—a mineralized layer of connective tissue that covers the root of the tooth; anatomically, cementum is part of the tooth; however, it also part of the periodontium.

Change talk—encouraging the expression of statements in the direction of change; evoking, facilitating, and strengthening a patient's desire for change. Change talk can be elicited with simple open-ended questions such as "What advantages do you see of cutting back on sugary foods?"

Chemokines—a major subgroup of cytokines that cause additional immune cells to be attracted to the site of infection or injury. Also see cytokines.

Chemotaxis—the process whereby leukocytes are attracted to an infection site in response to biochemical compounds released by invading microorganisms.

Chronic gingivitis—long-lasting gingivitis; gingivitis may exist for years without ever progressing to periodontitis. Also see gingivitis and acute gingivitis.

Chronic inflammation— a long-lived, out-of-control inflammatory response that continues for more than a few weeks; it is a pathological condition characterized by active inflammation, tissue destruction, and attempts at repair. Also see inflammation and acute inflammation.

Chronic periodontitis—a bacterial infection of the periodontium resulting in inflammation within the supporting tissues of the teeth, progressive destruction of the periodontal ligament, and loss of supporting alveolar bone; involves irreversible loss of attachment and bone and is the most frequently occurring form of periodontitis. Also see localized chronic periodontitis, generalized chronic periodontitis, and aggressive periodontitis.

Circumscribed—localized or confined to a specific site.

Clenching—the continuous or intermittent forceful closure of the maxillary teeth against the mandibular teeth.

Clinical attachment level (CAL)—an estimate of the true periodontal support around the tooth as measured with a periodontal probe. This measurement is only an estimation of the actual histologic level of attachment still present. It is a means of estimating the level of the junctional epithelium.

Clinical attachment loss—an estimate of the extent that the tooth-supporting structures have been destroyed around a tooth. Also see attachment loss.

Clinical periodontal assessment—a fact-gathering process designed to provide a comprehensive picture of the patient's periodontal health status. Also see comprehensive periodontal assessment and periodontal screening examination.

Coaggregation—the cell-to-cell adherence of one oral bacterium to another; the ability to adhere and coaggregate is an important determinant in the development of oral bacterial biofilms.

Coated tongue—see tongue coating.

Cochrane Database of Systematic Reviews—a database of systematic reviews of healthcare interventions.

Collaborate—to work together, such as a patient and healthcare provider working together to obtain the best possible health for the patient.

Collagen fibers—fibers that form a dense network of strong, rope-like cables that secure and hold the gingival connective tissues together.

Communicable—a disease that may be passed from one person to another by direct or indirect contact via substances such as inanimate objects; there is little or no evidence that periodontal infections are communicable.

Complement system—a complex series of proteins circulating in the blood that works to facilitate phagocytosis or kill bacteria directly by puncturing bacterial cell membranes.

Compliance—the extent to which a person's behavior coincides with health advice. Examples of compliant patients would be a patient who faithfully takes antihypertensive medications as prescribed by a physician or a patient who cooperates in meeting regularly scheduled periodontal maintenance appointments as recommended by the dental team. Also see noncompliant patients.

Comprehensive periodontal assessment—an intensive evaluation used to gather information about the periodontium; normally includes clinical features such as probing depth measurements, bleeding on probing, presence of exudate, level of the free gingival margin and the mucogingival junction, tooth mobility, furcation involvement, presence of calculus and bacterial plaque biofilm, gingival inflammation, radiographic evidence of alveolar bone loss, and presence of local contributing factors.

Concavity—a trench-like depression in the root surface; commonly occur on the proximal surfaces of anterior and posterior teeth and the facial and lingual surfaces of molar teeth.

Confirmation bias—a human tendency to look for or interpret information that confirms our beliefs.

Connective tissue papillae—finger-like extensions of connective tissue that extend up into the epithelium.

Connective tissue—tissue that fills the spaces between the tissues and organs in the body; it consists of cells separated by abundant extracellular substance.

Controlled-release delivery device—in dentistry, usually consists of an antibacterial chemical that is imbedded in a carrier material; it is designed to be placed directly into the periodontal pocket where the carrier material attaches to the tooth surface and dissolves slowly, producing a steady release of the antimicrobial agent over a period of several days within the periodontal pocket.

Conventional mechanical periodontal therapy—a term that refers to self-care, periodontal instrumentation, and control of local contributing factors.

Coronally positioned flap—a periodontal plastic surgical procedure that can be used to repair gingival recession if the recession is not advanced; the coronally positioned flap is a displaced flap (displaced in a coronal direction in this case). Also see laterally positioned flap and semilunar flap.

Cortical bone—a layer of compact bone that forms the hard, outside wall of the mandible and maxilla on the facial and lingual aspects; cortical bone surrounds the alveolar bone proper and gives support to the socket.

Cratered papillae—a papilla that appears to have been "scooped out" leaving a concave depression in the midproximal area. Cratered papillae are associated with necrotizing ulcerative periodontal disease.

C-reactive protein—a special type of plasma protein that is present during episodes of acute inflammation or infection: CRP is an important cardiovascular risk predictor.

Crestal irregularities—the appearance on a dental radiograph of breaks or fuzziness instead of a nice clean line at the crest of the interdental alveolar bone.

Crevicular fluid—see gingival crevicular fluid.

Crevicular incision—one type of horizontal incision employed during periodontal flap surgery in which the surgical scalpel is simply placed into the gingival crevice or sulcus and the tissues are incised apically to bone. Also see horizontal incision and internal bevel incision.

Crown lengthening surgery—a periodontal plastic surgical procedure designed to create a longer clinical crown for a tooth by removing some of the gingiva and usually by removing some alveolar bone from the necks of the teeth. Also see functional crown lengthening and esthetic crown lengthening.

Cyclosporine—an immunosuppressive agent used for prevention of transplant rejection as well as for management of a number of autoimmune conditions such as rheumatoid arthritis; associated with drug-influenced gingival enlargement.

Cytokines—a general name for powerful regulatory proteins released by immune cells that influence the behavior of other nearby cells: cytokines signal the immune system to send additional phagocytic cells to the site of an infection.

D

Databases—online indexes that list all articles published in a given period of time by journals in a particular profession or group of professions, such as PubMed, MEDLINE, or CINAHL (Cumulative Index of Nursing and Allied Health Literature).

Dental calculus—mineralized bacterial plaque biofilm, covered on its external surface by nonmineralized, living bacterial plaque biofilm.

Dental implant—a nonbiologic (artificial) device surgically inserted into the jawbone to replace a missing tooth or provide support for a prosthetic denture.

Dental prosthesis—see prosthesis.

Dental water jet—a generic term for a device that delivers a pulsed irrigation of water or other solution around and between teeth and into the gingival sulcus or periodontal pocket.

Dentinal hypersensitivity—a short, sharp painful reaction that occurs when some areas of exposed dentin are subjected to mechanical, thermal, or chemical stimuli.

Dentinal tubule—a microscopic tube within the dentin that spreads outward from the pulp throughout the dentin.

Dentogingival unit—composed of the junctional epithelium and the gingival fibers; the dentogingival unit acts to provide structural support to the gingival tissue.

Deplaquing—the disruption or removal of subgingival microbial plaque biofilm and its by-products from cemental surfaces and the pocket space.

Desmosome—a specialized cell junction that connects two neighboring epithelial cells and their cytoskeletons together.

Diabetes mellitus—a disease in which the body does not produce or properly use insulin. Insulin is a hormone that is needed to convert sugar, starches, and other food into energy that the body uses to sustain life. Also see type I diabetes mellitus and type II diabetes mellitus.

Dilantin—see phenytoin.

Disease progression—the change or advancement of periodontal destruction. Also see intermittent disease progression.

Disease site—an area of tissue destruction. A disease site may involve only a single surface of a tooth, for example, the distal surface of a tooth. The disease site may involve several surfaces of the tooth or all four surfaces (mesial, distal, facial, and lingual). Also see inactive disease site and active disease site.

Displaced flap—a periodontal flap that is sutured with the margin of the flap placed at a position other than its original position in relationship to the CEJ of the tooth; a displaced flap can be positioned apically, coronally, or laterally in relationship to its original position. Also see nondisplaced flap.

Dissection—the process of cutting apart or separating tissue. Also see blunt dissection and sharp dissection.

Doxycycline—an antibiotic drug that is used to treat a variety of infections. Doxycycline at low doses is used as a host-modulating agent to inhibit part of the destruction occurs in periodontitis. See subantibacterial dose.

Drug-influenced gingival enlargement—an esthetically disfiguring overgrowth of the gingiva that is a side effect associated with certain medications such as anticonvulsants, calcium channel blockers, and immunosuppressants.

Dry mouth—see xerostomia.

E

Elevation—separating the surface tissues from the underlying tooth root and alveolar bone during periodontal surgery; the term elevation is used to convey the concept of lifting the surface tissues away from the tooth roots and away from the alveolar bone.

Elicit—encouraging the patient to talk about his or her opinions, behaviors, attitudes.

Embrasure space—see gingival embrasure space.

Empathy—the ability to identify with and understand another person's feelings or difficulties.

Enamel matrix derivative (EMD)—a preparation of proteins extracted from porcine tooth buds; enamel matrix derivative has been used to enhance periodontal regeneration.

Endothelium—the thin layer of epithelial cells that line the interior surface of the blood vessels.

Epidemiology—the study of the health and disease within the total population (rather than an individual) and the risk factors that influence health and disease.

Epithelial tissue—the tissue that makes up the outer surface of the body (skin) and lines the body cavities such as the mouth, stomach, and intestines.

Epithelial-connective tissue interface—the boundary where the epithelial and connective tissues meet.

Essential oil—an active ingredient in some mouth rinses such as thymol, menthol, eucalyptol, and methyl salicylate.

Esthetic crown lengthening—a crown lengthening performed on teeth to improve the appearance of the teeth where there is excessive gingiva or a "gummy smile" as it is sometimes called. Also see functional crown lengthening.

Evidence levels—see levels of evidence.

Evidence-based healthcare—the conscientious, explicit, and judicious use of current best evidence in making decisions about the care of individual patients; requires the integration of individual clinical expertise and patient preferences with the best available external clinical evidence from systematic research.

Exotoxins—harmful proteins released from the bacterial cell that act on the body's host cells at a distance.

Extent—the degree or amount of periodontal destruction; can be characterized based on the number of sites that have experienced tissue destruction. Also see severity.

External basal lamina—a thin mat of extracellular matrix between the epithelial cells of the junctional epithelium and the gingival connective tissue. Also see internal basal lamina.

Extracellular matrix—a mesh-like material that surrounds the cells; this material helps to hold cells together and provides a framework within which cells can migrate and interact with one another.

Extracellular slime layer—a protective barrier that surrounds the mushroom-shaped bacterial microcolonies of a biofilm; protects the bacterial microcolonies from antibiotics, antimicrobials, and the body's immune system. Also see biofilm and fluid channels.

Exudate—pus that can be expressed from a periodontal pocket; sometimes called suppuration.

F

Facultative anaerobic bacteria—bacteria that can exist either with or without oxygen. Also see aerobic bacteria and anaerobic bacteria.

Fimbriae—hair-like structures possessed by some bacteria that enable them to attach rapidly upon contact with the tooth surface.

Flap curettage—see open flap debridement.

Flap for access—a periodontal surgical technique used to provide access to the tooth roots for improved root preparation. In this surgical procedure, the gingival tissue is incised and temporarily elevated (lifted away) from the tooth roots. Also see open flap debridement.

Flap—see periodontal flap

Fluid channels—a series of channels that penetrate the extracellular slime layer of a biofilm that provide nutrients and oxygen for the bacterial microcolonies and facilitate movement of bacterial metabolites, waste products, and enzymes within the biofilm structure. Also see biofilm and extracellular slime layer.

Food impaction—forcing food (such as pieces of tough meat) between teeth during chewing, trapping the food in the interdental area.

Free gingival graft—a type of periodontal plastic surgery that was one of the first procedures used to augment the width of attached gingiva. The free gingival graft requires harvesting a donor section of tissue, usually from the palate, so there are two intraoral wounds that are created during this surgery: the donor site and the recipient site.

Free gingival groove—a shallow linear depression that separates the free and attached gingiva; this line may be visible clinically but is not obvious in many instances.

Free gingiva—the unattached portion of the gingiva that surrounds the tooth in the region of the cementoenamel junction; also known as the unattached gingiva or the marginal gingiva.

Fremitus—a palpable or visible movement of a tooth when in function.

Frenectomy—a periodontal plastic surgical procedure that results in removal of a frenum, including removal of the attachment of the frenum to bone.

Full-thickness flap—a periodontal surgical procedure that includes elevation of the entire thickness of the soft tissue (including epithelium, connective tissue, and periosteum); the full-thickness flap provides the complete access to underlying bone that might be needed when bone replacement grafting or periodontal regeneration procedures are anticipated.

Functional crown lengthening—a periodontal plastic surgical procedure performed on a tooth where the remaining tooth structure is inadequate to support a needed restoration; can be used to make a restorative dental procedure (such as a crown) possible when the only sensible alternative might be to remove the tooth. Also see esthetic crown lengthening.

Functional occlusal forces—normal occlusal forces produced during the act of chewing food. Also see parafunctional occlusal forces.

Furcation involvement—an osseous defect that results in a loss of alveolar bone between the roots of a multirooted tooth.

G

Generalized chronic periodontitis—chronic periodontitis in which more than 30% of the sites in the mouth have experienced attachment loss and bone loss. Also see chronic periodontitis.

Genetic test—see PST genetic susceptibility test.

Gestational diabetes—a form of diabetes that occurs during pregnancy in women who have never had diabetes before pregnancy. Also see diabetes mellitus.

Gingival abscess—an abscess of the periodontium that is primarily limited to the gingival margin or interdental papilla without involvement of the deeper structures of the periodontium. Also see periodontal abscess, pericoronal abscess.

Gingival crevicular fluid—a fluid that flows into the sulcus from the adjacent gingival connective tissue; the flow is slight in health and increases in disease.

Gingival curettage—an older type of periodontal surgical procedure that involves an attempt to scrape away the lining of the periodontal pocket usually using a periodontal curet, often a Gracey curet. Research has demonstrated that normally the same benefits from gingival curettage can be derived from thorough periodontal instrumentation by the clinician plus meticulous self-care by the patient. Thus, curettage is rarely needed as a separate periodontal surgical procedure in modern dentistry.

Gingival diseases—a category of periodontal diseases that usually involve inflammation of the gingival tissues, most often in response to bacterial plaque biofilm. Also see gingivitis, plaque-induced gingivitis, non–plaque-induced gingivitis, acute gingivitis, and chronic gingivitis.

Gingival embrasure space—the small triangular open space (apical to the contact area) between the curved proximal surfaces of two teeth. In health, the interdental papilla fills the gingival embrasure space. Also see type I, type II, and type III gingival embrasure.

Gingival epithelium—a specialized stratified squamous epithelium that functions well in the wet environment of the oral cavity; the microscopic anatomy of the gingival epithelium is similar to the epithelium of the skin. Also see oral epithelium, sulcular epithelium, and junctional epithelium.

Gingival fibers—see supragingival fiber bundles.

Gingival margin—the thin, rounded edge of free gingiva that forms the coronal boundary, or upper edge, of the gingiva. In health, the gingival margin contacts the tooth slightly coronal to the cementoenamel junction.

Gingival pocket—a deepening of the gingival sulcus as a result of swelling or enlargement of the gingival tissue. Also see periodontal pocket.

Gingival sulcular fluid—see gingival crevicular fluid.

Gingival sulcus—the *space* between the free gingiva and the tooth surface.

Gingiva—the part of the mucosa that surrounds the cervical portions of the teeth and covers the alveolar processes of the jaws.

Gingivectomy—a resective periodontal surgical procedure designed to excise (cut away) and to remove some of the gingival tissue. Historically, the gingivectomy was used for many years in periodontics as a primary treatment modality, but it plays a greatly reduced role in modern dentistry. Also see gingivoplasty.

Gingivitis—an inflammation of the periodontium that is confined to the gingiva resulting in damage to the gingival tissue that is reversible. Also see gingival diseases, acute gingivitis, chronic gingivitis, and periodontitis.

Gingivoplasty—a periodontal surgical procedure used to reshape the surface of the gingiva to create a natural form and contour to the gingiva. Unlike the gingivectomy, gingivoplasty implies reshaping the surface of the gingiva without removing any of the gingiva actually attached to the tooth surface. Also see gingivectomy.

Glycemic control—a medical term referring to the typical levels of blood sugar (glucose) in a person with diabetes mellitus; optimal management of diabetes involves patients measuring and recording their own blood glucose levels.

Gram staining—a laboratory method that reveals differences in the chemical and physical properties of bacterial cell walls that divides bacteria into Gram-positive (purple color) and Gram-negative (red color) bacterial cell wall types. See Gram-positive bacteria and Gram-negative bacteria.

Gram-negative bacteria—bacteria with double cell walls that show a red stain under the microscope; believed to play an important role in inflammatory periodontitis. See Gram staining and Gram-positive bacteria.

Gram-positive bacteria—bacteria with thick, single cell walls that show a purple stain under the microscope; most of the bacteria associated with a healthy periodontium are Gram-positive. See gram staining and Gram-negative bacteria.

Growth factors—naturally occurring proteins that regulate both cell growth and development. Several growth factors are being studied for their effect in enhancing the predictability of periodontal regeneration.

Guided tissue regeneration (GTR)—a periodontal surgical procedure employed to encourage regeneration of lost periodontal structures (i.e., to regrow lost cementum, lost periodontal ligament, and lost alveolar bone).

H

Halitophobia—a fear of having bad breath, whether a valid concern or not.

Halitosis—a clinical name for bad breath. There are many causes of halitosis such as poor oral hygiene, tobacco and/or alcohol, and possibly a medical condition such as a respiratory infection or diabetes. Also see oral malodor and halitophobia.

Heat shock proteins—a group of proteins that are induced when a cell undergoes various types of environmental stresses like heat, cold, and oxygen deprivation.

Hemidesmosome—a specialized cell junction that connects the epithelial cells to the basal lamina.

Histology—a branch of anatomy concerned with the study of the microscopic structures of tissues.

HIV-associated gingivitis—see linear gingival erythema.

HIV—human immunodeficiency virus. Also see acquired immunodeficiency syndrome.

Horizontal bone loss—a common pattern of bone loss resulting in a fairly even, overall reduction in the height of the alveolar bone with the margin of the alveolar crest more or less perpendicular to the long axis of the tooth. Also see alveolar bone loss and vertical bone loss.

Horizontal incision—an incision that runs parallel to the gingival margins in a mesiodistal direction. Also see incision and vertical incision.

Hospital-acquired pneumonia—an infection of the lungs contracted during a stay in a hospital or long-term care facility. Hospital-acquired pneumonia is not caused by the same organisms that cause community-acquired pneumonia.

Host modulation—in dentistry, altering the host's (patient's) defense responses to help the body limit damage to the periodontium from infections such as periodontitis.

Host response—the way that an individual's body responds to an infection. Also see immune system and inflammation.

Host—a human in or on which another organism lives; in the case of periodontal disease, bacterial pathogens infect the host (individual with periodontal disease).

Hydrokinetic activity—the energy created by fluids in motion; in dentistry, the pulsating fluid delivered by dental water jet creates two zones of fluid movement.

I

Immune system—a collection of responses that protects the body against infections by bacteria, viruses, fungi, toxins, and parasites; the immune system defends the body against invading microorganisms, as well as toxins in the environment.

Immunoglobulins—Y-shaped proteins; the five major classes of immunoglobulin are immunoglobulin M (IgM), immunoglobulin D (IgD), immunoglobulin G (IgG), immunoglobulin A (IgA), and immunoglobulin E (IgE)

Implant abutment—a titanium post that attaches to the implant body and protrudes partially or completely through the gingival tissue into the mouth.

Implant body—the portion of the implant system that is surgically placed into the living alveolar bone; sometimes referred to as the implant fixture or implant.

Implant fixture—see implant body.

Implant—see dental implant and implant body.

Inactive disease site—an area of tissue destruction that is stable, with the attachment level of the junctional epithelium remaining the same over time.

Incidence—the number of new disease cases in a population that occur over a given period of time. Also see prevalence.

Incision—a cut into a body tissue or organ, especially one made during surgery. Also see horizontal incision, crevicular incision, internal bevel incision, and vertical incision.

Inflammation—the body's reaction to injury or invasion by disease-producing organisms that focuses host defense components at the site of the infection to eliminate microorganisms and heal damaged tissue. Inflammation is part of the immune response. Also see acute inflammation and chronic inflammation.

Inflammatory biochemical mediators—biologically active compounds secreted by cells that activate the body's inflammatory response; inflammatory mediators of importance in periodontitis are the cytokines, prostaglandins, and matrix metalloproteinases.

Informed consent—a patient's voluntary agreement to proposed treatment after achieving an understanding of the relevant facts, benefits, and risks involved. Also see informed refusal.

Informed refusal—a person's right to refuse all or a portion of the proposed treatment after the recommended treatment, alternate treatment options, and the likely consequences of declining treatment have been explained in a language understood by the patient. Also see informed consent.

Infrabony defect—an osseous defect in the alveolar bone resulting in bone resorption that occurs in an uneven, oblique direction.

Infrabony pocket—a periodontal pocket in which there is vertical bone loss and the junctional epithelium, forming the base of the pocket, is located *apical* to the crest of the alveolar bone. The base of the pocket is located within the cratered-out area of the bone alongside of the root surface. Also see periodontal pocket and suprabony pocket.

Innervation—nerve supply; innervation to the periodontium occurs via the branches of the trigeminal nerve.

Innocuous—species of bacteria that are not harmful. Also see pathogenic bacteria.

Insurance codes—numeric codes used by insurance companies and the government to classify different dental procedures. For example, periodontal maintenance procedures are designated by the insurance code D4910.

Intentional torts—actions designed to injure another person or that person's property.

Interdental gingiva—the portion of the gingiva that fills the interdental embrasure between two adjacent teeth apical to the contact area. The interdental gingiva consists of two interdental papillae.

Intermittent disease progression theory—states that periodontal disease is characterized by periods of disease activity and inactivity (remission).

Internal basal lamina—a thin mat of extracellular matrix between the epithelial cells of the junctional epithelium and the tooth surface. Also see external basal lamina.

Internal bevel incision—one type of horizontal incision employed during periodontal flap surgery in which the surgical scalpel enters the marginal gingiva but is not placed directly into the crevice or sulcus; the scalpel blade enters the gingival margin approximately 0.5–1.0 mm away from the margin and follows the general contour of the scalloped marginal gingiva. Also see horizontal incision and crevicular incision.

Irrigation—see oral irrigation.

J

Junctional epithelium (JE)—the specialized epithelium that forms the base of the sulcus and joins the gingiva to the tooth surface. Also see gingival epithelium.

Juvenile periodontitis—See aggressive periodontitis.

K

Keratinized epithelial cells—cells that have no nuclei and form a tough, resistant layer on the surface of the skin.

Kernatization—the process by which epithelial cells on the surface of the skin become stronger and waterproof. Also see keratinized epithelial cells and nonkeratinized epithelial cells.

Kwashiorkor—a severe protein deficiency that can result in a shift in subgingival oral bacteria to include more periodontal pathogens.

L

Laterally positioned flap—a periodontal plastic surgery technique that can be used to cover root surfaces with gingiva in isolated sites of gingival recession. Also see coronally positioned flap and semilunar flap.

Leukemia—a type of cancer that begins in blood cells in which the bone marrow produces a large number of abnormal white blood cells that do not function properly.

Leukocytes—white blood cells that act much like independent single-cell organisms able to move and capture microorganisms on their own.

Levels of evidence—a ranking system used in evidence-based healthcare to describe the strength of the results measured in a clinical trial or research study.

Liability—a healthcare provider's obligation or responsibility to provide services to another person (the patient). The healthcare provider's liability entails the possibility of being sued if the person receiving the services feels as if he has been treated improperly or negligently.

Linear gingival erythema (LGE)—a gingival manifestation of immunosuppression characterized by a distinct linear erythematous (red) band that is limited to the free gingiva; formerly known as HIV-associated gingivitis.

Lipopolysaccharide (LPS)—a major component of the cell membranes of Gram-negative bacteria (also known as endotoxin). LPS was previously thought to play a role in the inflammation seen in periodontal disease; however, recent research has shown that this theory is not correct. Also see peptides.

Localized chronic periodontitis—chronic periodontitis in which 30% or less of the sites in the mouth have experienced attachment loss and bone loss. Also see chronic periodontitis.

Lymph nodes—small, bean-shaped structures located on either side of the head, neck, armpits, and groin; these nodes filter out and trap bacteria, fungi, viruses, and other unwanted substances to safely eliminate them from the body.

Lymphatic system—a network of lymph nodes connected by lymphatic vessels that plays an important role in the body's defense against infection.

Lymphocytes—small leukocytes that play an important role in recognizing and controlling foreign invaders; two main types of lymphocytes are important in defense against periodontal pathogens are B lymphocytes and T lymphocytes. Also see B lymphocytes and T lymphocytes.

Lysosomes—granules found in the cytoplasm of PMNs that are filled with strong bactericidal and digestive enzymes; these granules can kill and digest bacterial cells after phagocytosis. Also see phagocytosis.

M

Macrophages—large phagocytic leukocytes (located in the tissue) that have one kidney-shaped nucleus and some granules. Also see monocytes.

Malodor—see oral malodor.

Malpractice—the improper or negligent treatment by a healthcare provider that results in injury or damage to the patient.

Matrix metalloproteinases (MMP)—a family of at least 12 different enzymes produced by various cells of the body that can act together to break down the connective tissue matrix; the presence of increased MMP levels causes extensive collagen destruction in the periodontal tissues.

MEDLINE (PubMed)—a free online index that enables quick access to locate relevant clinical evidence in the published medical, dental, and allied health literature; hosted by the National Library of Medicine.

Membrane attack complex—a protein unit created by the complement system that is capable of puncturing the cell membranes of certain bacteria. Also see complement system.

Memory B cells—see B lymphocytes.

Menopausal gingivostomatitis—decreased levels of circulating hormones in women who are menopausal or postmenopausal that may result in oral changes, such as thinning of the oral mucosa, dry mouth, burning sensations, altered taste, gingival recession, and alveolar bone loss.

Microbial reservoir—a niche or secure place in the oral cavity that can allow periodontal pathogens to live undisturbed during routine therapy and subsequently repopulate periodontal pockets quickly.

Mobility—the loosening of a tooth in its socket that may result from loss of bone support to the tooth. **Horizontal tooth mobility** is the ability to move the tooth in a facial-lingual direction in its socket. **Vertical tooth mobility** is the ability to depress the tooth in its socket.

Modified Widman flap surgery—see flap for access.

Monocytes—phagocytic leukocytes located in the bloodstream. Also see macrophages.

Morphology—the study of the anatomic surface features of the teeth.

Motivational interviewing (MI)—a patient-centered method for enhancing a patient's motivation for behavior change by exploring the patient's mixed feelings about change.

Mouth breathing—the process of inhaling and exhaling air primarily through the mouth, rather than the nose; often occurs during sleep.

Mucogingival junction—the clinically visible boundary where the pink attached gingiva meets the red, shiny alveolar mucosa.

Mucogingival surgery—terminology used in the past to describe periodontal surgical procedures that alter the relationship between gingiva and mucosa. Some of the periodontal plastic surgical procedures utilized in modern dentistry were previously described as mucogingival surgical procedures, and this older terminology can still be encountered. Also see periodontal plastic surgery.

Mucoperiosteal flap—see full-thickness flap.

N

Necrosis—cell death. For example, in the case of necrotizing ulcerative gingivitis, necrosis refers to the death of the cells comprising the gingival epithelium.

Necrotizing periodontal diseases—a unique type of periodontal disease that involves tissue necrosis (localized tissue death); characterized by painful infection with ulceration, swelling, and sloughing off of dead epithelial tissue from the gingiva. Also see necrotizing ulcerative gingivitis and necrotizing ulcerative periodontitis.

Necrotizing ulcerative gingivitis (NUG)—tissue necrosis that is limited to the gingival tissues. Also see necrotizing periodontal diseases and necrotizing ulcerative periodontitis.

Necrotizing ulcerative periodontitis (NUP)—tissue necrosis of the gingival tissues combined with loss of attachment and alveolar bone loss. Also see necrotizing periodontal diseases and necrotizing ulcerative periodontitis.

Negligence—a failure to exercise reasonable care to avoid injuring others. It is the failure to do something that a reasonable person would do under the same circumstances or the doing of something a reasonable person would not do. Negligence is characterized by carelessness, inattentiveness, and neglectfulness rather than by a positive intent to cause injury.

Neutropenia—a polymorphonuclear leukocyte (PMN) count of less than 1,000 cells/mL of blood; indicates an increased risk of infection.

Neutrophils—phagocytic cells that actively engulf and destroy microorganisms; play a vital role in combating the pathogenic bacteria responsible for periodontal disease; also known as polymorphonuclear leukocytes.

New attachment—a term used to describe the union of a *pathologically exposed root* with connective tissue or epithelium. Also see reattachment.

NHANES—abbreviation for the National Health and Nutrition Examination Survey.

Nifedipine—a calcium channel blocker used as a coronary vasodilator in the treatment of hypertension, angina, and cardiac arrhythmias; associated with drug-influenced gingival enlargement.

Nonabsorbable suture—a suture made from a material that does not dissolve in body fluids; a clinician must remove the nonabsorbable sutures after some healing of the wound has occurred.

Noncompliant patients—patients who do not follow recommendations for healthcare advice. Examples of noncompliant patients would be a patient who does not take medications daily to control diabetes as prescribed by a physician or a patient who does not follow instructions for performing daily self-care. Also see compliance.

Nondisplaced flap—a periodontal flap that is sutured with the margin of the flap at its original position in relationship to the CEJ on the tooth. Also see displaced flap.

Nonkeratinized epithelial cells—cells that have nuclei and act as a cushion against mechanical stress and wear. Nonkeratinized epithelial cells are softer and more flexible.

Non–plaque-induced gingival lesions—periodontal diseases that are not caused by bacterial plaque biofilm and do not disappear after plaque biofilm removal; however, the presence of dental plaque biofilm could increase the severity of the gingival inflammation in non–plaque-induced lesions. See plaque-induced gingival diseases.

Nonresponsive disease sites—areas in the periodontium that show deeper probing depths, continuing loss of attachment, or continuing clinical signs of inflammation in spite of thorough nonsurgical therapy.

Nonsteroidal anti-inflammatory drugs (NSAIDs)—medications used for many years in medical care to treat pain, acute inflammation, and chronic inflammatory conditions. NSAIDs have been evaluated for their effect on periodontitis (a disease intimately associated with inflammation). NSAIDs can reduce tissue inflammation by inhibiting prostaglandins including PGE_2 and, when administered daily over 3 years, have been shown to slow the rate of alveolar bone loss associated with periodontitis.

Nonsurgical periodontal therapy—a phase of periodontal therapy that includes self-care measures, periodontal instrumentation, and use of chemical agents to prevent or control plaque-induced gingivitis or chronic periodontitis.

O

Occlusal adjustment—a clinical therapy involving minor adjustments in an individual's bite that can be used to help control the damage from trauma from occlusion.

Odontoblastic process—a thin tail of cytoplasm from a cell in the tooth pulp called an odontoblast.

Omega-3 fatty acids—a type of polyunsaturated fat found in leafy green vegetables, vegetable oils, and cold-water fish; are capable of reducing serum cholesterol levels and having anticoagulant properties.

Open flap debridement—a periodontal surgical procedure that is quite similar in concept and execution to flap for access surgery; usually includes more extensive flap elevation than flap for access—providing access not only to the tooth roots but also to all of the alveolar bone defects. Also see flap for access.

Open-ended questions—questions that cannot be answered with a simple yes or no response.

Operculum—a flap of gingival tissue covering part of the occlusal surface of a partially erupted tooth. This tissue flap can become infected and this type of infection under the flap of tissue is referred to as a pericoronal abscess.

Opsonization—coating of the surface of a microorganism by complement components to facilitate the engulfment and destruction by phagocytes.

Oral epithelium (OE)—portion of the gingival epithelium that covers the outer surface of the free gingiva and attached gingiva; it extends from the crest of the gingival margin to the mucogingival junction. The oral epithelium is the only part of the periodontium that is visible to the unaided eye. Also see gingival epithelium.

Oral irrigation—the in-home use of a pulsating water stream created by a mechanized device. Also see dental water jet.

Oral malodor—a clinical term for bad breath that has its origin within the oral cavity. Also see halitosis.

Organoleptic evaluation—a technique for quantifying breath malodor that involves having a trained judge smell a patient's expired air and make an assessment whether or not it is unpleasant.

Osseointegration—the direct contact of living alveolar bone with the surface of the dental implant body (with no intervening periodontal ligament). Osseointegration is a major requirement for implant success.

Osseous crater—a bowl-shaped osseous defect in the interdental alveolar bone with bone loss nearly equal on the roots of two adjacent teeth. Also see infrabony defect.

Osseous defect—a deformity in the tooth-supporting alveolar bone usually resulting from periodontitis. Also see infrabony defect, osseous crater, and furcation involvement.

Osseous resective surgery—a periodontal surgical procedure employed to correct many of the strange deformities of the alveolar bone that often result from advancing periodontitis. Also see ostectomy and osteoplasty.

Osseous surgery—see osseous resective surgery.

Ostectomy—removal of alveolar bone that is actually attached to the tooth (i.e., still providing some support for the tooth). The removal of small amounts of supporting bone is justified by the attainment of alveolar bone contours that are compatible with the natural contours of the gingiva. Also see osteoplasty.

Osteoconductive grafting materials—grafting materials that form a framework for bone cells. Also see osteoinductive grafting materials.

Osteoectomy—see ostectomy.

Osteogenesis—the production of new bone; in periodontal surgery, osteogenesis is the potential for new bone cells and new bone to form following bone grafting.

Osteoinductive grafting materials—grafting materials with cells that convert into bone-forming cells. Also see osteoconductive grafting materials.

Osteonecrosis of the jaw—a rare condition in which there are painful areas of exposed bone in the mouth that fail to heal after an extraction or oral surgery procedure.

Osteopenia—a condition in which there is a decrease in bone density but not necessarily an increase in the risk or incidence of bone fracture; most commonly seen in people over the age of 50 who have lower than average bone density but do not have osteoporosis. Also see osteoporosis.

Osteoplasty—reshaping the surface of alveolar bone without actually removing any of the supporting bone. Also see ostectomy.

Osteoporosis—a reduction in bone mass that causes an increased susceptibility to fractures; occurs most frequently in postmenopausal women, in sedentary or bedridden individuals, and in patients receiving long-term steroid therapy. Also see osteopenia.

Overhanging restoration—a dental restoration that is not smoothly contoured with the tooth surfaces (also called an overhang).

P

Palatogingival groove—a developmental defect that forms on the palatal surface of a tooth and is most frequently seen on maxillary lateral incisors. Plaque biofilm retention is a common problem associated with a palatogingival groove since the groove is often difficult or impossible to clean effectively.

Papilla—see interdental gingiva.

Parafunctional occlusal forces—occlusal forces that result from tooth-to-tooth contact made when not in the act of eating. Also see functional occlusal forces.

Partial-thickness flap (or split-thickness flap)—includes elevation of only the epithelium and a thin layer of the underlying connective tissue rather than the entire thickness of the underlying soft tissues.

Pathogenesis—the sequence of events that occur during the development of a disease or abnormal condition.

Pathogenic—a species of bacteria that are capable of causing disease; also called virulent bacteria.

Pathogenicity—the ability of the dental plaque biofilm to cause periodontal disease.

Patient centered—a philosophy of healthcare that recognizes the patient's dignity and right of choice in all matters, without exception, related to healthcare; for example, consideration of behavior change and treatment planning is viewed from the patient's perspective rather than the clinician's perspective.

Peer-reviewed journal—a journal that uses a panel of experts to review research articles for study design, statistics, and conclusions.

Pellicle—a thin, bacteria-free membrane that forms on the surface of the tooth during the late stages of eruption.

Peptide—short chains of amino acids found in living bacterial cell membranes that control the transport of molecules in and out of the bacterial cell. T cells recognize these peptides and alert the immune system to the presence of bacteria.

Pericoronal abscess—an abscess of the periodontium that involves tissues around the crown of a partially erupted tooth. The pericoronal abscess is also referred to as pericoronitis.

Pericoronitis—see pericoronal abscess.

Peri-implant gingivitis—see peri-implant mucositis.

Peri-implant mucositis (also called peri-implant gingivitis)—plaque-induced gingivitis that is localized in the gingival tissues surrounding a dental implant. Also see peri-implantitis.

Peri-implant tissues—the periodontal tissues that surround the dental implant.

Peri-implantitis—chronic periodontitis in the tissues surrounding an osseointegrated dental implant, resulting in loss of alveolar bone. Also see peri-implant mucositis.

Periodontal abscess—a localized collection of pus that forms in a circumscribed area of the periodontal tissues that affects the deeper structures of the periodontium as well as the gingival tissues. Also see gingival abscess, pericoronal abscess.

Periodontal assessment—see clinical periodontal assessment.

Periodontal debridement—the removal or disruption of bacterial plaque biofilm, its by-products, and calculus deposits from coronal tooth surfaces and tooth root surfaces to the extent needed to reestablish periodontal health and restore a balance between the bacterial flora and the host's immune responses.

Periodontal disease—inflammation of the periodontium.

Periodontal dressing—a protective material applied over a periodontal surgical wound and used somewhat like using a bandage to cover a finger wound. Periodontal flaps that are well adapted to the alveolar bone and tooth roots may not always require a periodontal dressing. Periodontal dressings can be placed to facilitate flap adaptation and are frequently indicated when the surgical procedures have created varying tissue levels or when displaced flaps are used.

Periodontal flap—a surgical procedure in which incisions are made in the gingiva or mucosa to allow for separation of the surface tissues (epithelium and connective tissue) from the underlying tooth roots and underlying alveolar bone. Also see full-thickness flap, partial-thickness flap, nondisplaced flap, and displaced flap.

Periodontal ligament (PDL)—a thin sheet of fibrous connective tissue that surrounds the roots of the teeth and joins the root cementum with the bone of the tooth socket.

Periodontal maintenance—continuing patient care provided by the dental team to help the periodontitis patient maintain periodontal health following complete nonsurgical or surgical periodontal therapy. The term periodontal maintenance applies specifically to treated periodontitis patients. It is normally not appropriate to use the term periodontal maintenance for patients treated for other conditions such as those treated for the various types of gingivitis.

Periodontal microsurgery—a periodontal surgical procedure performed with the aid of a surgical microscope.

Periodontal osseous surgery—see osseous resective surgery.

Periodontal pack—see periodontal dressing.

Periodontal plastic surgery—directed toward correcting problems with attached gingiva, aberrant frenum, or vestibular depth; includes an array of periodontal surgical procedures that can be used to improve esthetics of the dentition and to enhance prosthetic dentistry as well as to deal with damage resulting from periodontitis. Also see free gingival graft, subepithelial connective tissue graft, coronally positioned flap, frenectomy, and crown lengthening surgery.

Periodontal pocket—a pathologic deepening of the gingival sulcus as the result of the apical migration of the junctional epithelium, destruction of the periodontal ligament fibers, and destruction of alveolar bone. Also see apical migration.

Periodontal Screening and Recording (PSR)—an efficient, easy-to-use screening system for the detection of periodontal disease.

Periodontal screening examination—a periodontal assessment used to determine the periodontal health status of the patient and identify patients needing a more comprehensive periodontal assessment.

Periodontitis as a manifestation of systemic diseases—a group of periodontal diseases that is associated with two general categories of systemic diseases: hematological (blood) disorders, such as leukemia or acquired neutropenia, and genetic disorders, such as Down syndrome or leukocyte adhesion deficiency syndrome.

Periodontitis associated with endodontic lesions—a category of periodontal disease that involves infection or death of the tissues of the dental pulp.

Periodontitis—a bacterial infection of the periodontium resulting in destruction of all parts of the periodontium including the gingiva, periodontal ligament, bone, and cementum; results in irreversible destruction to the tissues of the periodontium. See chronic periodontitis and aggressive periodontitis.

Periodontium—the functional system of tissues that surrounds the teeth and attaches them to the jaw bone. The periodontium is also called the "supporting tissues of the teeth" and "the attachment apparatus".

Periosteum—a dense membrane composed of fibrous connective tissue that closely wraps the outer surface of the alveolar bone; it consists of an outer layer of collagenous tissue and an inner layer of fine elastic fibers.

Phagocytosis—the process by which leukocytes engulf and digest microorganisms.

Phenytoin—one of the most commonly used anticonvulsant medications used to control convulsions or seizures in the treatment of epilepsy; associated with drug-influenced gingival enlargement.

PICO process—a structure for formulating questions; the PICO entails four critical components: Patient, Intervention, Comparison, and Outcome.

Plaque-induced gingival diseases—are periodontal diseases involving inflammation of the gingiva in response to bacteria located at the gingival margin; gingivitis associated with plague biofilm formation is the most common form of gingival disease. See non–plaque-induced gingival lesions.

Plasma B cells—see B lymphocytes.

Plastic surgery—see periodontal plastic surgery.

Polymorphonuclear leukocytes (PMNs)—phagocytic cells that actively engulf and destroy microorganisms; PMNs play a vital role in combating the pathogenic bacteria responsible for periodontal disease; also known as neutrophils.

Porphyromonas gingivalis—an important periodontal pathogen.

Postmenopausal osteoporosis—a disorder caused by the cessation of estrogen production and is characterized by bone fractures.

Pregnancy gingivitis—gingival inflammation initiated by plaque biofilm and exacerbated by hormonal changes in the second and third trimesters of pregnancy.

Pregnancy tumor—see pregnancy-associated pyogenic granuloma.

Pregnancy-associated pyogenic granuloma—a localized, mushroom-shaped gingival mass projecting from the gingival margin or more commonly from a gingival papilla during pregnancy.

Prevalence—the number of all cases (both old and new) of a disease that can be identified within a specified population at a given point in time. Also see incidence.

Primary herpetic gingivostomatitis—a painful oral condition that results from the initial infection with the herpes simplex virus (HSV).

Primary intention—healing that occurs when wound margins or edges are closely adapted to each other; an example of primary intention healing would be seen in a small wound in a finger that required stitches. Also see secondary and tertiary intention.

Primary trauma from occlusion—excessive occlusal forces on a sound (healthy) periodontium.

Professional subgingival irrigation—the in-office flushing of pockets performed by the dental hygienist or dentist using one of three systems: a blunt-tipped irrigating cannula, an ultrasonic unit equipped with a fluid reservoir, or a specialized air-driven handpiece.

Proinflammatory mediators—biologically active compounds secreted by immune cells that can damage the periodontium; such as prostaglandin E_2, IL-1α (interleukin-1 alpha), IL-1β (interleukin-1 beta), IL-6 (interleukin-6), and tumor necrosis factor alpha. Also see biochemical mediators.

Prostaglandins—a series of powerful biochemical mediators, of which prostaglandins D, E, F, G, H, and I are the most important biologically; prostaglandins of the E series (PGE) play an important role in the bone destruction seen in periodontitis.

Prosthesis—an appliance used to replace missing teeth. Also see removable prosthesis.

Pseudomembrane—a yellowish white or grayish tissue slough that covers the necrotic areas of the gingiva in necrotizing periodontal diseases. Also see necrotizing periodontal diseases.

PST genetic susceptibility test—a test for genetic susceptibility to periodontal disease.

Pulpal abscess—an abscess that results from an infection of the tooth pulp. A pulpal abscess can be caused by death of the tooth pulp from trauma to the tooth or from deep dental decay.

Pus—collections of dead white blood cells that can result when body defense mechanisms are involved in attempting to control an infection.

Pyogenic granuloma—see pregnancy-associated pyogenic granuloma.

R

Radiolucent—materials and structures that are easily penetrated by x-rays and appear as dark gray to black on the radiograph; examples of radiolucent structures are the tooth pulp, periodontal ligament space, a periapical abscess, marrow spaces in the bone, and bone loss defects.

Radiopaque—materials and structures that absorb or resist the passage of x-rays and appear light gray to white on the radiograph; examples of radiopaque structures and materials are metallic silver (amalgam restorations) and newer composite restorations, enamel, dentin, pulp stones, and compact or cortical bone.

Reattachment—healing of a periodontal wound by the reunion of the connective tissue and roots where these two tissues have been separated by incision or injury but *not by disease*. Also see the new attachment.

Recurrence of periodontitis—the return of periodontitis in a patient who has been previously successfully treated for periodontitis. The term recurrence implies that the periodontitis was brought under control during nonsurgical periodontal therapy (or nonsurgical periodontal therapy plus periodontal surgery) and that the periodontitis is once again resulting in progressive attachment loss.

Recurrent disease—new signs and symptoms of destructive periodontitis that reappear after periodontal therapy because the disease was not adequately treated and/or the patient did not practice adequate self-care.

Reevaluation—a formal step at the completion of nonsurgical therapy. During the reevaluation appointment, the members of the dental team perform another periodontal assessment to gather information about the patient's periodontal status.

Refereed journal—see peer-reviewed journal.

Reflective listening—the process in which the healthcare provider listens to the patient's remarks and then paraphrases what the clinician heard the patient say. This allows the clinician to check with the patient that he or she is "getting the patient's message right," ensuring that the clinician is developing a good picture of the patient's perspective.

Refractory disease—destructive periodontitis in a patient who, when monitored over time, exhibits additional attachment loss at one or more sites, despite appropriate, repeated professional periodontal therapy and a patient who practices satisfactory self-care and follows the recommended program of periodontal maintenance visits.

Refractory periodontitis—resistant to control even with what appears to be appropriate therapy. Referral to a periodontal practice is indicated when refractory periodontitis is suspected.

Regeneration—the biologic process by which the architecture and function of lost tissue is *completely* restored. Also see repair.

Relative contraindications—conditions that may make periodontal surgery inadvisable for some patients when the conditions or situations are severe or extreme; these same conditions may not be contraindications when the conditions are mild.

Removable prosthesis—an appliance used to replace missing teeth that the patient can remove for cleaning and before going to bed; commonly called a partial denture.

Repair—the healing of a wound by formation of tissues that do not precisely restore the original architecture or original function of the body part. Also see regeneration.

Resective periodontal surgery—periodontal surgical procedures that simply cut away and remove damaged periodontal tissues.

Risk assessment—the process of identifying risk factors that increase an individual's probability of disease.

Risk factors—factors that modify or amplify the likelihood of developing periodontal disease; major established risk factors for periodontitis are specific bacterial pathogens, cigarette smoking, and diabetes mellitus.

Rolling with resistance—when the healthcare provider listens carefully and explores the patient's perspective rather than attempting to persuade or provide counter arguments.

Root caries—tooth decay that occurs on the tooth root surfaces.

Root concavity—a trench-like depression in the root surface; commonly occur on the proximal surfaces of anterior and posterior teeth and the facial and lingual surfaces of molar teeth.

S

Scurvy—a systemic disorder caused by severe and prolonged deprivation of vitamin C; can be accompanied by changes in the periodontium.

Secondary intention—healing that takes place when the margins or edges of the wound are not closely adapted (i.e., the two wound edges are not in close contact with each other). When healing by secondary intention takes place, granulation tissue must form to close the space between the wound margins prior to growth of epithelial cells over the surface of the wound. Also see primary intention and tertiary intention.

Secondary trauma from occlusion—defined as normal occlusal forces on an unhealthy periodontium previously weakened by periodontitis.

Self-efficacy—a person's belief in his or her ability to perform specific tasks (e.g., public speaking, studying, etc.) to attain a goal.

Semilunar flap—a periodontal plastic surgical procedure that can be used to cover gingival recession where the recession is not far advanced and where the keratinized tissues have an adequate thickness. The semilunar flap is a variation of a coronally positioned flap.

Sequestrum—a fragment of necrotic (dead) alveolar bone. Necrotizing ulcerative periodontitis can be accompanied by the formation of bone sequestra.

Severity—the seriousness of periodontal tissue destruction as determined by the rate of disease progression over time and the response of the tissues to treatment; may be described as slight (mild), moderate, or severe. Also see extent.

Sharp dissection—elevation of a flap by incising the underlying connective tissue in such a manner as to separate the epithelial surface plus a small portion of the connective tissue from the periosteum; use of this technique would leave the periosteal tissues covering the bone.

Sharpey fibers—the ends of the periodontal ligament fibers that are embedded in the cementum and alveolar bone.

Sialometry—a diagnostic test used to measure salivary flow rate that usually involves placing a collection device over the parotid gland duct orifice or the submandibular/sublingual gland duct orifices and measuring saliva flow per minute with glands stimulated and with the glands unstimulated.

Signs—the features of a disease that can be observed or are measurable by a clinician such as gingival redness, bleeding on gentle probing, tooth mobility. Also see symptoms.

Sjögren syndrome—an inflammatory autoimmune disease that is the most common systemic condition associated with xerostomia; pronounced "show-grins."

Smear layer—crystalline debris from the tooth surface that covers or plugs the dentinal tubules and inhibits fluid flow, thus preventing the sensitivity.

Split-thickness flap—see partial-thickness flap.

Stippling—the dimpled appearance, similar to an orange peel, that may be visible on the surface of the attached gingiva.

Stratified squamous epithelium—a type of epithelium that is composed of flat cells arranged in several layers that makes up the skin and the mucosa of the oral cavity.

Subantibacterial doses—doses of an antibiotic that are below the normal bacterial killing or inhibiting doses. Doxycycline at low doses is used as a host-modulating agent to inhibit part of the destruction that occurs in periodontitis.

Subepithelial connective tissue graft—a periodontal plastic surgical procedure that can also be used to augment the width of attached gingiva and to cover areas of gingival recession. In addition to gingival augmentation, the subepithelial connective tissue graft is used to alter the contour of alveolar ridges to improve the esthetics of some types of dental prostheses.

Sulcular epithelium (SE)—the epithelial lining of the gingival sulcus; it extends from the crest of the gingival margin to the coronal edge of the junctional epithelium. Also see gingival epithelium.

Sulcular fluid—see gingival crevicular fluid.

Sulcular incision—see crevicular incision.

Suppuration—see exudate.

Suprabony pocket—a periodontal pocket in which there is horizontal bone loss and the junctional epithelium, forming the base of the pocket, is located *coronal* to the crest of the alveolar bone. Also see periodontal pocket and infrabony pocket.

Supragingival fiber bundles (gingival fibers)—a network of rope-like collagen fiber bundles in the gingival connective tissue located coronal to the crest of the alveolar bone.

Suture—a stitch; a device placed by a surgeon to hold tissues together during healing. Also see nonabsorbable suture and absorbable suture.

Symptoms—the features of a disease that can be noticed by the patient such as itching gums, blood on the bed pillow, or a bad taste in the mouth. Also see signs.

Systematic review—a concise summary of individual research studies on a treatment or device to determine the overall validity and clinical applicability of that treatment or device.

Systemic delivery—in dentistry, usually refers to administering chemical agents in the form of a tablet or capsule. When a tablet is taken by the patient, the chemical agent is released as the tablet dissolves, and the agent subsequently enters the blood stream; thus, the chemical agent is circulated "systemically" throughout the body.

Systemic risk factors—conditions or diseases that increase an individual's susceptibility to periodontal infection by modifying or amplifying the host response to the bacterial infection; proven systemic risk factors include diabetes mellitus, osteoporosis, hormone alteration, medications, tobacco use, and genetic influences.

T

Tannerella forsythia—an important periodontal pathogen.

T cells—see T lymphocytes.

Tertiary intention—healing of a wound that is temporarily left open with the specific intent of surgically closing that wound at a later date; healing by tertiary intention is not normally a type of healing that applies to healing of periodontal surgical procedures. Also see primary intention and secondary intention.

Therapeutic mouth rinse—a mouth rinse that has some actual benefit (provides some therapeutic action) to the patient in addition to the simple goal of making the breath smell a bit better.

Tissue—a group of interconnected cells that perform a similar function within an organism. For example, muscle cells group together to form muscle tissue that functions to move parts of the body. Also see connective tissue and epithelial tissue.

Tissue-associated plaque biofilm—bacteria that adhere loosely to the epithelium of the pocket wall that can invade the gingival connective tissue and be found within the periodontal connective tissues and on the surface of the alveolar bone.

Titanium—a biocompatible metal that is used in dental implant systems.

T lymphocytes—small leukocytes whose main function is to intensify the response of other immune cells—such as B lymphocytes and macrophages—to the bacterial invasion.

Tongue coating—an accumulation of bacteria, food debris, and desquamated epithelial cells on the dorsal surface of the tongue and is a source of oral malodor.

Tongue thrusting—the application of forceful pressure against the anterior teeth with the tongue.

Tooth-associated plaque biofilm—bacteria that attach to an area of the tooth surface that extends from the gingival margin almost to the junctional epithelium at the base of the pocket.

Topical delivery—in dentistry, usually refers to placing a chemical agent into the mouth or even into a periodontal pocket where the chemical agent then comes into contact with plaque biofilm forming either on the teeth or in the periodontal pocket.

Transendothelial migration—the process of immune cells exiting the vessels and entering the tissues.

Transmission—the transfer of periodontal pathogens from the oral cavity of one person to another.

Trauma from occlusion—excessive occlusal forces that cause damage to the periodontium. Also see primary trauma from occlusion and secondary trauma from occlusion.

Treatment plan—a sequential outline of the measures to be carried out by the dentist, the dental hygienist and the patient to eliminate disease and restore a healthy periodontal environment.

Triangulation—the appearance on a dental radiograph of widening of the periodontal ligament space; triangulation is caused by the resorption of bone along either the mesial or distal aspect of the interdental (interseptal) crestal bone.

TRIP database—one of the Internet's leading resources for evidence-based medicine—allows users to rapidly identify the highest quality clinical evidence for clinical practice.

Type I diabetes mellitus—a type of diabetes mellitus caused by destruction of the insulin-producing cells of the pancreas. Also see diabetes mellitus and type II diabetes mellitus.

Type I gingival embrasure—space filled by the interdental papilla. Also see type II gingival embrasure and type III gingival embrasure.

Type II diabetes mellitus—a type of diabetes mellitus that occurs when the body does not make enough insulin hormone and/or the body cells ignore the insulin and fail to use it to help bring glucose into the cells; the most common form of diabetes. Also see diabetes mellitus and type I diabetes mellitus.

Type II gingival embrasure—height of interdental papilla is reduced so that there is some open space visible between two teeth. Also see type I gingival embrasure and type III gingival embrasure.

Type III gingival embrasure—interdental papilla is missing so that there is an open triangular space visible between two teeth. Also see type I gingival embrasure and type II gingival embrasure.

U

Ulceration—the loss of the epithelium normally covering underlying connective tissue.

Unattached plaque—bacteria that are free floating within the pocket environment.

V

Vertical bone loss—a less common pattern of bone loss resulting in an uneven reduction in the height of the alveolar bone. In vertical bone loss, the resorption progresses *more rapidly* in the bone next to the root surface leaving a trench-like area of missing bone alongside the root. Also see alveolar bone loss and horizontal bone loss.

Vertical incision—an incision that runs perpendicular to the gingival margin in an apico-occlusal direction; primarily used to allow elevation of the flap during the surgical procedure without stretching or damaging the soft tissues during flap elevation. Also see incision and crevicular incision.

Virulence factors—the mechanisms that enable biofilm bacteria to colonize, invade, and damage the tissues of the periodontium.

Virulent—species of bacteria that are capable of causing disease; another term for pathogenic.

Volatile sulfur compounds—a family of gases that is responsible for oral malodor.

X

Xenografts—bone replacement grafts taken from another species, such as bovine bone replacement graft material; these materials must be modified to eliminate the potential for rejection. Also see autografts, allografts, and alloplasts.

Xerostomia—dry mouth that results from a reduction in salivary flow.

Index